Pulmonary Hypertension: Diagnosis and Treatment

Pulmonary Hypertension: Diagnosis and Treatment

Edited by Carter Moore

hayle
medical

New York

Hayle Medical,
750 Third Avenue, 9ᵗʰ Floor,
New York, NY 10017, USA

Visit us on the World Wide Web at:
www.haylemedical.com

ISBN: 978-1-63241-754-1

Cataloging-in-Publication Data

Pulmonary hypertension : diagnosis and treatment / edited by Carter Moore.
     p. cm.
Includes bibliographical references and index.
ISBN 978-1-63241-754-1
1. Pulmonary hypertension. 2. Pulmonary hypertension--Diagnosis. 3. Pulmonary hypertension--Treatment.
4. Lungs--Diseases. 5. Hypertension. 6. Pulmonary circulation. I. Moore, Carter.
RC776.P87 P85 2019
616.24--dc23

Table of Contents

Preface

The purpose of the book is to provide a glimpse into the dynamics and to present opinions and studies of some of the scientists engaged in the development of new ideas in the field from very different standpoints. This book will prove useful to students and researchers owing to its high content quality.

A medical condition involving an increase in the pressure of blood within the arteries of the lungs is known as pulmonary hypertension. Its common symptoms include shortness of breath, fast heartbeat, chest pain, syncope, tiredness and swelling of the legs. A detailed analysis of the person's family history and physical examination are required for diagnosing pulmonary hypertension. Other diagnostic techniques include echocardiography, electrocardiography, chest X-rays, arterial blood gas tests and computed tomography scans. Prostacyclin, treprostinil, sildenafil, calcium channel blockers, etc. are some medications that may be used for the management of pulmonary hypertension. This condition can also be surgically addressed via atrial septostomy, pulmonary thromboendarterectomy and lung transplantation. This book explores all the important aspects of the diagnosis and treatment of pulmonary hypertension in the present day scenario. The various advancements in its diagnosis and treatment are glanced at and their applications as well as ramifications are looked at in detail. This book, with its detailed analyses and data, will prove immensely beneficial to professionals and students.

At the end, I would like to appreciate all the efforts made by the authors in completing their chapters professionally. I express my deepest gratitude to all of them for contributing to this book by sharing their valuable works. A special thanks to my family and friends for their constant support in this journey.

Editor

Pulmonary Hypertension in Wild Type Mice and Animals with Genetic Deficit in $K_{Ca}2.3$ and $K_{Ca}3.1$ Channels

Christine Wandall-Frostholm[1][*][◑], Lykke Moran Skaarup[1][◑], Veeranjaneyulu Sadda[1,2], Gorm Nielsen[2], Elise Røge Hedegaard[1], Susie Mogensen[1], Ralf Köhler[2,3], Ulf Simonsen[1]

1 Department of Biomedicine, Aarhus University, Aarhus, Denmark, 2 Institute for Molecular Medicine, Cardiovascular and Renal Research, University of Southern Denmark, Odense, Denmark, 3 Aragon Institute of Health Sciences I+CS and ARAID, Zaragoza, Spain

Abstract

Objective: In vascular biology, endothelial $K_{Ca}2.3$ and $K_{Ca}3.1$ channels contribute to arterial blood pressure regulation by producing membrane hyperpolarization and smooth muscle relaxation. The role of $K_{Ca}2.3$ and $K_{Ca}3.1$ channels in the pulmonary circulation is not fully established. Using mice with genetically encoded deficit of $K_{Ca}2.3$ and $K_{Ca}3.1$ channels, this study investigated the effect of loss of the channels in hypoxia-induced pulmonary hypertension.

Approach and Result: Male wild type and $K_{Ca}3.1^{-/-}/K_{Ca}2.3^{T/T(+DOX)}$ mice were exposed to chronic hypoxia for four weeks to induce pulmonary hypertension. The degree of pulmonary hypertension was evaluated by right ventricular pressure and assessment of right ventricular hypertrophy. Segments of pulmonary arteries were mounted in a wire myograph for functional studies and morphometric studies were performed on lung sections. Chronic hypoxia induced pulmonary hypertension, right ventricular hypertrophy, increased lung weight, and increased hematocrit levels in either genotype. The $K_{Ca}3.1^{-/-}/K_{Ca}2.3^{T/T(+DOX)}$ mice developed structural alterations in the heart with increased right ventricular wall thickness as well as in pulmonary vessels with increased lumen size in partially- and fully-muscularized vessels and decreased wall area, not seen in wild type mice. Exposure to chronic hypoxia up-regulated the gene expression of the $K_{Ca}2.3$ channel by twofold in wild type mice and increased by 2.5-fold the relaxation evoked by the $K_{Ca}2.3$ and $K_{Ca}3.1$ channel activator NS309, whereas the acetylcholine-induced relaxation - sensitive to the combination of $K_{Ca}2.3$ and $K_{Ca}3.1$ channel blockers, apamin and charybdotoxin - was reduced by 2.5-fold in chronic hypoxic mice of either genotype.

Conclusion: Despite the deficits of the $K_{Ca}2.3$ and $K_{Ca}3.1$ channels failed to change hypoxia-induced pulmonary hypertension, the up-regulation of $K_{Ca}2.3$-gene expression and increased NS309-induced relaxation in wild-type mice point to a novel mechanism to counteract pulmonary hypertension and to a potential therapeutic utility of $K_{Ca}2.3/K_{Ca}3.1$ activators for the treatment of pulmonary hypertension.

Editor: Tim Lahm, Indiana University, United States of America

Funding: NovoNordisk Foundation supported Ulf Simonsen and Ralf Köhler. Ulf Simonsen is supported by the Danish Heart Foundation and he is member of LiPhos (Living Photonics: Monitoring light propagation through cells), which is funded by the EC Seventh Framework programme. Ralf Köhler is supported by a grant of the Deutsche Forschungsgemeinschaft (KO1899/11-1) and the Fondo de Investigación Sanitaria (Red HERACLES RD12/0042/0014). The funders had no role in study design, data collection and analysis, decision to publish, or preparation of the manuscript.

Competing Interests: The authors have declared that no competing interests exist.

* E-mail: cwf@farm.au.dk

◑ These authors contributed equally to this work.

Introduction

Pulmonary hypertension is a disabling disease with increased blood pressure in the pulmonary circulation, resulting in shortness of breath, dizziness, edema, right ventricular hypertrophy, heart failure, and premature death. Pulmonary hypertension involves endothelial dysfunction, vasoconstriction, and remodeling of the pulmonary vasculature. The current treatment options are unsatisfactory [1].

The endothelium participates in regulating vascular tone by releasing vasoactive autacoids. Endothelium-dependent relaxation involves the release of a variety of diffusible relaxing factors such as nitric oxide (NO) [2,3], prostacyclin [4], CYP450-generated epoxyeicosanoids acids (11,12-EET and 14,15-EET) [5–7], and an electrical mechanism known as endothelium-derived hyperpolarization (EDH) [8–10] that produces hyperpolarization of the underlying smooth muscle and closure of voltage-gated calcium channels. The resulting reduction of intracellular calcium leads to relaxation. The small-conductance and intermediate-conductance calcium-activated potassium channels, $K_{Ca}2.3$ and $K_{Ca}3.1$ channel, respectively [11], have been demonstrated to play a significant role in EDH-type relaxation, as a combination of the $K_{Ca}2.3$ and $K_{Ca}3.1$ channel blockers (apamin plus charybdotoxin or apamin plus TRAM-34) inhibits EDH-type relaxation [8,12–14]. Impaired EDH-mediated relaxation involving the $K_{Ca}2.3$ and $K_{Ca}3.1$ channels have been reported to contribute to endothelial dysfunction associated with various human and experimental cardiovascular disease such as hypertension, diabetes, and restenosis [15–18]. In line with the roles of the two channels in endothelial function, $K_{Ca}3.1^{-/-}$ mice have been reported to have moderately elevated blood pressure [19] and to develop mild left ventricular hypertrophy, as well as a pronounced defect of endothelium-dependent acetylcholine-induced relaxation in both carotid artery and resistance vessels [19,20]. Likewise, suppression of $K_{Ca}2.3$ gene expression in $K_{Ca}2.3^{T/T(+DOX)}$ mice has been shown to elevate blood pressure and increase pressure- and phenylephrine-induced constrictions [21]. Combined $K_{Ca}3.1$- and $K_{Ca}2.3$ channel deficiency in transgenic doxycycline-treated $K_{Ca}3.1^{-/-}/K_{Ca}2.3^{T/T(+DOX)}$ mice has been reported to increase blood pressure, reduce hyperpolarization of endothelial cells, and to reduce acetylcholine-induced relaxation in carotid arteries and resistance arteries, although the combined deficiency of the two channels has no additive effects on blood pressure [22]. While the roles of the $K_{Ca}2.3$- and the $K_{Ca}3.1$ channels have been at least partially elucidated for systemic blood pressure control [19,21–23], the precise role of the channels in the pulmonary circulation is still unclear.

Thus far, $K_{Ca}2.3$ and $K_{Ca}3.1$ expression have been found in human, porcine, and rat pulmonary artery endothelial cells [24–27], as well as in the bronchial epithelium [26,27]. In pulmonary arteries relaxation sensitive to blockers of the $K_{Ca}2.3$ and $K_{Ca}3.1$ channels has been observed in several studies [26,28–30]. Moreover, the potent $K_{Ca}2.3$- and $K_{Ca}3.1$ channel activator NS309 (6,7-dichloro-1H-indole-2,3-dione 3-oxime) has been shown to induce relaxation being sensitive to $K_{Ca}2.3$- and $K_{Ca}3.1$ blockade in rat and human pulmonary arteries [26,27], rat mesenteric arteries [31], and in porcine retinal arterioles [32]. In addition, $K_{Ca}3.1$ expression has also been found in proliferating vascular smooth muscle cells [33,34], and it may also be increased in the smooth muscle of the hypertrophied arteries in pulmonary hypertension.

In this study, we used $K_{Ca}3.1^{-/-}/K_{Ca}2.3^{T/T(+DOX)}$ mice to study the physiological role of $K_{Ca}2.3$ and $K_{Ca}3.1$ channels in the pulmonary arteries from mice with hypoxia-induced pulmonary hypertension. Our hypothesis was that $K_{Ca}2.3$ and $K_{Ca}3.1$ channels participate in maintaining endothelial function in the pulmonary vasculature, whereas deficiency of $K_{Ca}2.3$- and $K_{Ca}3.1$ channels aggravates endothelial dysfunction, and thereby contributes to pulmonary hypertension and the associated structural pathologies. Moreover, we tested whether activation of the channels by NS309 improves endothelium-dependent vasodilation in pulmonary arteries of mice with hypoxia-induced pulmonary hypertension.

Materials and Methods

Ethics statement

This study followed the recommendations in the Guide for the Care and Use of Laboratory Animals of the National Institutes of Health and the ARRIVE Guidelines. The animal studies were approved by the Animal Ethical Committee according to Danish legislation (permit no. 2011/561-2011).

Animal model

The mice were housed in standard cages and had free access to water and food. $K_{Ca}3.1^{-/-}/K_{Ca}2.3^{T/T}$ mice were generated by interbreeding of $K_{Ca}3.1^{-/-}$ [19] and $K_{Ca}2.3^{T/T}$ [35] mice as previously described [22]. 32 Male C57Bl/6 mice and $K_{Ca}3.1^{-/-}/K_{Ca}2.3^{T/T}$ mice, with an age between 15–25 weeks, were given doxycycline (DOX) (Piggidox, 2 mg/kg) in the drinking water, six days before the start of the experiment and throughout the experiment for the suppression of the $K_{Ca}2.3$ channel in the $K_{Ca}3.1^{-/-}/K_{Ca}2.3^{T/T}$ mice. Each genotype was divided into normoxic and hypoxic groups. The hypoxic groups were placed

in hypobaric chambers and exposed to hypoxia for four weeks to induce pulmonary hypertension. The hypobaric chambers were connected to a vacuum pump and depressurized to 560 mbar corresponding to an atmospheric oxygen tension of 10%, as previously described for rats [36].

Hemodynamic measurements

The animal was weighed and anaesthetized by an intraperitoneal injection with a combination of fentanyl (3.313 mg/kg), fluanisone (104.8 mg/kg), and midazolam (52.44 mg/kg), and if necessary the anesthesia was maintained every 30 min. The neck area was shaved and the animal was placed on a heating pad. A 1 cm incision was made on the right side of the neck. By blunt dissection, the right external jugular vein was located and isolated. A hole was cut in the vein and through this, a catheter (SPC-1000, Millar Instruments Inc, USA) was inserted and secured by a suture. The catheter was led into the right ventricle and the position was confirmed by observing the characteristic ventricular waveform. The pressure profile was recorded over a three minute period using a Quad Bridge amplifier connected to a PowerLab device (ADInstruments, Oxfordshire, England) and recorded with Chart 5.5 (ADInstruments). The animal was euthanized after blood pressure measurement by cervical dislocation.

Assessment of right ventricular hypertrophy

Immediately after the mice were sacrificed, heart, lungs, and liver were removed and kept in cold (5° C) physiological saline solution (PSS). A blood sample was collected in a microcapillary tube and centrifuged (International equipment company, microcapillary centrifuge model M B) for three hours as previously described [36].

The hematocrit value was calculated as the length of the erythrocyte layer divided by the length of the entire blood sample. Wet weight of liver and left lung were determined and expressed as percentage of body weight. The heart was isolated and both atria were removed. The free wall of the right ventricle (RV) was separated from left ventricle and septum (LV+S). Each part was weighed and the ratios of right ventricle to left ventricle plus septum (RV/(LV+S)) were calculated and used to assess right ventricular hypertrophy. The thickness of the right ventricular free wall, as well as the septum was measured with a Zeiss Eyepiece calibrating reticule at three different points, at the middle of the wall, and each half then bisected in a cranial and caudal direction, respectively.

QPCR

Samples of lung tissue were dissected and placed in RNAlater filled Eppendorff tubes at 4°C for 24 hours and then stored at −20°C. RNA was extracted using Trizol reagent (Invitrogen, Naerum, Denmark), and genomic DNA was eliminated using DNAse I (Qiagen Germantown, MD). The concentration of RNA was determined densitometrically at 260 nm. Reverse transcription of RNA was performed using iScript cDNA synthesis kit (Bio-Rad, Copenhagen, Denmark). A standard PCR protocol was used with initial denaturing at 95°C for 3 min and subsequently 40 cycles of denaturing at 95°C for 25 sec, annealing at 57°C for 20 sec and extending at 72°C for 40 sec. A final step of extension was done at 72°C for 3 min. The PCR-products were analyzed by gel electrophoresis using 1.5% agarose in Tris-borate-EDTA buffer and staining with GelRed™ (Biotium, Hayward, CA). Semiquantitative RT-PCR was done using iQ™ CYBR® Green Supermix (Bio-Rad) and a Stratagene MX3000p cycler (Stratagene, La Jolla, CA) with an initial denaturing at 95°C for 10 min followed by 40 cycles of denaturing at 95°C for 20 sec, annealing at 60°C for 20 sec and an extension step at 72°C for 20 sec. Thereafter, a three-step series of 95°C for 60 sec, 55°C for 30 sec, and a gradual increase to 95°C was run to determine melting points of qPCR products. Signals were normalized to expression of the house keeping gene clathrin (CLCT) and are given as % CLCT. The identity of all PCR products was verified by sequencing. Specific RT-PCR primers were designed to span intronic sequences. The expected product lengths were 226 bp for $K_{Ca}2.1$, 250 bp for $K_{Ca}2.2$, 70 bp for $K_{Ca}2.3$, 217 bp for $K_{Ca}3.1$, 349 for $K_{Ca}1.1$, 416 bp for endothelial nitric oxide synthase (eNOS), 152 bp for smooth muscle actin (SMA), 176 bp for collagen-1, and 150 bp for transforming growth factor β (TGFβ). Primer sequences were as follows (5′ → 3′): $K_{Ca}2.1$ FP, TCAAAAATGCTGCTGCAAAC; $K_{Ca}2.1$ RP, TCATATGCGATGCTCTGGTGC; $K_{Ca}2.2$ FP, GGTCATTGAGACCGAGCTGT; $K_{Ca}2.2$ RP, ATTCCCAGG-TATGGGATGGA; $K_{Ca}2.3$ FP, CCATGCCAAAGTCAGGAA-AC; $K_{Ca}2.3$ RP, CATCTTGACACCCCGAAGTT; $K_{Ca}3.1$ FP, CTGAGAGGCAGGCTGTCAATG; $K_{Ca}3.1$ RP, ACGTGTT-TCTCCGCCTTGTT; $K_{Ca}1.1$ FP, ACACTTGGACGCCTC-TTCAT; $K_{Ca}1.1$ RP, CTCTGGCAAGATCATGTGGA; eNOS FP, GGTGTCCCTAGAGCACGA; eNOS RP, CTCGGAAAG-CCTCCTCCT; SMA FP, AATGGCTCTGGGCTCTGTAA; SMA RP, CTCTTGCTCTGGGCTTCATC; Collagen-1 FP, GAACCCCAAGGAAAAGAAGC; Collagen-1 RP, GCTACGC-TGTTCTTGCAGTG; TGFβ FP, ACCGGAGAGCCCTGGA-TAC; TGFβ RP, AGGGTCCCAGACAGAAGTTG; CLCT FP, AAGGAGGCGAAACTC ACAGA; CLCT RP, GAGCAGTCA ACATCCAGCAA.

In previous studies we have performed immunoblotting of lungs from rat and man [26,27], but unfortunately we were unable to validate the gene expression results in this study with protein quantification in mouse lung using western blotting, as we experienced a series of difficulties (e.g. lack of specificity and multiple bands) with the mouse antibodies for the $K_{Ca}2.3$ and $K_{Ca}3.1$ channels, despite trying several types ($K_{Ca}2.3$: SC-28621 (Santa Cruz Biotechnology, Santa Cruz, CA); APC-025 (Alamone Labs, Jerusalem, Israel); H00003782-A01 (Abnova, Taiwan). $K_{Ca}3.1$: P4997, AV35098 (Sigma-Aldrich, St. Louis, MO); SC-32949 (Santa Cruz Biotechnology); CA1788 (Cell Applications, San Diego, CA). All mice were genotyped and QPCR performed as stated above.

Genotyping

All animals were tested for the presence of the $K_{Ca}3.1^{-/-}$ and $K_{Ca}2.3^{T/T}$ alleles by polymerase chain reaction (PCR) on DNA extracts from tail tips. The reaction was carried out in a thermal cycler (ABI system, Applied Biosystems, Carlsbad, CA) using the following protocol, an initial denaturation step at 94°C for 3 min, followed by 10 cycles consisting of 35 sec at 94°C, 35 sec at 58°C and 50 sec at 72°C, proceeded by 25 cycles of the same three steps at the same temperature but with additional 5 sec prolongation at the extension step per cycle, and a final extension step (10 min at 72°C). The reaction product was analysed on a 1% agarose gel. The primer sequence were as follows $K_{Ca}2.3^{T/T}$: Forward primer (FP) 5′-ATGGACACTTCTGGGCACTT-3′, Reverse Primer (RP) 5′-AGAGTGCAACAGACCAGGAT; $K_{Ca}3.1^{+/+}/K_{Ca}3.1^{-/-}$: FP 5′-CTTTGGATCCAGATGTTTCTTGGTG- 3′, $K_{Ca}3.1^{+/+}$ RP 5′-GCCACAGTGTGTCTGTGAGG-3′; $K_{Ca}3.1^{-/-}$ RP 5′- CGT-GCAATCCATCTTGTTCA-3′.

Lung perfusion and immunohistochemistry

Catheters with heparin (0.1 ml 100 IU, LEO Pharma, Copen-hagen, Denmark) were inserted into the truncus pulmonalis as well as in the trachea and secured by sutures. The left lung lobe was first perfused with a perfusion mixture (calcium free PSS, 2% albumin, 10% heparin (100 IU), and papaverin (10^{-4} M; Sigma-Aldrich)) and then with 4% formaldehyde. The perfusion pressure was maintained at 12–14 mmHg using fluid columns. The left lung lobe was weighed and fixed in 4% formaldehyde for two days and was kept afterwards in ethanol (70%) until embedding in paraffin. The paraffin-embedded left lung lobe was cut in transverse sections of 5 μm. The sections were de-paraffinized and rehydrated by washing 2×5 min each in: xylene, a decreasing ethanol series (99, 96, 76%), and distilled water. Antigen retrieval was performed using a Tris/EDTA pH 9.0 buffer and heating in a microwave for 2×5 min/600 W. Endogenous peroxidase activity was blocked by incubation with 3% H_2O_2 for 20 min, followed by washing for 2×5 min in PBS. To avoid non-specific binding of primary antibodies, sections were incubated with 10% calf serum for 10 min. Thereafter, sections were incubated at 4°C overnight with anti-Von Willebrand factor (1:500, Dako, Denmark). After washing 2×5 min in PBS, sections were incubated in HRP-conjugated secondary antibody (goat-anti rabbit, 1:3000, Zymed laboratories, USA) for one hour at room temperature and washed again 2×5 min in PBS. DAB chromogen (Sigma, USA) was added and sections were incubated for 5 min. Sections were washed again 4×5 min in PBS and incubated with 10% calf serum for 10 min before incubating with primary anti-α-smooth muscle actin (1:250, Abcam, UK) for 75 min at room temperature. After wash 2×5 min in PBS, sections were incubated in AP-conjugated secondary antibody (donkey-anti goat, 1:500, Abcam, UK) one hour at room temperature and washed again 2×5 min in PBS. Stay red chromogen (Sigma-Aldrich) was added and incubated for 5–10 min. After 5 min wash in distilled water, sections were incubated with Mayer's hematoxylin for 20 sec, washed again in water and mounted using **Flourmount mounting media** (Sigma-Aldrich).

Morphometric measurements

At 400× magnification small pulmonary vessels of each animal ranging from 10 to 80 μm in internal diameter were counted in a blinded manner. Non-muscular arterioles were detected by the endothelial anti-Von Willebrand staining. To assess the degree of muscularization, the amount of α-SMA-positive vessel wall area was determined. Arteries that contained α-SMA-positive vessel area between 4 and 69% were defined as partially-muscularized. Arteries that contained 70% and above were defined as fully-muscularized. Wall area was expressed as percentage of the vessel using the following formulae: % wall area = ([area$_{outer}$ − area$_{inner}$) / area$_{outer}$) ×100. The area was calculated using the two perpendicular diameters for both vessel (diameter$_{outer}$) and lumen (diameter$_{inner}$) and applying the area formulae for ellipses (area$_{ellipse}$ = π × the two perpendicular radiuses) to account for deviations from the perfect circle form. To avoid oblique sections, vessels with an area difference of more than 20% between the areal calculated as ellipse and circle (area$_{circle}$ = π × radius^2) were excluded.

Functional studies

Segments of 2nd and 3rd order pulmonary artery (approximately 2 mm in length) with an internal diameter of 564±28 μm (n = 55) in wild type mice and of 534±20 μm (n = 58) in $K_{Ca}3.1^{-/-}/K_{Ca}2.3^{T/T(+DOX)}$ mice (n.s. vs. wt) were dissected from the right lung lobes and mounted on two 40 μm wires in microvascular myographs (Danish Myotechnology, Aarhus, Denmark) for isometric tension recordings. The myograph chamber filled with PSS was heated to 37° C and equilibrated with 5% CO_2 in artificial air (20.9% O_2, 74% N_2). The artery segments were stepwise stretched to 2.4 kPa, corresponding to a transmural pressure of 18 mmHg. The segments were allowed to equilibrate for about 10 min. The viability of the segments was confirmed by their ability to contract to first potassium-rich PSS (KPSS, 60 mM) and subsequently to phenylephrine (PE, 1 μM). All arteries were incubated with the cyclooxygenase inhibitor indomethacin (3 μM) for 30 min before concentration-response curves were constructed. One artery segment from each mouse was incubated with the eNOS inhibitor N^G-nitro-L-arginine (L-NNA, 10^{-4} M) for 30 min, another segment was incubated with a combination of apamin ($5*10^{-7}$ M) and charybdotoxin (ChTx, 10^{-7} M) for 15 min, and a third artery segment was kept as a control with no additional inhibitors. The arteries were contracted with PE (10^{-7} M) and upon stable contraction, acetylcholine ($3*10^{-7}$ M) was added. After a washout and incubation with the respective blockers, the arteries were contracted with PE (10^{-7} M) and when stable contraction was obtained, NS309 concentration-response curves (10^{-8}–$3*10^{-5}$ M) were performed. After a washout and incubation with the blockers, the arteries were contracted to PE (10^{-7} M) and when the contraction was stable, sodium nitroprusside (SNP) concentration-response curves (10^{-10}–10^{-5} M) were performed. The response of the artery segments was measured as the change in force. The data on relaxation are given as percentage (% relaxation) of the contraction induced by PE.

Drugs and solutions

Doxycycline (Piggidox Vet.) was obtained from Boehringer Ingelheim Danmark A/S. Hypnorm (fentanyl citrate 0.315 mg/ml, fluanisone 10 mg/ml) was purchased from VetaPharma Ltd (Leeds, UK) and dormicum (midazolam, 5 mg/ml) from Hoffmann-La Roche (Basel, Switzerland).

For myograph experiments. The PSS was of the following composition (mM): $CaCl_2$ 1.6, NaCl 119, KCl 4.7, glucose 5.5, $MgSO_4$ H_2O 1.17, $NaHCO_3$ 25, KH_2PO_4 1.18, and EDTA 0.026. The calcium-free PSS solution was of the same composition without $CaCl_2$ 1.6, and potassium-rich PSS (KPSS) solution was of the same composition with NaCl exchanged with KCl to give a final concentration 60 mM. Acetylcholine, indomethacin,PE; L-NNA, and SNP were purchased from Sigma-Aldrich (St. Louis, MO). Apamin and charybdotoxin were purchased from Latoxan (Valence, France). NS309 was kindly donated from Neurosearch (Ballerup, Denmark). For preparation of stock solutions, all drugs were dissolved in distilled water, with the exception of indomethacin and NS309 that were dissolved in DMSO and further diluted in PSS to achieve the final concentration. Apamin and ChTx were prepared in albumin-coated tubes. All solutions were kept at $-20°$ C until use.

Statistics

The computer program GraphPad Prism (San Diego, CA, USA) was used for statistical analysis. Data were expressed as means $\pm$SEM and differences between groups were analyzed by using two-way ANOVA followed by Bonferroni post hoc test. A probability value of P<0.05 was considered significant. The data from a vessel was excluded from the dataset due to technical reasons.

Results

Basic characteristics of normoxic and hypoxic strains

Body weight, heart rate, hematocrit, heart weight-, wet lung weight- and liver weight normalized to body weight are presented in Table 1. Age matched $K_{Ca}3.1^{-/-}/K_{Ca}2.3^{T/T(+ DOX)}$ mice were smaller than wild type mice. The body weight of chronic hypoxic

mice of either genotype was smaller compared to normoxic mice. Exposure to chronic hypoxia increased hematocrit levels, wet lung weight and liver weight. The chronic hypoxic $K_{Ca}3.1^{-/-}/K_{Ca}2.3^{T/T(+DOX)}$ mice however had a significantly smaller increase in liver weight than the chronic hypoxic wild type mice. The heart weight remained unaltered in the normoxic/chronic hypoxic wild type- and $K_{Ca}3.1^{-/-}/K_{Ca}2.3^{T/T(+DOX)}$ mice.

Hemodynamics

Exposure to chronic hypoxia increased the right ventricular systolic blood pressure in normoxic mice of either genotype by 10 to 12 mm Hg (from 24.3$\pm$1.8 mmHg to 37.4$\pm$1.9 mmHg in wild type mice and from 26.4$\pm$2.6 mmHg to 36.0$\pm$2.4 mmHg in $K_{Ca}3.1^{-/-}/K_{Ca}2.3^{T/T(+DOX)}$ mice) and there were no differences between genotypes (Fig. 1A for means and Fig. 1B for tracings). Heart rate was not affected by chronic hypoxia in either genotype and there were no differences between genotypes (Table 1).

Right ventricular hypertrophy

Right ventricular hypertrophy was assessed by determining the weight ratio of the right ventricle over the left ventricle plus septum (RV/LV+S). The chronic hypoxic mice developed right ventricular hypertrophy compared to normoxic mice (Fig. 1C). There was no difference in the degree of right ventricular hypertrophy between wild type- and $K_{Ca}3.1^{-/-}/K_{Ca}2.3^{T/T(+DOX)}$ mice in hypoxia. However, hypoxic $K_{Ca}3.1^{-/-}/K_{Ca}2.3^{T/T(+DOX)}$ mice had an increased right ventricular wall thickness compared to wild type mice (Fig. 1D).

mRNA expression studies

As shown in Fig. 2A, quantitative RT-PCR confirmed the loss of $K_{Ca}3.1$-exon 4 transcripts and reduced $K_{Ca}2.3$ mRNA expression in the $K_{Ca}3.1^{-/-}/K_{Ca}2.3^{T/T(+DOX)}$ mice as expected. In wild type mice, exposure to chronic hypoxia up-regulated $K_{Ca}2.3$ and $K_{Ca}1.1$ mRNA expression, whereas $K_{Ca}2.1$ channel expression was down-regulated. With the exception of $K_{Ca}2.3$, mRNA expression of $K_{Ca}1.1$ was also increased in the $K_{Ca}3.1^{-/-}/K_{Ca}2.3^{T/T(+DOX)}$ and $K_{Ca}2.1$ expression was down-regulated in a similar fashion. Neither genotype nor hypoxia affected mRNA expression of $K_{Ca}2.2$ or eNOS.

As shown in Fig. 2B, expression of α-smooth muscle actin (α-SMA) was increased in hypoxic wild type- and $K_{Ca}3.1^{-/-}/K_{Ca}2.3^{T/T(+DOX)}$ mice if compared to the respective normoxic controls. Expression levels of collagen-1 were not altered by hypoxia but were down-regulated in $K_{Ca}3.1^{-/-}/K_{Ca}2.3^{T/T(+DOX)}$ mice compared to wild type mice. TGFβ expression was not altered by hypoxia or genotype.

Morphological alterations

The pulmonary vessels were stained for Von Willebrandt factor and α-smooth muscle actin and non-muscularized, partially-muscularized, and muscularized vessels were counted and measured (Fig. 3). Chronic hypoxic mice of either genotype had significantly decreased lumen diameters of non-muscularized vessels when compared to normoxic mice of either genotype (Fig. 4A). In contrast, chronic hypoxia did not alter the lumen diameters of partially-muscularized- or fully-muscularized vessels of either genotype. However, the partially-muscularized as well as the fully-muscularized vessels in $K_{Ca}3.1^{-/-}/K_{Ca}2.3^{T/T(+DOX)}$ mice had larger lumen diameter compared to wild type mice.

As shown in Fig. 4B, the wall/lumen ratio for non-muscularized vessels in $K_{Ca}3.1^{-/-}/K_{Ca}2.3^{T/T(+DOX)}$ mice was significantly different from the wild type mice. There was a tendency towards

Table 1. Characteristics of the animals.

		Wild type	$K_{Ca}3.1^{-/-}/K_{Ca}2.3^{T/T(+DOX)}$
Initial	Normoxia	33±1.68	25±0.61*
body weight (g)	Hypoxia	32±1.35	23±0.65*
End	Normoxia	34±1.11	25±0.77*
body weight (g)	Hypoxia	30±0.76#	21±0.56*#
Heart rate	Normoxia	466±33	393±30
(BPM)	Hypoxia	413±48	402±27
Hematocrit	Normoxia	39±3.01	38±3,20
(%)	Hypoxia	54±2.38#	55±3.64#
Heart weight	Normoxia	0.5±0.026	0.5±0.017
(% of BW)	Hypoxia	0.5±0.015	0.5±0.020
RV	Normoxia	0.10±0.003	0.11±0.005
(% of BW)	Hypoxia	0.14±0.006#	0.14±0.006#
LV+S	Normoxia	0.40±0.027	0.39±0.011
(% of BW)	Hypoxia	0.36±0.012	0.36±0.018
Lung weight	Normoxia	0.3±0.047	0.4±0.062
(% of BW)	Hypoxia	0.5±0.059#	0.5±0.063#
Liver weight	Normoxia	4.9±0.69	4.9±0.14
(% of BW)	Hypoxia	6.0±0.21#	5.5±0.16#

Selected morphological and functional characteristics and hematocrit of the normoxic and hypoxic strains. Values are means ±SEM, n=7–8. BPM = beats per minute. BW = body weight. *P<0.05 vs. wild type; #P<0.05 vs. normoxia; 2-way ANOVA (n=7–8 per group).

an increased wall/lumen ratio in chronic hypoxic wild type mice if compared to normoxic wild type mice, whereas the ratio was lower in chronic hypoxic $K_{Ca}3.1^{-/-}/K_{Ca}2.3^{T/T(+DOX)}$ mice if compared to normoxic $K_{Ca}3.1^{-/-}/K_{Ca}2.3^{T/T(+DOX)}$ mice. The wall/lumen ratio was decreased in partially-muscularized vessels in $K_{Ca}3.1^{-/-}/K_{Ca}2.3^{T/T(+DOX)}$ mice when compared to wild type mice. Exposure to chronic hypoxia reduced the wall/lumen ratio in muscularized vessels of either genotype.

The numbers of partially and fully muscularized vessels were increased in both wild type and $K_{Ca}3.1^{-/-}/K_{Ca}2.3^{T/T(+DOX)}$ mice (Fig. 4C).

For the analysis of wall area, the data were grouped according to vessel lumen categories (lumen diameters (μm): 10–19; 20–29; 60–69; Fig. 4C) as previously described [37]. In the vessels with a lumen from 20–29 μm the wall area was larger in hypoxic than in normoxic wild type mice. In contrast, the wall area of the vessels from $K_{Ca}3.1^{-/-}/K_{Ca}2.3^{T/T(+DOX)}$ mice was unaltered in response to chronic hypoxia. The wall area was less in vessels with lumen diameters of 20–39 μm in lung sections from $K_{Ca}3.1^{-/-}/K_{Ca}2.3^{T/T(+DOX)}$ mice (Fig. 4D).

Functional studies

Precontracted pulmonary arteries from chronic hypoxic wild type mice exhibited significantly impaired acetylcholine-induced ($3*10^{-7}$ M) relaxation if compared to normoxic wild type mice (Fig. 5A). Chronic hypoxia also reduced acetylcholine-induced relaxation in arteries from $K_{Ca}3.1^{-/-}/K_{Ca}2.3^{T/T(+DOX)}$ mice and responses under either conditions were similar to those in the wild type mice (Fig. 5A). The $K_{Ca}2.3$- and $K_{Ca}3.1$ channel inhibitors, apamin and charybdotoxin reduced the acetylcholine-induced relaxation in both normoxic and chronic hypoxic wild type mice (Fig. 5B). In contrast to wild type mice, apamin and charybdotoxin did not reduce the acetylcholine-induced relaxation in normoxic

$K_{Ca}3.1^{-/-}/K_{Ca}2.3^{T/T(+DOX)}$ mice (Fig. 5B). However, acetylcholine-induced relaxation became sensitive to apamin and charybdotoxin in the hypoxic $K_{Ca}3.1^{-/-}/K_{Ca}2.3^{T/T(+DOX)}$ mice (Fig. 5B, columns on the right). This might be explained by the up-regulation of mRNA expression of $K_{Ca}1.1$ as described above. Inhibition of NO synthesis by L-NNA almost abolished acetylcholine-evoked relaxation in both normoxic and chronic hypoxic wild type mice as well as in $K_{Ca}3.1^{-/-}/K_{Ca}2.3^{T/T(+DOX)}$ mice (Fig. 5C), still suggesting that NO is the major endothelium-derived vasodilator in pulmonary arteries of both strains.

NS309 at 10^{-6} M induced similar relaxations of precontracted pulmonary arteries, in both normoxic and hypoxic wild type mice and $K_{Ca}3.1^{-/-}/K_{Ca}2.3^{T/T(+DOX)}$ mice. However, NS309-evoked relaxations were significantly increased in the chronic hypoxic mice of either genotype (Fig. 5D). Incubation with apamin and charybdotoxin did not significantly reduced NS309-induced relaxations of pulmonary arteries from normoxic wild type and $K_{Ca}3.1^{-/-}/K_{Ca}2.3^{T/T(+DOX)}$ mice (Fig. 5E). However, the larger NS309-induced relaxation in hypoxic wild type mice was significantly reduced by apamin and charybdotoxin (Fig. 5E). In contrast, apamin and charybdotoxin failed to reduce the larger NS309-induced relaxations of pulmonary arteries from $K_{Ca}3.1^{-/-}/K_{Ca}2.3^{T/T(+DOX)}$ mice. This suggested that the larger NS309-induced relaxation observed in pulmonary arteries from hypoxic wild mice was mediated by $K_{Ca}3.1$ and $K_{Ca}2.3$ channels. L-NNA reduced NS309-evoked relaxations by trend in both wild type and $K_{Ca}3.1^{-/-}/K_{Ca}2.3^{T/T(+DOX)}$ mice and abolished the difference between normoxic and hypoxic mice (Fig. 5F).

Exposure to chronic hypoxia did not alter the concentration-response curve for SNP (Figure S1). These findings suggest that the smooth muscle response to NO was unaltered.

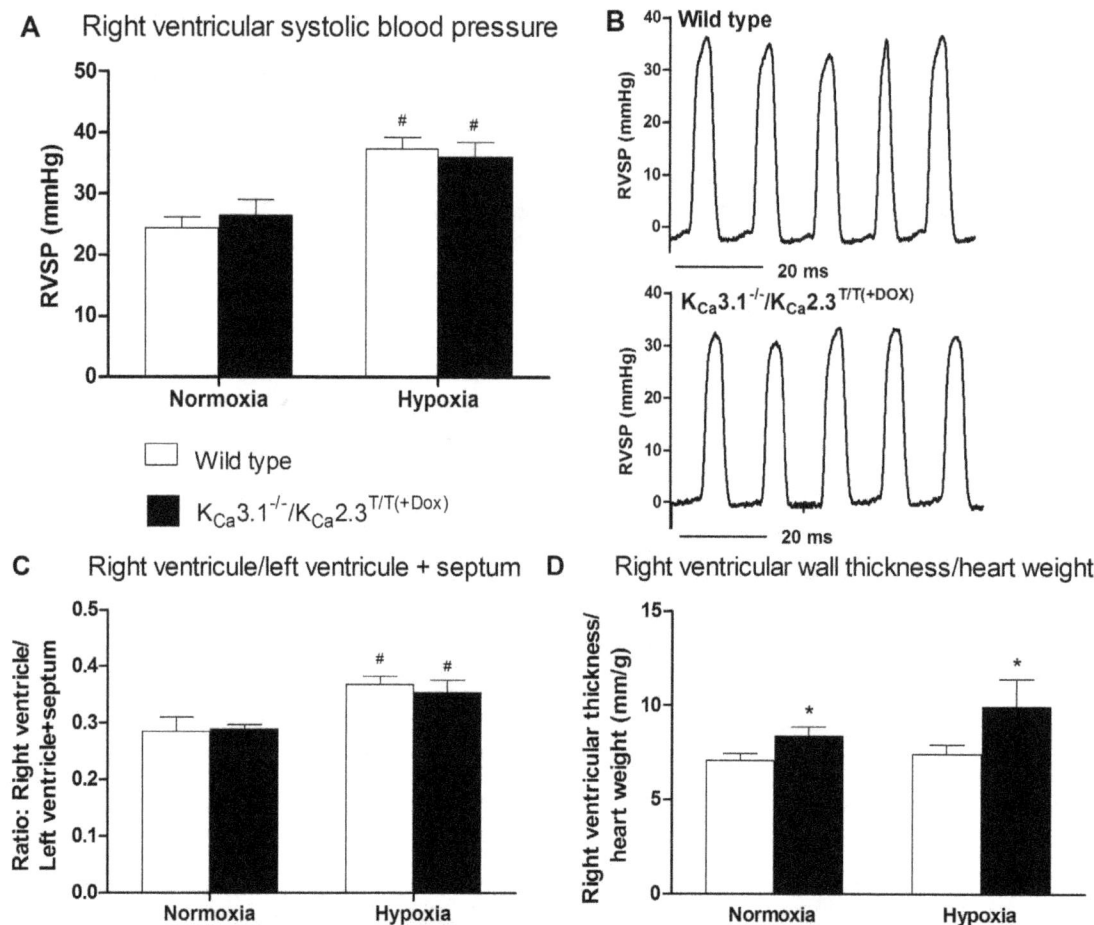

Figure 1. Right ventricular systolic blood pressure and hypertrophy. A) The effect of chronic hypoxia on right ventricular systolic blood pressure (RVSBP) in wild type and $K_{Ca}3.1^{-/-}/K_{Ca}2.3^{T/T(+Dox)}$ mice. Values are means $\pm$SEM, normoxic wild type (n = 8) and $K_{Ca}3.1^{-/-}/K_{Ca}2.3^{T/T(+Dox)}$ mice (n = 7). B) Representative trace of right ventricular pressure measurements in normoxic wild type mice (top) and normoxic $K_{Ca}3.1^{-/-}/K_{Ca}2.3^{T/T(+Dox)}$ mice (bottom). C) Hypoxia induced right ventricular hypertrophy as indicated by alterations of the weight ratio of right ventricle/left ventricle + septum, in wild type and $K_{Ca}3.1^{-/-}/K_{Ca}2.3^{T/T(+Dox)}$ mice, n = 8. D) The effect of hypoxia on right ventricular wall thickness/heart weight (HW) in wild type and $K_{Ca}3.1^{-/-}/K_{Ca}2.3^{T/T(+Dox)}$ mice. Values are mean $\pm$SEM, n = 8. Data were analyzed by 2$-$way ANOVA and differences were considered significant when *$P<0.05$ vs. wild type, $^{\#}$ $P<0.05$ vs. normoxia.

Discussion

The main findings of the present study are that the deficits of the $K_{Ca}2.3$ and $K_{Ca}3.1$ channels failed to change hypoxia-induced pulmonary hypertension, and that chronic hypoxia up-regulated $K_{Ca}2.3$-gene expression (and also of $K_{Ca}1.1$) and increased NS309-induced relaxation in wild type mice. The latter finding points to a novel mechanism to counteract pulmonary hypertension and implicates a potential therapeutic usage of $K_{Ca}2.3/$ $K_{Ca}3.1$ activators for the treatment of pulmonary hypertension. Moreover, genetic deficit of $K_{Ca}3.1$ channels and partial suppression of $K_{Ca}2.3$ channels caused a significant increase of right ventricular wall thickness and alteration in the pulmonary vessels with reduced wall area of pulmonary vessels and increased lumen diameter in partially-muscularized and fully-muscularized vessels.

The effects of hypoxia-induced pulmonary hypertension in wild type mice

The hypoxic model of pulmonary hypertension mimics the changes in pulmonary circulation seen in high altitude. Mice exposed to chronic hypoxia develop pulmonary vasoconstriction, pulmonary vascular remodeling, and right ventricular hypertrophy [38].

In this study, the right ventricular systolic blood pressure was significantly increased in the chronic hypoxic mice reflecting pulmonary hypertension. Right ventricular hypertrophy measured as the right ventricle over left ventricle and septum weight ratio, was significantly increased in chronic hypoxic mice, indicating development of pulmonary hypertension in the chronic hypoxic mice.

Our qRT-PCR studies revealed that exposure to chronic hypoxia increased the mRNA expression of $K_{Ca}2.3$ channels by twofold in the lung of wild type mice. Although it appears a limitation of the present study that the increased $K_{Ca}2.3$ expression is found in the lung, it support our previous studies showing up-regulation of $K_{Ca}2.3$ protein expression in pulmonary arteries without alteration in expression in bronchioles from chronic hypoxic rats [39]. Regarding mRNA expression of $K_{Ca}3.1$ channels in animal models of pulmonary hypertension, previous results have been inhomogeneous: $K_{Ca}3.1$ mRNA expression have been found to be up-regulated in rats with monocrotaline-induced

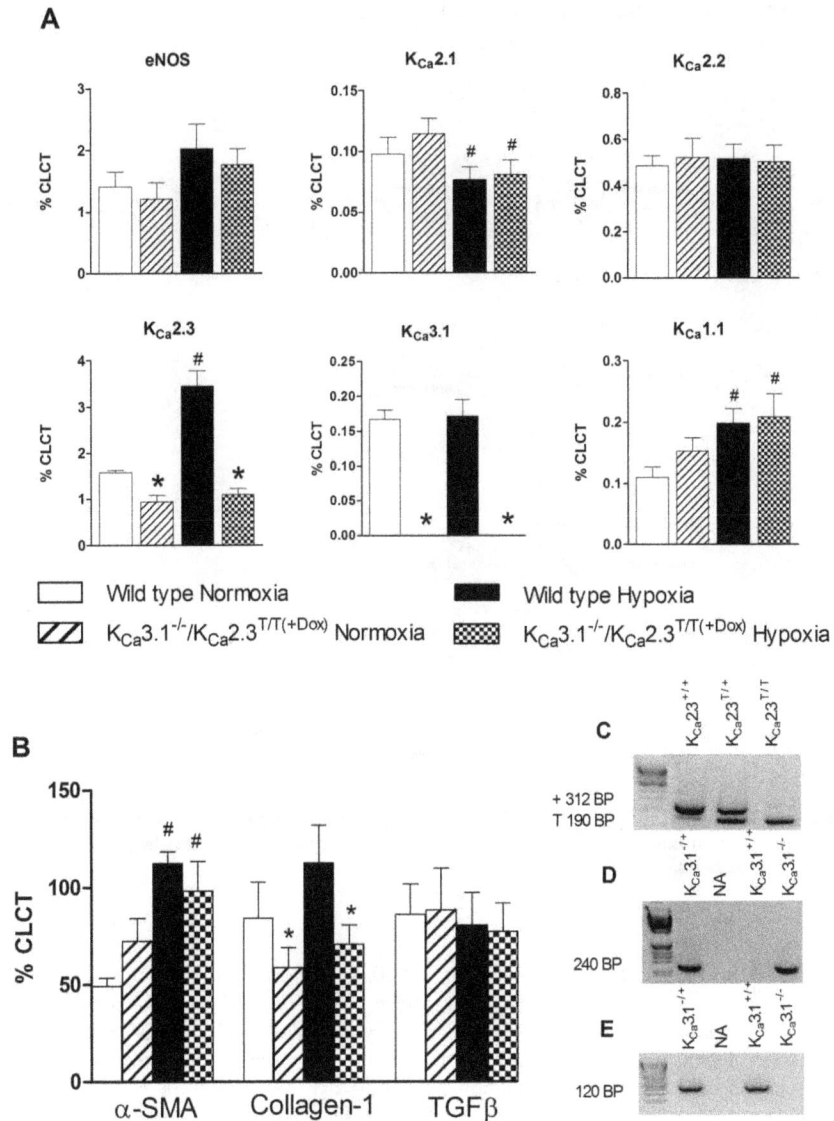

Figure 2. Lung mRNA expression levels of A) eNOS, $K_{Ca}2.1$, $K_{Ca}2.2$, $K_{Ca}2.3$, $K_{Ca}3.1$, and $K_{Ca}1.1$; B) α-Smooth muscle actin (α-SMA), collagen-1, and TGFβ. Data are given as means ±SEM, n = 7–8. Data were analyzed by two-way ANOVA and differences were considered significant when *$P<0.05$ from wild type, # $P<0.05$ from normoxia. Statistical interaction (£) was observed in $K_{Ca}2.3$ expression (A). C–E) Genotyping: C:Gel electrophoresis shows that polymerase chain reacton (PCR) detected the $K_{Ca}2.3$-wild type allele (wild type (+)) and the tTA allele (T) in $K_{Ca}2.3^{T/+}$, and $K_{Ca}2.3^{T/T}$. D and E: PCR detected the targeted allele in $K_{Ca}3.1^{-/+}$ and in $K_{Ca}3.1^{-/-}$ as well as the wild type allele in $K_{Ca}3.1^{+/-}$ and $K_{Ca}3.1^{+/+}$. A DNA ladder was used to determine products sizes.

pulmonary hypertension [40] or unaltered in chronic hypoxic rats [39]. In the present study on mice, chronic hypoxia did not change the $K_{Ca}3.1$ channel mRNA expression. These discrepancies might be explained by a higher degree of lung fibrosis in monocrotaline-induced pulmonary hypertension than in hypoxia-induced pulmonary hypertension. Development of fibrosis was shown to be accompanied by a higher expression of $K_{Ca}3.1$ [22,41].

Regarding the NO system, a decrease in production or activity of NO was previously found in chronic hypoxic animals. Several studies demonstrated an increase in eNOS mRNA but a decrease in NO activity [42–46], while other studies found that the decreased plasma- and lung perfusate NO^-_x in piglets was related to a decrease in eNOS mRNA rather than decreased activity [47]. In this study, the mRNA expression of eNOS was not significantly

changed in the hypoxic mice albeit NO-mediated relaxation of pulmonary arteries in chronically hypoxic mice was reduced as detailed below. This indicates endothelial dysfunction at the level of NO activity and in the absence of compensatory up-regulation of eNOS-mRNA expression.

Hypoxia-induced pulmonary hypertension is associated with vascular remodeling in pulmonary arteries, including the appearance of smooth muscle-like cells in previously non-muscularized vessels, thickening of the media and increased accumulation of smooth muscle cells as well as increased deposition of extracellular matrix proteins, predominantly collagen and elastin [38]. Here we found increased mRNA levels of α-SMA but not of collagen-1 or TGFβ indicating vascular remodeling and media thickening as

| Non-muscularized | Partially-muscularized | Muscularized |

Wild type Normoxia

Wild type Hypoxia

$K_{Ca}3.1^{-/-}/K_{Ca}2.3^{T/T(+Dox)}$ Normoxia

$K_{Ca}3.1^{-/-}/K_{Ca}2.3^{T/T(+Dox)}$ Hypoxia

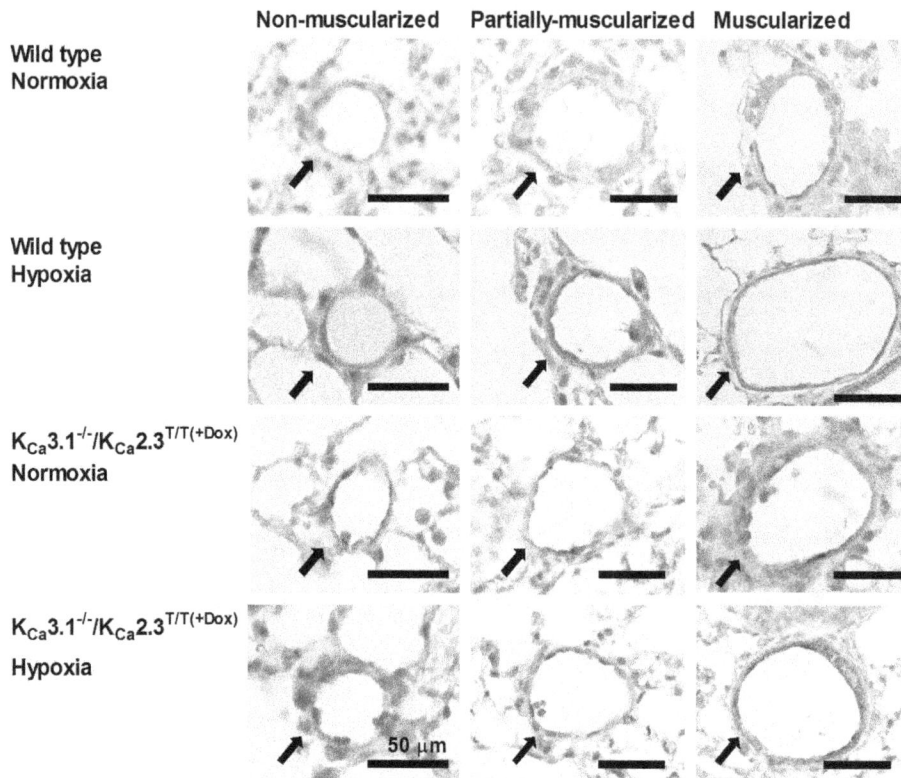

Figure 3. Images of mouse lung showing pulmonary vessels stained for von-Willebrand factor and α-smooth muscle actin from $K_{Ca}3.1^{-/-}/K_{Ca}2.3^{T/T(+Dox)}$ - and wild type mice under normoxic and hypoxic conditions, identifying non-muscularized vessels, partially-muscularized vessels, and fully-muscularized vessels.

outlined above but no substantial pulmonary fibrosis in this murine model.

In agreement with previous studies, exposure to chronic hypoxia and the subsequent development of pulmonary hypertension and of endothelial dysfunction were associated with impaired acetylcholine-induced relaxation in wild type mice [48,49]. The acetylcholine-induced relaxations predominantly involved the NO-pathway as indicated by a full blockade of the response by a blocker of NO-synthesis in hypoxic and normoxic wild type mice. However, also $K_{Ca}2.3$ and $K_{Ca}3.1$ channels contributed to the response in normoxic and hypoxic mice since blockers of the channels clearly reduced the response under either condition.

Regarding the effects of pharmacological activation of the $K_{Ca}2.3$ and $K_{Ca}3.1$ channels in pulmonary arteries, a previous study showed that exposure to chronic hypoxia reduced the relaxations in pulmonary arteries induced by the $K_{Ca}3.1/K_{Ca}2.3$ channel activator NS4591[39]. In contrast, in our study, chronic hypoxia increased the relaxation to the activator NS309 by 3-fold. This discrepancy might be explained by the 10-fold higher potency of NS4591 on the $K_{Ca}3.1$ channel over the $K_{Ca}2.3$ channel and that in our study NS309 preferentially used the up-regulated $K_{Ca}2.3$ channel expression, as described above, to produce a stronger relaxation. However, NS309 in the present study produced a $K_{Ca}2.3/K_{Ca}3.1$-independent relaxation. These small dilator effects could be related to the fact that NS309 at concentrations above 10 μM blocks voltage-dependent Ca^{2+} channels [50] further corroborating substantial unspecific vasodilator effects of this compound. This is further supported by our observation that the NS309-induced relaxation in normoxic wild type mice was insensitive to the $K_{Ca}2.3$ and $K_{Ca}3.1$ channel blockers, apamin and charybdotoxin, which contrasts with earlier findings in rat arteries [26,39]. Nevertheless, the increased NS309-evoked relaxation in chronic hypoxic mice were sensitive to the $K_{Ca}2.3$ and $K_{Ca}3.1$ channel blockers, suggesting that under these conditions and in keeping with the up-regulation of $K_{Ca}2.3$ in the hypoxic mice, a substantial portion of vasodilator capacity is now carried by activation of the $K_{Ca}2.3$ channel and EDH-vasodilator pathways. This interpretation is further supported by the notion that NS309-induced relaxations were not reduced by L-NNA in these hypoxic mice.

Pulmonary hypertension in mice with genetic deficit of $K_{Ca}2.3$ and $K_{Ca}3.1$ channels

The $K_{Ca}3.1^{-/-}/K_{Ca}2.3^{T/T(+DOX)}$ mice developed increased right ventricular systolic blood pressure as well as increased right ventricular hypertrophy ratio to a similar degree as the hypoxic wild type mice. Furthermore, increased ratios of right ventricular wall thickness/heart weight was found in normoxic and hypoxic $K_{Ca}3.1^{-/-}/K_{Ca}2.3^{T/T(+DOX)}$ mice. This may suggest that the down-regulation of the channels caused hypertrophy of the right heart. In addition, previous studies found that the $K_{Ca}2.3^{T/T}$ mice had structural alterations, including enhancement of arteries and enlargement of other hollow organs [21,51], thus the life-long overexpression of the channel in this genetic model of channel overexpression(-Dox)/suppression(+Dox) may influence cardiac development and morphology.

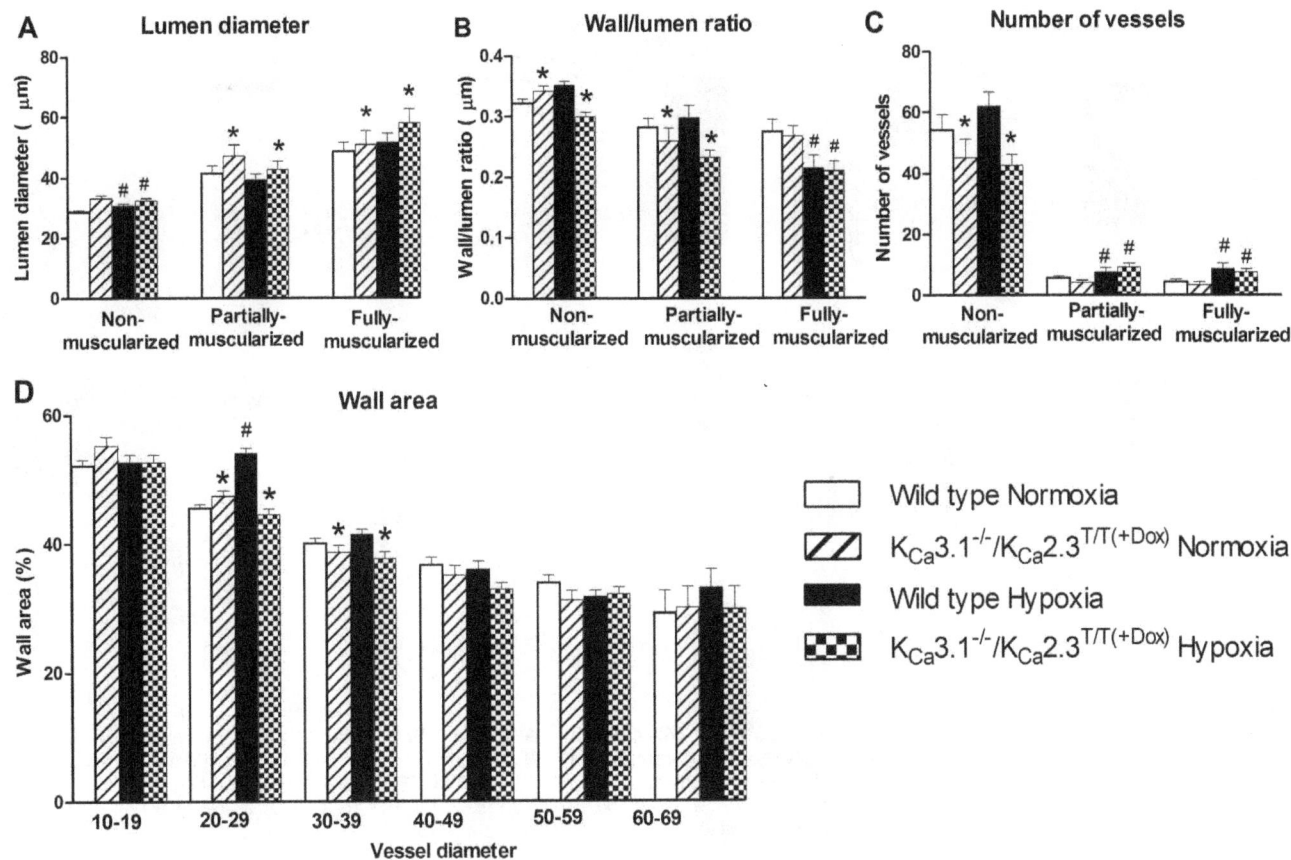

Figure 4. Morphometric measurements. A: Lumen diameter (μm) in vessels divided in groups of non-muscularized-, partially- and fully-muscularized vessels. B: Wall/lumen ratio divided in groups of non-muscularized-, partially- and fully-muscularized vessels. C: Number of non-muscularized-, partially- and muscularized vessels in each experimental group. D: Wall area of the vessels divided in groups of vessel diameter. * P< 0.05 vs. wild type and # P<0.05 vs. normoxia. Statistical interaction was observed in Figure (B) for non-muscularized vessels.

$K_{Ca}2.3$ mRNA expression was present in Dox-treated $K_{Ca}3.1^{-/-}/K_{Ca}2.3^{T/T}$ mice though expression was significantly lower than in wild types, reflecting the fact that the $K_{Ca}2.3$ channel was suppressed rather than knocked out. $K_{Ca}3.1$ channel expression was almost abolished in $K_{Ca}3.1^{-/-}/K_{Ca}2.3^{T/T(+DOX)}$ mice. It is noteworthy that the genetic alterations did not affect the mRNA expression of the other Ca^+-activated K^+ channels ($K_{Ca}2.1$, $K_{Ca}2.2$, and $K_{Ca}1.1$) compared to wild type mice and, thus, there was no evident compensation caused by increased channel expression of these related K_{Ca} channels.

Genetic deficit of $K_{Ca}2.3$ and $K_{Ca}3.1$ channels in normoxic and hypoxic $K_{Ca}3.1^{-/-}/K_{Ca}2.3^{T/T(+DOX)}$ mice increased lumen diameter in partially muscularized- and muscularized vessels compared to normoxic and chronic hypoxic wild type mice. This could be due to the structural alterations previously seen in the $K_{Ca}2.3^{T/T}$ mice [21]. Furthermore, the wall area was significantly decreased in $K_{Ca}3.1^{-/-}/K_{Ca}2.3^{T/T(+DOX)}$ mice compared to wild type mice in vessels of 20–39 μm. Intuitively, one would expect that these structural alterations decrease pulmonary pressure. However pulmonary vascular remodeling by itself is not necessarily sufficient for altering pulmonary pressure in chronic hypoxic mice [52]. In the present study the blood pressure was also not altered in the $K_{Ca}3.1^{-/-}/K_{Ca}2.3^{T/T(+DOX)}$ mice compared to wild type mice regardless of normoxic or chronic hypoxic conditions. This can probably be explained by early developmental alterations in this model.

In a previous study, $K_{Ca}3.1^{-/-}$ mice had reduced acetylcholine-induced relaxation in carotid arteries [19]. Similarly, transgenic $K_{Ca}3.1^{-/-}/K_{Ca}2.3^{T/T(+DOX)}$ mice exhibited defective acetylcholine-induced relaxation in carotid- and systemic resistance arteries [22]. Contrary to these previous findings, $K_{Ca}3.1^{-/-}/K_{Ca}2.3^{T/T(+DOX)}$ mice in the present study did not show impaired acetylcholine-induced relaxation in pulmonary arteries compared to wild type mice. However, this might be explained by the fact that the acetylcholine-induced relaxation in the murine pulmonary arteries was almost entirely mediated by NO and insensitive to blockers of $K_{Ca}2.3$ and $K_{Ca}3.1$ channels, while in other vascular beds the $K_{Ca}3.1/K_{Ca}2.3$-EDH-system and a possible interaction of the EDH with the NO system were found to be more important [22,53].

Surprisingly, exposure to chronic hypoxia converted the acetylcholine-induced relaxation in these mice into an apamin- and charybdotoxin-sensitive relaxation. This could be due to an up-regulation of an apamin-sensitive K^+ channel and/or a charybdotoxin-sensitive K^+ channel (such as $K_{Ca}1.1$), as an adaptation to the hypoxic condition in the $K_{Ca}3.1^{-/-}/K_{Ca}2.3^{T/T(+DOX)}$ mice.

In conclusion, chronic hypoxia increased expression of $K_{Ca}2.3$ and $K_{Ca}1.1$ genes, decreased the expression of $K_{Ca}2.1$, and improved the endothelium-dependent vasodilatation to pharmacological activation of the channels. Such a mechanism could be of help to compensate for the loss of NO-activity in pulmonary

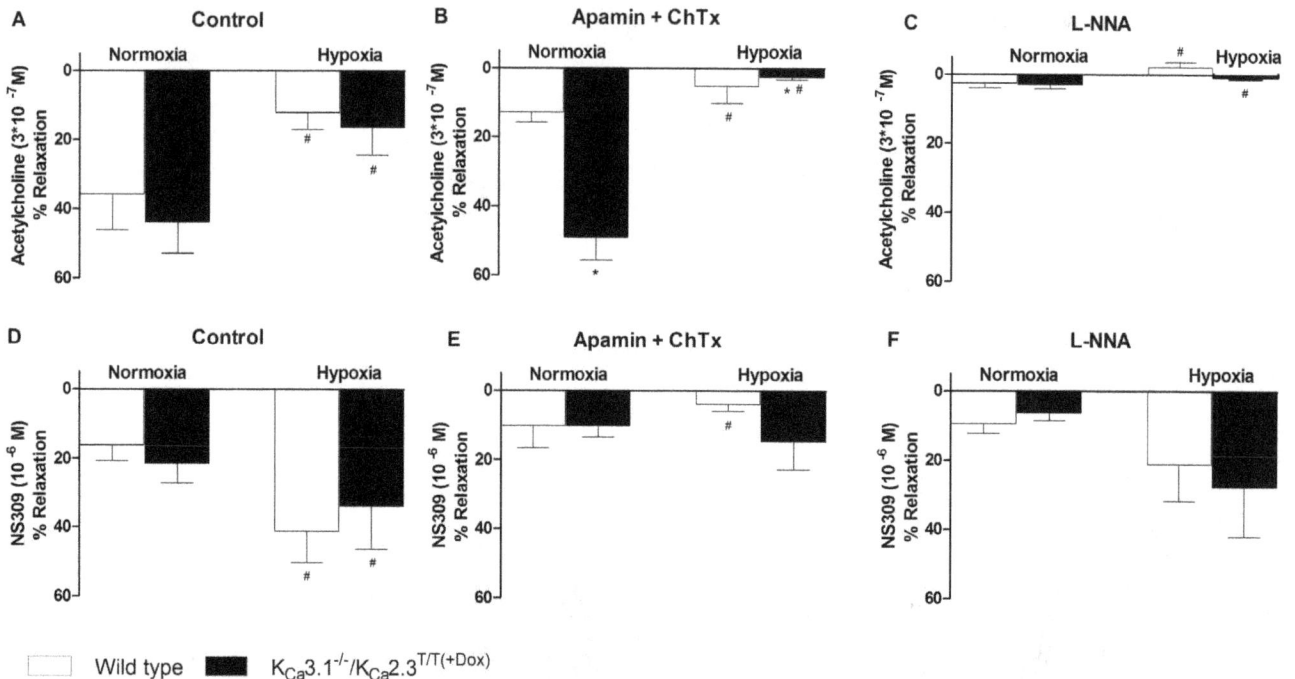

Figure 5. Functional studies of acetylcholine-induced ($3*10^{-7}$ M) relaxation (A–C) and NS309-induced (10^{-6} M) relaxation (D–F) in wild type and $K_{Ca}3.1^{-/-}/K_{Ca}2.3^{T/T(+Dox)}$ mice. A) Acetylcholine-induced relaxation. B) Acetylcholine-evoked relaxation in the presence of apamin ($5*10^{-7}$ M) and ChTx (10^{-7} M). C) Acetylcholine-evoked relaxation in the presence of L-NNA (10^{-4} M). D) NS309-induced relaxation. E) NS309-induced relaxation in the presence of apamin ($5*10^{-7}$ M) and ChTx (10^{-7} M). F) NS309-evoked relaxation in the presence of L-NNA (10^{-4} M). Data were analyzed by 2-way ANOVA and * $P<0.05$ vs. wild type and # $P<0.05$ vs. normoxia; n=6-7 per group.

hypertension and could be pharmacologically targeted to counteract pulmonary hypertension. Genetic deficit of $K_{Ca}3.1$ and $K_{Ca}2.3$ did not worsen pulmonary hypertension or endothelial dysfunction, though it prevented structural vascular remodelling in chronic hypoxia-induced pulmonary hypertension.

Supporting Information

Figure S1 Relaxation to SNP-induced (10^{-10}–10^{-5} M) in PE (10^{-7} M) pre-contracted arteries, in normoxic wild type and $K_{Ca}3.1^{-/-}/K_{Ca}2.3^{T/T(+Dox)}$ mice (left) and hypoxic wild type and $K_{Ca}3.1^{-/-}/K_{Ca}2.3^{T/T(+Dox)}$ mice.

Acknowledgments

We acknowledge laboratory technician Henriette Gram Johanson for excellent technical assistance and Thomas Dalsgaard for helpful discussions.

Author Contributions

Conceived and designed the experiments: CWF ERH RK US. Performed the experiments: CWF LMS VS GN SM. Analyzed the data: CWF LMS VS GN ERH SM RK US. Contributed reagents/materials/analysis tools: RK US. Wrote the paper: CWF RK US. Obtained permission for the animal experiments: US.

References

1. Benza RL, Miller DP, Barst RJ, Badesch DB, Frost AE, et al. (2012) An evaluation of long-term survival from time of diagnosis in pulmonary arterial hypertension from the REVEAL Registry. Chest 142: 448–456.
2. Ignarro LJ, Burke TM, Wood KS, Wolin MS, Kadowitz PJ (1984) Association between cyclic GMP accumulation and acetylcholine-elicited relaxation of bovine intrapulmonary artery. J Pharmacol Exp Ther 228: 682–690.
3. Palmer RM, Ferrige AG, Moncada S (1987) Nitric oxide release accounts for the biological activity of endothelium-derived relaxing factor. Nature 327: 524–526. doi:10.1038/327524a0
4. Moncada S, Vane JR (1978) Pharmacology and endogenous roles of prostaglandin endoperoxides, thromboxane A2, and prostacyclin. Pharmacol Rev 30: 293–331.
5. Campbell WB, Gebremedhin D, Pratt PF, Harder DR (1996) Identification of epoxyeicosatrienoic acids as endothelium-derived hyperpolarizing factors. Circ Res 78: 415–423.
6. Fisslthaler B, Popp R, Kiss L, Potente M, Harder DR, et al. (1999) Cytochrome P450 2C is an EDHF synthase in coronary arteries. Nature 401: 493–497.
7. Hercule HC, Schunck WH, Gross V, Seringer J, Leung FP, et al. (2009) Interaction between P450 eicosanoids and nitric oxide in the control of arterial tone in mice. Arterioscler Thromb Vasc Biol 29: 54–60.

8. Edwards G, Dora KA, Gardener MJ, Garland CJ, Weston AH (1998) K+ is an endothelium-derived hyperpolarizing factor in rat arteries. Nature 396: 269–272.
9. Busse R, Edwards G, Félétou M, Fleming I, Vanhoutte PM, et al. (2002) EDHF: bringing the concepts together. Trends Pharmacol Sci 23: 374–380.
10. Félétou M, Vanhoutte PM (2006) Endothelium-derived hyperpolarizing factor: where are we now? Arterioscler Thromb Vasc Biol 26: 1215–1225.
11. Wei AD, Gutman GA, Aldrich R, Chandy KG, Grissmer S, et al. (2005) International Union of Pharmacology. LII. Nomenclature and molecular relationships of calcium-activated potassium channels. Pharmacol Rev 57: 463–472.
12. Corriu C, Félétou M, Canet E, Vanhoutte PM (1996) Endothelium-derived factors and hyperpolarization of the carotid artery of the guinea-pig. Br J Pharmacol 119: 959–964.
13. Petersson J, Zygmunt PM, Hogestatt ED (1997) Characterization of the potassium channels involved in EDHF-mediated relaxation in cerebral arteries. Br J Pharmacol 120: 1344–1350.
14. Yamanaka A, Ishikawa T, Goto K (1998) Characterization of endothelium-dependent relaxation independent of NO and prostaglandins in guinea pig coronary artery. J Pharmacol Exp Ther 285: 480–489.

15. Grgic I, Kaistha BP, Hoyer J, Köhler R (2009) Endothelial Ca+-activated K+ channels in normal and impaired EDHF-dilator responses—relevance to cardiovascular pathologies and drug discovery. Br J Pharmacol 157: 509–526.

16. Félétou M (2009) Calcium-activated potassium channels and endothelial dysfunction: therapeutic options? Br J Pharmacol 156: 545–562.

17. Köhler R, Kaistha BP, Wulff H (2010) Vascular KCa-channels as therapeutic targets in hypertension and restenosis disease. Expert Opin Ther Targets 14: 143–155.

18. Dalsgaard T, Kroigaard C, Simonsen U (2010) Calcium-activated potassium channels - a therapeutic target for modulating nitric oxide in cardiovascular disease? Expert Opin Ther Targets 14: 825–837.

19. Si H, Heyken WT, Wölfle SE, Tysiac M, Schubert R, et al. (2006) Impaired endothelium-derived hyperpolarizing factor-mediated dilations and increased blood pressure in mice deficient of the intermediate-conductance Ca2+-activated K+ channel. Circ Res 99: 537–544.

20. Wölfle SE, Schmidt VJ, Hoyer J, Köhler R, de WC (2009) Prominent role of KCa3.1 in endothelium-derived hyperpolarizing factor-type dilations and conducted responses in the microcirculation in vivo. Cardiovasc Res 82: 476–483.

21. Taylor MS, Bonev AD, Gross TP, Eckman DM, Brayden JE, et al. (2003) Altered expression of small-conductance Ca2+-activated K+ (SK3) channels modulates arterial tone and blood pressure. Circ Res 93: 124–131.

22. Brähler S, Kaistha A, Schmidt VJ, Wölfle SE, Busch C, et al. (2009) Genetic deficit of SK3 and IK1 channels disrupts the endothelium-derived hyperpolarizing factor vasodilator pathway and causes hypertension. Circulation 119: 2323–2332.

23. Damkjaer M, Nielsen G, Bodendiek S, Staehr M, Gramsbergen JB, et al. (2012) Pharmacological activation of KCa3.1/KCa2.3 channels produces endothelial hyperpolarization and lowers blood pressure in conscious dogs. Br J Pharmacol 165: 223–234.

24. Burnham MP, Bychkov R, Félétou M, Richards GR, Vanhoutte PM, et al. (2002) Characterization of an apamin-sensitive small-conductance Ca(2+)-activated K(+) channel in porcine coronary artery endothelium: relevance to EDHF. Br J Pharmacol 135: 1133–1143.

25. Bychkov R, Burnham MP, Richards GR, Edwards G, Weston AH, et al. (2002) Characterization of a charybdotoxin-sensitive intermediate conductance Ca2+-activated K+ channel in porcine coronary endothelium: relevance to EDHF. Br J Pharmacol 137: 1346–1354.

26. Kroigaard C, Dalsgaard T, Simonsen U (2010) Mechanisms underlying epithelium-dependent relaxation in rat bronchioles: analogy to EDHF-type relaxation in rat pulmonary arteries. Am J Physiol Lung Cell Mol Physiol 298: L531–L542.

27. Kroigaard C, Dalsgaard T, Nielsen G, Laursen BE, Pilegaard H, et al.(2012) Activation of endothelial and epithelial K(Ca) 2.3 calcium-activated potassium channels by NS309 relaxes human small pulmonary arteries and bronchioles. Br J Pharmacol 167: 37–47.

28. Guerard P, Goirand F, Fichet N, Bernard A, Rochette L, et al. (2004) Arachidonic acid relaxes human pulmonary arteries through K+ channels and nitric oxide pathways. Eur J Pharmacol 501: 127–135.

29. Fuloria M, Smith TK, Aschner JL (2002) Role of 5,6-epoxyeicosatrienoic acid in the regulation of newborn piglet pulmonary vascular tone. Am J Physiol Lung Cell Mol Physiol 283: L383–L389.

30. Karamsetty MR, Nakashima JM, Ou L, Klinger JR, Hill NS (2001) EDHF contributes to strain-related differences in pulmonary arterial relaxation in rats. Am J Physiol Lung Cell Mol Physiol 280: L458–L464.

31. Stankevicius E, Dalsgaard T, Kroigaard C, Beck L, Boedtkjer E, et al. (2011) Opening of small and intermediate calcium-activated potassium channels induces relaxation mainly mediated by nitric-oxide release in large arteries and endothelium-derived hyperpolarizing factor in small arteries from rat. J Pharmacol Exp Ther 339: 842–850.

32. Dalsgaard T, Kroigaard C, Bek T, Simonsen U (2009) Role of calcium-activated potassium channels with small conductance in bradykinin-induced vasodilation of porcine retinal arterioles. Invest Ophthalmol Vis Sci 50: 3819–3825.

33. Neylon CB, Lang RJ, Fu Y, Bobik A, Reinhart PH (1999) Molecular cloning and characterization of the intermediate-conductance Ca(2+)-activated K(+) channel in vascular smooth muscle: relationship between K(Ca) channel diversity and smooth muscle cell function. Circ Res 85: e33–e43.

34. Köhler R, Wulff H, Eichler I, Kneifel M, Neumann D, et al. (2003) Blockade of the intermediate-conductance calcium-activated potassium channel as a new therapeutic strategy for restenosis. Circulation 108: 1119–1125.

35. Bond CT, Sprengel R, Bissonnette JM, Kaufmann WA, Pribnow D, et al. (2000) Respiration and parturition affected by conditional overexpression of the Ca2+-activated K+ channel subunit, SK3. Science 289: 1942–1946.

36. Baandrup JD, Markvardsen LH, Peters CD, Schou UK, Jensen JL, et al. (2011) Pressure load: the main factor for altered gene expression in right ventricular hypertrophy in chronic hypoxic rats. PLoS One 6: e15859.

37. Cahill E, Costello CM, Rowan SC, Harkin S, Howell K, et al. (2012) Gremlin plays a key role in the pathogenesis of pulmonary hypertension. Circulation 125: 920–930.

38. Stenmark KR, Fagan KA, Frid MG (2006) Hypoxia-induced pulmonary vascular remodeling: cellular and molecular mechanisms. Circ Res 99: 675–691.

39. Kroigaard C, Kudryavtseva O, Dalsgaard T, Wandall-Frostholm C, Olesen SP, et al. (2013) KCa3.1 channel downregulation and impaired EDH-type relaxation in pulmonary arteries from chronic hypoxic rats. Exp Physiol 98 (4):957–69.

40. Morio Y, Homma N, Takahashi H, Yamamoto A, Nagaoka T, et al. (2007) Activity of endothelium-derived hyperpolarizing factor is augmented in monocrotaline-induced pulmonary hypertension of rat lungs. J Vasc Res 44: 325–335.

41. Huang C, Shen S, Ma Q, Chen J, Gill A, et al. (2013) Blockade of KCa3.1 Ameliorates Renal Fibrosis Through the TGF-beta1/Smad Pathway in Diabetic Mice. Diabetes 62: 2923–2934.

42. Shaul PW, North AJ, Brannon TS, Ujiie K, Wells LB, et al. (1995) Prolonged in vivo hypoxia enhances nitric oxide synthase type I and type III gene expression in adult rat lung. Am J Respir Cell Mol Biol 13: 167–174.

43. Le Cras TD, Xue C, Rengasamy A, Johns RA (1996) Chronic hypoxia upregulates endothelial and inducible NO synthase gene and protein expression in rat lung. Am J Physiol 270: L164–L170.

44. Le Cras TD, Tyler RC, Horan MP, Morris KG, Tuder RM, et al. (1998) Effects of chronic hypoxia and altered hemodynamics on endothelial nitric oxide synthase expression in the adult rat lung. J Clin Invest 101: 795–801.

45. Xue C, Johns RA (1996) Upregulation of nitric oxide synthase correlates temporally with onset of pulmonary vascular remodeling in the hypoxic rat. Hypertension 28: 743–753.

46. Resta TC, Gonzales RJ, Dail WG, Sanders TC, Walker BR (1997) Selective upregulation of arterial endothelial nitric oxide synthase in pulmonary hypertension. Am J Physiol 272: H806–H813.

47. Fike CD, Kaplowitz MR, Thomas CJ, Nelin LD (1998) Chronic hypoxia decreases nitric oxide production and endothelial nitric oxide synthase in newborn pig lungs. Am J Physiol 274: L517–L526.

48. Adnot S, Raffestin B, Eddahibi S, Braquet P, Chabrier PE (1991) Loss of endothelium-dependent relaxant activity in the pulmonary circulation of rats exposed to chronic hypoxia. J Clin Invest 87: 155–162.

49. Mam V, Tanbe AF, Vitali SH, Arons E, Christou HA, et al. (2010) Impaired vasoconstriction and nitric oxide-mediated relaxation in pulmonary arteries of hypoxia- and monocrotaline-induced pulmonary hypertensive rats. J Pharmacol Exp Ther 332: 455–462.

50. Morimura K, Yamamura H, Ohya S, Imaizumi Y (2006) Voltage-dependent Ca2+-channel block by openers of intermediate and small conductance Ca2+-activated K+ channels in urinary bladder smooth muscle cells. J Pharmacol Sci 100: 237–241.

51. Herrera GM, Pozo MJ, Zvara P, Petkov GV, Bond CT, et al. (2003) Urinary bladder instability induced by selective suppression of the murine small conductance calcium-activated potassium (SK3) channel. J Physiol 551: 893–903.

52. Littler CM, Wehling CA, Wick MJ, Fagan KA, Cool CD, et al. (2005) Divergent contractile and structural responses of the murine PKC-epsilon null pulmonary circulation to chronic hypoxia. Am J Physiol Lung Cell Mol Physiol 289: L1083–L1093.

53. Feletou M, Kohler R, Vanhoutte PM (2012) Nitric oxide: orchestrator of endothelium-dependent responses. Ann Med 44: 694–716.

2

Longitudinal *In Vivo* SPECT/CT Imaging Reveals Morphological Changes and Cardiopulmonary Apoptosis in a Rodent Model of Pulmonary Arterial Hypertension

Michael L. Paffett[1]*, Jacob Hesterman[2], Gabriel Candelaria[3], Selita Lucas[1], Tamara Anderson[3], Daniel Irwin[3], Jack Hoppin[2], Jeffrey Norenberg[3], Matthew J. Campen[1]

1 Department of Pharmaceutical Sciences, University of New Mexico Health Sciences Center, Albuquerque, New Mexico, United States of America, **2** inviCRO, Boston, Massachusetts, United States of America, **3** Radiopharmaceutical Sciences Program, College of Pharmacy and Keck-UNM Small-Animal Imaging Resource, University of New Mexico Health Sciences Center, Albuquerque, New Mexico, United States of America

Abstract

Pulmonary arterial hypertension (PAH) has a complex pathogenesis involving both heart and lungs. Animal models can reflect aspects of the human pathology and provide insights into the development and underlying mechanisms of disease. Because of the variability of most animal models of PAH, serial *in vivo* measurements of cardiopulmonary function, morphology, and markers of pathology can enhance the value of such studies. Therefore, quantitative *in vivo* SPECT/CT imaging was performed to assess cardiac function, morphology and cardiac perfusion utilizing ^{201}Thallium (^{201}Tl) in control and monocrotaline-treated rats. In addition, lung and heart apoptosis was examined with ^{99m}Tc-Annexin V (^{99m}Tc-Annexin) in these cohorts. Following baseline imaging, rats were injected with saline or monocrotaline (50 mg/kg, i.p.) and imaged weekly for 6 weeks. To assess a therapeutic response in an established pulmonary hypertensive state, a cohort of rats received resveratrol in drinking water (3 mg/kg/day) on days 28–42 post-monocrotaline injection to monitor regression of cardiopulmonary apoptosis. PAH in monocrotaline-treated rats was verified by conventional hemodynamic techniques on day 42 (right ventricular systolic pressure (RSVP) = 66.2 mmHg in monocrotaline vs 28.8 mmHg in controls) and in terms of right ventricular hypertrophy (RV/LVS = 0.70 in monocrotaline vs 0.32 in controls). Resveratrol partially reversed both RVSP (41.4 mmHg) and RV/LVS (0.46), as well as lung edema and RV contractility $+dP/dt_{max}$. Serial ^{99m}Tc-Annexin V imaging showed clear increases in pulmonary and cardiac apoptosis when compared to baseline, which regressed following resveratrol treatment. Monocrotaline induced modest changes in whole-heart perfusion as assessed by ^{201}Tl imaging and cardiac morphological changes consistent with septal deviation and enlarged RV. This study demonstrates the utility of functional *in vivo* SPECT/CT imaging in rodent models of PAH and further confirms the efficacy of resveratrol in reversing established monocrotaline-induced PAH presumably by attenuation of cardiopulmonary apoptosis.

Editor: James West, Vanderbilt University Medical Center, United States of America

Funding: This study was supported in part by an internally funded pilot project, Translational Cardiopulmonary Functional Assessment in a Rat Model of Pulmonary Arterial Hypertension (CMDP2010), by a grant from the National Institutes of Health (ES014369), and Small-Animal SPECT/CT images in this article were generated at the Keck-University of New Mexico Small-Animal Imaging Resource (KUSAIR) established through a grant from the W.M. Keck Foundation, and supported by the NCI-designated University of New Mexico Cancer Center Support Grant (P30CA118100-06). The funders had no role in study design, data collection and analysis, decision to publish, or preparation of the manuscript.

Competing Interests: J. Hesterman and J. Hoppin work for inviCRO and their roles are technical support related to image acquisition and analysis.

* E-mail: mpaffett@salud.unm.edu

Introduction

Idiopathic pulmonary artery hypertension (PAH) is a devastating lung vascular disease mainly afflicting women in their fourth decade of life [1]. PAH is associated with an extremely poor prognosis, with an estimated median survival of 2.8 years from time of diagnosis to death [2]. Despite significant advancements in disease management, there is no known cure for PAH and treatment regimens remain palliative. The pathobiology of PAH is characterized as an obliterative vascular disease of the small pulmonary arteries in which excessive proliferation of pulmonary artery endothelial and smooth muscle cells lead to remodeling of pulmonary arteries, increased pulmonary vascular resistance, and eventually right heart failure. Furthermore, right ventricular failure is the major cause of mortality in patients diagnosed with idiopathic or severe secondary varieties of PAH [3].

Because the disease is difficult to diagnose until later stages, much of what is known about PAH comes from animal models. Numerous models exist, with varying coherence to the human disease. Such models provide an opportunity to observe factors that may contribute to the early stages of pulmonary arterial remodeling, lesion formation, and right ventricular hypertrophy, as in humans we are mostly knowledgeable regarding outcomes of fulminant disease. Thus, a key advantage of animal disease models coupled with *in vivo* imaging techniques is the unique capacity to conduct serial, non-invasive studies that allow for a better understanding of disease progression and response to therapeutic intervention. Recent findings by Marsboom et al. [4]

utilize ^{18}F-fluorodeoxyglucose positron emission tomography in both monocrotaline and Sugen models of PAH to monitor the shift toward glycolytic metabolism lung vascular cells as well as therapeutic responses to dichloroacetate or imatinib. In a different study, therapeutic efficacy of the angiotensin II receptor antagonist varlsartan has been demonstrated by serial *in vivo* measurements of cardiac apoptosis utilizing ^{99m}Tc-Annexin-V (^{99m}Tc-Annexin) scintigraphy in the monocrotaline model of PAH [5]. With respect to conventional physiological assessment of classical indices of PAH, we established a time-course reflecting the development of increasing RSVP and right ventricular hypertrophy in the monocrotaline model [6]. Moreover, we found that oral administration of resveratrol attenuates these pathologic variables after the development of monocrotaline-induced PAH. Although controversial, allosteric activation of SIRT1 by resveratrol may be one of several protective mechanisms in addition to its anti-inflammatory and anti-oxidant related mechanisms [7]. In terms of cardiac function, resveratrol has been shown to improve contractility, diastolic function and attenuate cardiomyocytes apoptosis in a number of experimental models of cardiac dysfunction [8,9,10]. Furthermore, resveratrol improves survival in rodent models of heart failure and myocardial infarction by modulating cardio-myocyte energetic phenotype [11] and reversing left ventricular hypertrophy [12].

The present study explores a SPECT/CT characterization of the major pathophysiological changes in response to monocrota-line, a toxin selectively injurious to the pulmonary vascular endothelium that leads to pulmonary artery and right ventricular remodeling. Quantitative *in vivo* ECG-gated [201]TI SPECT/CT imaging was performed to assess longitudinal changes in cardiac function, morphology and perfusion. Additionally, cardiac and pulmonary vascular apoptosis was assessed by ^{99m}Tc-Annexin in control and monocrotaline-treated rats. Furthermore, parallel longitudinal studies examined the effects of chronic oral resveratrol administration on monocrotaline-induced cardiac and pulmonary vascular apoptosis by ^{99m}Tc-Annexin radiographic imaging. Findings from the study highlight the value of longitudinal analysis in observing monocrotaline-induced RV dysfunction and the efficacy of chronic oral resveratrol administration on pulmonary as well as cardiac apoptosis.

Results

Similar to our previous report [6], a moderate monocrotaline dose (50 mg/kg) induced significant increases in peak and mean right ventricular pressure (Fig. 1A-B) when compared to saline injected rats. No effects of oral resveratrol administration (day 28–42) were seen in saline injected controls. However, resveratrol led to a significant attenuation in systolic and mean right ventricular pressures in monocrotaline injected rats which was consistent with our previous findings [6]. Interestingly, $+dP/dt_{max}$ was elevated in the monocrotaline-saline group compared to controls (saline-saline) and resveratrol normalized the magnitude of $+dP/dt_{max}$ to the level of controls (Fig. 1C). In an effort to determine whether anesthesia had a disproportional impact on these hemodynamic measures, heart rates were calculated and were found to be consistent between groups indicating a consistent level of anesthesia (Fig. 1D).

In addition to blood pressure measurements, the changes in mass of the right ventricular and left ventricular plus septa were examined across these cohorts. As expected, monocrotaline-induced PAH led to hypertrophy of the RV relative to the left ventricle plus septal wall (RV/LVS) as indicated in Figure 2A.

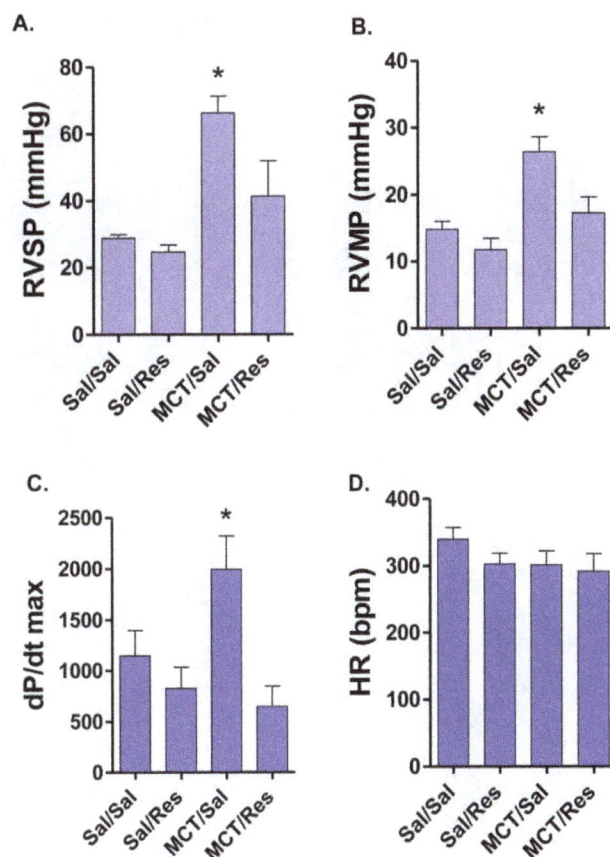

Figure 1. Monocrotaline induced significant changes in right ventricular systolic (A) and mean (B) pressure, which were alleviated by late treatment with resveratrol in the drinking water. Right-sided cardiac contractility, as assessed by $+dP/dt_{max}$ from the RV pressure wave, was significantly elevated in the MCT-treated rats, and again reduced to control levels by resveratrol (C). No heart rate (HR) differences among the groups were noted, confirming a consistent level of anesthetic depth between groups during hemodynamic assessment (D). Asterisks indicate significant (P<0.05) elevation over other groups by ANOVA with Newman-Keuls Posthoc Comparison Test.

Additionally, a slight increase in lung edema was noted (Fig. 2B), but was not significant in this moderate model of monocrotaline PAH. *In vivo* SPECT imaging revealed pronounced leftward septal wall deviation at week 4 in the monocrotaline-treated rats (Fig. 2C &D); however, radiologic analysis of RV morphology was limited to overt RV hypertrophy due to disproportionate ^{201}Tl uptake in the left ventricle compared to the thinner walled RVs in the control rats. In a manner consistent with reduced RV systolic pressures (Fig. 1), resveratrol reversed both RV hypertrophy (Fig. 2A) and septal deviation (Fig. 2B & C) in monocrotaline-treated rats, demonstrating therapeutic efficacy.

Given the overt changes on RV hypertrophy and cardiac wall morphology by monocrotaline, we set forth to examine left ventricle diastolic and systolic volumes from ECG-gated ^{201}Tl SPECT images. Monocrotaline induced progressive reductions in LV residual volume, which is consistent with the notion of ventricular interdependence (Fig. 3A). As mentioned above, the SPECT image analysis software algorithm was unable to reliably compute RV diastolic and systolic volumes in control rats because of disproportional ^{201}Tl signal from the LV, which consistently obscured RV ^{201}Tl signal except in extreme cases of RV

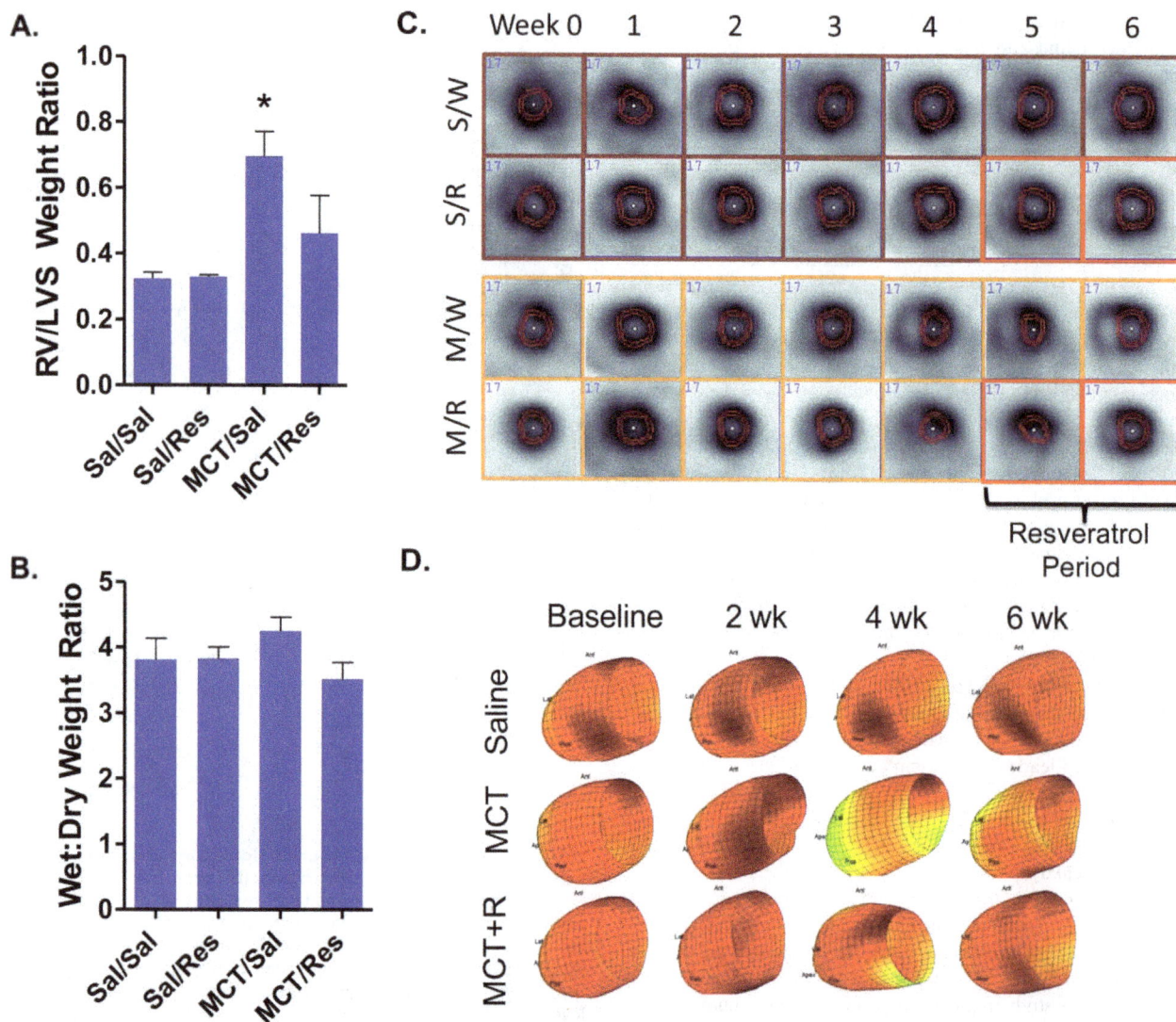

Figure 2. Right ventricular remodeling following MCT injection was evident from the ratio of right ventricular mass to left ventricular plus septal mass (RV/LVS); this effect was diminished by resveratrol treatment (A). No obvious effect on lung remodeling or edema formation was noted at 42 days post-MCT injection (B). Right ventricular enlargement was evident at 3–4 weeks in MCT/water-treated rats (M/W), with some resolution in MCT/resveratrol rats (M/R) from SPECT images of ^{201}Thallium (C). No apparent changes were noted in saline/water (S/W) or saline/resveratrol (S/R) control rats. Notably, septal indentation, a result of increased right ventricular pressure, was evident as early as 2 weeks post-MCT (D). Asterisks indicate significant (P<0.05) elevation over other groups by ANOVA with Newman-Keuls Posthoc Comparison Test.

hypertrophy. Further *post hoc* analysis of ejection fraction (%) and stroke volume (μL) was derived from diastolic-systolic filling curves (Fig. 3B & C). Interestingly, ejection fraction was elevated in monocrotaline-treated rats at weeks 4–5 and then returned to baseline at week 6, whereas ejection fraction was unchanged in saline controls. Moreover, stroke volume was not changed in either group suggesting an increase in contractility. Therefore, we assessed RV contractility (+dP/dt_{max}) and found a significant increase in +dP/dt_{max} 6 weeks following monocrotaline treatment compared to saline controls, which resolved in the monocrotaline-treated rats receiving resveratrol (Fig. 1C). In addition to cardiac function utilizing ECG-gated ^{201}Tl imaging, we were able to longitudinally evaluate net cardiac perfusion (Fig. 4). No consistent changes in net cardiac perfusion were observed as a result of monocrotaline, although a slight non-significant trend occurred at week 5.

Longitudinal *in vivo* quantification of pulmonary and cardiac ^{99m}Tc-Annexin SPECT imaging was performed in saline- and monocrotaline-treated rats receiving either tap water or resveratrol. Thoracic SPECT/CT images illustrate this increase in ^{99m}Tc-Annexin binding in monocrotaline-treated rats and the sparing effect of resveratrol on lung apoptosis (Fig. 5A). Monocrotaline induced a progressive increase in ^{99m}Tc-Annexin binding in the lung compared to saline controls (Figure 5B). This elevation in ^{99m}Tc-Annexin began in the lungs of some monocrotaline-treated rats as early as 3 weeks post injection and was consistently elevated at weeks 5 and 6. Specifically, 2 premature lethalities were observed in the early onset of increased ^{99m}Tc-Annexin binding *(data not shown)*. Similar to these pulmonary findings, monocrotaline induced a corresponding increase in ^{99m}Tc-Annexin binding in the heart in which these elevations were only observed during weeks 5–6 post monocrotaline (Fig. 6A). Furthermore, resveratrol treatment abrogated this increase in ^{99m}Tc-

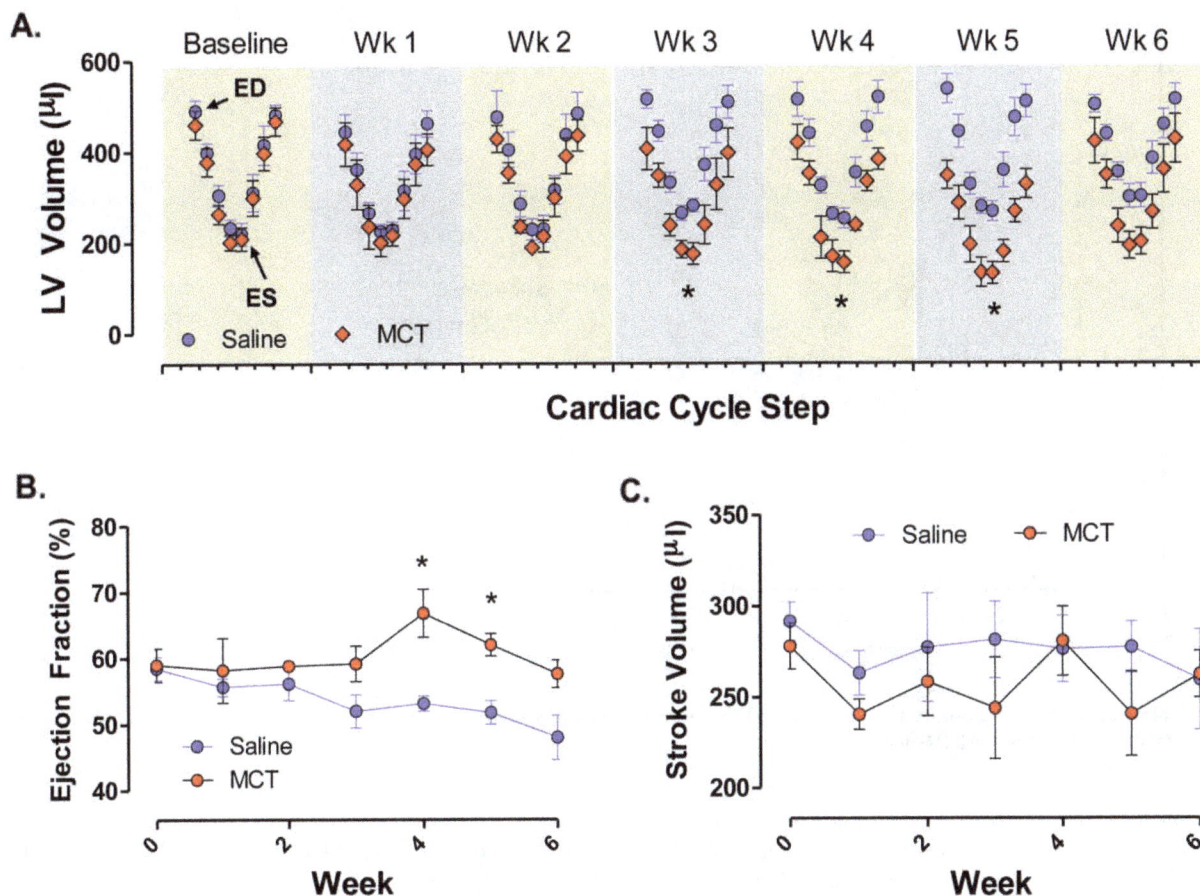

Figure 3. Left-sided cardiac cycle changes over the 6-week period of MCT-induced PAH pathogenesis (A). ECG-gating methods enabled the distribution of [201]Thallium decay detections into 8 bins between electrocardiographic R waves. Cardiac cycles from end diastole (ED) to subsequent end diastole are shown, with end systole (ES) in the middle. Both treatment groups showed nearly identical left ventricular function at baseline and up until week 3 post-MCT injection. At week 3, and progressing through week 5, a significant reduction in the overall volume of the left ventricle was noted. This corresponded with increased ejection fraction (B) and no net change in stroke volume (C) over the same time period. Asterisks indicate significant (P<0.05) elevation over other groups by 2-way (time, treatment) ANOVA.

Annexin in monocrotaline-treated rats and had no measureable effect of altering apoptosis in saline control rats.

Discussion

The present study confirms the ability of orally-administered resveratrol to provide therapeutic effects in an established model of pulmonary hypertension. The use of non-invasive, *in vivo* SPECT-CT imaging offered the ability to examine functional, morphological, and biomolecular changes longitudinally in this model, which revealed an important role of resveratrol in blocking the development of apoptosis in the hearts and lungs of monocrotaline-treated subjects.

In vivo SPECT/CT imaging revealed a number of pathophysiological changes in the cardiopulmonary system over a 6-week period of PAH development. Most prominent were changes in the diastole/systole filling curves (Fig. 2A), evidenced by a significant reduction in LV filling volumes during the cardiac cycle developed from weeks 3–5 in monocrotaline-treated rats. Furthermore, volumetric SPECT assessment of LV function corroborated the development of septal deviation, as evidenced by the reduced ventricular reserve volume and morphological findings, which nicely illustrates the concept of ventricular interdependence. Under normal physiological conditions, the right ventricular force

generation and diastolic behavior is influenced by the left ventricle [13], whereas when RV pressure increases there is an impingement on left ventricular diastolic filling. Importantly, and consistent with what is found in compensated RV dysfunction, LV function was unimpaired in terms of overall output [14]. However, in scenarios where the right ventricular function is compromised, such as in Cor Pulmonale, secondary LV diastolic dysfunction is likely and the impairment of cardiac output is of clinical concern.

Interestingly, we observed an increase in ejection fraction without increases in stroke volume, which could potentially be explained in part by increases in contractility (illustrated by compensatory increases in $+dP/dt_{max}$) along with the reduction in end-diastolic volumes. Although we did observe an increase in ejection fraction in monocrotaline-treated rats, this parameter appeared to resolve due to spontaneous disease regression or secondary to RV failure. Indeed, in a slightly more severe model of monocrotaline-induced PAH (using 60 mg/kg instead of 50 mg/kg), Correia-Pinto et al. [15] demonstrated substantial LV diastolic dysfunction and biomolecular changes at week 6 post-injection. Similar findings were also reported by Campian et al. [5], where echocardiographic assessment of RV failure was evident in monocrotaline-treated rats and was significantly delayed with

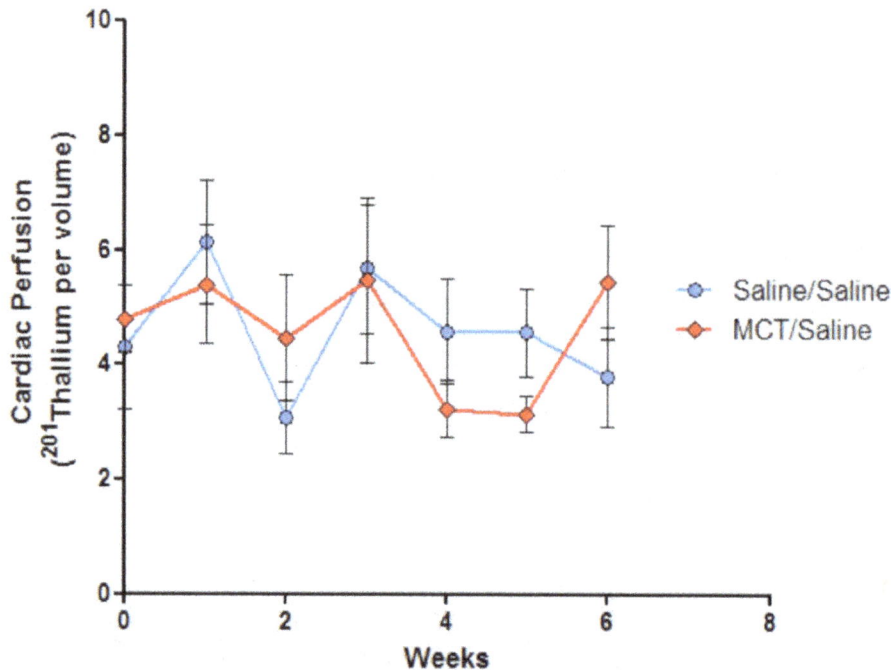

Figure 4. Global cardiac perfusion, as assessed by 201Thallium detection, showed no significant differences between groups or trends across the 42-day imaging period.

long-term administration of valsartan, although losartan proved to have little therapeutic benefit in secondary human forms of PAH [16]. Aside from this caveat related to the discrepancy between the monocrotaline model and various forms of human PAH, this report documented the progression of RV dysfunction in rats. This was attributed to, in part, by an increase in early stage myocardial apoptosis and highlights the importance of *in vivo* longitudinal study design in order to better identify temporal events and how these markers relate to cardiac function during disease progression.

The plant-derived phytoalexin, resveratrol, has recently been shown to prevent [7] as well as reverse monocrotaline-induced PAH [6]. It has not clear if the principle therapeutic action resides within the pulmonary vasculature and/or the myocardium. The present study provides robust support for inhibition of cell death, both in the heart and lungs, as a major therapeutic outcome of resveratrol treatment, however we cannot be certain whether these effects are entirely the result of resveratrol; an oxidation product of resveratrol or metabolite of this poorly bioavailable phytoalexin. While Csiszar et al. [7] did not show significant increases in pulmonary endothelial apoptosis, this was possibly due to assessments of PAH endpoints at an earlier stage of disease. They examined tissues at 14 and 21 days post-monocrotaline, while we did not observe increased annexin signals until day 28 in some subjects, with consistently-elevated apoptosis at day 35 post-monocrotaline. Using ^{99m}Tc-Annexin scintigraphy, Campian et al. [5] showed that the 60 mg/kg monocrotaline-treated model could induce right ventricular apoptosis as early as the third week post-injection and reaching a maximum at day 28, with confirmation by TUNEL staining and autoradiography. Vascular TUNEL staining has been shown to increase at day 28 in the monocrotaline-treated model [17] and other groups using different methods (i.e. Caspase-3 staining) have observed indications of vascular apoptosis at earlier time points [18]. In addition, Yang et al. [19] observed a histological improvement in right ventricular apoptosis

by resveratrol at day 21 post-monocrotaline treatment although the resveratrol was administered prior to the development of PAH.

Taken together, these studies are consistent with regard to the onset of either cardiac or vascular apoptosis, despite discrepancies in monocrotaline dosing, and reinforce the utility of longitudinal *in vivo* studies designed to assess the efficacy of resveratrol to reverse established monocrotaline-induced PAH. In addition to the potential contribution of myocardial apoptosis to RV failure, increases in myocardial fibrosis also appear to influence disease progression in a number of heart failure models. Specifically, myocardial collagen deposition has been documented in a compensatory RV hypertrophy monocrotaline model [20] as well as overt failure (60 mg/kg) with the toxic pyrrole [5]. Although speculative, alternative therapeutic actions of resveratrol in the current study may be related to anti-inflammatory and/or anti-fibrotic effects described by Chan et al. [21], where this dietary compound decreased inflammatory cell infiltration, decreased cardiac fibrosis and improved both cardiac and vascular function.

One notable caveat is that the monocrotaline-treated model of PAH is associated with a substantial inflammatory response. Specifically, monocrotaline-enhanced IL-6 response and reduction in the clinically-relevant marker BMPR2 are known to contribute to the development of PAH [22]. In addition to these findings, Wang et al. [23] demonstrated monocrotaline-induced PAH is associated with differential perivascular T-helper activation. With respect to phosphatidylserine externalization as an early marker of apoptosis, activated macrophages also externalize these residues; thus, annexin may also serve as an inflammatory marker [24]. Resveratrol potentially mitigates components of the secondary inflammation caused by monocrotaline [7]. However, in the present study there was a 5-week delay in monocrotaline-induced ^{99m}Tc-Annexin signal in the heart and lungs (Fig. 5 & 6) which was completely nullified with resveratrol. In previous work, we found that monocrotaline-associated inflammation was minimal at 6-

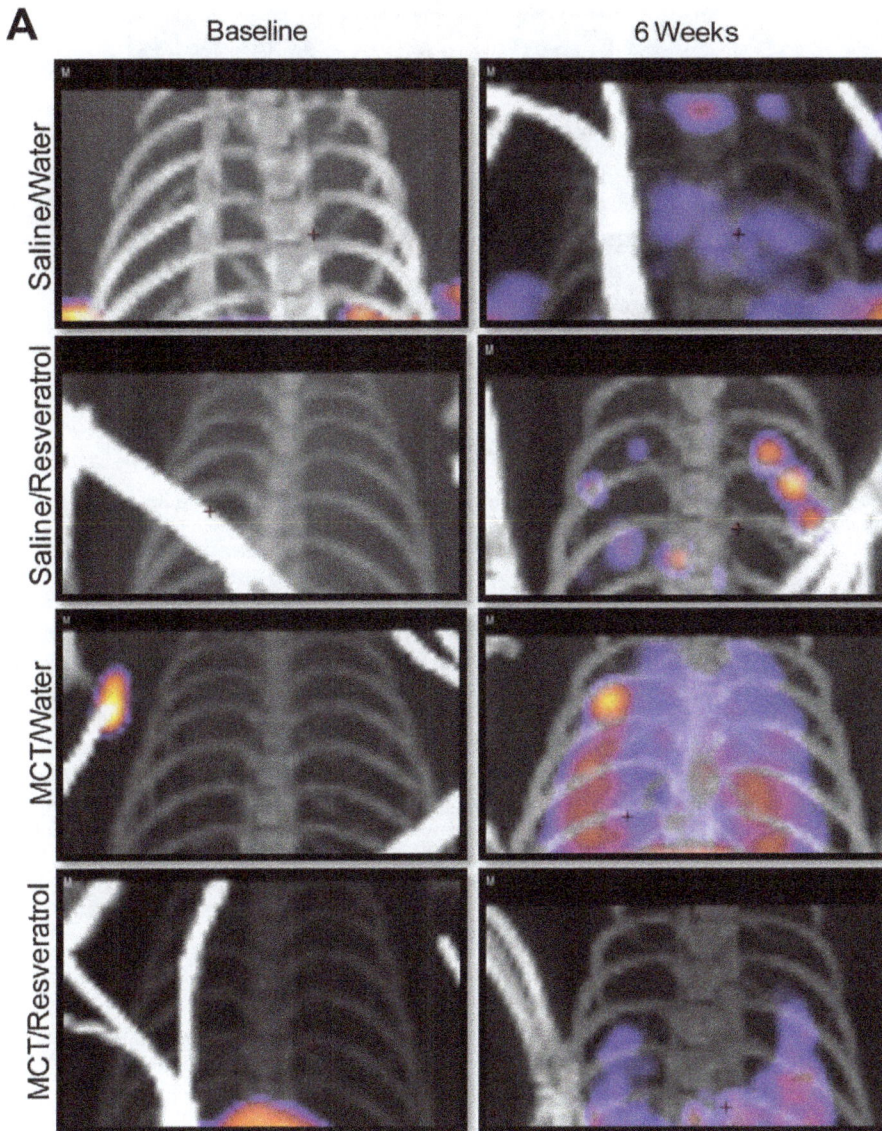

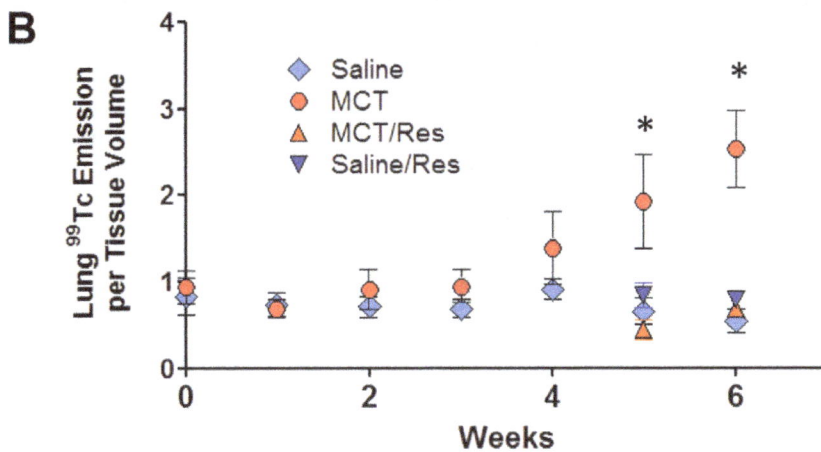

Figure 5. Representative SPECT/CT images of lung ^{99}Tc-annexin at day 0 and day 42 from one subject per group. CT images include the ECG wires in various positions. Quantitative assessments of ^{99}Tc energy from the lung region, with cardiac region subtracted out, are shown graphically, below. Asterisks indicate significant (P<0.05) elevation in the MCT-only group compared to other groups by 2-way (time, treatment) ANOVA.

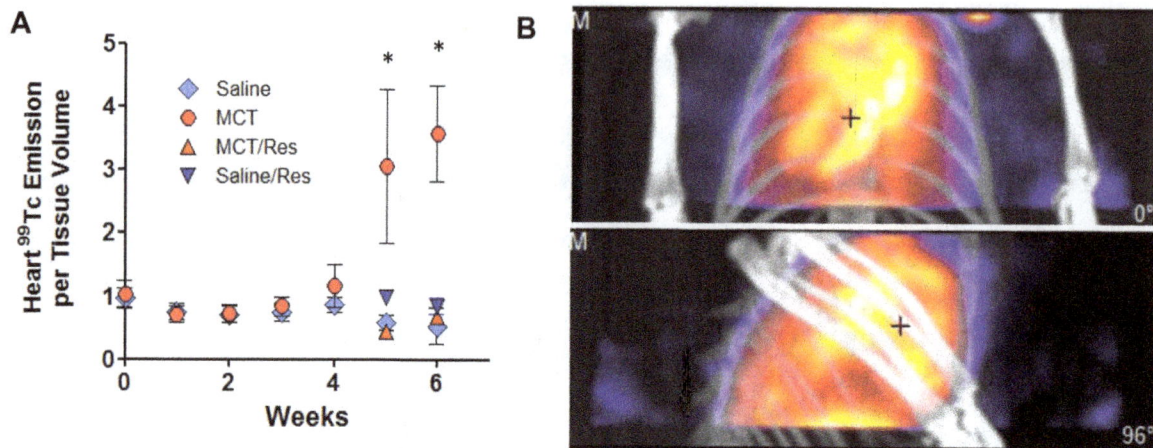

Figure 6. Quantitative assessments of ^{99}Tc-annexin energy from the cardiac region, without consideration of pulmonary signals, are shown graphically. A severe induction of cardiac apoptosis was observed in one MCT-only rat, depicted from two positions in the figure to the right. Asterisks indicate significant ($P<0.05$) elevation in the MCT-only group compared to other groups by 2-way (time, treatment) ANOVA.

weeks post-injection [6], thus the present findings strongly suggest that apoptosis is indicated by the annexin labeling.

Another distinct challenge with this imaging technology was the difficulty in assessing RV function and morphology in healthy animals. With a minor modification of the detection criteria, we were able to assess RV function in severe cases of PAH, but as these could not be compared with control animals, therefore we excluded these data. However, the potential exists to conduct efficacy studies on the reversal of RV dysfunction in models of established PAH. Finally, the monocrotaline-treatment model, while commonly used, has a number of limitations with regard to human disease. The major differences relate to the remodeling of the pulmonary arterioles, where in humans the development of plexiform lesions and myoendothelial transition can be observed, while monocrotaline causes hypertrophy of conduit and resistance vessels without the obliterative pathology in the capillaries. However, organ-level changes are quite consistent, especially with regard to right ventricular enlargement. Perhaps more importantly for the present application, imaging analysis of several related models, such as chronic hypoxia or hypoxia plus a VEGF inhibitor, would be readily conducted mirroring the present study design.

Conclusion

Longitudinal *in vivo* SPECT/CT dual isotope imaging in a commonly used model of pulmonary hypertension revealed dynamic changes in cardiac function and cardiopulmonary apoptosis. The utility of this serial imaging technique could be applied to pharmacotherapy and efficacy assessment related to drug development across a broad range of experimental disease models.

Materials and Methods

Study Design

All procedures were approved by the University of New Mexico Office of Animal Care Compliance. Male Sprague-Dawley rats were obtained from a commercial vendor (Charles River) at approximately 300 g body weight. Rats were maintained in AAALAC-approved facilities with food and water available ad libitum.

Following a baseline imaging session, induction of pulmonary hypertension was achieved by a single intraperitoneal injection of monocrotaline at a concentration reported to cause modest disease (50 mg/kg, N = 12) (6), or an equivalent volume of sterile saline. At 28 days post monocrotaline injection, a cohort of rats (N = 12) was given resveratrol (Sigma Aldrich) in the drinking water (3 mg/kg/day). Resveratrol was administered via non-translucent water bottles and dosing was determined by average daily water intake which continued until the end of the study at Day 42. Fresh water containing resveratrol was changed every day to avoid problems with stability and solubility.

Radiolabeling and Incorporation Yield

Thallium-201 chloride, USP, a sterile, isotonic, aqueous injectate, pH = 4.5–7.5 was obtained from a commercial nuclear pharmacy. The volumes injected were adjusted using 0.9% NaCl, USP (Hospira). Hynic-Annexin V kit preparation vials were supplied by the NIH National Cancer Institute. Hynic-Annexin V kit vials were stored at −80°C prior to use.

A Hynic-Annexin V vial containing 0.275 mg and containing a lyophilized stannous tricine buffer were thawed at room temperature (22°C) for 5 to 8 minutes. Approximately 30–50 mCi of ^{99m}Tc (sodium pertechnetate) in 0.5 mL were added to the Hynic-Annexin V vial and gently swirled. Three mL of normal saline (Hospira) were added to the stannous tricine. After mixing the solution, 300 µL of the tin solution w withdrawn and added to the annexin solution. The solution was mixed and allowed to incubate at room temperature for 15 minutes.

The radionuclide incorporation yield was determined using a citrate-dextrose solution (Sigma). The radiolabeled compound (2–5 mL) was spotted on an iTLC chromatographic strip (Silica Gel Impregnated Glass Fiber Sheets, Varian). The iTLC strips were scanned on an AR2000 (Bioscan Inc.). The radioactivity at the origin (Rf = 0–4.25 cm), middle (Rf = 4.25–4.75 cm), and solvent front (Rf = 4.75–9 cm) were analyzed to determine the radiolabeling yield. based on incorporation yield, impurities and free/reduced-hydrolyzed ^{99m}Tc radioactivities, respectively. The percent incorporation yields were calculated by taking the origin divided by the sum of the origin, middle and solvent times 100. Greater than 90% radiolabeling incorporation yield was required for acceptance. In addition, the middle section of the strip (impurities) had to contain ≤5% of the total radioactivity. The pH of the solution was measured to ensure it was in the specified range of 5.5 to 6.5. The final volume was adjusted according to injection volumes needed following quality assurance end-product testing.

Radioimaging Studies

SPECT/CT studies were performed utilizing a NanoSPECT/CT® dedicated small-animal imaging system (Bioscan, Inc. Washington, DC). Imaging of a limited cohort of resveratrol- or saline-treated rats (n = 3/group) was performed at baseline, then again on days 7, 14, 21, 28, 35, and 42 post-monocrotaline injection. Thirty (30) minutes prior to imaging, rats were injected with ^{201}Tl (540 µCi, mean activity) via tail vein to evaluate cardiac perfusion and morphology and ^{99m}Tc-Annexin (608 µCi, mean activity) to assess heart and lung apoptosis. Thoracic imaging studies were performed on anesthetized rats (1.5%–2.0% isoflurane) using a temperature-controlled bed. A dual-isotope protocol was used to acquire ECG-gated and static ^{201}Tl and ^{99m}Tc-Annexin images simultaneously. A crosstalk removal procedure was used prior to image reconstruction to account for spillover of counts between the ^{201}Tl and ^{99m}Tc energy windows. Due to a larger proportion of LV to RV mass and correspondingly greater LV ^{201}Tl signal, analysis of LV volume was performed to compute ejection fraction, stroke volume and myocardial perfusion polar maps (FlowQuant, University of Ottawa Heart Institute). An automated analysis routine was developed to identify heart and lung regions of interest (ROIs) from the ^{201}Tl static reconstruction. These ROIs were applied to the ^{99m}Tc-Annexin static reconstruction to assess heart and lung apoptosis. Qualitative perfusion mapping images and reported values for ^{201}Tl and ^{99m}Tc-Annexin were normalized to injected dose of each radionuclide.

Hemodynamics

Rats were anesthetized with isoflurane and following a media-lateral incision, the right external jugular vein was exposed by blunt dissection. RSVP measurements were made via a fluid-filled pressure transducer (Becton Dickinson, DTXplus) where a heparinized (0.01%), saline filled Micro-Renathane catheter (0.050 OD X 0.040 ID) was placed in the right jugular vein. Catheter advancement preceded until strong positive-negative deflections were observed, indicating catheter placement in the right ventricle, then secured with 4-0 silk suture. Pressure data was collected for 1 minute using a conventional data acquisition system (AD Instruments). Following mid-line thoracotomy, rats were euthanized by exsanguination and visual confirmation of catheter placement in either right ventricle or PA was examined. In addition to RV systolic pressure, post hoc analysis of RV mean pressure, heart rate and $+dP/dt_{max}$ was performed by using PowerLab software suite 4/30 (AD Instruments).

Statistics

All data were tested for normal distributions prior to analysis. ^{201}Tl and ^{99m}Tc-Annexin image generation/analysis as well as assessments of hemodynamics were performed in a blinded fashion. As RV hypertrophy developed in the MCT cohort, modest to moderate detection of the ^{210}Tl signal in the RV became observable, thus unintentional un-blinding of the ^{201}Tl analysis within experimental PAH cohort developed. Despite this longitudinal observation, assumed to be associated with the development of right ventricular hypertrophy, post hoc (off-line) analysis of ^{201}Tl and ^{99m}Tc-Annexin imaging was performed in a blinded fashion. Hemodynamic and organ weight data were assessed by Analysis of Variance (ANOVA) with Newman-Keuls Multiple Comparison Test to establish group differences (Graph-Pad Prism, v5.02). Time-course and cardiac cycle data derived from imaging was analyzed with a 2-way ANOVA with Bonferroni post hoc testing. Probability values less than 0.05 were considered significant.

Author Contributions

Conceived and designed the experiments: MLP JH JN MJC. Performed the experiments: MLP JH GC TA DI MJC. Analyzed the data: MLP JH JN MJC. Contributed reagents/materials/analysis tools: JH GC SL DI. Wrote the paper: MLP MJC.

References

1. Humbert M, Morrell NW, Archer SL, Stenmark KR, MacLean MR, et al. (2004). Cellular and molecular pathobiology of pulmonary arterial hypertension. *J Am Coll Cardiol*. 43: 13S–24S.
2. D'Alonzo GE, Barst RJ, Ayres SM, Bergofsky EH, Brudage BH, et al. (1991) Survival in patients with primary pulmonary hypertension: results from a national prospective registry. *Ann Intern Med* 115: 343–349.
3. Voelkel NF, Quaife RA, Leinwand LA, Barst RJ, McGoon MD, et al. (2006) National Heart, Lung, and Blood Institute Working Group on Cellular and Molecular Mechanisms of Right Heart Failure. Right ventricular function and failure: report of a National Heart, Lung, and Blood Institute working group on cellular and molecular mechanisms of right heart failure. *Circulation* 114: 1883–91.
4. Marsboom G, Wieholt C, Haney CR, Toth PT, Ryan JJ, et al. (2012) Lung ^{18}F-fluorodeoxyglucose positron emission tomography for diagnosis and monitoring of pulmonary arterial hypertension. *Am J Respir Crit Care Med*. 185: 670–9.
5. Campian ME, Verberne HJ, Hardziyenka M, de Bruin K, Selwaness M, et al. (2009) Serial noninvasive assessment of apoptosis during right ventricular disease progression in rats. *J Nucl Med*. 50: 1371–7.
6. Paffett ML, Lucas SL, Campen MJ (2012) Resveratrol Reverses Monocrotaline-Induced Pulmonary Vascular and Cardiac Dysfunction: A Potential Role for Atrogin-1 in Smooth Muscle. *Vascular Pharmacology*, 56: 64–73.
7. Csiszar A, Labinskyy N, Olson S, Pinto JT, Gupte S, et al. (2009) Resveratrol Prevents Monocrotaline-Induced Pulmonary Hypertension in Rats. Hypertension 54: 668–675.
8. Jian B, Yang S, Chaudry IH, Raju R (2011) Resveratrol improves cardiac contractility following trauma-hemorrhage by modulating SIRT1. *Mol Med*. 18: 209–14.
9. Louis XL, Thandapilly SJ, Mohankumar SK, Yu L, Taylor CG, et al. (2011) Treatment with low-dose resveratrol reverses cardiac imparment in obese prone but not obese resistant rats. *J Nutr Biochem*. http://dx.doi.org/10.1016/j.jnutbio.2011.06.010 [Epub ahead of print].
10. Zhang C, Feng Y, Qu S, Wei X, Zhu H, et al. (2011) Resveratrol attenuates doxorubicin-induced cardiomyocytes apoptosis in mice through SIRT1-mediated deacetylation of p53. Cardiovasc Res. 90: 538–45.
11. Rimbaud S, Ruiz M, Piquereau J, Mateo P, Fortin D, et al. (2011) Resveratrol improves survival, hemodynamics and energetics in a rat model of hypertension leading to heart failure. PloS ONE. 6: 1–12.
12. Chen YR, Yi FF, Li XY, Wang CY, Chen L, et al. (2008) Resveratrol attenuates ventricular arrhythmias and improves the long-term survival in rats with myocardial infarction. Cardiovasc Drugs Ther. 22: 479–485.
13. Santamore WP, Dell'Italia LJ (1998) Ventricular interdependence: significant left ventricular contributions to right ventricular function. Prog Cardiovasc Dis. 40: 289–308.
14. Vizza CD, Lynch JP, Ochoa LL, Richardson G, Trulock EP (1998) Right and left ventricular dysfunction in patients with severe pulmonary disease. Chest 113: 576–83.
15. Correia-Pinto J, Henriques-Coelho T, Roncon-Albuquerque R Jr, Lourenco AP, Melo-Rocha G, et al. (2009) Time course and mechanisms of left ventricular systolic and diastolic dysfunction in monocrotaline-induced pulmonary hypertension. Basic Res Cardiol. 104: 535–45.
16. Morrell NW, Higham MA, Phillips PG, Shakur BH, Robinson PJ, et al. (2005) Pilot study of losartan for pulmonary hypertension in chronic obstructive pulmonary disease. Respir Res. 6: 88.
17. Guerard P, Rakotoniaina Z, Goirand F, Rochette L, Dumas M, et al. (2006) The HMG-CoA reductase inhibitor, pravastatin, prevents the development of monocrotaline-induced pulmonary hypertension in the rat through reduction of endothelial cell apoptosis and overexpression of eNOS. Naunyn Schmiedebergs Arch Pharmacol. 373: 401–14.
18. Zaiman AL, Podowski M, Medicherla S, Gordy K, Xu F, et al. (2008) Role of the TGF-beta/Alk5 signaling pathway in monocrotaline-induced pulmonary hypertension. Am J Respir Crit Care Med. 177: 896–905.

19. Yang DL, Zhang HG, Xu YL, Gao YH, Yang XJ, et al. (2010) Resveratrol inhibits right ventricular hypertrophy induced by monocrotaline in rats. *Clin Exp Pharmacol Physiol*. 37: 150–155.

20. Lamberts RR, Caldenhoven E, Lansink M, Witte G, Vaessen RJ, et al. (2007) Preservation of diastolic function in monocrotaline-induced right ventricular hypertrophy in rats. *Am J Physiol Heart Circ Physiol*. 293: H1869–76.

21. Chan V, Fenning A, Iyer A, Hoey A, Brown L (2011) Resveratrol improves cardiovascular function in DOCA-salt hypertensive rats. *Curr Pharm Biotechnol*. 12: 429–36.

22. Price LC, Montani D, Tcherakian C, Dorfmuller P, Souza R, et al. (2011) Dexamethasone reverses monocrotaline-induced pulmonary arterial hypertension in rats. *Eur Respir J*. 37: 813–22.

23. Wang W, Wang YL, Chen XY, Li YT, Hao W, et al. (2011) Dexamethasone attenuates development of monocrotaline-induced pulmonary arterial hypertension. *Mol Biol Rep*. 38: 3277–84.

24. Laufer EM, Reutelingsperger CPM, Narula J, Hofstra L (2008) Annexin V: an imaging biomarker of cardiovascular risk. *Basic Res Cardiol*. 103: 95–14.

3

Phosphodiesterase 10A Upregulation Contributes to Pulmonary Vascular Remodeling

Xia Tian[1], Christina Vroom[1], Hossein Ardeschir Ghofrani[1], Norbert Weissmann[1], Ewa Bieniek[1], Friedrich Grimminger[1], Werner Seeger[1,2], Ralph Theo Schermuly[1,2], Soni Savai Pullamsetti[1,2]*

1 Medical Clinic II/V, University Hospital, Giessen, Germany, 2 Max-Planck-Institute for Heart and Lung Research, Bad Nauheim, Germany

Abstract

Phosphodiesterases (PDEs) modulate the cellular proliferation involved in the pathophysiology of pulmonary hypertension (PH) by hydrolyzing cAMP and cGMP. The present study was designed to determine whether any of the recently identified PDEs (PDE7-PDE11) contribute to progressive pulmonary vascular remodeling in PH. All *in vitro* experiments were performed with lung tissue or pulmonary arterial smooth muscle cells (PASMCs) obtained from control rats or monocrotaline (MCT)-induced pulmonary hypertensive (MCT-PH) rats, and we examined the effects of the PDE10 inhibitor papaverine (Pap) and specific small interfering RNA (siRNA). In addition, papaverine was administrated to MCT-induced PH rats from day 21 to day 35 by continuous intravenous infusion to examine the *in vivo* effects of PDE10A inhibition. We found that PDE10A was predominantly present in the lung vasculature, and the mRNA, protein, and activity levels of PDE10A were all significantly increased in MCT PASMCs compared with control PASMCs. Papaverine and PDE10A siRNA induced an accumulation of intracellular cAMP, activated cAMP response element binding protein and attenuated PASMC proliferation. Intravenous infusion of papaverine in MCT-PH rats resulted in a 40%–50% attenuation of the effects on pulmonary hypertensive hemodynamic parameters and pulmonary vascular remodeling. The present study is the first to demonstrate a central role of PDE10A in progressive pulmonary vascular remodeling, and the results suggest a novel therapeutic approach for the treatment of PH.

Editor: Wael El-Rifai, Vanderbilt University Medical Center, United States of America

Funding: This work was supported by the Deutsche Forschungsgemeinschaft, Sonderforschungsbereich 547 "Kardiopulmonales Gefäßsystem", Projekt C6 and by the European Commission under the Sixth Frame work Programme (contract No. LSHM-CT-2005-018725, PULMOTENSION). The funders had no role in study design, data collection and analysis, decision to publish, or preparation of the manuscript.

Competing Interests: The authors have declared that no competing interests exist.

* E-mail: soni.pullamsetti@mpi-bn.mpg.de

Introduction

Pulmonary arterial hypertension (PAH) is a fatal disease characterized by progressively elevated pulmonary vascular resistance, which results from vasoconstriction, vascular remodeling and *in situ* thrombosis. These events lead to right ventricular hypertrophy and right heart failure [1]. All cell types of the vessel wall, including pulmonary arterial smooth muscle cells (PASMCs), endothelial cells and adventitial fibroblasts, are involved in this remodeling process [2]. Although the underlying mechanisms of pulmonary vascular remodeling in PAH are not completely understood, therapies targeting reduced prostacyclin synthesis, increased endothelin signaling and increased cyclic nucleotide phosphodiesterase (PDE) levels have been approved for the treatment of PAH [3–5].

Phosphodiesterases comprise a family of 11 isoforms (PDE1-PDE11) that each have different capacities for hydrolyzing cAMP, cGMP, or both. Because cAMP and cGMP are ubiquitous second messengers, PDEs are involved in many important signaling pathways that regulate proliferation, migration, and differentiation [6,7]. Current evidence suggests that individual isozymes modulate distinct regulatory pathways in the cell, which are mainly determined by their sub-cellular localization [7]. PDE1A has been reported to translocate to the nucleus in synthetic proliferating vascular smooth muscle cells (SMCs) [8]. In addition, sub-isoforms of PDE4 have been shown to have diverse functions in subcellular pools of cAMP that result from compartmentalization [9].

Interestingly, the expression and activities of PDEs have been reported to be altered in both experimental and human PAH [10]. Expression profiling of single members of the PDE superfamily in healthy and remodeled pulmonary vasculature revealed that the PDE1, PDE3 and PDE5 isoforms are differentially regulated [11–13]. In preclinical and clinical studies, we have shown that the inhibition of PDE1 by 8-methoxymethyl-IBMX (8MM-IBMX) [11] and PDE5 by sildenafil [4,12] stabilizes second messenger signaling and regulates vascular remodeling, vascular tone and optimization of gas exchange. Moreover, in monocrotaline (MCT)-induced PH (MCT-PH) rats, inhibition of PDE3 and PDE4 has been shown to partly reverse the pathological inward remodeling of PAH [14,15].

The roles of the recently identified PDEs (PDE7-PDE11) in PAH are complicated and not well understood. Among them, PDE7 and PDE8 are cAMP-specific, PDE9 is cGMP-specific, and PDE10A and PDE11 are dual-substrate PDEs [16]. The cellular- and subcellular-specific distribution and substrate specificity of these newly identified PDEs may provide important insights into the pathology and pathophysiology of PAH.

The aim of the present study was to characterize the expression pattern of newly identified PDEs (PDE7-PDE11) in lung tissue and primary PASMCs from control and MCT-PH rats to identify potential therapeutic targets in the PDE family that are involved in the pathogenesis of PAH. Because the results showed a significant increase of PDE10A in the pulmonary hypertensive vasculature, we addressed the specific contribution of PDE10A to the vascular remodeling in PAH by employing small interfering RNA (siRNA) or an inhibitor in our *in vitro* and *in vivo* studies.

Methods

Patients

Human lung tissue was obtained from 4 donors and 4 patients with idiopathic PAH (IPAH) who underwent lung transplantation. The study protocol for human tissue donation was approved by the ethics committee (Ethik Kommission am Fachbereich Humanmedizin der Justus Liebig Universität Giessen) of the University Hospital Giessen (Giessen, Germany) in accordance with national law and "Good Clinical Practice/International Conference on Harmonisation" guidelines (AZ 31/93). Written informed consent was obtained from each individual patient or the patient's next of kin.

Animals

Adult male Sprague Dawley rats (250–300 g in body weight; Charles River Laboratories, Germany) were randomized for a subcutaneous injection of saline or 60 mg/kg MCT (Sigma-Aldrich) to induce pulmonary hypertension (PH) [17]. Both the University Animal Care Committee and the Federal Authorities for Animal Research of the Regierungspräsidium Giessen (Hessen, Germany) approved the study protocols (AZ GI 20/10 Nr. 52/2009).

Surgical preparation and hemodynamic measurement

The animals were classified into the following three groups: 1) rats injected with saline (Control, n = 9); 2) MCT-injected rats subjected to mini-pump implantation from day 21 to day 35 with saline (MCT [35 d], n = 8) or 3) MCT-injected rats subjected to mini-pump implantation from day 21 to day 35 with 1 µg/kg/min papaverine (Sigma-Aldrich) (MCT [35 d]/papaverine, n = 8). 3 weeks after MCT injection, rats were subjected to treatment for 2 weeks by implantation of osmotic mini-pumps (Alzet Model 2ML2, Durect). On day 21, after the rats were anesthetized, a mini-pump filled with 2 ml of saline or papaverine (5 mg/ml) was implanted in the dorsal subcutaneous region under sterile conditions, and a tunneled catheter (PE 50 tubing) was inserted into the left jugular vein. After wounds were closed with sutures, the rats were recovered from anesthesia by an intraperitoneal injection of naloxone and atipazemole (50 and 100 µg/kg, respectively). At the end of the treatment, the rats were anesthetized with an intraperitoneal injection of ketamine (9 mg/kg body mass) and medetomidine (100 µg/kg body mass), which was followed by an intramuscular injection of heparin (50 IU/kg body mass) to measure the hemodynamic parameters. The rats were then tracheotomized and ventilated at a frequency of 60 breaths/min with positive end expiratory pressure at 1 cm H_2O. To measure right ventricular pressure, a right heart PE 50 catheter was inserted through the right jugular vein, and a polyethylene catheter was inserted into the left carotid artery to measure arterial pressure. After measurements, the left lung was fixed for histology in 3% paraformaldehyde solution, and the right lung was snap frozen in liquid nitrogen after exsanguinations [18].

Histological assessment of the degree of muscularization of small pulmonary arteries

Three-µm lung sections from blocks fixed in 3% paraformaldehyde solution were used for double staining with anti-von Willebrand factor antibody (1:900 dilution, Dako) and anti α-smooth muscle actin antibody (1:900 dilution, Sigma-Aldrich) to analyze small peripheral pulmonary artery muscularization. In each rat, 80 to 100 intra-acinar arteries (20–50 µm) were categorized as fully muscularized, partially muscularized, or nonmuscularized, as previously described [18].

Isolation of pulmonary arterial smooth muscle cells (PASMCs)

Rat PASMCs were cultured from peripheral small pulmonary artery explants as previously described [19]. Small pulmonary arteries were freshly obtained from rats and maintained in Hank's balanced salt solution (HBSS, Gibco) supplemented with penicillin (100 units/ml, PAN) and streptomycin (100 units/ml, PAN). Under a dissecting microscope, the adventitia layer was removed by microdissection. Arterial segments were cut open along the longitudinal axis, and the endothelium was gently removed by scraping the luminal surface. The arteries were minced into 1 mm^2 explant pieces and maintained in Dulbecco's modified Eagle's medium/F12 (DMEM/F12, Gibco) supplemented with 10% fetal bovine serum (FBS, Biowest), penicillin (100 units/ml), streptomycin (100 units/ml), and 2 mM L-glutamine (PAN). After 5 days, PASMCs started to migrate from the explants, and this was followed by 10 days of subculturing. Early-passage (passages 2–5) PASMCs were used for all experiments. Cells were positively stained for α-smooth muscle actin by immunocytochemistry, and the expression of vascular smooth muscle cell (VSMC) phenotypic genes (α-smooth muscle actin, smooth muscle-myosin heavy chain, and calponin) was confirmed by polymerase chain reaction (PCR) (data not shown). Every experiment was performed with primary PASMCs isolated from at least 3 individual rats.

RNA isolation and cDNA synthesis

For cDNA synthesis, total RNA from tissues or cells was extracted using Trizol® (Invitrogen) according to the manufacturer's instructions. One µm of RNA was used for reverse transcriptase polymerase chain reaction (RT-PCR) in a total volume of 20 µl with oligo(dT)$_{15}$ primer using the ImProm-II reverse transcription system (Promega) according to the manufacturer's instructions.

Quantitative real-time polymerase chain reaction (qRT-PCR)

The intron-spanning primer pairs (Metabion) were designed using the Primer3 program, and these primer pairs are shown in Table 1. qRT-PCR was performed on an Mx3000P® QPCR System machine (Stratagene) using SYBR® GreenER™ qPCR SuperMix Universal kits (Invitrogen). Using the MxPro™ QPCR software, a dissociation curve was generated for each gene to ensure single product amplification, and we determined the threshold cycle (Ct value) for each gene. The comparative $2^{-\Delta\Delta Ct}$ method was used to analyze mRNA fold changes between control and MCT group, which was calculated as ratio $= 2^{-(\Delta Ct\ control-\Delta Ct\ MCT)}$, where Ct is the cycle threshold and ΔCt (Ct target - Ct reference) is the Ct value normalized to the reference gene porphobilinogen deaminase (PBGD) obtained for the same cDNA samples. Each reaction was run in duplicate and repeated in three independent experiments. The calculated $2^{-\Delta\Delta Ct}$ was transformed into a percentage using the control value as 100% to indicate the mRNA expression.

Immunohistochemistry

Three-µm lung sections were cut from lung blocks fixed in 3% paraformaldehyde solution. After deparaffinization in xylene and rehydration in a series of grade-decreasing ethanol solutions, the

Table 1. Primer pairs of rat PDEs for quantitative realtime-PCR.

Gene	Forward Primer	Reverse Primer
PDE1A	5'- ATCAGCCACCCAGCCAAA -3'	5'- GGAGAAAACGGAAGCCCTAA -3'
PDE3A	5'- CACAAGCCCAGAGTGAACC -3'	5'- TGGAGGCAAACTTCTTCTCAG -3'
PDE3B	5'- GTCGTTGCCTTGTATTTCTCG -3'	5'- AACTCCATTTCCACCTCCAGA -3'
PDE4A	5'- CGACAAGCACACAGCCTCT -3'	5'- CTCCCACAATGGATGAACAAT -3'
PDE7A	5'- GAAGAGGTTCCCACCCGTA -3'	5'- CTGATGTTTCTGGCGGAGA -3'
PDE7B	5'- GGCTCCTTGCTCATTTGC -3'	5'- GGAACTCATTCTGTCTGTTGATG-3'
PDE8A	5'- TGGCAGCAATAAGGTTGAGA -3'	5'- GAATGTTTCCTCCTGTCTTT -3'
PDE8B	5'- TCGGTCCTTCCTCTTCTCC -3'	5'- AACTTCCCCGTGTTCTATTTGA -3'
PDE9A	5'- GTGGGTGGACTGTTTACTGGA -3'	5'- TCGCTTTGGTCACTTTGTCTC -3'
PDE10A	5'- GACTTGATTGGCATCCTTGAA -3'	5'- CCTGGTGTATTGCTACGGAAG -3'
PDE11A	5'- CCCAGGCGATAAATAAGGTTC -3'	5'- TGCCACAGAATGGAAGATACA -3'
PBGD	5'- CAAGGTTTTCAGCATCGCTAC -3'	5'- ATGTCCGGTAACGGCGGC -3'

slides were washed in phosphate-buffered saline (PBS). For PDE10A, antigen retrieval was achieved using 0.25% trypsin for 15 min at 37°C; and for proliferating cell nuclear antigen (PCNA), antigen retrieval was achieved by cooking in citrate buffer (pH 6.0) buffer followed by a 15-min incubation in proteinase K at room temperature. The sections were treated with 3% hydrogen peroxide to block endogenous peroxidases prior to serum blocking. Then, a NovaRED horseradish peroxidase (HRP) kit (Vector) was used for PDE10A staining, and a ZymedChem-plus alkaline phosphatase (AP) Polymer kit (Zymed) was used for PCNA staining according to the manufacturer's instructions. The sections were incubated with anti-PDE10A polyclonal antibody (1:200 in 10% bovine serum albumin, Scottish Biomedical) or anti-PCNA polyclonal antibody (1:100 in 10% bovine serum albumin) at 4°C overnight. After being washed, slidses were incubated with the corresponding secondary antibody conjugated with HRP or AP for 1 h. After slides were washed, color development was performed with a substrate/chromogen mixture followed by counterstaining with hematoxylin. The sections were examined under a Leica DM 2500 microscope using Leica QWin imaging software (Leica). Sections from 4–5 rats in each group were stained with each antibody. PCNA positive pulmonary vascular cells were counted throughout the entire section and expressed as fold changes of the control lung by calculating the number of PCNA-positive cells per pulmonary vessel [20].

Immunocytochemistry

Rat PASMCs grown on 8-well chamber slides were fixed with −20°C-cooled acetone-methanol mix (1:1) for 10 min at 4°C. After being washed 3 times with PBS, the fixed cells were sequentially incubated with blocking buffer (3% bovine serum albumin in PBS) for 1 h at room temperature, primary antibody against PDE10A (1:200 in blocking buffer, Novus) overnight at 4°C, and FITC-conjugated anti-rabbit secondary antibody (Alexa Fluor® 488 1:1000 in blocking buffer, Invitrogen) for 1 h at room temperature. Cells were counterstained for nuclei with DAPI and visualized using a Leica DMLA fluorescence microscope and Leica QWin imaging software (Leica). PASMCs from 3 individual rats of each group were stained.

Immunoblotting

Protein extracted with RIPA buffer (Santa Cruz) was resolved with SDS-PAGE (10% acrylamide) and transferred onto nitrocellulose membranes. After being blocked with 5% non-fat milk for 1 h at room temperature, membranes were probed with rabbit polyclonal anti-PDE10A antibody (1:2000, Scottish Biomedical), rabbit polyclonal anti-CREB antibody (1:1000, Millipore), rabbit polyclonal anti-phospho-CREB (Ser133) antibody (1:1000, Millipore) or mouse monoclonal anti-GAPDH antibody (1:5000, Novus) overnight at 4°C. Following washing with TBS containing 0.1% Triton X-100, HRP-conjugated secondary antibodies (1:50000; anti-rabbit, Pierce; anti-mouse, Sigma-Aldrich) were applied for 1 h. After washing, the blots were developed with an enhanced chemiluminescence (ECL) kit (Amersham) followed by film exposure. Blots were repeated three times independently.

PDE activity assay

3-Isobutyl-1-methylxanthine (IBMX), erythro-9-(2-hydroxy-3-nonyl) adenine (EHNA), rolipram and papaverine were purchased from Sigma-Aldrich. 8MM-IBMX and milrinone were purchased from Calbiochem. Phosphodiesterase enzyme activity was measured using modifications of the methods of Thompson and Appleman [21] and Bauer and Schwabe [22]. Protein was extracted from PASMCs with RIPA buffer (Santa Cruz) and normalized to the same concentration for use. The reactions were performed with 10 μg of protein in 100 μl of HEPES buffer (40 mM; pH 7.6), which consisted of $MgCl_2$ (5 mM), bovine serum albumin (1 mg/ml), cAMP (1 μM) and [^{3}H]-cAMP (1 μCi/ml, Amersham), at 37°C for 15 min. The samples were boiled for 3 min, subsequently cooled for 5 min and incubated with 25 μl of *Crotalus atrox* snake venom (20 mg/ml, Sigma-Aldrich) for 15 min at 37°C. After being chilled on ice, the samples were applied to QAE Sephadex A-25 (Amersham) mini-chromatography columns and eluted with 1 ml of ammonium formate (30 mM, pH 7.5). The eluents were collected in 2 ml of scintillation solution (Roth), and counts per minute (CPM) were measured by a beta-counter. Each assay was performed in triplicate and repeated twice independently. Data are expressed as pmol cAMP/min/mg protein.

cAMP enzyme immunoassay (EIA)

At the end of culture, cells were washed twice with PBS and lysed in 0.1 M HCl at room temperature for 10 min. After centrifugation, the supernatants were normalized to the same protein concentration for use. Fifty-µl of protein samples, which were pre-diluted to 0.3 µg/µl, and standard solutions were incubated with 50 µl of tracer and 50 µl of antibody in the dark at 4°C overnight. After washing 5 times, plates were incubated with Ellman's solution for 90–120 min at room temperature with gentle shaking. The plates were read at a wavelength of 405 nm, and the concentration was calculated by the ready-made Cayman EIA Double workbook. The standard curve was generated as a plot of the percent bound/maximum bound (%B/B0) vs concentration of a series of known standards using linear (y) and log (x) axes. Using the 4-parameter logistic equation obtained from the standard curve, the cAMP concentrations of samples were determined, which are given as nmol/mg protein. Each sample was determined in duplicate and repeated twice.

Proliferation assay

PASMC proliferation was evaluated using the [³H]-thymidine incorporation assay. PASMCs (1×10^4 cells/well) were seeded on 48-well plates and grown overnight. The next day, the medium was substituted with DMEM/F12 containing 0.1% FBS with or without siRNA to render the cells quiescent. After 24-h serum starvation, cells were induced to reenter the cell cycle by 10% FBS, and the cells were incubated with or without papaverine for 24 h. The final 4 h of the incubation included the incorporation of [³H]thymidine (0.4 µCi/ml, Amersham). Cells were then washed twice with 500 µl of chilled HBSS, fixed with 250 µl of ice-cold methanol and precipitated by 250 µl of 10% trichloroacetic acid. Finally, samples were lysed in 0.1 M NaOH, transferred to 4 ml of scintillation solution (Roth) and counted by a beta-counter to determine CPM values. All labeling was performed on quadruplicate cultures and repeated twice independently. The proliferation of PASMCs is shown as a percentage (taking the CPM of unstimulated PASMCs under 0.1% FCS as 100%).

RNA interference

siRNA oligonucleotides specific for PDE10A (sense: 5'-GGA CAGCUUGGAUUCUACA-3'; anti-sense: 5'-UGUAGAAUC CAAGCUGUCC-3') and scramble siRNA (dTdT 3' overhang) were purchased from Eurogentec and transient transfection of siRNA was performed with X-tremeGENE siRNA Transfection Reagent (Roche) according to the manufacturer's protocols. PASMCs were subcultured to 40% confluence in antibiotic-free DMEM supplemented with 10% FBS and 2 mM L-glutamine. Transfection of 100 nM siRNA (ratio of siRNA to transfection reagent, 1 µg/4 µl) was performed in Opti-MEM (Gibco) for 5 h, which was followed by culturing in DMEM supplemented with 10% FBS and 2 mM L-glutamine for up to 24 h (RNA isolation) or 48 h (protein isolation and enzyme immunoassay, respectively). The RNA interference was well established and repeated three times.

Statistical analysis

Data are expressed as the mean and standard error of the mean (SEM). All statistical analyses were performed with Student's t test for comparisons between two groups or with one-way ANOVA and Newman-Keuls post-hoc test for multiple comparisons. Differences between groups were considered significant at P<0.05.

Results

Expression of PDE7-11 in rat lung tissues and PASMCs

The expression of PDE7-11 was investigated by qRT-PCR. In the lungs of MCT-treated rats, we observed upregulation of PDE7A, PDE7B, and PDE10A and downregulation of PDE8B. The other PDEs were expressed at similar levels as the controls

(Figure 1A). In the isolated PASMCs at passage 2, we only observed the presence of PDE7A, PDE7B, PDE8A, PDE10A and PDE11A, and we found a 2.5-fold increase in PDE7A and PDE10A mRNA expression in MCT PASMCs compared with control PASMCs (Figure 1B). However, the translational regulation of PDE7A in lung vasculature is beyond the scope of our study due to the fact that PDE7A protein signal was not detectable with the antibodies we possess (data not shown); therefore, we focused on PDE10A.

PDE10A is selectively upregulated in pulmonary vasculature and in PASMCs from MCT-PH rats

Because the present study was the first to report PDE10A expression in the lung, immunohistochemistry was performed to verify the PDE10A expression pattern. Figure 2A shows that a stronger immunoreactivity of PDE10A was observed in lung specimens from MCT-PH rats, which suggests that the site-specific change of PDE10A expression was induced in pulmonary hypertensive lungs, especially in the medial layers of pulmonary arteries. In contrast, only weak expression of PDE10A was detected in pulmonary vessels of control rat lungs. In addition, immunoreactivity against PDE10A was also noted in bronchial SMCs in the small airways. To investigate whether PDE10A induction is specific in remodeled pulmonary vasculature, we examined PDE10A expression in pulmonary and systemic arteries, including the aortic and femoral artery. qRT-PCR data showed a 2-fold increase in PDE10A mRNA expression in the pulmonary arteries of MCT-PH rats compared to control rats, which showed no changes in either the aortic artery or the femoral artery (Figure 2B). In corroboration, immunoblotting demonstrated a significant increase in PDE10A expression in MCT PASMCs compared with control (Figure 3A and 3B). In addition, immunofluorescence staining showed a predominant presence of PDE10A in the nuclei of PASMCs (Figure 3C). Similar localization was observed with two additional anti-PDE10A antibodies (data not shown).

Higher contribution of PDE10A to the total cAMP PDE activity in MCT PASMCs compared with control PASMCs

In addition to the expression level, the enzyme activity of PDE10A was also determined by the PDE activity assay. The total cAMP hydrolyzing PDE activity was increased in MCT PASMCs compared to control PASMCs (8.72 vs 7.66 pmol cAMP/min/mg protein), and this activity was suppressed by a non-selective PDE inhibitor, IBMX, to a similar basal level (1.9 pmol cAMP/min/mg protein) (Figure 4A). Interestingly, the PDE10A accounted for 53% of the total cAMP PDE activity in MCT PASMCs as opposed to 38% in control PASMCs (Figure 4B and 4C). In contrast, the contribution of other cAMP hydrolyzing PDEs (PDE1, PDE2, PDE3 and PDE4) declined from 70% in control PASMCs to 52% in MCT PASMCs. Taken together, these data suggest that PDE10A is one of the major cAMP hydrolyzing PDEs in PASMCs, and the cAMP hydrolyzing activity contributed by PDE10A was significantly increased in PASMCs from MCT-PH rats.

PDE10A knockdown by siRNA inhibits PASMC proliferation

The immunoblotting results in Figure 5A show that endogenous PDE10A protein expression in control and MCT PASMCs was strongly suppressed by PDE10A siRNA (100 nM), whereas no change occurred after transfection with scramble siRNA. In addition, to examine the isoform-specific effects of PDE10A siRNA, the expression of other cAMP-PDE isoforms was analyzed after

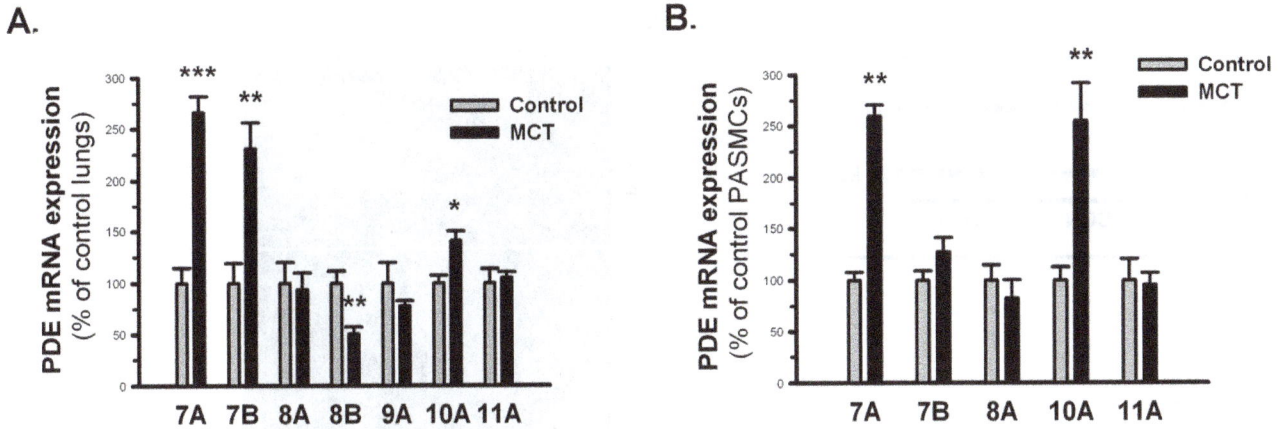

Figure 1. Expression of PDE7-PDE11 isoforms in rat lung tissue and rat PASMCs. A) mRNA expression of PDE7-PDE11 in lung homogenates from control rats (gray bars) and MCT-PH rats (black bars) as shown by qRT-PCR after normalization to PBGD. *P<0.05, **P<0.01, ***P<0.001 vs control lungs. n=4 in each group. **B)** Relative mRNA levels of PDE7-PDE11 in control (gray bars) and MCT (black bars) PASMCs demonstrated by qRT-PCR after normalization to PBGD. **P<0.01 vs control PASMCs. n=4 in each group. Values are expressed as the mean ± SEM.

PDE10A siRNA transfection. Quantitative RT-PCR results suggest that PDE10A siRNA suppressed PDE10A mRNA expression by 75% without affecting PDE1A, PDE3A, PDE3B and PDE4A expression (Figure S1). [³H]-thymidine incorporation stimulated by 10% FBS indicated that MCT PASMCs were 80% more proliferative than control PASMCs (Figure 5B). Furthermore, the proliferation of MCT PASMCs was reduced by 40% of the original level after PDE10A knockdown, whereas proliferation was only reduced by 25% of the original level in control PASMCs (Figure 5B).

Pharmacological inhibition of PDE10A *in vitro* suppresses PASMC proliferation, accumulates intracellular cAMP and activates cAMP response element binding protein (CREB)

Administration of the PDE10 inhibitor papaverine (Pap, 25 μM) resulted in a 40% reduction in [³H]-thymidine incorporation in MCT PASMCs compared to a 25% reduction in control

PASMCs (Figure 6A). The cAMP EIA assay data suggested that intracellular cAMP levels were increased 2.1-fold in MCT PASMCs after Pap (25 μM) treatment (Figure 6B), whereas there was only a 1.5-fold increase in cAMP levels in control PASMCs. Because CREB is an important downstream target of cAMP, we investigated whether CREB was activated by increased cAMP levels following PDE10 inhibition by determining the phosphorylation of serine 133 (Ser133) via immunoblotting. Figure 6C shows that control PASMCs exhibited high levels of CREB phosphorylation, which increased slightly after PDE10A inhibition by Pap (25 μM). In contrast, Pap (25 μM) dramatically increased the phosphorylation of CREB (Ser33) in MCT PASMCs.

Therapeutic effects of papaverine in MCT-PH rats *in vivo*

We performed *in vivo* experiments with an MCT-PH rat model to examine the therapeutic efficacy and anti-remodeling potential

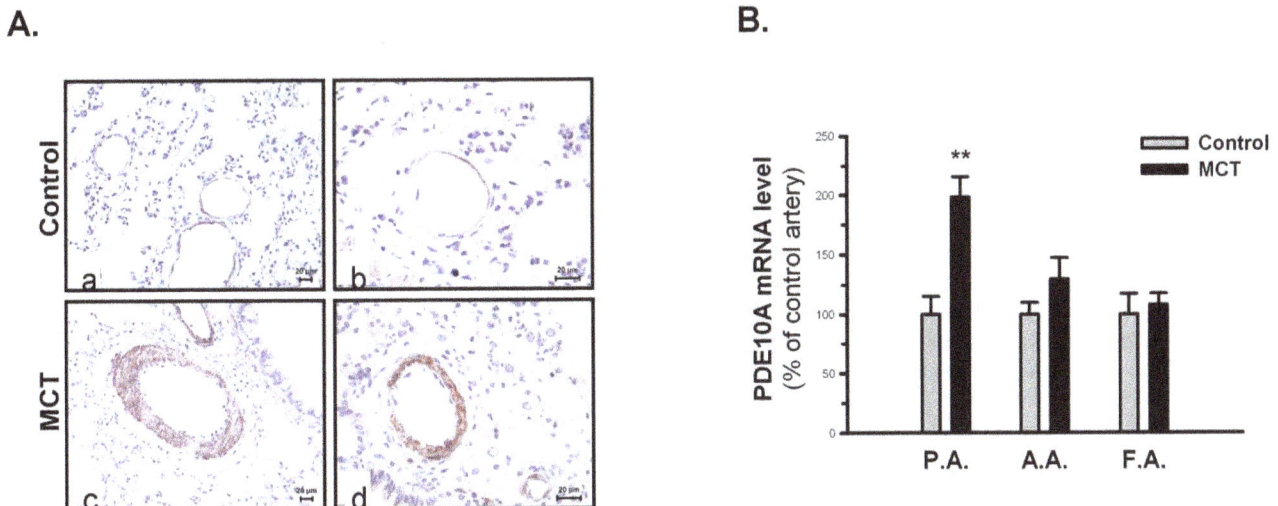

Figure 2. PDE10A expression and localization in rat pulmonary vasculature. A) Immunohistochemistry staining of PDE10A in lung sections from control (a, b) and MCT (c, d) rats. Scale bar: 20 μm. **B)** PDE10A mRNA expression in the pulmonary artery (P.A.), aortic artery (A.A.) and femoral artery (F.A.) from control rats (gray bars) and 4-week MCT-PH rats (black bars) are shown as a percentage of control by qRT-PCR after normalization to PBGD. **P<0.01 vs control PASMCs. n=4 in each group. Values are expressed as the mean ± SEM.

A.

B.

C.

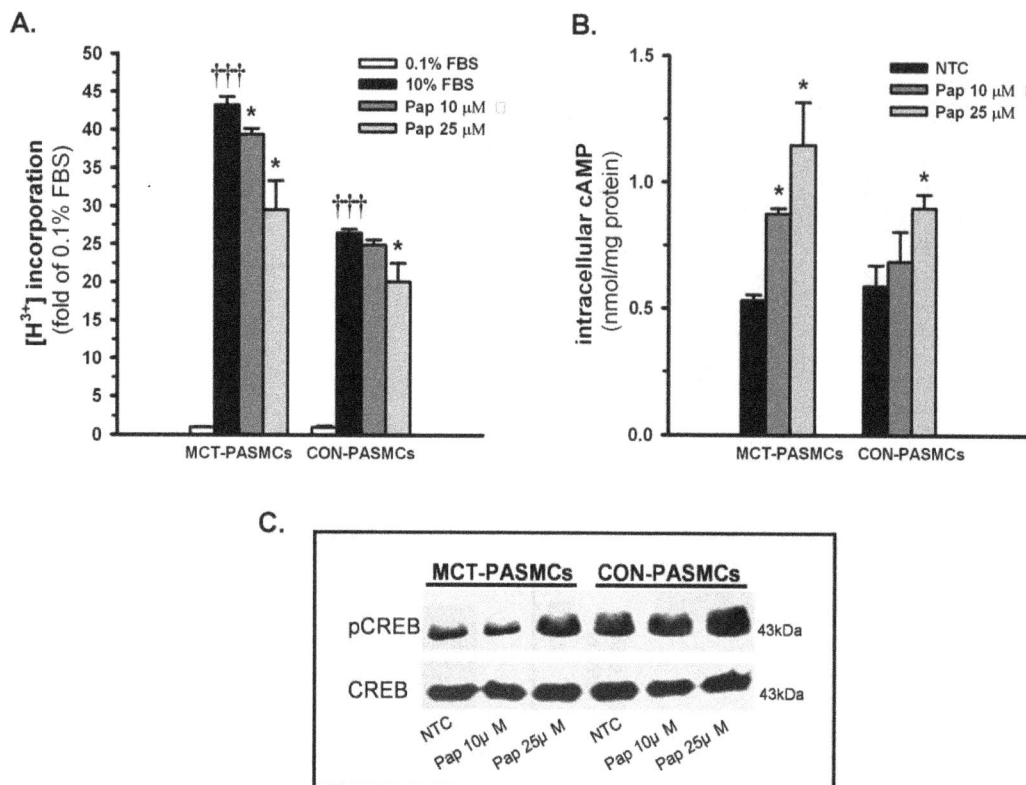

Figure 6. Effects of the PDE10A inhibitor papaverine (Pap) on PASMC proliferation, intracellular cAMP accumulation and CREB activation. A) FBS stimulated PASMC proliferation after Pap (10 μM, 25 μM) treatment for 24 h. [^{3}H]thymidine incorporation was used to evaluate cell proliferation. †††$P<0.001$ vs 0.1% FBS, *$P<0.05$ vs 10% FBS, n = 4 in each group. **B)** Intracellular cAMP levels in PASMCs after Pap treatment measured by a cAMP enzyme immunoassay. The cAMP content of PASMC lysates is given as nmol/mg protein. *$P<0.05$, ***$P<0.001$ vs NTC (negative control), n = 4 in each group. **C)** CREB phosphorylation after Pap (10 μM, 25 μM) treatment. Representative immunoblots are shown in the figure, Values are expressed as the mean ± SEM.

approach against pulmonary vascular remodeling for the treatment of PAH.

PDE10A is one of the most recently described PDEs, and it was characterized as a dual-substrate gene in 1999 in mouse and in human brain [23–25]. PDE10A has the capacity to hydrolyze both cAMP and cGMP; however, the K_m for cAMP is approximately 0.05 μM compared with 3 μM for cGMP. Interestingly, the V_{max} for cAMP hydrolysis is fivefold lower than that for cGMP. Because of this kinetic pattern, PDE10A-mediated cGMP hydrolysis is potently inhibited by cAMP *in vitro*, which suggests that PDE10A may function as a cAMP-PDE and a cAMP-inhibited cGMP-PDE *in vivo* [23–25]. Furthermore, the cGMP-binding regulatory (GAF) domain of PDE10A is unique compared to the GAF domains of other PDE families because it is the only one that binds to cAMP instead of cGMP, which may contribute to the preferential hydrolysis of Camp [26]. The unique distribution of PDE10A in the brain and its enrichment in the striatum indicate that PDE10A inhibitors are potential therapeutic agents for the treatment of neurological and psychiatric disorders [27]. Recently, PDE10A-selective inhibitors have also been suggested to be useful in the treatment of diabetes and obesity [24,28]. In the present studies, we observed a higher expression of PDE10A in the MCT-PH rat pulmonary arteries and isolated PASMCs, which suggests that PDE10A may contribute to the proliferative phenotype of PASMCs. Although the specific functional role of PDE10A in lung tissue needs to be characterized in more detail, the present study also suggests a reactivation of PDE10A signaling in

abnormal proliferative lung disease tissues, such as the tissues observed in pathological vascular remodeling. Moreover, PDE10A immunoreactivity was markedly increased in pulmonary arteries of IPAH patient lungs compared to the donor lungs, which indicates the clinical relevance of the findings obtained from the MCT-PH rat model.

Vascular remodeling, which includes the proliferation and hypertrophy of SMCs, is a characteristic feature of PAH. Recent studies have reported that targeting abnormal PASMC proliferation in the vascular media blocks the development of PAH and attenuates pulmonary arterial remodeling in rodents and humans [17,29]. In our studies, downregulation of PDE10A by siRNA led to a greater suppression of PASMC proliferation among hyperproliferative cells than among healthy control cells, which suggests that PDE10A could be a useful therapeutic target for pulmonary vascular remodeling and other disorders characterized by increased PASMC proliferation. Furthermore, applying the selective PDE10A inhibitor papaverine also suppressed the proliferation of MCT PASMCs to a greater extent than control PASMCs. These anti-proliferative effects are largely due to an increase in intracellular cAMP levels that may stimulate the activity of protein kinase A (PKA) [30,31]. In line with this notion, several studies from our group and others have reported that compounds that activate adenylate cyclase or inhibit PDE counteract several pathways involved in SMC proliferation [11,15,32]. For example, cAMP in vascular SMCs was shown to decrease the expression of cyclin D1 and cdk2 as well as the

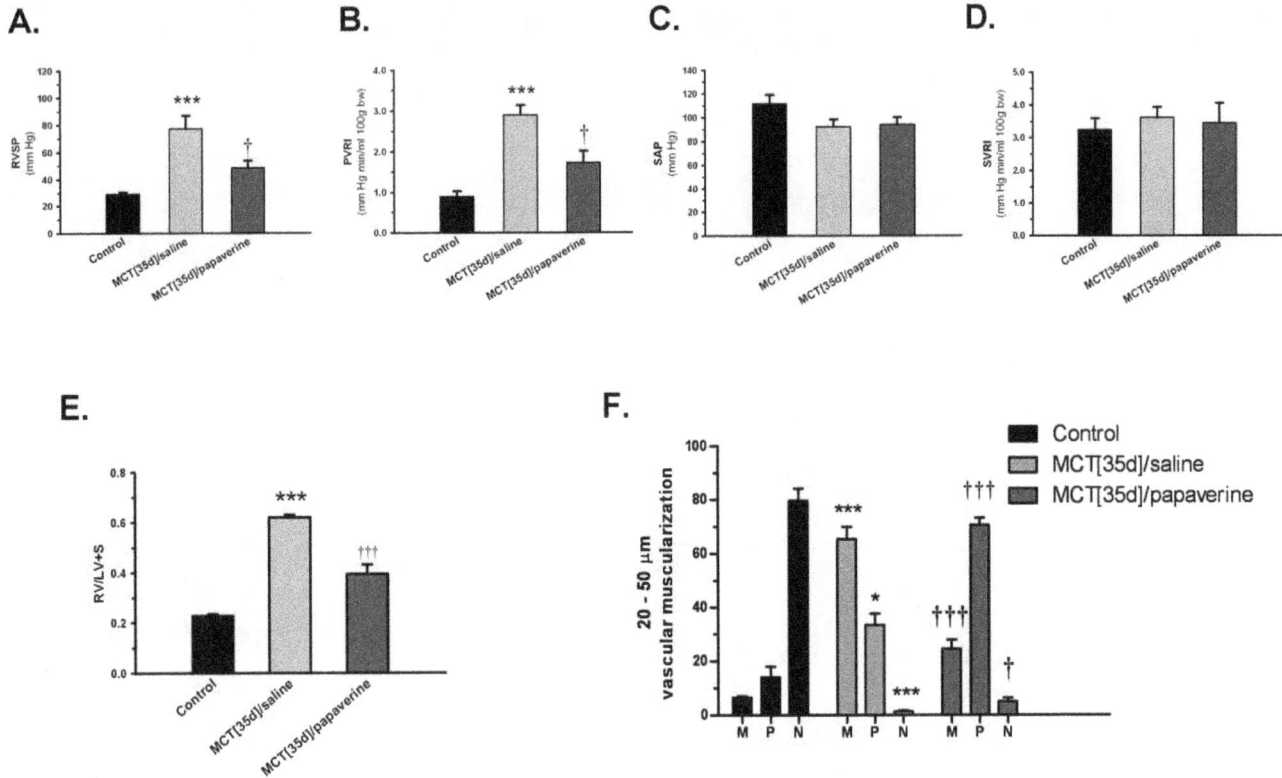

Figure 7. Effects of papaverine on MCT-PH rats *in vivo*. Papaverine was applied by continuous intravenous infusion with osmotic minipumps from days 21 to 35. A) RVSP (mm Hg), B) SAP (mm Hg), C) PVRI (mm Hg min/ml 100 g body), and D) SVRI (mm Hg min/ml 100 g body) are given as the mean ± SEM. ***P<0.001 vs control; †P<0.05 vs. MCT [35 d]/saline. Control: n = 9; MCT [35 d]/saline: n = 8; MCT [35 d]/papaverine: n = 8. E) Right heart mass, which was measured by the ratio of RV/LV+S. F) Effect of papaverine on the extent of muscularization of peripheral pulmonary arteries. The percentage of nonmuscularized (N), partially muscularized (P), or fully (M) muscularized pulmonary arteries related to the total number of pulmonary arteries is given as the mean ± SEM. A total of 80 to 100 intra-acinar vessels were analyzed in the lung of each rat from each group. ***P<0.001 vs control; †P<0.05 vs MCT [35 d]/saline. Values are expressed as the mean ± SEM.

activation of extracellular signal-regulated kinase (ERK). In addition, cAMP in vascular SMCs has been shown to increase the expression of the anti-proliferative molecules p53 and p21 [33–35]. Furthermore, there is now substantial evidence that cAMP/PKA signaling acts as a molecular gate to block cell cycle progression, primarily via occupancy of the cAMP response elements (CREs) in the promoter region of the cyclin A gene and increases in the level and phosphorylation status of the transcription factor CREB [36]. In accordance, we found that CREB phosphorylation was markedly increased in MCT PASMCs after PDE10A inhibition by papaverine. We only observed a minor increase in control PASMCs, which suggested that hyperproliferative PASMCs were more sensitive to PDE10A inhibition. This may have important consequences for pulmonary media wall remodeling in PAH *in vivo* because CREB content has been shown to be diminished in smooth muscle cells in remodeled pulmonary arteries with PAH [37].

More importantly, numerous studies have demonstrated that the compartmentalization and dynamics of cAMP signaling are crucial for cAMP-triggered cellular responses [38]. In contrast to the conventional transmembrane adenylyl cyclase, soluble adenylyl cyclase (sAC) is distributed in specific subcellular compartments, including mitochondria, centrioles, mitotic spindles, and nuclei. sAC has been proved to be an alternative source of intracellular cAMP pools regulated in a temporary and spatial manner [39]. Furthermore, the direct activation of nuclear PKA by nuclear-localized cAMP was demonstrated to be a more

efficient signaling pathway leading to CREB activation compared to activation of cytoplasmic PKA [40]. Notably, the subcellular distribution of PDE proteins may regulate the specific intracellular localization of cAMP by compartmentalized hydrolysis of cAMP [41]. As we showed in the present study, PDE10A was localized in the nuclei of PASMCs with great abundance. Furthermore, PDE10 inhibition led to cAMP accumulation and significant activation of the transcriptional factor CREB, which was followed by cAMP accumulation. PDE10 inhibition may lead to increased cAMP in the nuclei of PASMCs and regulate cell growth responses by activating CREB. Further investigations on the subcellular distribution of cAMP after PDE10 inhibition, however, are required to prove this finding.

Recently, Murray et al. demonstrated that the total PDE activity levels are increased in PAH PASMCs compared to control PASMCs [42]. In agreement with these findings, an increase in the total cAMP-PDE activity was observed in our experimental model of PAH. Notably, the relative contribution of PDE10A to the total cAMP-PDE activity was increased in MCT PASMCs compared to control PASMCs, which indicated that PDE10A inhibition was more effective in increasing cAMP generation and inhibiting the hyperproliferation of PASMCs from MCT-PH rats. This suggests that PDE inhibitors that increase cAMP levels in general, as well as PDE10A-selective inhibitors, offer new possibilities for therapeutic intervention for pulmonary vascular remodeling in PH. In line with these findings, treatment of MCT-PH rats with the PDE10A inhibitor papaverine for 14 days markedly improved their

A.

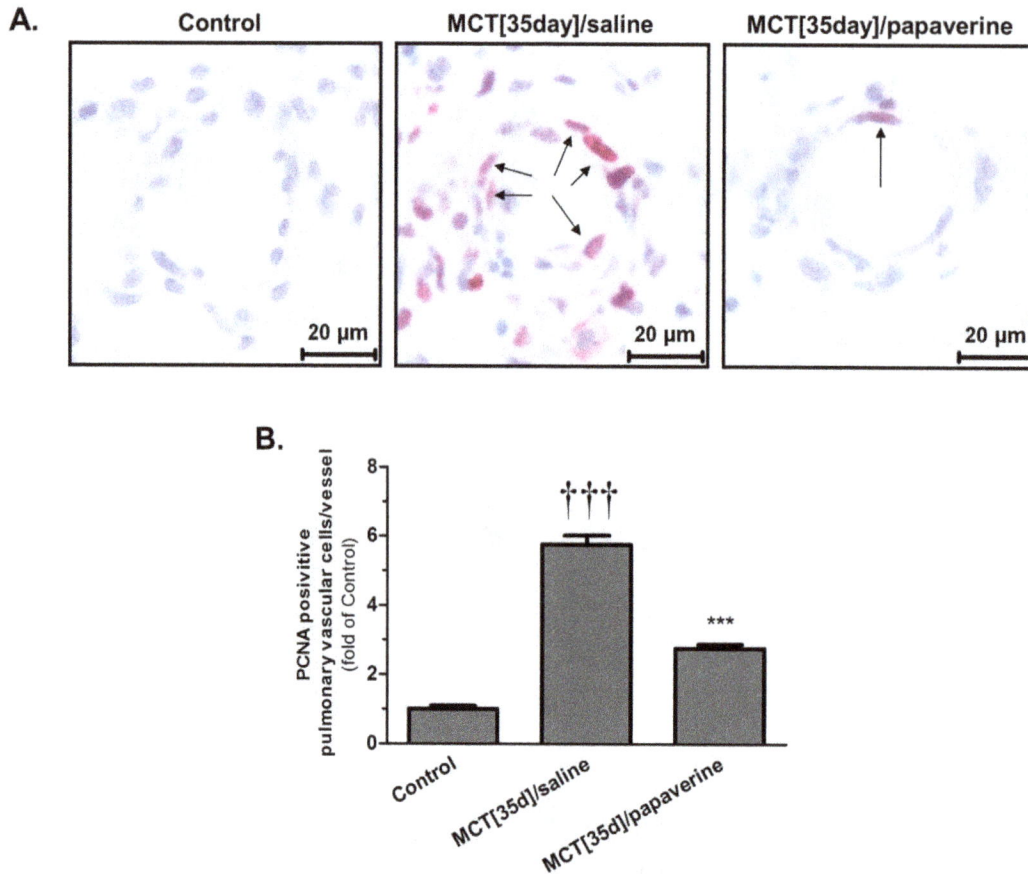

Figure 8. Anti-proliferative effects of papaverine *in vivo*. Proliferating cell nuclear antigen (PCNA) staining was performed to identify proliferating pulmonary vascular cells. **A**) Representative PCNA immunostaining microphotographs of the rat lung sections from control (left), MCT [35 day]/saline placebo (middle) and MCT [35 day]/papaverine (right), with black arrows indicating the PCNA-positive vascular cells in red. Scale bar: 20 μm. **B**) Effects of papaverine on pulmonary vascular cell proliferation are expressed as fold changes compared to control lungs, n = 5 in each group. ***P<0.001 vs control; †††P<0.001 vs MCT [35 d]/saline. Values are expressed as the mean ± SEM.

hemodynamics. Indeed, RVSP and PVRI values were significantly lowered after papaverine treatment. The structural changes of the lung vasculature, such as the high percentage of fully muscularized peripheral pulmonary arteries and proliferating vascular cells, were significantly decreased after papaverine treatment. In addition, right heart hypertrophy was significantly reduced by papaverine. Because papaverine is used as a potent vasodilator in the systemic and cerebral vasculature, we could not eliminate the possibility that it may exert vasodilatory effects on pulmonary vessels [43]. Papaverine-induced vasorelaxation is believed to be related to reduced calcium influx following PKA activation after cAMP levels increase [44,45]. Nevertheless, the present study

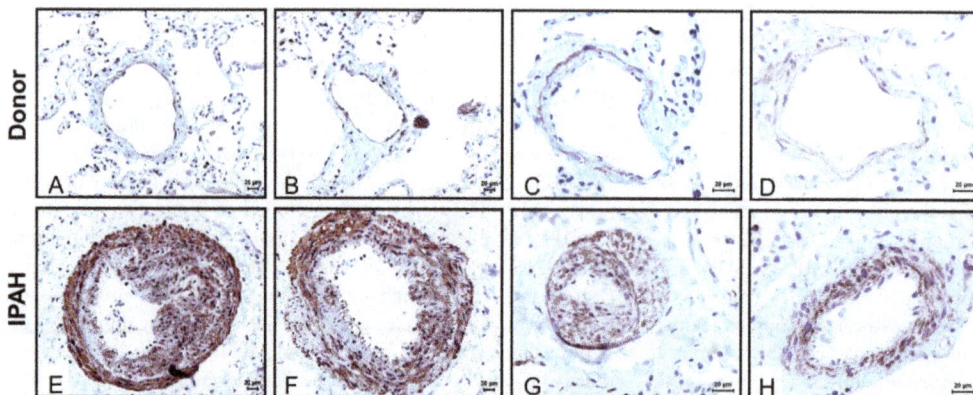

Figure 9. Pulmonary vascular expression and localization of PDE10A in lung tissues from donor and IPAH patients. Representative PDE10A immunostaining microphotographs of the human lung sections from donors (A–D) and IPAH patients (E–H). Scale bar: 20 μm.

showed that the systemic pressures of papaverine-treated rats are similar to those of healthy rats. The effects of papaperine may not be exclusively targeted to PDE10A, although a continuous intravenous infusion of papaverine should not result in high plasma levels of this compound. Based on our previous experience in the field of *in vivo* siRNA mediated knockdown, we believe that *in vivo* siRNA targeting of PDE10A in pulmonary arterial SMCs is not feasible because the cells are present between endothelial and fibroblast cells in pulmonary vasculature. Within published literature in the field of PH, only two manuscripts have addressed the siRNA mediated knockdown of endothelial specific genes [46,47]. Hence, new PDE10 inhibitors with higher selectivity and potency are required to explore these therapeutic aspects in more detail.

In conclusion, PDE10A expression and activity are increased in PASMCs of experimental MCT-PH rats. Using PDE10A-targeted siRNA and the PDE10 inhibitor papaverine, we demonstrated that PDE10A plays a major role in the hyperproliferation of PASMCs. Furthermore, papaverine significantly improved pulmonary hemodynamics and significantly reversed the structural abnormalities underlying the MCT-PH rat model. To the best of our knowledge, this was the first study addressing a central role of PDE10A in progressive pulmonary vascular remodeling, and we propose the inhibition of PDE10A as a novel therapeutic approach to the treatment of PAH.

Supporting Information

Figure S1 mRNA expression of cAMP-PDEs (PDE10A, PDE1A, PDE3A, PDE3B and PDE4A) after PDE10A siRNA transfection. To examine the isoform-specific effects of PDE10A siRNA, cAMP-PDEs were analyzed by qRT-PCR after a 24-h transfection of 100 nM scramble siRNA (gray bars) or PDE10A siRNA (black bars). PASMCs treated with transfection reagent alone were used as a negative control (NTC), n = 3 in each group. Values are expressed as the mean ± SEM.

Figure S2 Representative double immunostaining microphotographs of the rat lung sections were used to assess the muscularization of small pulmonary arteries. Staining was undertaken for von Willebrand factor (brown; endothelial cells) and α-smooth muscle actin (purple; smooth muscle cells).

Author Contributions

Conceived and designed the experiments: SSP RTS XT WS FG. Performed the experiments: XT CV EB. Analyzed the data: XT SSP. Contributed reagents/materials/analysis tools: HAG NW. Wrote the paper: XT SSP.

References

1. Rubin LJ (1997) Primary pulmonary hypertension. N Engl J Med 336: 111–117.
2. Stenmark KR, Mecham RP (1997) Cellular and molecular mechanisms of pulmonary vascular remodeling. Annu Rev Physiol 59: 89–144.
3. Olschewski H, Simonneau G, Galie N, Higenbottam T, Naeije R, et al. (2002) Inhaled iloprost for severe pulmonary hypertension. N Engl J Med 347: 322–329.
4. Galie N, Ghofrani HA, Torbicki A, Barst RJ, Rubin LJ, et al. (2005) Sildenafil citrate therapy for pulmonary arterial hypertension. N Engl J Med 353: 2148–2157.
5. Rubin LJ, Badesch DB, Barst RJ, Galie N, Black CM, et al. (2002) Bosentan therapy for pulmonary arterial hypertension. N Engl J Med 346: 896–903.
6. Conti M, Beavo J (2007) Biochemistry and physiology of cyclic nucleotide phosphodiesterases: essential components in cyclic nucleotide signaling. Annu Rev Biochem 76: 481–511.
7. Lugnier C (2006) Cyclic nucleotide phosphodiesterase (PDE) superfamily: a new target for the development of specific therapeutic agents. Pharmacol Ther 109: 366–398.
8. Nagel DJ, Aizawa T, Jeon KI, Liu W, Mohan A, et al. (2006) Role of nuclear Ca²⁺/calmodulin-stimulated phosphodiesterase 1A in vascular smooth muscle cell growth and survival. Circ Res 98: 777–784.
9. Baillie GS, Houslay MD (2005) Arrestin times for compartmentalised cAMP signalling and phosphodiesterase-4 enzymes. Curr Opin Cell Biol 17: 129–134.
10. Maclean MR, Johnston ED, Mcculloch KM, Pooley L, Houslay MD, et al. (1997) Phosphodiesterase isoforms in the pulmonary arterial circulation of the rat: changes in pulmonary hypertension. J Pharmacol Exp Ther 283: 619–624.
11. Schermuly RT, Pullamsetti SS, Kwapiszewska G, Dumitrascu R, Tian X, et al. (2007) Phosphodiesterase 1 upregulation in pulmonary arterial hypertension: target for reverse-remodeling therapy. Circulation 115: 2331–2339.
12. Schermuly RT, Kreisselmeier KP, Ghofrani HA, Yilmaz H, Butrous G, et al. (2004) Chronic sildenafil treatment inhibits monocrotaline-induced pulmonary hypertension in rats. Am J Respir Crit Care Med 169: 39–45.
13. Wharton J, Strange JW, Moller GM, Growcott EJ, Ren X, et al. (2005) Antiproliferative effects of phosphodiesterase type 5 inhibition in human pulmonary artery cells. Am J Respir Crit Care Med 172: 105–113.
14. Pullamsetti S, Krick S, Yilmaz H, Ghofrani HA, Schudt C, et al. (2005) Inhaled tolafentrine reverses pulmonary vascular remodeling via inhibition of smooth muscle cell migration. Respir Res 6: 128.
15. Phillips PG, Long L, Wilkins MR, Morrell NW (2005) cAMP phosphodiesterase inhibitors potentiate effects of prostacyclin analogs in hypoxic pulmonary vascular remodeling. Am J Physiol Lung Cell Mol Physiol 288: L103–L115.
16. Soderling SH, Beavo JA (2000) Regulation of cAMP and cGMP signaling: new phosphodiesterases and new functions. Curr Opin Cell Biol 12: 174–179.
17. Schermuly RT, Dony E, Ghofrani HA, Pullamsetti S, Savai R, et al. (2005) Reversal of experimental pulmonary hypertension by PDGF inhibition. J Clin Invest 115: 2811–2821.
18. Schermuly RT, Kreisselmeier KP, Ghofrani HA, Samidurai A, Pullamsetti S, et al. (2004) Antiremodeling effects of iloprost and the dual-selective phosphodiesterase 3/4 inhibitor tolafentrine in chronic experimental pulmonary hypertension. Circ Res 94: 1101–1108.
19. Lai YJ, Pullamsetti SS, Dony E, Weissmann N, Butrous G, et al. (2008) Role of the prostanoid EP4 receptor in iloprost-mediated vasodilatation in pulmonary hypertension. Am J Respir Crit Care Med 178: 188–196.
20. Dahal BK, Kosanovic D, Pamarthi PK, Sydykov A, Lai YJ, et al. (2010) Therapeutic efficacy of azaindole-1 in experimental pulmonary hypertension. Eur Respir J 36: 808–818.
21. Thompson WJ, Appleman MM (1971) Characterization of cyclic nucleotide phosphodiesterases of rat tissues. J Biol Chem 246: 3145–3150.
22. Bauer AC, Schwabe U (1980) An improved assay of cyclic 3′,5′-nucleotide phosphodiesterases with QAE-Sephadex columns. Naunyn Schmiedebergs Arch Pharmacol 311: 193–198.
23. Soderling SH, Bayuga SJ, Beavo JA (1999) Isolation and characterization of a dual-substrate phosphodiesterase gene family: PDE10A. Proc Natl Acad Sci U S A 96: 7071–7076.
24. Fujishige K, Kotera J, Michibata H, Yuasa K, Takebayashi S, et al. (1999) Cloning and characterization of a novel human phosphodiesterase that hydrolyzes both cAMP and cGMP (PDE10A). J Biol Chem 274: 18438–18445.
25. Loughney K, Snyder PB, Uher L, Rosman GJ, Ferguson K, et al. (1999) Isolation and characterization of PDE10A, a novel human 3′, 5′-cyclic nucleotide phosphodiesterase. Gene 234: 109–117.
26. Gross-Langenhoff M, Hofbauer K, Weber J, Schultz A, Schultz JE (2006) cAMP is a ligand for the tandem GAF domain of human phosphodiesterase 10 and cGMP for the tandem GAF domain of phosphodiesterase 11. J Biol Chem 281: 2841–2846.
27. Hebb AL, Robertson HA (2007) Role of phosphodiesterases in neurological and psychiatric disease. Curr Opin Pharmacol 7: 86–92.
28. Cantin LD, Magnuson S, Gunn D, Barucci N, Breuhaus M, et al. (2007) PDE-10A inhibitors as insulin secretagogues. Bioorg Med Chem Lett 17: 2869–2873.
29. Merklinger SL, Jones PL, Martinez EC, Rabinovitch M (2005) Epidermal growth factor receptor blockade mediates smooth muscle cell apoptosis and improves survival in rats with pulmonary hypertension. Circulation 112: 423–431.
30. Koyama H, Bornfeldt KE, Fukumoto S, Nishizawa Y (2001) Molecular pathways of cyclic nucleotide-induced inhibition of arterial smooth muscle cell proliferation. J Cell Physiol 186: 1–10.
31. Iyengar R (1996) Gating by cyclic AMP: expanded role for an old signaling pathway. Science 271: 461–463.
32. Rybalkin SD, Bornfeldt KE, Sonnenburg WK, Rybalkina IG, Kwak KS, et al. (1997) Calmodulin-stimulated cyclic nucleotide phosphodiesterase (PDE1C) is induced in human arterial smooth muscle cells of the synthetic, proliferative phenotype. J Clin Invest 100: 2611–2621.
33. Vadiveloo PK, Filonzi EL, Stanton HR, Hamilton JA (1997) G1 phase arrest of human smooth muscle cells by heparin, IL-4 and cAMP is linked to repression of cyclin D1 and cdk2. Atherosclerosis 133: 61–69.

34. Bornfeldt KE, Krebs EG (1999) Crosstalk between protein kinase A and growth factor receptor signaling pathways in arterial smooth muscle. Cell Signal 11: 465–477.

35. Hayashi S, Morishita R, Matsushita H, Nakagami H, Taniyama Y, et al. (2000) Cyclic AMP inhibited proliferation of human aortic vascular smooth muscle cells, accompanied by induction of p53 and p21. Hypertension 35: 237–243.

36. Kothapalli D, Stewart SA, Smyth EM, Azonobi I, Pure E, et al. (2003) Prostacylin receptor activation inhibits proliferation of aortic smooth muscle cells by regulating cAMP response element-binding protein- and pocket protein-dependent cyclin a gene expression. Mol Pharmacol 64: 249–258.

37. Klemm DJ, Watson PA, Frid MG, Dempsey EC, Schaack J, et al. (2001) cAMP response element-binding protein content is a molecular determinant of smooth muscle cell proliferation and migration. J Biol Chem 276: 46132–46141.

38. Saucerman JJ, Zhang J, Martin JC, Peng LX, Stenbit AE, et al. (2006) Systems analysis of PKA-mediated phosphorylation gradients in live cardiac myocytes. Proc Natl Acad Sci U S A 103: 12923–12938.

39. Zippin JH, Chen Y, Nahirney P, Kamenetsky M, Wuttke MS, et al. (2003) Compartmentalization of bicarbonate-sensitive adenylyl cyclase in distinct signaling microdomains. FASEB J 17: 82–84.

40. Zippin JH, Farrell J, Huron D, Kamenetsky M, Hess KC, et al. (2004) Bicarbonate-responsive "soluble" adenylyl cyclase defines a nuclear cAMP microdomain. J Cell Biol 164: 527–534.

41. Lugnier C (2006) Cyclic nucleotide phosphodiesterase (PDE) superfamily: a new target for the development of specific therapeutic agents. Pharmacol Ther 109: 366–398.

42. Murray F, Patel HH, Suda RY, Zhang S, Thistlethwaite PA, et al. (2007) Expression and activity of cAMP phosphodiesterase isoforms in pulmonary artery smooth muscle cells from patients with pulmonary hypertension: role for PDE1. Am J Physiol Lung Cell Mol Physiol 292: L294–L303.

43. Christensen CW, Rosen LB, Gal RA, Haseeb M, Lassar TA, et al. (1991) Coronary vasodilator reserve. Comparison of the effects of papaverine and adenosine on coronary flow, ventricular function, and myocardial metabolism. Circulation 83: 294–303.

44. Aoki H, Nishimura J, Kobayashi S, Kanaide H (1994) Relationship between cytosolic calcium concentration and force in the papaverine-induced relaxation of medial strips of pig coronary artery. Br J Pharmacol 111: 489–496.

45. Torres-Flores V, Hernandez-Rueda YL, Neri-Vidaurri PC, Jimenez-Trejo F, Calderon-Salinas V, et al. (2008) Activation of protein kinase A stimulates the progesterone-induced calcium influx in human sperm exposed to the phosphodiesterase inhibitor papaverine. J Androl 29: 549–557.

46. Miyawaki-Shimizu K, Predescu D, Shimizu J, Broman M, Predescu S, et al. (2006) siRNA-induced caveolin-1 knockdown in mice increases lung vascular permeability via the junctional pathway. Am J Physiol Lung Cell Mol Physiol 290: L405–413.

47. Izikki M, Guignabert C, Fadel E, Humbert M, Tu L, et al. (2009) Endothelial-derived FGF2 contributes to the progression of pulmonary hypertension in humans and rodents. J Clin Invest 119: 512–523.

4

Erythroid-Specific Transcriptional Changes in PBMCs from Pulmonary Hypertension Patients

Chris Cheadle[1]*, Alan E. Berger[1], Stephen C. Mathai[2], Dmitry N. Grigoryev[3], Tonya N. Watkins[1], Yumiko Sugawara[1], Sangjucta Barkataki[1], Jinshui Fan[1], Meher Boorgula[1], Laura Hummers[4], Ari L. Zaiman[2], Reda Girgis[2], Michael A. McDevitt[5], Roger A. Johns[6], Frederick Wigley[4], Kathleen C. Barnes[1], Paul M. Hassoun[2]*

1 Division of Allergy and Clinical Immunology, Johns Hopkins University School of Medicine, Baltimore, Maryland, United States of America, 2 Division of Pulmonary/ Critical Care Medicine, Johns Hopkins University School of Medicine, Baltimore, Maryland, United States of America, 3 Medical Genetic Core, Children's Mercy Hospitals and Clinics, Kansas City, Missouri, United States of America, 4 Division of Rheumatology, Johns Hopkins University School of Medicine, Baltimore, Maryland, United States of America, 5 Division of Hematology, Johns Hopkins University School of Medicine, Baltimore, Maryland, United States of America, 6 Department of Anesthesiology and Critical Care Medicine, Johns Hopkins University School of Medicine, Baltimore, Maryland, United States of America

Abstract

Background: Gene expression profiling of peripheral blood mononuclear cells (PBMCs) is a powerful tool for the identification of surrogate markers involved in disease processes. The hypothesis tested in this study was that chronic exposure of PBMCs to a hypertensive environment in remodeled pulmonary vessels would be reflected by specific transcriptional changes in these cells.

Methodology/Principal Findings: The transcript profiles of PBMCs from 30 idiopathic pulmonary arterial hypertension patients (IPAH), 19 patients with systemic sclerosis without pulmonary hypertension (SSc), 42 scleroderma-associated pulmonary arterial hypertensio patients (SSc-PAH), and 8 patients with SSc complicated by interstitial lung disease and pulmonary hypertension (SSc-PH-ILD) were compared to the gene expression profiles of PBMCs from 41 healthy individuals. Multiple gene expression signatures were identified which could distinguish various disease groups from controls. One of these signatures, specific for erythrocyte maturation, is enriched specifically in patients with PH. This association was validated in multiple published datasets. The erythropoiesis signature was strongly correlated with hemodynamic measures of increasing disease severity in IPAH patients. No significant correlation of the same type was noted for SSc-PAH patients, this despite a clear signature enrichment within this group overall. These findings suggest an association of the erythropoiesis signature in PBMCs from patients with PH with a variable presentation among different subtypes of disease.

Conclusions/Significance: In PH, the expansion of immature red blood cell precursors may constitute a response to the increasingly hypoxic conditions prevalent in this syndrome. A correlation of this erythrocyte signature with more severe hypertension cases may provide an important biomarker of disease progression.

Editor: Lisa Ng Fong Poh, Agency for Science, Technology and Research – Singapore Immunology Network, Singapore

Funding: Supported by NHLBI P50 Grant HL084946 (Specialized Center for Clinically- Oriented Research, to P.M.H.). Supported in part by the Mary Beryl Patch Turnbull Scholar Program (to K.C.B.). The Scleroderma Research Foundation has provided support for the Johns Hopkins Scleroderma Center. The funders had no role in study design, data collection and analysis, decision to publish, or preparation of the manuscript.

Competing Interests: The authors have declared that no competing interests exist.

* E-mail: ccheadl1@jhmi.edu (CC); phassou1@jhmi.edu (PMH)

Introduction

Pulmonary arterial hypertension (PAH) is a vascular disease that carries significant morbidity and mortality [1,2,3]. Morbidity and mortality rates vary and depend on the age, the degree of pulmonary hypertension, and the response to vasodilator therapy. Death as a result of both acute and chronic right heart failure may occur. PAH is currently characterized by uncontrolled cell proliferation and inflammation involving the pulmonary vascular resistive vessels, leading to a progressive increase in pulmonary vascular resistance, right ventricle hypertrophy, and eventual heart failure.

PAH can complicate connective tissue diseases such as scleroderma [4,5] as well as other autoimmune diseases such as systemic lupus erythematosus and rheumatoid arthritis [6,7]. Scleroderma, or systemic sclerosis (SSc), is a chronic multisystem autoimmune disease characterized by a vasculopathy, diffuse fibrosis of skin and various internal organs, and immune abnormalities. Up to 10–15% of SSc patients eventually develop PAH [8]. While the factors which lead a subset of SSc patients to go on to develop PAH are unclear, it is of great clinical interest to develop early markers of SSc-associated PAH (SSc-PAH) disease in order to provide more aggressive treatment to the "at risk" patient population. The early phase of the disease process has been difficult to study rigorously because of the delay in the diagnosis of

SSc-PAH and the lack of reliable biomarkers for early disease. Lung biopsy is avoided since it is invasive and unsafe in these patients. For this reason we chose to use gene expression profiling of peripheral blood mononuclear cells (PBMCs) as a surrogate tissue which is readily obtainable from patients and provides a large pool of gene transcripts shown to have the potential to be highly sensitive to the disease microenvironments on a systems wide basis [9,10]. Previous studies using PBMCs have demonstrated an ability to discriminate between PAH, in general, and healthy controls, identify PAH-specific genes [11], as well as distinguish between IPAH and SSc-PAH gene signatures [12]. However, more recent studies have shown considerable heterogeneity when examining directly the contrast in gene expression profiles in PBMCs from SSc-PAH and SSc patients [13,14,15]. For example, while Pendergrass et al. [13] focused on the increased expression of 9 genes that distinguished SSc-PAH from SSc, Risbano et al. [14] describe 5 genes which when down-regulated distinguish SSc-PAH from SSc patients. We hypothesized that chronic exposure of PBMCs to elevated pulmonary pressures in remodeled pulmonary vessels will be reflected by specific transcriptional changes in these cells and distinguish PH of various etiologies from both SSc and normal controls.

Results

Expression Profiling

The transcript profiles of PBMCs from 42 SSc associated PAH (SSc-PAH) patients, 30 IPAH patients, 19 patients with SSc, and 8 patients with SSc complicated by interstitial lung disease and PH (SSc-PH-ILD) were compared to the transcript profiles of PBMCs from 41 healthy individuals (see Table 1 for a summary of demographic and clinical patient descriptions, see Table S3 for all relevant clinical data and descriptions, on a patient-by-patient basis). In our initial data analysis we compared the gene expression for each disease group versus that of the controls (as described in Methods) and found large numbers of significantly regulated genes between patients and controls (Figure 1). Among the 89 genes significantly up-regulated in common among IPAH and SSc with or without accompanying PH were components of the Toll-like receptor (TLR) signaling pathway including the STAT1, TLR7, and TLR8 genes. An expanded search of all genes in the TLR signaling pathway revealed a broad general trend (Figure 2A) of up-regulation of these genes in each disease group (ttest p-values of the average expression of these pathway genes by group versus controls were p = 0.04 for IPAH, p = 0.0006 for SSc-PAH, and p = 0.004 for SSc, SSc-PH-ILD was not significant at p = 0.09) altogether suggesting a chronic activation of the innate immune system in these patients. Scleroderma patients with or without PAH demonstrated a pattern of 30 distinct immune response genes (DAVID [NIH Database for Annotation, Visualization, and Integrated Discovery]: defense response; $p < 7 \times 10^{-4}$) up-regulated in common including CXCL10, FCGR1A, HCK, MX2, NCF1C, PARP4, and TLR4 (see Table S1 for all cited genes, enrichment results, and complete group comparison results).

Interestingly, PH patients (IPAH and SSc-PAH) shared a large number of distinct genes (118) (Figure 1A) that were significantly up-regulated in these PH groups but not in SSc including a total of seven genes CA2, HBA2, HBD, HBG1, HBG2, HBM, HBQ1 shown to be highly enriched for blood gas transport (DAVID: gas transport: $p < 7 \times 10^{-10}$). This same group of 118 genes also contained a sub-group of genes involved in platelet biology (DAVID: platelet alpha granule: $p < 1 \times 10^{-6}$), a finding seen as well using MsigDB (Broad Institute Molecular Signatures Data Base) (platelet specific genes: $p < 1.6 \times 10^{-12}$).

The 136 genes down-regulated for all disease groups relative to healthy controls were significantly enriched for apoptosis (DAVID: apoptosis: $p < 1.4 \times 10^{-4}$), a trend that extended to the additional 170 down-regulated genes in common between SSc-PAH and IPAH (DAVID: regulation of apoptosis: $p < 3.0 \times 10^{-6}$). Further examination of down-regulated changes in gene expression individually in each condition using the methods of gene set analysis (webPAGE [16]) revealed a common trend of down-regulation of multiple pathways involved in T cell function (Table 2). Examination of several of these pathways in detail (Figure 2B) demonstrated a clear pattern of down-regulation of genes in these pathways across all patient groups relative to controls.

Signature Identification

Unsupervised clustering of 296 genes (chosen from a pool of the 500 most variable genes and which displayed distinct clustering patterns) across all samples shows a clear trend of multiple clusters of correlated gene expression (Figure 3). Many of these clusters overlap the groups noted above. For example, in the first cluster, Immune Response genes down-regulated (IR-DR), 56 of the 58 genes depicted in this cluster are members of the group of the statistically down-regulated genes shared by all three major disease groups (IPAH, SSc-PAH, and SSc). Conversely, over half of the genes (41/81) in the Immune Response genes up-regulated (IR-UR) cluster are members of the group of the statistically up-regulated genes shared by all three major disease groups (IPAH, SSc-PAH, and SSc). Additional clusters included a gene expression signature originally identified in neutrophils [17] and found as an immature neutrophil signature (INS) in the PBMC fraction of blood from both vasculitis related to Wegener's granulomatosis [18] and systemic lupus erythematosus [19] patients relative to healthy controls, presumably as part of an aggravated chronic immune response. In this study the INS signature, when present, appears to be distributed nonspecifically among all samples. Although these three signatures (IR-UR, IR-DR, and INS) were clearly identified and annotated they were of less interest to this study either because of their general non-specificity (INS) or because of their inability to distinguish among separate disease groups (IR-UR, IR-DR). Two other signatures, however, both of which had been identified by functional annotation during our initial analysis (the gas transport and platelet specific genes), were represented by clusters shown here also to be related. The average expression levels for the Illumina probes in these two distinct groups have a Pearson correlation r = 0.6 across all subjects (see Table S2 for a complete listing of the genes in these two clusters). A distinctive feature of the gene expression of these two signatures (Erythroid Differentiation Signature – EDS; and Platelet derived – PI) is that they are specific primarily to disease groups of patients with PH studied in this cohort (IPAH, SSc-PAH, SSc-PH-ILD).

Signature Characterization

In order to further characterize disease specific gene expression, all patient and control samples (see Methods) were directly evaluated by the methods of gene set analysis using gene lists derived from the Mouse Genome Informatics (MGI) database [20]. The file used for mouse phenotypic information contains 5011 distinct genes and 5142 phenotypic terms derived from information from specific gene mutations in multiple mouse strains, including an extensive library of specific gene knock-in and knock-out strains. In this analysis, patterns of gene expression among the PH, control and SSc groups were visualized across the entirety of the dataset by displaying the average gene expression for every mouse gene set for each human sample (Figure 4A). Patterns of disease specific gene set expression were detected

Table 1. Demographic and clinical characteristics of the patients with PH.

Variable	Overall (n=140)	Control (n=41)	SSc (n=19)	IPAH (n=30)	SSc-PAH (n=42)	SSc-PH-ILD (n=8)
Age (mean ± SD years)	53±13	45±12	55±10	52±12	60±13	61±11
Gender n (%)						
Female	117 (83.6)	34 (82.9)	19 (100)	25 (83.3)	33 (78.6)	6 (75.0)
Male	23 (16.4)	7 (17.0)	0 (0)	5 (16.7)	9 (21.4)	2 (25.0)
Race n (%)						
African American	20 (14.3)	7 (17.1)	0 (0)	5 (16.7)	8 (19.0)	0 (0)
Asian	4 (2.9)	1 (2.4)	0 (0)	1 (3.3)	1 (2.4)	1 (12.5)
Caucasian	115 (82.1)	33 (80.5)	19 (100)	23 (76.7)	33 (78.6)	7 (87.5)
Hispanic	1 (0.7)	0 (0)	0 (0)	1 (3.3)	0 (0)	0 (0)
NYHA functional class n (% of the PAH subjects)						
I	9 (11.3)	NA	NA	7 (23.3)	2 (4.8)	0 (0)
II	39 (48.7)	NA	NA	16 (53.3)	22 (52.4)	1 (12.5)
III	30 (37.5)	NA	NA	6 (20.0)	17 (40.4)	7 (87.5)
IV	2 (2.5)	NA	NA	1 (3.3)	1 (2.4)	0 (0)
NA (# for which value is not available)	60 (the non-PAH subjects)	41	19	0	0	0
6MWD (mean ± SD (# missing values))	1174±395 (64)	NA	NA	1383±392 (3)	1091±340 (1)	891±378 (0)
RA mean (mean ± SD (# missing values))	7.7±4.2 (61)	NA	NA	7.7±4.2 (0)	7.9±4.4 (1)	7.5±3.8 (0)
CI (mean ± SD (# missing values))	2.66±0.72 (61)	NA	NA	2.61±0.69 (0)	2.66±0.74 (1)	2.88±0.80 (0)
PVRI (mean ± SD (# missing values))	1062±573 (61)	NA	NA	1214±573 (0)	955±556 (1)	1042±610 (0)
PA saturation (mean ± SD (# missing values))	66.7±8.2 (65)	NA	NA	66.1±9.1 (2)	67.1±8.0 (2)	66.9±6.7 (1)

Except where indicated otherwise, values are the number (%).

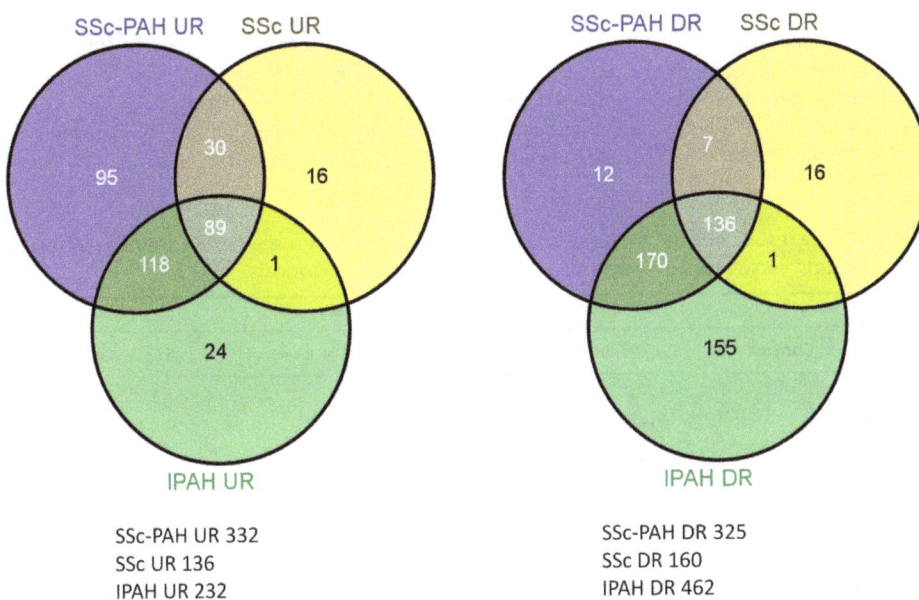

Figure 1. Venn diagrams illustrating the distribution of statistically significant disease-specific changes in gene expression. A) up-regulated and B) down-regulated gene expression for comparisons between SSc, SSc-PAH, and IPAH patients versus healthy controls. Total number of calculated differentially expressed genes for each comparison are as indicated below each diagram.

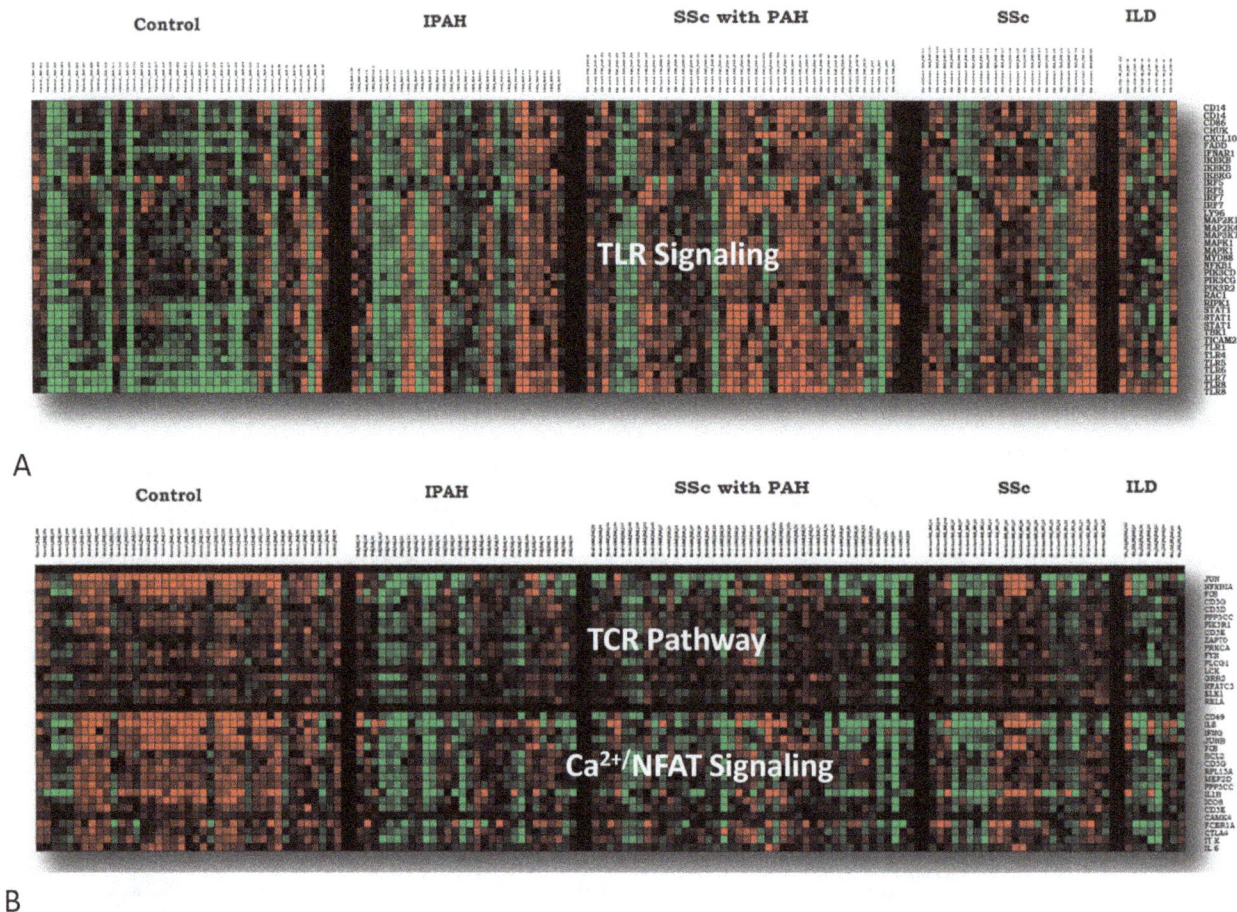

Figure 2. Heat map illustration of the distribution of gene expression among all samples for genes selected by pathways. A) TLR (Toll-like Receptor) Signaling, B) TCR (T cell receptor) Pathway, Ca^{2+}/NFAT Signaling. Red indicates increase and green indicates decrease in relative gene expression for each gene calculated individually across all samples.

which mapped to mouse gene lists involved in multiple phenotypes of blood disorders (Figure 4A, as indicated by arrows in the right panel). A summary of the differential expression p-value scores for these six blood disorder pathways when the individual disease groups were compared to controls shows a marked elevation of

gene expression in the SSc-PH-ILD, IPAH, and SSc-PAH groups but not for SSc patients (Figure 4B). In particular, the contrast between SSc-PAH and SSc patients is striking.

The combination of elevated hemoglobin gene expression in patients with PH and the preliminary evidence that many

Table 2. Gene Set Analysis – selected pathway results illustrate a strong downward regulation of the adaptive immune response across multiple pathways for all disease groups versus healthy controls regardless of patient diagnosis.

GeneSet	Annotation	IPAH_v_Control	SSc-PH-ILD_v_Control	SSc-PAH_v_Control	SSc_v_Control
TOB1 PATHWAY	BioCarta	−4.620	−4.205	−5.096	−6.653
CA²⁺NFAT SIGNALING	GEArray	−5.695	−3.866	−5.047	−5.395
IL12 PATHWAY	BioCarta	−3.757	−3.740	−4.826	−6.919
TCR PATHWAY	BioCarta	−4.963	−4.673	−5.085	−4.813
CCR5 PATHWAY	BioCarta	−4.488	−3.189	−5.027	−5.916
ARE/NRF2 PATHWAY	BioCarta	−4.174	−2.190	−4.210	−5.027
IL2PATHWAY	BioCarta	−3.685	−3.575	−2.811	−3.572
TH1-TH2-TH3 GENES	SABiosciences	−3.263	−3.289	−1.938	−4.736

Enrichment scores are derived using the PAGE technique (see Methods) and are equivalent to (gene set size adjusted) Gaussian distributed z scores. The negative sign direction of the scores indicates that for each of the indicated pathways and comparisons the average gene expression is lower in the disease group than in controls. Shaded pathways (Ca2+NFAT signaling and the TCR Pathway) are broken out on a gene by gene and sample by sample basis in Figure 2.

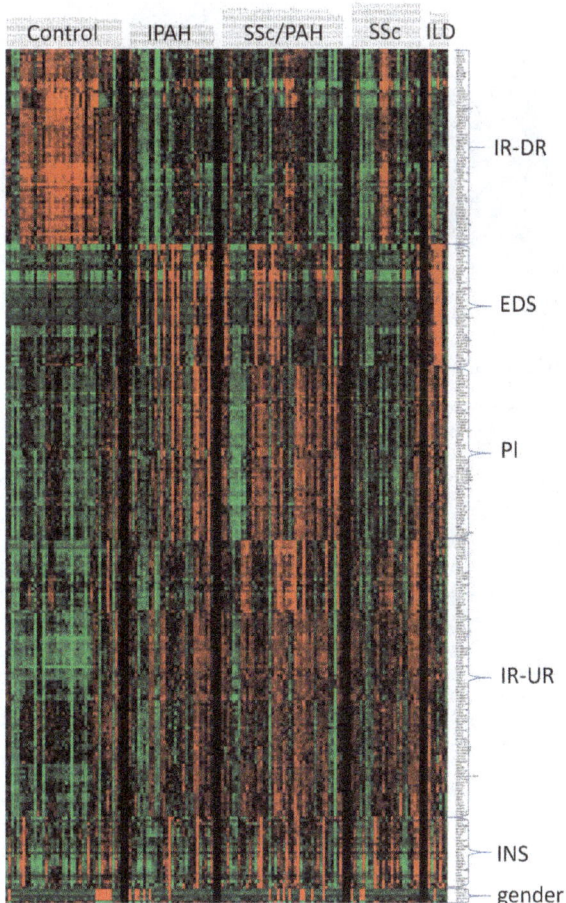

Figure 3. Heat map of unsupervised clustering (genes only) of 296 genes selected for both high variance (from a set of 500 most variant genes) and also as representative of six major patterns of distinctly correlated genes across the dataset. These patterns included an Immune Response signature (up- or down-regulated between controls and disease: IR-UR and IR-DR, respectively), the Erythroid Differentiation Signature (EDS) a Platelet specific signature (PI), and an Immature Neutrophil Signature (INS). The gender specific cluster acts as a positive control, the specific signatures are discussed in detail in the text, particularly that of the EDS.

differentially regulated genes in these disease groups mapped by gene set analysis to mouse blood disorder phenotypes suggested that human PH patients may be distinguished from healthy controls and SSc patients by a programmatic shift in gene expression in PBMCs, perhaps related to conditions of tissue hypoxia such as induced by PH. In order to further explore the functional implications of these regulated gene groups, a comprehensive list of genes was derived for the EDS and for the PI groups by selecting all microarray probes in the complete dataset whose expression levels have a Pearson Correlation ≥ 0.7 with the average expression for the probes in each cluster (EDS; 42 Illumina probes, 40 unique genes, and PI; 60 probes, 54 unique genes) as initially shown in Figure 3, across all the samples. This resulted in the identification of 169 Illumina probes representing 149 unique genes for the EDS, and 456 probes covering 384 unique genes for the PI signatures, respectively (Table S2). These are the sets of probes and genes used for further analysis of these signatures.

Tissue specificity of the EDS

The full gene list for the EDS signature (149 unique genes) was next tested against the Gene Expression Barcode, a web-based tool [21] which allows for highly accurate estimates of tissue specific gene expression. Inspection of the EDS gene expression across a catalog of over 130 curated human tissue types derived from the GEO (Gene Expression Omnibus) and the ArrayExpress public repositories demonstrated that the expression of EDS genes as a group is highly restricted to a few distinctive cell types (Figure 5) of the hematopoietic lineage including a very high level of enrichment in reticulocytes and in bone marrow. Reticulocytes from cord blood were particularly enriched relative to reticulocytes from circulation. It is interesting to note in this context that cord blood has been well characterized as having a less mature reticulocyte population than adult blood [22].

Inspection of the EDS specific gene list showed markedly increased levels of expression for two genes in particular, ALAS2 (aminolevulinate, delta-, synthase2) (Illumina Probe ID [ILMN 2367126]) and ERAF (erythroid differentiation associated factor; recently renamed to AHSP [alpha hemoglobin stabilizing protein]) (Illumina Probe ID [ILMN 1696512]), (Figure 6 A&B) both essential for the terminal differentiation of erythroid cells [23]. The specific overexpression of ALAS2 and ERAF in hypertension samples was confirmed by RT-PCR (Figure 6C). The expression levels of these two genes track so well with the EDS gene expression signature overall (Pearson's correlation coefficient of $r = 0.92$ for ERAF and $r = 0.95$ for ALAS2 versus the average EDS gene expression across all samples) that we are using them as single gene candidate biomarkers to track EDS-specific gene expression elevation in patients currently enrolled in ongoing longitudinal studies. The tissue specific expression of both of these genes is restricted, primarily to fetal liver, bone marrow (in adults), and most abundantly in CD71+ early erythroid cells in the circulation (BioGPS http://biogps.gnf.org). We note that hemoglobin production in erythroid cells is one of the most important stages in their terminal differentiation [24], the induction of ALAS2 is essential for hemoglobin production [25] and ERAF/AHSP is essential for proper assembly of nascent alpha globin incorporation into hemoglobin-A [26]. In addition, conditions of hypoxia have been shown to directly result in elevated levels of ALAS2 in a human model of erythroid terminal differentiation [27].

External Validation of the Association of the EDS with Pulmonary Hypertension

In order to examine the extent of EDS association with PH, in general, beyond this current study, a survey was carried out of other published PH microarray studies (with and without SSc) in which PBMCs were the target tissue and for which full datasets were available through GEO (NCBI – Gene Expression Omnibus) [31]. A total of four datasets were identified, three of them recently published (in 2010), each of which contained at least one phenotype for PH (Table 3). Two of these datasets also included phenotypes for SSc both with and without accompanying PH (Risbano et al. [14] and Pendergrass et al. [13]). Each dataset was queried using the methods of gene set analysis using the EDS gene expression signature gene list embedded in a background of over 550 pathway gene lists derived from multiple sources. The strongest overall enrichment scores for the EDS were, not surprisingly, generated from the PH phenotypes of our own study (JHU; SSc-PH-ILD-33.3, IPAH-21.1, and SSc-PAH-17.9). The slightly positive enrichment score for the JHU SSc group reflects several patients who are EDS positive (and who may be progressing towards PH).

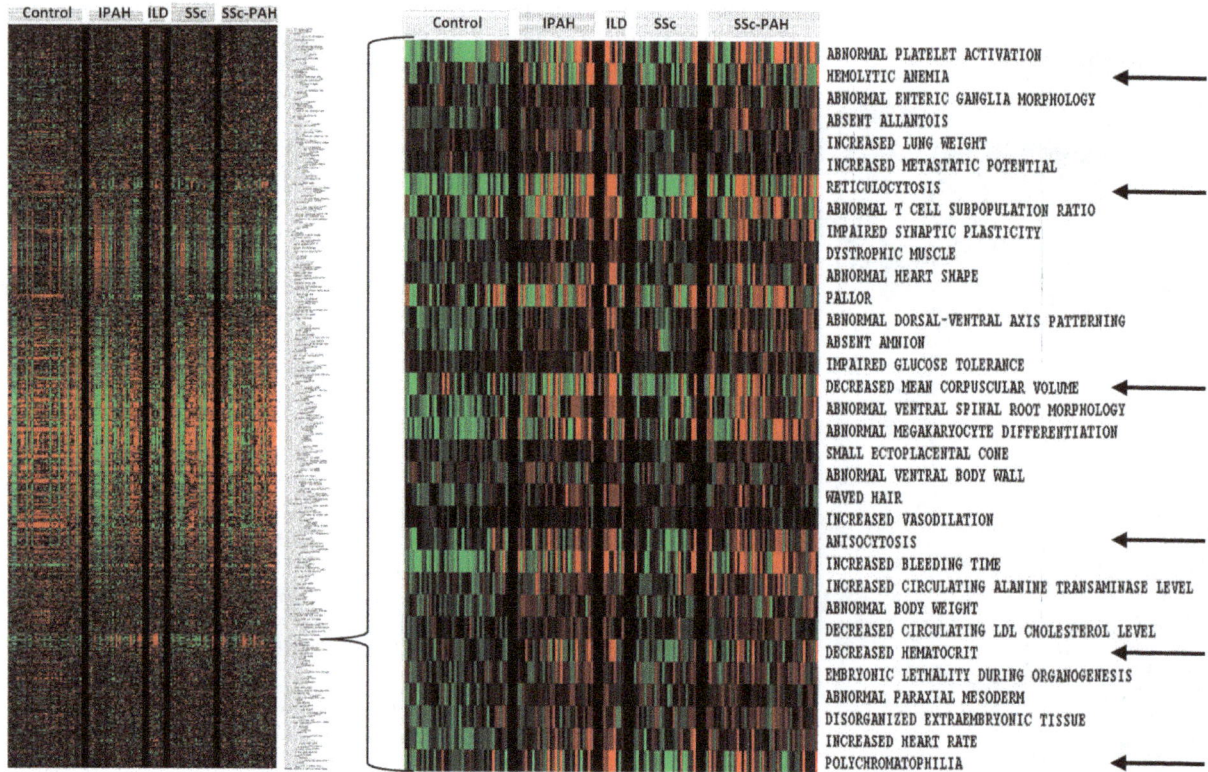

A

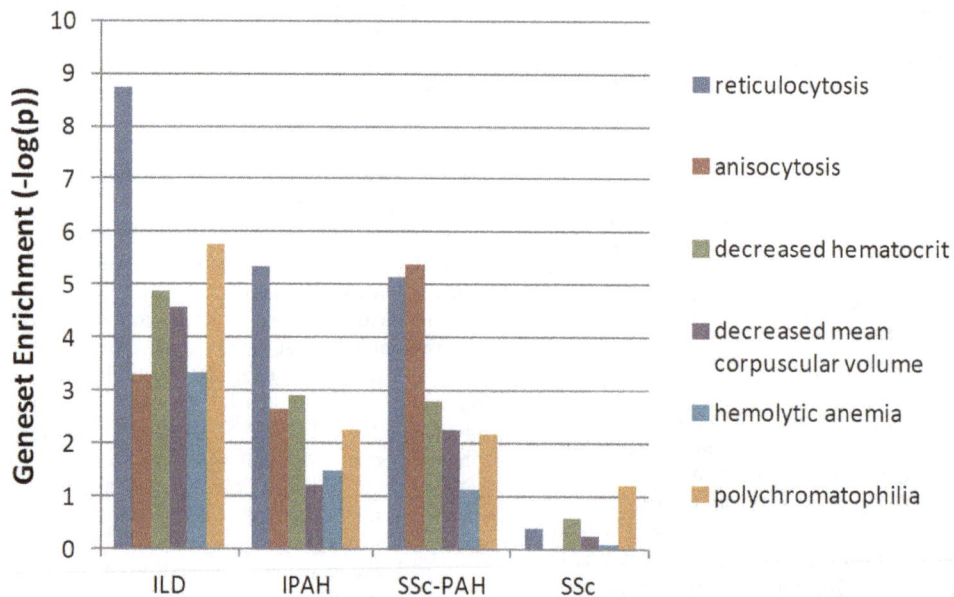

Human gene expression in subjects with hypertension maps specifically to mouse phenotypes of blood disorders

B

Figure 4. Results from gene set analysis of all gene expression data versus gene lists derived from the Mouse Genome Informatics (MGI) database. A) Gene set enrichment scores were calculated by the PAGE method using row normalized data for all (filtered) genes and samples. The scores were averaged by group and are normalized in the sense that that the average gene expression as scored by PAGE for any one gene set is expressed as the z transformation ((gene set size adjusted) of the average gene expression for that set. Disease specific patterns of gene set enrichment are as shown in the zoomed image. B) Average gene set expression in disease groups versus controls for various blood disorder-specific gene sets (as indicated by arrows in Fig. 4A) were tested by Students t test, the results being reported as the negative log (base 10) of the derived p-value ($-$ log(p)).

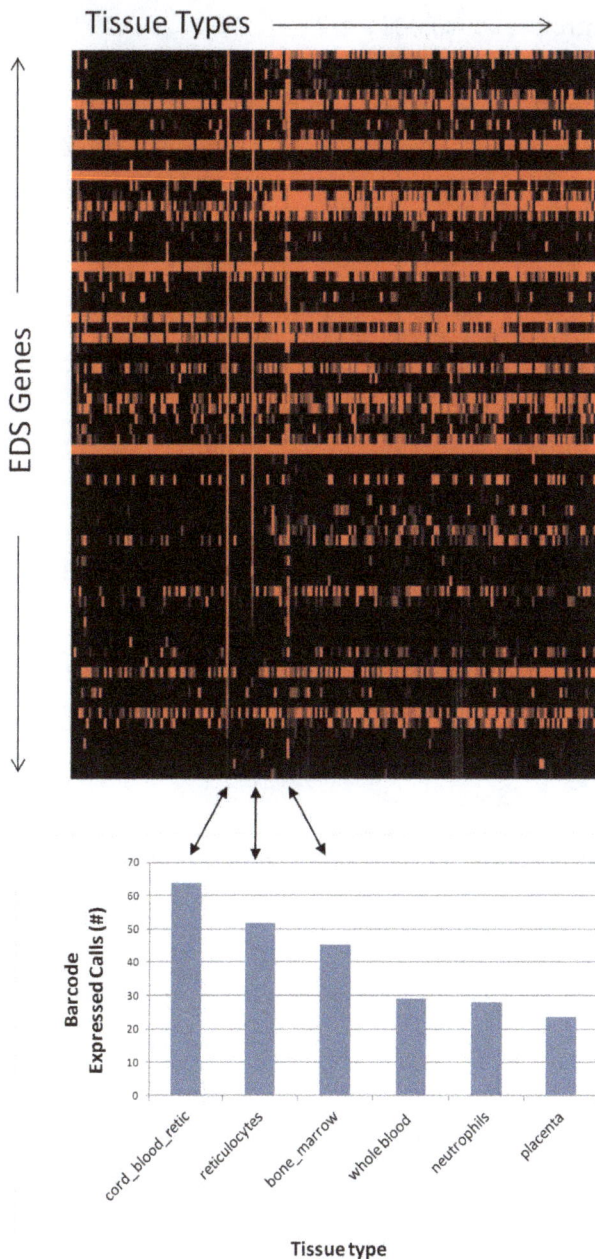

Figure 5. Gene Expression Barcode for EDS signature genes. The heat map is derived from individual barcode scores from zero (black) to one (red) with red indicating an increased likelihood that the gene is present in all samples in the experiment from which the tissue specific expression estimate is derived (see McCall et al. for complete description of the barcode algorithm [21]). As shown, the genes for the EDS signature were overrepresented for three tissues, in particular (cord blood reticulocytes, adult blood reticulocytes, and bone marrow), and their respective number of barcode expression calls are as indicated in the barchart directly below the corresponding areas of the barcode heatmap.

In every external study examined, the PH phenotypes were significantly enriched for the EDS signature relative to controls and other non-PH phenotypes. In many cases the EDS gene list was the top scorer above all other pathways and signatures. In Risbano et al. [14] IPAH and SSc-PAH had scores of 26 and 7.6, respectively, while the SSc phenotype showed a strong negative enrichment of -15.5. An explanation for this anomaly can be seen by a sample by sample analysis using the gene expression of both ALAS2 and ERAF/AHSP as surrogate EDS biomarkers (Figure S1). In the Risbano et al. study [14], for reasons unclear, the EDS is suppressed in SSc patients relative to controls, while both the IPAH and the SSc-PAH groups contain patients with elevated biomarker levels relative to either controls or SSc groups. Conversely, in Pendergrass et al [13], patients with a diagnosis of SSc-PAH are clearly enriched for the EDS (PAGE enrichment score = 15) but so also, albeit to a lesser degree, are patients diagnosed with SSc (PAGE enrichment score = 9.25). A possible explanation for this, once again, becomes clear upon the examination of gene expression sample by sample (Figure S1). In the Pendergrass data at least three patients scored as SSc have a high EDS score perhaps indicating, as within our own cohort, a further, as yet undetected, progression to the PH state. In datasets examining only PH (Bull et al. [11] and Rajkumar et al. [32] there is a clear and unambiguous enrichment (Table 3. Bull et al.; IPAH-7.7 and Rajkumar et al.; PAH-4.1, respectively) in their PH groups relative to controls. In the Rajkumar data, patients with idiopathic pulmonary fibrosis (IPF), a lung disease group not associated with PH did not display the EDS.

Interestingly, the platelet specific signature (Pl), while distinct in terms of gene content from the EDS (less than 5% gene overlap), was present in some patients with high EDS (Figure 3, Table S2), but did not show as much specificity for hypertension in our study or others (Figure S2) and for this reason was not pursued further. An additional data set was also evaluated which compared the gene expression between reticulocytes from cord blood and in the circulation [33]. The EDS was highly over-expressed in cord blood reticulocytes relative to peripheral blood supporting previous observations characterizing the presence of a less mature reticulocyte population in cord blood [22,33] and supporting the identification of the EDS with reticulocyte development.

Correlation of the EDS with Hemodynamic Measurements

It should be noted that despite the strong association of the EDS signature with the PH phenotype in our data and in others, only a subset of the patients in each group actually display elevated EDS levels. In order to better understand the association of EDS positive patients with disease progression, EDS gene expression regulation was examined for those patients for whom hemodynamic measurements were available within four months of the date of blood draw for the PBMC isolations used in this study (12 IPAH; 23 SSc-PAH). The clinical parameters of mean right atrial pressure (RAmean), cardiac index (CI), pulmonary vascular resistance index (PVRI), and pulmonary artery saturation (PA sat) were used. ALAS2 gene expression was taken as a primary biomarker representing the entire EDS (note the Pearson correlation r between ALAS2 and ERAF/AHSP gene expression, among the subjects used for this analysis, was 0.987, and 0.957 for

ALAS2

Comparison	p-Value
ILD-Control	0.0103
IPAH-Control	<0.0001
SSc/PAH-Control	<0.0001
SSc-Control	0.4215

A

ERAF

Comparison	p-Value
ILD-Control	0.0122
IPAH-Control	<0.0001
SSc/PAH-Control	<0.0001
SSc-Control	0.3771

B

	RT-PCR ALAS2	Microarray ALAS2	RT-PCR ERAF	Microarray ERAF
fold change	338.7	135.9	188.9	42.5
ttest p-val	6.2E-16	9.6E-20	1.4E-14	2.3E-14

C

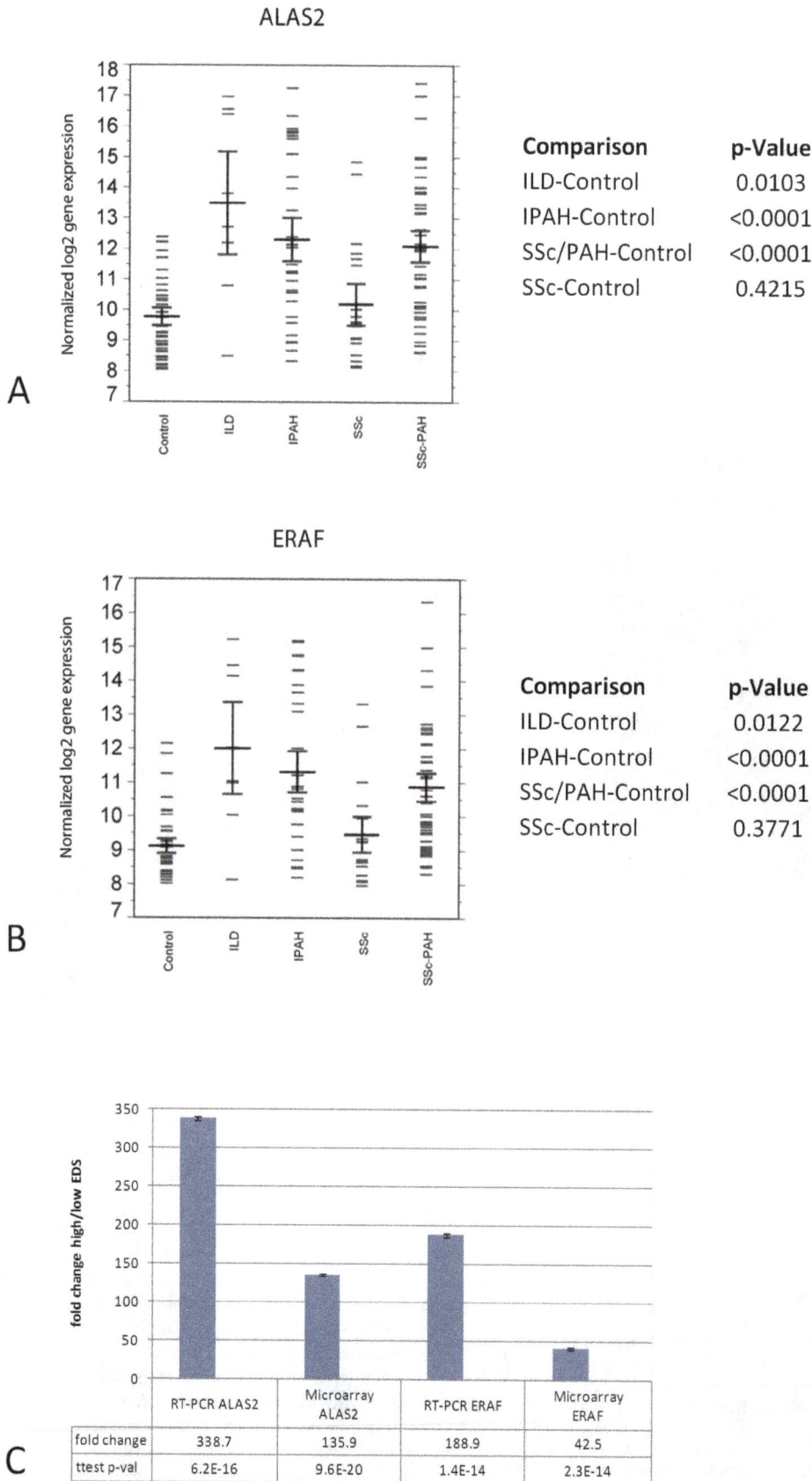

Figure 6. Statistically significant differential expression of erythroid CD71+ specific genes. A) ALAS2 and B) ERAF/AHSP genes in hypertension groups (SSc-PH-ILD, IPAH, and SSc-PAH) versus healthy controls and scleroderma (SSc). The box plots give the mean (horizontal black line), sample values (short blue lines), and 84% confidence interval (CI) (red lines) for each group, (non-overlap of the 84% CIs of two groups is an

approximate indicator of significant difference between their means at the 0.05 level of significance). C) Individual ALAS2 and ERAF gene expression microarray results were validated by RT-PCR for high and low EDS patients across all hypertension classes (SSc-PAH, IPAH, SSc-PH-ILD). Further inspection of the EDS gene list also showed the inclusion of genes for both the GATA1 and KLF transcription factors which are both essential for erythroid development [28,29]. A test by gene set analysis of the entire dataset comparing each PH group directly versus the SSc group as the baseline group showed a significant and specific enrichment among genes which contain three different GATA transcription factor binding sites in their upstream promoter regions (TRANSFAC [30]) (Figure 7A). Interestingly, the genes up-regulated in each of the GATA transcription factor binding site gene sets were mostly non-overlapping either with each other (an average of 59–62% unique genes for each gene list) or with the EDS gene expression signature itself (95% unique non-overlapping genes) (Figure 7B) indicating that the effects of elevated GATA1 gene expression are both pervasive in the PH groups and are supplemental to the EDS gene expression signature itself. The observation that downstream regulatory events are related directly to EDS elevation (through the up-regulation of the GATA1 transcription factor gene) and are associated with PH groups, taken together with the previously demonstrated strong association of the EDS with reticulocyte maturation (Figure 5), led us to the identification of this signature as the Erythroid Development Signature (EDS).

IPAH and SSc-PAH, respectively), and was hence used for the purpose of computing correlations of the EDS with hemodynamic measurements (Figure 8). Disease severity in IPAH patients as indicated by increasing RAmean and PVRI were strongly correlated with increasing ALAS2 gene expression ($r = 0.776$, $p = 0.003$; $r = 0.752$, $p = 0.0048$, respectively). Conversely, measures of healthy lung and cardiac function such as PA saturation and Cardiac Index (CI) were negatively correlated with decreasing ALAS2 gene expression ($r = -0.71$, $p = 0.0098$; $r = -0.449$, $p = 0.14$, respectively). The consistency of these measurements suggests that there is indeed a direct correlation between disease severity and EDS gene expression in IPAH patients. Surprisingly, there were no corresponding significant correlations for any of these four hemodynamic parameters among the SSc-PAH patients (Figure S3) despite the clear and significant enrichment for EDS genes (see Figure 6A&B) in this group. The level of EDS gene over-expression among SSc-PAH patients was thus not seen to be directly related to the markers of PH disease status examined here and distinguishes IPAH and SSc-PAH for that reason.

Discussion

Previous studies using PBMC have been used to identify PH-specific genes [11] as well as distinguishing between IPAH and SSc-PAH [12]. In general, however, these studies have shown considerable heterogeneity when examining directly the contrast in gene expression profiles in PBMC from SSc-PAH and SSc patients [13,14]. For example, while Pendergrass et al. [13] focused on the increased expression of 9 genes that distinguished SSc-PAH from SSc, Risbano et al. [14] described 5 genes which when down-regulated distinguish SSc-PAH from SSc patients. In a comparison of the complete datasets from these studies in combination with results from this current study we found one gene, in particular, ALAS2, which is significantly over-expressed in SSc-PAH versus SSc in all three datasets. We present data here in support of the finding that one of the distinguishing molecular phenotypes in terms of gene expression between patients with PAH versus either healthy controls or patients with SSc alone, involves a distinctive signature uniquely associated with erythrocyte development. This signature was also present in patients with IPAH and SSc-PH-ILD in the current study and segregates with PH in multiple published clinical studies for which data is publicly available [11,13,14,32]. We have demonstrated here that the EDS signature is quantitatively enriched and validated in at least four independently published datasets derived from microarray studies across multiple microarray platforms (Affymetrix, Illumina, and Agilent) in which the PBMCs from PH patients were tested.

In all cases (our data and others) only a subset of PH patients in the affected groups were EDS positive and in our data, at least, the presence of the EDS was associated with increasingly severe disease (as judged by hemodynamic parameters) for IPAH but not for SSc-PAH patients (Figure 8, Figure S3). The presence of the

EDS signature induced by PAH may be indicative of increased red blood cell recruitment as part of a systemic response to severe chronic local hypoxia. An increase of up-regulated genes selectively expressed in erythrocytes/reticulocytes (including ALAS2 and ERAF/AHSP, and many other EDS genes) in whole blood was also noted to be consistent with previous observations of higher red blood cell counts (hematocrit) in obesity [34]. An increase in RBC trafficking may constitute a useful marker of PH disease, in general, and serve as a useful marker of increased disease severity specifically in IPAH patients. The lack of correlation of the EDS genes with hemodynamic measurements in the SSc-PAH patients is puzzling, particularly, as the signature as a whole is similarly enriched in patients from both disease groups. This perhaps reflects the different etiologies of these two different types of PH and emphasizes their distinct origins. Furthermore, we have previously reported that hemodynamic alterations are distinct between IPAH and SSc-PAH patients and do not always reflect, in the latter group, the severity of PAH [35,36].

The cell specific source of the EDS remains an open question. In order to eliminate the likelihood that direct RBC contamination in the PBMC preparations used in this current study might account for the presence of the EDS, PBMC samples from both high and low EDS patients were subjected to multiple rounds of isotonic ammonium chloride hemolysis. This treatment lyses mature red blood cells with minimal effect on lymphocytes and does not appreciably affect nucleated red cells. In our test samples high EDS gene expression was not affected by this treatment (Figure S4).

High levels of gene expression for ALAS2 and ERAF are found almost exclusively in CD71+ erythroid progenitor cells, and the complete EDS signature (as defined here) appears to correlate especially well with genes known to be expressed in reticulocytes and particularly well in cell populations enriched for less mature reticulocytes (as in cord blood – Figure 5). Our hypothesis is that the EDS gene expression signature is derived from a population of nucleated reticulocytes which co-sediment with lymphocytes and monocytes in the PBMC fraction of Ficoll gradients.

The identity of the EDS corresponds closely to a gene expression signature reported by Ebert et al., [37] where the authors provide detailed gene expression information for an in vitro experiment in which bone marrow CD34+ cells were expanded under conditions which induced erythroid differentiation and major changes in gene expression were recorded pre- and post- induction. Our EDS gene list overlapped the induced erythroid gene list by over 50% including both the ALAS2 and ERAF genes (ALAS2, CA1, EPB42, ERAF, FECH, GLRX5, GSPT1, GYPB, GYPE, HBA2, MYL4, SELENBP1, SLC25A37, SNCA, TMCC2, and TSPAN5). Interestingly, a major difference between the Ebert induced erythroid signature and the PAH EDS is the very strong upregulation of IL8 recorded in the Ebert

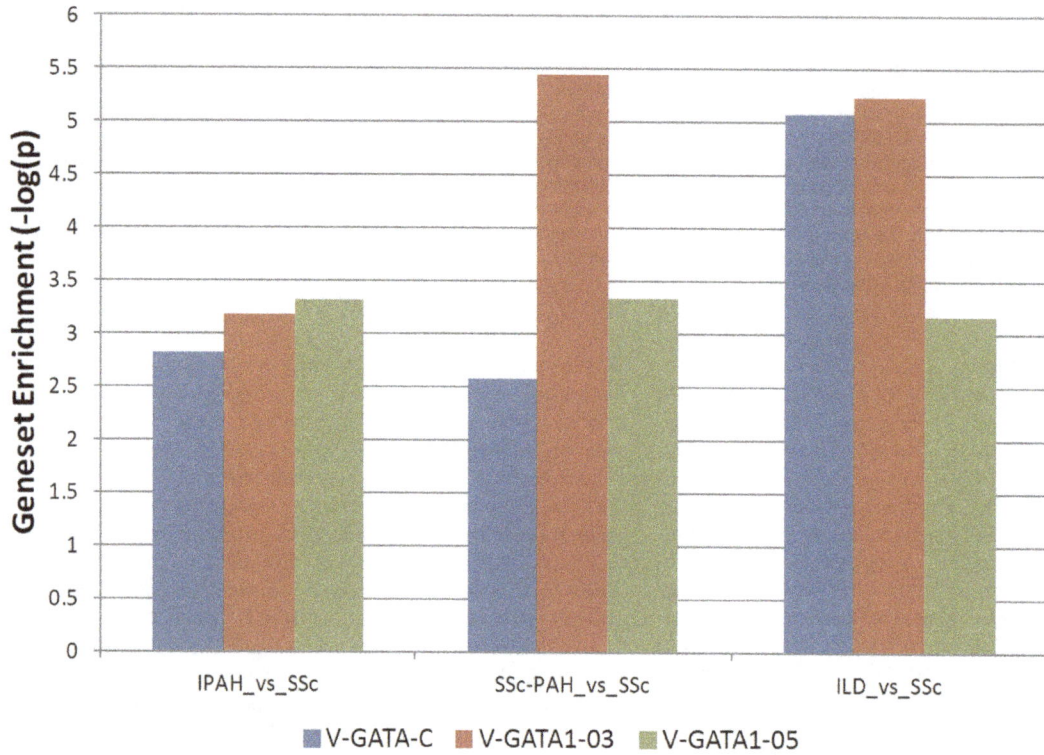

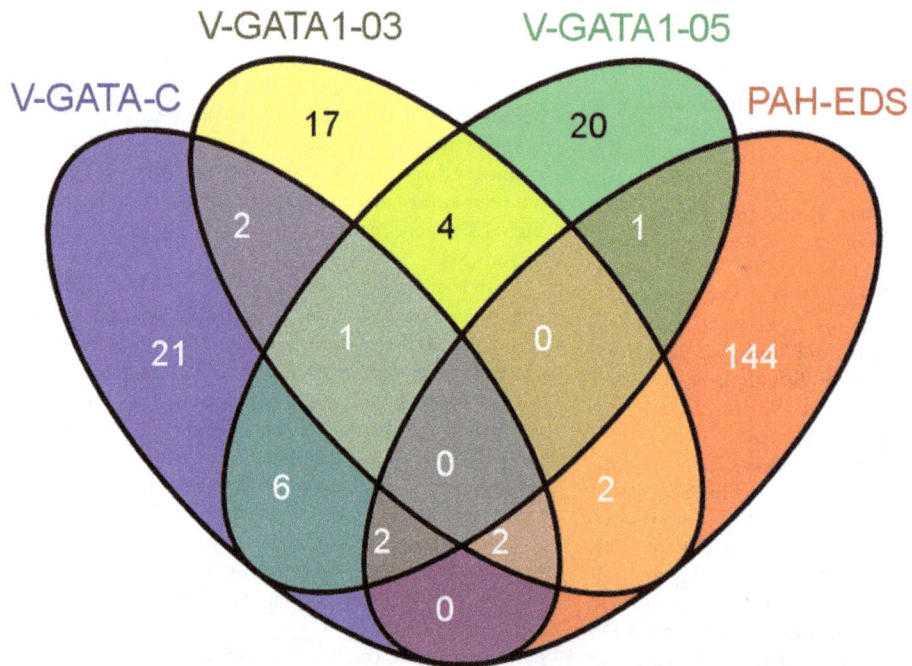

Figure 7. Results from gene set analysis using gene lists derived from the TransFac (gene associated transcription factor binding sites) database. A). The average changes in gene expression for patients with SSc-PH-ILD, IPAH, and SSc-PAH were tested versus patients with SSc. The p-values associated with the gene set enrichment scores are reported here as −log(p). B). Venn diagram illustrating overlap between the average up-regulated gene expression associated with the presence of 3 distinct GATA transcription factor binding sites. The EDS gene signature is included for comparison.

Table 3. Results from gene set analysis using the EDS as the query gene list. Enrichment scores are as described above.

Dataset	GEO #	SSc-PH-ILD	IPAH	SSc-PAH	SSc	PAH	IPF-PH	CBvAB
JHU	GSE33463	33.327	21.082	17.886	2.688	-	-	-
Risbano et al.[14]	GSE22356	-	26.019	7.553	−15.476	-	-	-
Pendergrass et al.[13]	GSE19617	-	-	15.004	9.247	-	-	-
Bull et al.[11]	GSE703	-	7.736	-	-	-	-	-
Rajkumar et al.[31]	GSE15197	-	-	-	-	4.083	−1.337	-
Goh et al.[32]	GSE6236	-	-	-	-	-	-	7.811

In all cases data was downloaded from the NCBI Gene Expression Omnibus (GEO) website as processed by the submitter and published by GEO as a Series Matrix File. Phenotype labels: Interstitial Lung Disease (SSC-PH-ILD), Idiopathic Arterial Hypertension (IPAH), Scleroderma with Pulmonary Arterial Hypertension (SSc-PAH), Scleroderma (SSc), Pulmonary Arterial Hypertension only (PAH), Idiopathic Pulmonary Fibrosis with Pulmonary Hypertension (IPF-PH), and human Cord Blood versus human Adult Blood (CBvAB).

signature but not in the PAH-EDS (IL8 was upregulated sporadically and non-specifically across the entire PAH dataset). The reason for this discrepancy is not clear but worth noting given the otherwise very strong correlation between the two signatures.

Additional evidence for the source of the EDS in PBMCs has recently been obtained indirectly by others. Researchers from the Children's Hospital in Cincinnati reported the up-regulation of the expression of genes involved in the processes of hemoglobin synthesis and oxygen transport in the PBMCs of systemic juvenile idiopathic arthritis (sJIA) patients relative to healthy controls [38]. They suggested (as we do here) that this cluster of genes might represent the signature of immature nucleated RBCs that can copurify with PBMCs isolated on Ficoll gradients. The PH and the sJIA erythropoiesis signatures are highly overlapping (Figure S5) suggesting a common PBMC cell source. The Cincinnati team also mapped their experimentally derived EDS using bioinfor-

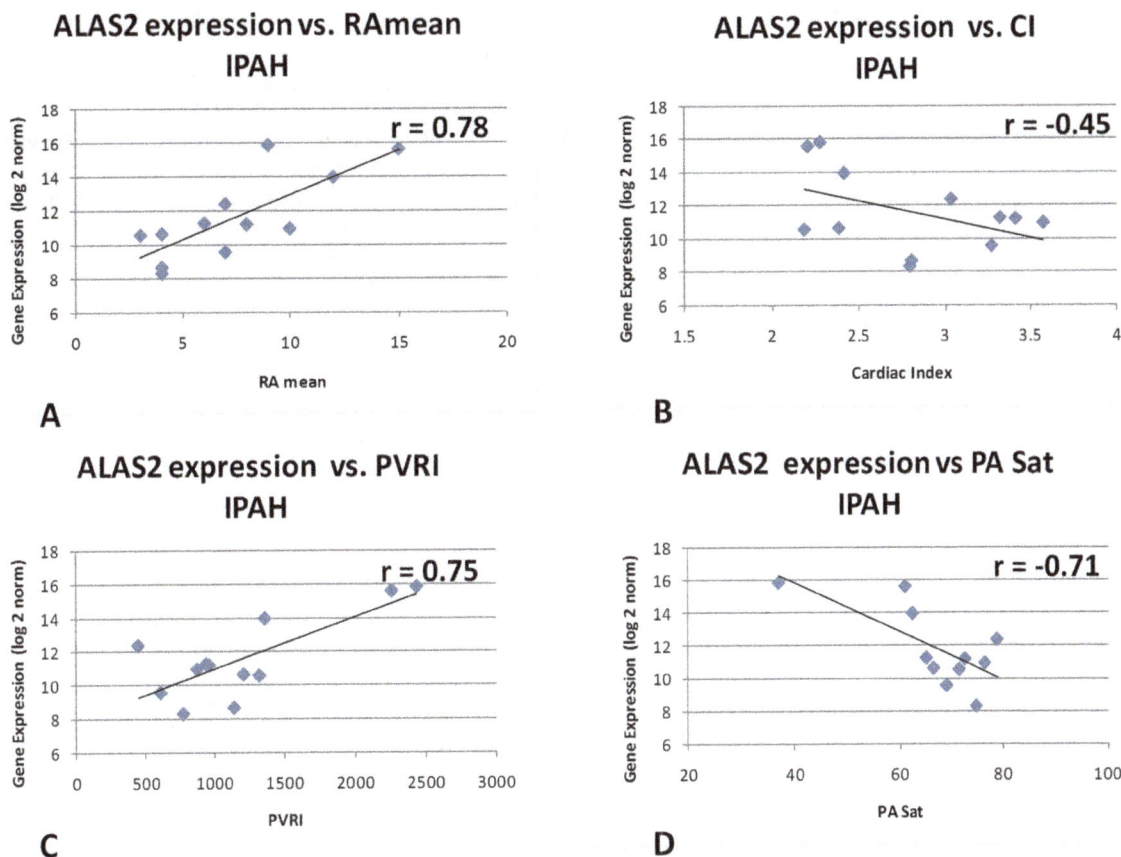

Figure 8. ALAS2 gene expression positively correlates with increasing disease severity in IPAH patients. EDS gene expression for 12 IPAH patients for whom hemodynamic measurements were available within four months of the date of blood draw. The clinical parameters of right atrial pressure (RAmean), cardiac index (CI), pulmonary vascular resistance index (PVRI), and pulmonary artery saturation (PA sat) were used. Disease severity in IPAH patients as indicated by increasing RAmean and PVRI are strongly correlated with increasing ALAS2 gene expression and negatively correlated with measures of healthy lung and coronary function such as PA saturation and Cardiac Index (CI).

matics methods to CD71+ immature erythroid precursor cells [39] and, in addition, they present data showing that patients with sJIA had significantly increased proportions of immature cell populations, including CD34+ cells, correlating highly with the strength of their measurements of the erythropoiesis signature. It has been independently demonstrated by *in vitro* expansion experiments that the potential, at least, for the production of large amounts of erythroid progenitor cells can be derived directly from PBMCs without additional purification [40], although whether the source of this expansion is derived from CD34+ cells remains uncertain [41]. Despite the strong indirect evidence presented by ourselves and others, the direct evidence for the expansion of CD71+ erythrocyte precursors in the periphery as the source of the EDS remains to be demonstrated.

The exact role of the EDS in specific disease states remains to be determined. Clearly there are strong associations between the EDS and PH and sJIA, but also the EDS has been observed in active lupus as well, and co-segregates with multiple additional immune-related signatures in a large asthma cohort study (unpublished data). In an ongoing longitudinal PAH study that we are currently conducting, it has become clear that the EDS as well as the immune response and platelet signatures are also variable in patients over time. Unfortunately, it is still too early for more than a speculative interpretation of these results. For now, it would appear that the EDS is an important new marker in chronic disease with the distinct property that in hypertension, at least, the expansion of immature precursor cells may actually constitute an active biological response to increasingly severe disease conditions.

Materials and Methods

Ethics Statement

All the samples used during this study were obtained following written informed consent from the donors. The Johns Hopkins University Institutional Review Board approved the conduct of this study.

Study subjects

The cohort was comprised of subjects identified from the Johns Hopkins Pulmonary Hypertension Program and the Johns Hopkins Scleroderma Center as part of our center's Specialized Center for Clinically-Oriented Research program. Consecutive outpatients with a diagnosis of IPAH, SSc-PAH, SSc-PH-ILD and SSc were recruited and enrolled in the study between 2007 and 2010. Controls subjects were family and friends who accompanied subjects to clinic visits and had no known cardiovascular, pulmonary, or renal disease.

Limited or diffuse SSc was as previously defined [42]. PAH was defined as a mean pulmonary artery pressure (mPAP) of >25 mmHg, pulmonary artery wedge pressure (PAWP) ≤15 mmHg, and pulmonary vascular resistance (PVR) >3 Wood units [43], in the absence of other known causes of pulmonary hypertension. Results of pulmonary function tests (PFT) and high-resolution computed tomography (HRCT) of the chest closest to the date of the diagnostic RHC (right heart catheterization) were recorded. Percent of predicted results for all PFT data were calculated according to Crapo [44]. Patients with significant obstructive lung disease, defined as a forced expiratory volume in one second over forced vital capacity ratio (FEV_1/FVC) <0.5 or 0.5–0.7 accompanied by radiographic evidence of emphysema, were excluded [45,46]. Interstitial lung disease was defined by a combination of PFT and HRCT criteria as previously described in epidemiologic studies and clinical trials of PAH therapy [47,48,49]. Patients were classified as having SSc-PH-ILD if they met all the above criteria, and had a total lung capacity (TLC) of <60% of predicted or a TLC between 60% and 70% of predicted combined with moderate to severe fibrosis (grade 3–4) on HRCT [50]. The onset of scleroderma was defined by the first non-Raynaud's phenomenon manifestation.

Severity of PAH was assessed by routine functional and hemodynamic measurements obtained closest to the date of blood collection for genomic analyses. Subjects were then stratified by cardiac index dichotomized at 2.2 L/min/m^2 based upon prior studies demonstrating poorer survival for PAH patients with a CI less than this value [51].

Isolation of Peripheral Blood Mononuclear Cells

Venous blood was collected by simple venipuncture under aseptic conditions. All samples were processed within two hours of collection to minimize gene expression variations associated with longer sample incubation times [52]. PBMCs were separated by Ficoll density gradient, immediately lysed in Trizol reagent (Invitrogen, Carlsbad, California), and stored at −80°C.

Purification of RNA

Total RNA was extracted using the Trizol Reagent method (Invitrogen, Carlsbad, California 92008, cat. no. 15596-026). Additional purification was performed on RNeasy columns (Qiagen, Valencia, CA 913555, cat. no. 74104). The quality of total RNA samples was assessed using an Agilent 2100 Bioanalyzer (Agilent Technologies, Palo Alto, CA).

Microarray Analysis

RNA samples were labeled according to the chip manufacturer's recommended protocols. In brief, for Illumina, 0.5 μg of total RNA from each sample was labeled by using the Illumina TotalPrep RNA Amplification Kit (Ambion, Austin, TX 78744-1832, cat. no. IL1791) in a two step process of cDNA synthesis followed by *in vitro* RNA transcription. Single stranded RNA (cRNA) was generated and labeled by incorporating biotin-16-UTP. 0.75 ugs of biotin-labeled cRNA was hybridized (16 hours) to Illumina Sentrix Human HT12_v3 BeadChips (Illumina, San Diego, CA 92121-1975, cat.no. BD-103-0203). The hybridized biotinylated cRNA was detected with streptavidin-Cy3 and quantitated using Illumina's BeadStation 500GX Genetic Analysis Systems scanner. The expression data discussed in this publication have been deposited in NCBI's Gene Expression Omnibus [53] and are accessible through GEO Series accession number GSE 33463 (http://www.ncbi.nlm.nih.gov/geo/query/acc.cgi?acc = GSE 33463).

Quantitative RT-PCR (QRT-PCR) Analysis

cDNA was obtained from total RNA using the cDNA Archive Kit according to the manufacturer's protocol (Applied Biosystems, Foster City, CA). Probes and primers were designed and synthesized by Applied Biosystems. All PCR amplifications were carried out in triplicate on an ABI Prism® 7300 Sequence Detection System, using a fluorogenic 5′ nuclease assay (Taq-Man® probes). Relative gene expressions were calculated by using the $2^{-\Delta\Delta Ct}$ method as described in [54]. The ΔCt value of each sample was calculated using 3 endogenous control genes (GAPDH, ACTB, and PGK1).

Analytical Methods and Statistical Analysis

A single intensity (expression) value for each Illumina probe on the array was obtained using Illumina BeadStudio software with standard settings and no background correction. The expression values for all the probes for each sample were scaled to have median 256 (2^8) and then log (base 2) transformed before performing statistical analysis. Analysis for differential expression between pairs of disease groups and between individual disease groups and the group of controls was carried out for each Illumina microarray probe.

Illumina probes (and consequently, the corresponding genes) considered to be significantly differentially expressed between two groups of samples were those satisfying the three criteria: (i) Two-sided Welch t-test p-values less than or equal to 0.01 [55]; (ii) a Benjamini-Hochberg false discovery rate (FDR) less than or equal to 0.1 [56]; and (iii) a fold change above 1.5 or below 1/1.5 (calculated using geometric means). Statistical testing for differences in expression levels of a given probe between two groups was not done unless at least 80% of the samples in the group with the higher average expression level for that probe had Illumina detection p-values <0.01 (thus avoiding false positives based on background noise and also reducing the number of statistical tests for the subsequent false discovery rate calculation). A comprehensive spreadsheet of group comparison results is given in Table S1.

Heat maps (and the ordering by hierarchical clustering of the samples and the genes in heat maps) were based on normalization of the expression values for each sample using z transformation [55,57,58] (utilizing only the probes which had an Illumina detection p-value <0.01 for least one sample, and for which there was an available gene symbol), followed by z-transformation of the normalized expression values for each Illumina probe across all samples. Hierarchical clustering was performed using the Cluster and TreeView software programs [59]. The clustering algorithm was set to complete linkage clustering using uncentered correlation.

Gene set analysis was carried out using the web-PAGE tool [16] (http://dpwebpage.nia.nih.gov/PAGE/index.html) with the p-value cutoff set to 0.01 and the minimum number of genes per gene set equal to 10. The input used was either a z ratio (z transformation of the difference between the means computed for two groups [60] (Table 2, Table 3-JHU data, Figure 7) for all internal data; or a simple difference metric was computed and used for all external data (Table 2). One exception was the use of all row normalized data on a sample by sample basis to generate the functional genomic landscape as illustrated in Figure 4A. In this variation of the gene set algorithm, gene sets are tested against the complete expression data for each sample, enrichment scores map the relative abundance levels of groups of genes which can then be compared for variation between samples and groups of samples as seen. The gene sets used are as described in the corresponding Table and Figure legends.

Evaluation of lists of differentially expressed genes for enrichment in predefined categories and functional groups of genes was carried out using the NIH functional analysis tool

DAVID [61], and the Broad Institute Molecular Signatures Database MSigDB facility [62].

Associating hemodynamic measurements with gene expression

Correlation between expression levels of a given gene and the values of a selected clinical variable for a specified group of n subjects was evaluated as the Pearson product-moment correlation coefficient r estimating the population correlation coefficient ρ. Tests of the null hypothesis $\rho = 0$ were conducted using the customary t-test depending on r and n.

Supporting Information

Table S1 PAH significance tests, gender specific EDS stats, siglists-unique, UR functional enrichment, DR functional enrichment.

Table S2 EDS and Platelet specific genes.

Table S3 Demographic and clinical data for subjects.

Figure S1 EDS genes in published PH gene expression datasets.

Figure S2 Platelet signature in published PH gene expression datasets.

Figure S3 Correlations of ALAS2 gene expression with clinical measurements in SSc-PAH patients.

Figure S4 RBC lysis treatment shows no effect on EDS gene expression.

Figure S5 EDS genes over-expressed in sJIA dataset.

Acknowledgments

We would like to thank Danielle Boyce from the JHU SOM Pulmonary Division for patient demographic and clinical data.

Author Contributions

Conceived and designed the experiments: CC SCM DNG ALZ REG RAJ MAM FMW KCB PMH. Performed the experiments: TW SB JF MB. Analyzed the data: CC AEB YS DNG. Contributed reagents/materials/analysis tools: SCM LH FMW. Wrote the paper: CC AEB SCM DNG PMH.

References

1. D'Alonzo GE, Barst RJ, Ayres SM, Bergofsky EH, Brundage BH, et al. (1991) Survival in patients with primary pulmonary hypertension. Results from a national prospective registry. Ann Intern Med 115: 343–349.

2. Gaine SP, Rubin LJ (1998) Primary pulmonary hypertension. Lancet 352: 719–725.

3. Rich S, Dantzker DR, Ayres SM, Bergofsky EH, Brundage BH, et al. (1987) Primary pulmonary hypertension. A national prospective study. Ann Intern Med 107: 216–223.

4. Hassoun PM (2009) Therapies for scleroderma-related pulmonary arterial hypertension. Expert Rev Respir Med 3: 187–196.

5. Hassoun P (2011) Lung involvement in systemic sclerosis. Presse Med 40: e3–e17.

6. Fagan KA, Badesch DB (2002) Pulmonary hypertension associated with connective tissue disease. Prog Cardiovasc Dis 45: 225–234.

7. Bendayan D, Shitrit D, Kramer MR (2006) Pulmonary arterial hypertension associated with autoimmune disease: a single medical center experience. Isr Med Assoc J 8: 252–254.

8. Steen VD (2005) The lung in systemic sclerosis. J Clin Rheumatol 11: 40–46.

9. Burczynski ME, Dorner AJ (2006) Transcriptional profiling of peripheral blood cells in clinical pharmacogenomic studies. Pharmacogenomics 7: 187–202.

10. Liew CC, Ma J, Tang HC, Zheng R, Dempsey AA (2006) The peripheral blood transcriptome dynamically reflects system wide biology: a potential diagnostic tool. J Lab Clin Med 147: 126–132.

11. Bull TM, Coldren CD, Moore M, Sotto-Santiago SM, Pham DV, et al. (2004) Gene microarray analysis of peripheral blood cells in pulmonary arterial hypertension. Am J Respir Crit Care Med 170: 911–919.

12. Grigoryev DN, Mathai SC, Fisher MR, Girgis RE, Zaiman AL, et al. (2008) Identification of candidate genes in scleroderma-related pulmonary arterial hypertension. Transl Res 151: 197–207.

13. Pendergrass SA, Hayes E, Farina G, Lemaire R, Farber HW, et al. (2010) Limited systemic sclerosis patients with pulmonary arterial hypertension show biomarkers of inflammation and vascular injury. PLoS One 5: e12106.

14. Risbano MG, Meadows CA, Coldren CD, Jenkins TJ, Edwards MG, et al. (2010) Altered immune phenotype in peripheral blood cells of patients with scleroderma-associated pulmonary hypertension. Clin Transl Sci 3: 210–218.

15. Christmann RB, Hayes E, Pendergrass S, Padilla C, Farina G, et al. (2011) Interferon and alternative activation of monocyte/macrophages in systemic sclerosis-associated pulmonary arterial hypertension. Arthritis Rheum 63: 1718–1728.

16. De S, Zhang Y, Garner JR, Wang SA, Becker KG (2010) Disease and phenotype gene set analysis of disease-based gene expression in mouse and human. Physiol Genomics 42A: 162–167.

17. Martinelli S, Urosevic M, Daryadel A, Oberholzer PA, Baumann C, et al. (2004) Induction of genes mediating interferon-dependent extracellular trap formation during neutrophil differentiation. J Biol Chem 279: 44123–44132.

18. Cheadle C, Berger AE, Andrade F, James R, Johnson K, et al. (2010) Transcription of proteinase 3 and related myelopoiesis genes in peripheral blood mononuclear cells of patients with active Wegener's granulomatosis. Arthritis Rheum 62: 1744–1754.

19. Bennett L, Palucka AK, Arce E, Cantrell V, Borvak J, et al. (2003) Interferon and granulopoiesis signatures in systemic lupus erythematosus blood. J Exp Med 197: 711–723.

20. Bult CJ, Eppig JT, Kadin JA, Richardson JE, Blake JA (2008) The Mouse Genome Database (MGD): mouse biology and model systems. Nucleic Acids Res 36: D724–728.

21. McCall MN, Uppal K, Jaffee HA, Zilliox MJ, Irizarry RA (2011) The Gene Expression Barcode: leveraging public data repositories to begin cataloging the human and murine transcriptomes. Nucleic Acids Res 39: D1011–1015.

22. Paterakis GS, Lykopoulou L, Papassotiriou J, Stamulakatou A, Kattamis C, et al. (1993) Flow-cytometric analysis of reticulocytes in normal cord blood. Acta Haematol 90: 182–185.

23. Harigae H, Suwabe N, Weinstock PH, Nagai M, Fujita H, et al. (1998) Deficient heme and globin synthesis in embryonic stem cells lacking the erythroid-specific delta-aminolevulinate synthase gene. Blood 91: 798–805.

24. Friend C, Scher W, Holland JG, Sato T (1971) Hemoglobin synthesis in murine virus-induced leukemic cells in vitro: stimulation of erythroid differentiation by dimethyl sulfoxide. Proc Natl Acad Sci U S A 68: 378–382.

25. Greer J, Wintrobe M (2009) Wintrobe's clinical hematology; Greer J, Foerster J, Rodgers G, Paraskevas F, Glader B, et al., editors. Philadelphia, PA: Lippincot Williams & Wilkins. 837 p.

26. Yu X, Mollan TL, Butler A, Gow AJ, Olson JS, et al. (2009) Analysis of human alpha globin gene mutations that impair binding to the alpha hemoglobin stabilizing protein. Blood 113: 5961–5969.

27. Kaneko K, Furuyama K, Aburatani H, Shibahara S (2009) Hypoxia induces erythroid-specific 5-aminolevulinate synthase expression in human erythroid cells through transforming growth factor-beta signaling. Febs J 276: 1370–1382.

28. Ohneda K, Yamamoto M (2002) Roles of hematopoietic transcription factors GATA-1 and GATA-2 in the development of red blood cell lineage. Acta Haematol 108: 237–245.

29. Nuez B, Michalovich D, Bygrave A, Ploemacher R, Grosveld F (1995) Defective haematopoiesis in fetal liver resulting from inactivation of the EKLF gene. Nature 375: 316–318.

30. Matys V, Fricke E, Geffers R, Gossling E, Haubrock M, et al. (2003) TRANSFAC: transcriptional regulation, from patterns to profiles. Nucleic Acids Res 31: 374–378.

31. Barrett T, Troup DB, Wilhite SE, Ledoux P, Evangelista C, et al. (2011) NCBI GEO: archive for functional genomics data sets–10 years on. Nucleic Acids Res 39: D1005–1010.

32. Rajkumar R, Konishi K, Richards TJ, Ishizawar DC, Wiechert AC, et al. (2010) Genomewide RNA expression profiling in lung identifies distinct signatures in idiopathic pulmonary arterial hypertension and secondary pulmonary hypertension. Am J Physiol Heart Circ Physiol 298: H1235–1248.

33. Goh SH, Josleyn M, Lee YT, Danner RL, Gherman RB, et al. (2007) The human reticulocyte transcriptome. Physiol Genomics 30: 172–178.

34. Ghosh S, Dent R, Harper ME, Gorman SA, Stuart JS, et al. (2010) Gene expression profiling in whole blood identifies distinct biological pathways associated with obesity. BMC Med Genomics 3: 56.

35. Le Pavec J, Humbert M, Mouthon L, Hassoun PM (2010) Systemic sclerosis-associated pulmonary arterial hypertension. Am J Respir Crit Care Med 181: 1285–1293.

36. Fisher MR, Mathai SC, Champion HC, Girgis RE, Housten-Harris T, et al. (2006) Clinical differences between idiopathic and scleroderma-related pulmonary hypertension. Arthritis Rheum 54: 3043–3050.

37. Ebert BL, Galili N, Tamayo P, Bosco J, Mak R, et al. (2008) An erythroid differentiation signature predicts response to lenalidomide in myelodysplastic syndrome. PLoS Med 5: e35.

38. Fall N, Barnes M, Thornton S, Luyrink L, Olson J, et al. (2007) Gene expression profiling of peripheral blood from patients with untreated new-onset systemic juvenile idiopathic arthritis reveals molecular heterogeneity that may predict macrophage activation syndrome. Arthritis Rheum 56: 3793–3804.

39. Hinze CH, Fall N, Thornton S, Mo JQ, Aronow BJ, et al. (2010) Immature cell populations and an erythropoiesis gene-expression signature in systemic juvenile idiopathic arthritis: implications for pathogenesis. Arthritis Res Ther 12: R123.

40. Filippone C, Franssila R, Kumar A, Saikko L, Kovanen PE, et al. (2010) Erythroid progenitor cells expanded from peripheral blood without mobilization or preselection: molecular characteristics and functional competence. PLoS One 5: e9496.

41. van den Akker E, Satchwell TJ, Pellegrin S, Daniels G, Toye AM (2010) The majority of the in vitro erythroid expansion potential resides in CD34(-) cells, outweighing the contribution of CD34(+) cells and significantly increasing the erythroblast yield from peripheral blood samples. Haematologica 95: 1594–1598.

42. LeRoy EC, Black C, Fleischmajer R, Jablonska S, Krieg T, et al. (1988) Scleroderma (systemic sclerosis): classification, subsets and pathogenesis. J Rheumatol 15: 202–205.

43. McLaughlin VV, Archer SL, Badesch DB, Barst RJ, Farber HW, et al. (2009) ACCF/AHA 2009 expert consensus document on pulmonary hypertension: a report of the American College of Cardiology Foundation Task Force on Expert Consensus Documents and the American Heart Association: developed in collaboration with the American College of Chest Physicians, American Thoracic Society, Inc., and the Pulmonary Hypertension Association. Circulation 119: 2250–2294.

44. Crapo RO, Morris AH, Gardner RM (1981) Reference spirometric values using techniques and equipment that meet ATS recommendations. Am Rev Respir Dis 123: 659–664.

45. Crapo RO, Morris AH (1981) Standardized single breath normal values for carbon monoxide diffusing capacity. Am Rev Respir Dis 123: 185–189.

46. Crapo RO, Morris AH, Clayton PD, Nixon CR (1982) Lung volumes in healthy nonsmoking adults. Bull Eur Physiopathol Respir 18: 419–425.

47. Hachulla E, Gressin V, Guillevin L, Carpentier P, Diot E, et al. (2005) Early detection of pulmonary arterial hypertension in systemic sclerosis: a French nationwide prospective multicenter study. Arthritis Rheum 52: 3792–3800.

48. Simonneau G, Barst RJ, Galie N, Naeije R, Rich S, et al. (2002) Continuous subcutaneous infusion of treprostinil, a prostacyclin analogue, in patients with pulmonary arterial hypertension: a double-blind, randomized, placebo-controlled trial. Am J Respir Crit Care Med 165: 800–804.

49. Girgis RE, Frost AE, Hill NS, Horn EM, Langleben D, et al. (2007) Selective endothelin A receptor antagonism with sitaxsentan for pulmonary arterial hypertension associated with connective tissue disease. Ann Rheum Dis 66: 1467–1472.

50. MacDonald SL, Rubens MB, Hansell DM, Copley SJ, Desai SR, et al. (2001) Nonspecific interstitial pneumonia and usual interstitial pneumonia: comparative appearances at and diagnostic accuracy of thin-section CT. Radiology 221: 600–605.

51. McLaughlin VV, Archer SL, Badesch DB, Barst RJ, Farber HW, et al. (2009) ACCF/AHA 2009 expert consensus document on pulmonary hypertension a report of the American College of Cardiology Foundation Task Force on Expert Consensus Documents and the American Heart Association developed in collaboration with the American College of Chest Physicians; American Thoracic Society, Inc.; and the Pulmonary Hypertension Association. J Am Coll Cardiol 53: 1573–1619.

52. Baechler EC, Batliwalla FM, Karypis G, Gaffney PM, Moser K, et al. (2004) Expression levels for many genes in human peripheral blood cells are highly sensitive to ex vivo incubation. Genes Immun 5: 347–353.

53. Edgar R, Domrachev M, Lash AE (2002) Gene Expression Omnibus: NCBI gene expression and hybridization array data repository. Nucleic Acids Res 30: 207–210.

54. Yuan JS, Reed A, Chen F, Stewart CN Jr. (2006) Statistical analysis of real-time PCR data. BMC Bioinformatics 7: 85.

55. Pan W (2002) A comparative review of statistical methods for discovering differentially expressed genes in replicated microarray experiments. Bioinformatics 18: 546–554.

56. Benjamini Y, Hochberg Y (1995) Controlling the false discovery rate: a practical and powerful approach to multiple testing. JRSS-B 57: 289–300.

57. Cheadle C, Vawter MP, Freed WJ, Becker KG (2003) Analysis of microarray data using Z score transformation. J Mol Diagn 5: 73–81.

58. Nadon R, Woody E, Shi P, Rghei N, Hubschle H, et al. (2002) Statistical inference in array genomics. In: Geschwind D, Gregg J, eds. Microarrays for the Neurosciences. Cambridge: MIT Press.

59. Eisen MB, Spellman PT, Brown PO, Botstein D (1998) Cluster analysis and display of genome-wide expression patterns. Proc Natl Acad Sci U S A 95: 14863–14868.

60. Cheadle C, Cho-Chung YS, Becker KG, Vawter MP (2003) Application of z-score transformation to Affymetrix data. Appl Bioinformatics 2: 209–217.

61. Huang da W, Sherman BT, Lempicki RA (2009) Systematic and integrative analysis of large gene lists using DAVID bioinformatics resources. Nat Protoc 4: 44–57.

62. Subramanian A, Tamayo P, Mootha VK, Mukherjee S, Ebert BL, et al. (2005) Gene set enrichment analysis: a knowledge-based approach for interpreting genome-wide expression profiles. Proc Natl Acad Sci U S A 102: 15545–15550.

5

Novel Mutations in *BMPR2, ACVRL1* and *KCNA5* Genes and Hemodynamic Parameters in Patients with Pulmonary Arterial Hypertension

Guillermo Pousada[1], Adolfo Baloira[2], Carlos Vilariño[3], Jose Manuel Cifrian[4], Diana Valverde[1]*

1 Department of Biochemistry, Genetics and Immunology, Faculty of Biology, University of Vigo, Instituto de Investigación Biomédica de Vigo (IBIV), Vigo, Spain, **2** Respiratory Division, Complejo Hospitalario Universitario de Pontevedra, Pontevedra, Spain, **3** Respiratory Division, Complejo Hospitalario Universitario de Vigo, Vigo, Spain, **4** Respiratory Division, Hospital Universitario Marqués de Valdecilla, Santander, Spain

Abstract

Background: Pulmonary arterial hypertension (PAH) is a rare and progressive vascular disorder characterized by increased pulmonary vascular resistance and right heart failure. The aim of this study was to analyze the Bone Morphogenetic Protein Receptor 2 (*BMPR2*), Activin A type II receptor like kinase 1 (*ALK1/ACVRL1*) and potassium voltage-gated channel, shakerrelated subfamily, member 5 (*KCNA5*) genes in patients with idiopathic and associated PAH. Correlation among pathogenic mutations and clinical and functional parameters was further analyzed.

Methods and Results: Forty one patients and fifty controls were included in this study. Analysis of *BMPR2, ACVRL1* and *KCNA5* genes was performed by polymerase chain reaction (PCR) and direct sequencing. Fifty one nucleotide changes were detected in these genes in 40 of the 41 patients; only 22 of these changes, which were classified as pathogenic, have been detected in 21 patients (51.2%). Ten patients (62.5%) with idiopathic PAH and 10 (40%) with associated PAH showed pathogenic mutations in some of the three genes. Several clinical and hemodynamics parameters showed significant differences between carriers and non-carriers of mutations, being more severe in carriers: mean pulmonary artery pressure (p = 0.043), pulmonary vascular resistence (p = 0.043), cardiac index (p = 0.04) and 6 minute walking test (p = 0.02). This differences remained unchanged after adjusting for PAH type (idiopathic vs non idiopathic).

Conclusions: Pathogenic mutations in *BMPR2* gene are frequent in patients with idiopathic and associated PAH group I. Mutations in *ACVRL1* and *KCNA5* are less frequent. The presence of these mutations seems to increase the severity of the disease.

Editor: Shama Ahmad, University of Colorado, Denver, United States of America

Funding: This study was supported by the grants IN-202-05 from SOGAPAR, CO-0085-10 from Actelion Pharmaceuticals and INBIOMED 2009-063 Xunta de Galicia. The funders had no role in study design, data collection and analysis, decision to publish, or preparation of the manuscript.

Competing Interests: The authors confirm that they received funding from a commercial source: "Actelion Pharmaceuticals". But, this does not alter their adherence to PLOS ONE policies on sharing data and materials.

* E-mail: dianaval@uvigo.es

Introduction

Pulmonary arterial hypertension (PAH; OMIM #178600) is a rare and progressive disorder characterized by obstruction of pre-capillary pulmonary arteries [1]. It is defined by a sustained increase in mean pulmonary artery pressure (mPaP) ≥25 mmHg at rest with normal wedge pressure [2]. Symptoms of PAH include dyspnea, syncope and chest pain, and eventually leads to right-sided heart failure and death [1]. Structural and functional changes in the vascular wall and thrombus formation are the main factors responsible for the increased pulmonary vascular resistance in these patients [3].

PAH can be inherited (FPAH), idiopathic (IPAH), or associated with other diseases, drug or toxin exposures (APAH) [4]. The disease is more frequent in women, with a ratio of at least 1.7:1 women to men [2]. Much of what is known about the genetic basis of PAH is related to mutations in bone morphogenetic protein receptor type 2 (*BMPR2*). This gene is located on chromosome 2q33 and mutations have been identified in over 80% of patients with FPAH, but are likely to be responsible for over 90% of the cases. However, only 20% of carriers developed the disease [5,6]. The frequency of mutations in *BMPR2* gene is not well defined in IPAH, but it has been reported a value of 9–26% in small cohorts of patients [6,7,8].

Some other genes have been implicated in the pathogenesis of the disease, including Activin A type II receptor like kinase 1 (*ALK1/ACVRL1*) and potassium voltage-gated channel, shakerrelated subfamily, member 5 (*KCNA5*). Mutations in *ACVRL1* gene, located in chromosome 12q13, are directly related to some cases of PAH associated with hereditary hemorrhagic telangiectasia (HHT) [9]. This receptor is also a member of the transforming growth factor beta (TGF-β) superfamily and plays a role in different tissues producing different responses, including proliferation, differentiation, migration, increase of cell survival and angiogenesis. *ACVRL1* is expressed mainly in the developing vascular system and plays a critical role in arteriogenesis and developing arterial endothelial cells [10,11]. *KCNA5* protein is situated in the cellular intermembrane space and is composed by four subunits. The *KCNA5* gene is located on chromosome 12p13 and is formed by a single exon of 2865 bp and 613 residues. Indeed, mutations in the exon or in the promoter region of *KCNA5* gene have been reported to be associated with IPAH and may underline the altered function and expression of voltage-gated K+ channel 1.5 (Kv1.5) observed in pulmonary arteriolar smooth muscle cells (PASMC) from these patients [12,13].

The aim of this study was to analyze *BMPR2*, *ACVRL1* and *KCNA5* genes in patients with idiopathic and associated PAH, characterize the changes found and correlate them with clinical and hemodynamic variables.

Materials and Methods

Patients and samples

Patients with idiopathic or associated PAH (group 1 of Dana Point) followed in our clinic of PAH were included in this study. Cardiac catheterization was performed using the latest consensus diagnostic criteria of the ERS-ESC (European Respiratory Society-European Society of Cardiology) (mean resting pulmonary pressure $\geq$25 mmHg, capillary pressure <15 mmHg) in all cases, [14]. PAH was considered idiopathic after exclusion of any of the possible causes associated with the disease. Clinical history included use of drugs, especially appetite suppressants, and screening for connective tissue diseases and hepatic disease. The study included serology for HIV, autoimmunity, thoracic CT scan and echocardiography. Patients with PAH that could be related to chronic lung disease were excluded. Fifty healthy individuals were used as controls. All patients and controls signed an informed consent. The Autonomic Ethics Committee approved the study (*Comité Autonómico de Ética da Investigación de Galicia - CAEI de Galicia*).

Genomic DNA was extracted from leukocytes isolated from venous blood using the FlexiGene DNA Kit (Qiagen, Germany) according to the manufacturer's protocol.

Genomic study

Amplification of the exons and intronic junctions of the genes was performed with 50 ng of genomic DNA from each individual. Changes in other regions were not analyzed. The primers used for the *BMPR2* gene were as described by Deng *et al* [15]. The amplification conditions were as follows: 95°C for 5 min, 35 cycles of 95°C for 30 s, 55°C for 30 s (for the exons 1, 3, 5, 6, 7, 8, 9, 10, 11 and 13) and 60°C for 30 s (for the exons 2 and 12), 72°C for 30 s and, finally, 72°C for 7 min. The PCR mix contained 1.5 mM Cl$_2$ Mg, with 0.2 U of Taq Polymerase (Biotaq, Bioline, UK).

The exons and intronic junctions of the *ACVRL1* gene were amplified using the conditions of 95°C for 1 min followed by 35 cycles of 95°C for 30 s, 55°C for 30 s (for the exons 5, 7, 8, 9 and 10), 56°C for 30 s (for the exon 4), 60°C for 30 s (for the exon 6), 62°C for 30 s (for the exon 2) and 64°C for the exon 3), 72°C for 30 s and, finally, 72°C for 7 min. The primers used to amplify this gene were described by Berg *et al* [16].

The single exon and intronic junctions of the *KCNA5* gene was amplified for the 4 validated amplicons spanning the coding sequence of *KCNA5* gene. The primers used were described by Tao Yang *et al* [17]. The amplification conditions were 95°C for 30 s, followed by 35 cycles of 95°C for 30 s, 66°C for 30 s, 72°C for 30 s and, finally, 72°C for 7 min.

PCR products were confirmed by electrophoresis on a 2% agarose gel containing ethidium bromide. PCR fragments were purified using the Nucleic Acid and Protein Purification kit (NucleoSpin Extract II; Macherey-Nagel, Germany) and sequenced with the BigDye Terminator version 1.1 Cycle Sequencing Kit (Applied Biosystems, California, USA). The reactions were performed on a GeneAmp PCR System 2700 (Applied Biosystems). The sequencing reactions were precipitated and finally analyzed on an ABI PRISM 3100 genetic analyzer (Applied Biosystems).

Sequence data was aligned to reference Ensembl cDNA sequence ENST00000374580 for *BMPR2* gene, ENST00000388922 for *ACVRL1* gene and ENST00000252321 for the *KCNA5* gene and examined for sequence variations. Detected mutations were confirmed by a second independent PCR reaction and were identified in both forward and reverse strands. To predict whether a rare missense variant was deleterious, we used the combined results of three different computer algorithms:

- The polymorphism phenotyping program, PolyPhen-2 (available at http://genetics.bwh.harvard.edu/pph/) uses sequence conservation, structure and SWISS-PROT annotation to characterize an amino acid substitution as benign, possibly damaging or probably damaging [18].
- Pmut (available at http://mmb2.pcb.ub.es:8080/PMut/) provides prediction by neural networks, which use internal databases, secondary structure prediction and sequence conservation. This program provides a binary prediction of "neutral" or "pathologic" [19].
- Sort Intolerant from Tolerant (SIFT) (available at http://sift.jcvi.org) uses sequence homology to predict whether a change is tolerated or damaging [20].

Intronic, isocoding and missense changes were analyzed using the programs *NNSplice* (http://fruitfly.org:9005/seq_tools/splice.html), *NetGene2* (http://www.cbs.dtu.dk/services/NetGene2/), *Splice View* (http://zeus2.itb.cnr.it/~webgene/wwwspliceview_ex.html) and *HSF Human* (http://www.umd.be/HSF/) in order to predict whether those changes could be affecting, creating or eliminating donor/acceptor splice sites.

Statistical analysis

Values are expressed as mean$\pm$SD (standard deviation). A non-parametric test was used for comparisons between patients and controls. Chi-square test was used to compare genotype with clinical and hemodynamic variables. These correlations were analyzed by the Spearman test. Values <0.05 were considered statistically significant. Analysis was carried out using the statistical package SPSS v19.

Results

Description of the cohort

Forty one unrelated PAH patients (16 idiopathic, 17 associated to connective tissue disease, 4 related to HIV and 4 portopulmonary) and fifty healthy controls without familial history of PAH were included. At the time of diagnosis 3 patients were in functional class (FC) I, 14 patients in FC II, 21 patients in FC III and 3 in FC IV. The clinical features of patients are showed in Table 1.

Mutations in *BMPR2*, *ACVRL1* and *KCNA5* genes

A total of 53 nucleotide changes in the *BMPR2*, *ACVRL1* and *KCNA5* genes were identified in 40 out of 41 patients. We found 30 changes in 33 patients in *BMPR2* gene, 11 variations in 24 patients

Table 1. Clinical features and hemodynamic parameters of patients.

	Carriers of mutations	Non-carriers of mutations	p-value	Idiopathic PAH	Associated PAH	p-value
Number	20	21		16	25	
Gender	10 F/10 M	10 F/11 M	0.216	8 F/8 M	13 F/12 M	0.552
Age at diagnosis (years)	53±15	51±16	0.437	52±21	53±12	0.552
mPaP (mmHg)	57±15	45±14	0.043	52±16	47±13	0.510
sPaP (mmHg)	69±22	73±19	0.448	74±20	70±21	0.490
PVR (mmHg.l^{-1}.m^{-1})	11.92±3.18	8.53±4.46	0.043	9.96±4.68	7.21±2.8	0.222
CI (l.m^{-1}.m^{-2})	2.05±0.68	3.75±0.44	0.040	2.6±0.74	2.54±0.45	0.346
6MWT (m)	314±130	428±103	0.020	370±136	374±127	0.308
PAH types	10 IPAH/10 APAH	6 IPAH/15 APAH	0,222	16 patients	25 patients	0,222

Values are expressed as mean ± standard deviation; F: female, M: male; mPaP: mean pulmonary artery pressure; sPaP: systolic pulmonary artery pressure; PVR: pulmonary vascular resistence; CI: cardiac index; 6MWT: 6 minute walking test; IPAH: idiopathic pulmonary arterial hypertension; APAH: associated pulmonary arterial hypertension.

in *ACVRL1* gene, and 12 changes in 15 patients in the case of *KCNA5* gene.

Thirty-one variations (60.8%) were located in coding regions. Missense variations accounted for 39.6% of total changes found in coding regions; nonsense variations only represented 5.7% and synonymous changes a 13%. The 26.4% of changes were located in intronic regions (two of them were heterozygous deletions) and a 9.4% in UTR regions of these genes. (Figure 1).

The three different computer algorithms used to classify the nucleotide changes showed different results. A missense mutation was considered pathogenic when at least two of the three programs (*PolyPhen-2*, *Pmut* and *SIFT*) classified it as pathogenic. These changes are summarized in Table 2. None of these mutations were detected in a panel of 100 chromosomes from controls. Furthermore, we used four programs to predict whether these changes could affect donor/acceptor splice sites. We consider a mutation as potentially pathogenic when the pathogenic score was equal or greater than 2 (Tables 3, 4, 5).

After the combination of all software, we found 22 pathological mutations in 21 patients, with a frequency of 51%. Most of the

mutations were found in *BMPR2* gene (41.5%), followed by *KCNA5* (7.3%) and, finally, *ACVRL1* (4.9%). These results are shown in Figure 2. IPAH patients were carriers of *BMPR2* mutations in 8 cases (50%), two cases for *KCNA5* gene (12.5%) and 2 cases for *ACVRL1* gene (12.5%) (Figure 2). The 62.5% of patients (10patients) with IPAH had at least one pathogenic mutation in some of these genes. On the other hand, 44% (11 patients) of APAH patients showed pathogenic mutations (36% in *BMPR2* gene, 4% in *ACVRL1* gene and 4% in *KCNA5* gene).

In our cohort of patients we found 5 patients with more than one pathogenic mutation in *BMPR2* or in combination with *KCNA5* or *ACVRL1* genes (Table 6). All of these mutations are described for first time in this study, except c.529+37C>G.

Association with clinical features and hemodynamic parameters

We analyzed clinical features and hemodynamic parameters comparing the group of patients harboring a pathogenic mutation with those patients with no mutation. The parameters included were: gender, age at diagnosis, mPaP (mean pulmonary pressure),

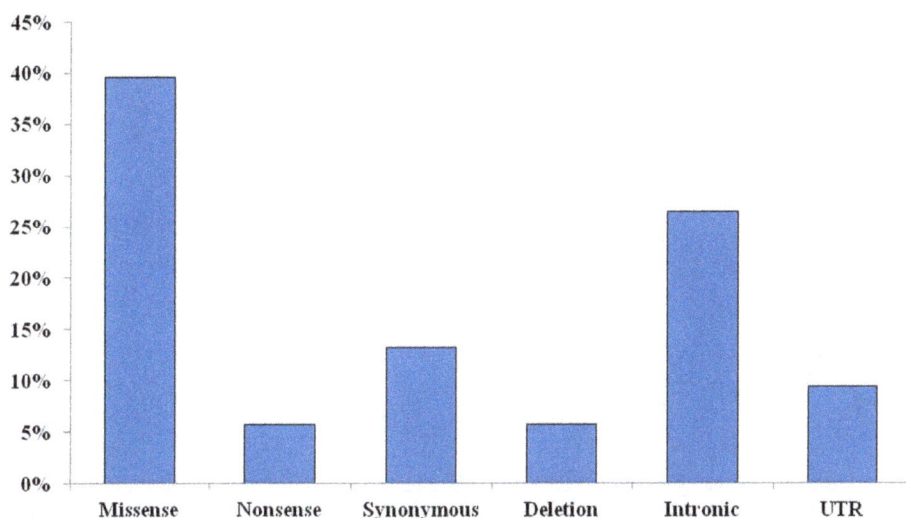

Figure 1. Total percentage of nucleotide changes found in this study for the analyzed genes. The variations that appear in greater proportion are missense, followed by those located in the intronic region.

Table 2. Missense changes found in the coding region of the *BMPR2*, *ACVRL1* and *KCNA5* genes and their classification according to three different computer algorithms (*PolyPhen-2*, *Pmut* and *SIFT*).

CLASSIFICATION MISSENSE VARIATIONS FOUND IN THE CODING REGION OF GENES

Gene	Nucleotide change	Amino-acid change	Times founded	PolyPhen-2	Pmut	Sift	Score
BMPR2 (Exon 2)	c.190A>C	p.(S64G)	1	Benign	Neutral	Tolerated	0
BMPR2 (Exon 2)	c.229A>T	p.(I77L)	1	Benign	Neutral	Damaging	1
BMPR2 (Exon 3)	c.251G>T	p.(C84F)	2	Probably damaging	Neutral	Damaging	2
BMPR2 (Exon 3)	c.259C>T	p.(H87Y)	1	Benign	Neutral	Damaging	1
BMPR2 (Exon 3)	c.275A>T	p.(Q92L)	1	Benign	Pathologic	Damaging	2
BMPR2 (Exon 4)	c.484G>C	p.(A162P)	1	Probably damaging	Neutral	Damaging	2
BMPR2 (Exon 6)	c.790G>A	p.(D264N)	1	Possibly damaging	Neutral	Damaging	2
BMPR2 (Exon 8)	c.1021G>A	p.(V341M)	3	Possibly damaging	Neutral	Damaging	2
BMPR2 (Exon 12)	c.2324G>A	p.(S775N)	2	Benign	Neutral	Tolerated	0
ACVRL1 (Exon 2)	c.24A>T	P.(K8N)	1	Benign	Neutral	Tolerated	0
ACVRL1 (Exon 3)	c.176A>T	p.(E59V)	1	Benign	Neutral	Tolerated	0
ACVRL1 (Exon 4)	c.476A>T	p.(E159V)	1	Benign	Neutral	Tolerated	0
ACVRL1 (Exon 6)	c.673A>T	p.(S225C)	1	Probably Damaging	Pathological	Damaging	3
ACVRL1 (Exon 8)	c.1186A>G	p.(T396A)	8	Benign	Neutral	Tolerated	0
KCNA5 (Exon 1)	c.125T>A	p.(L42H)	1	Benign	Neutral	Tolerated	0
KCNA5 (Exon 1)	c.253C>A	p.(L85M)	1	Benign	Neutral	Tolerated	0
KCNA5 (Exon 1)	c.340A>C	p.(T114P)	1	Benign	Neutral	Tolerated	0
KCNA5 (Exon 1)	c.385C>G	p.(L119V)	2	Benign	Neutral	Damaging	1
KCNA5 (Exon 1)	c.509C>G	p.(P170R)	1	Probably Damaging	Pathological	Damaging	3
KCNA5 (Exon 1)	c.551G>C	p.(R184P)	1	Probably Damaging	Pathological	Damaging	3
KCNA5 (Exon 1)	c.1733G>A	p.(R577K)	1	Benign	Neutral	Tolerated	0

These results are considered damaging if the score is equal or greater than two.

Table 3. Results from four different bioinformatic programs used to predict the effect on the splicing process in *BMPR2* gene (NNSplice, NetGene2, Splice View and HSF Human).

Sequence variants	NNSplice	NetGene2	Splice View	HSF Human	Score
c.1-301G>A	The WT consensus sequence is not recognized	Score for the aceptor site increases from 25 to 26	The WT consensus sequence is not recognized	Neutral	1
c.190A>C (p.(S64G))	Neutral	The WT consensus sequence is not recognized	A new donor site is created	Score for donor and acceptor site decreases	2
c.229A>T (p.(I77L))	The WT consensus sequence is not recognized	Score for the main donor site increases from 31 to 34	Neutral	A new acceptor site is created	2
c.251G>T (p.(C84F))	Score for the aceptor site increases from 87 to 89	Score for the main acceptor site decreases from 33 to 27	Neutral	The main donor site is not recognized	3
c.259C>T (p.(H87Y))	Score for the aceptor site decreases from 87 to 86	Score for the main acceptor site decreases from 33 to 30	Neutral	The main donor site is not recognized and the acceptor increase	3
c.275A>T (p.(Q92L))	Neutral	Score for the main acceptor site decreases from 33 to 25	Neutral	Score for donor and acceptor site increases	2
c.327G>C (p.(Q109Q))	Neutral	Score for the main donor site decreases from 79 to 76	Neutral	The main donor site is not recognized	2
c.419-43delT	Neutral	Neutral	Neutral	Neutral	0
c.484G>C (p.(A162P))	Score for the aceptor site decreases from 80 to 66	Neutral	Neutral	The main donor site is not recognized	2
c.529+37C>G	A new acceptor site is created	Neutral	Neutral	A new acceptor site is created	2
c.529+53A>G	Neutral	Neutral	Neutral	A new acceptor site is created	1
c.529+139A>T	Neutral	Neutral	Neutral	Score for donor site decreases and the acceptor site increase	1
c.530-24G>T	Neutral	Score for the main donor site increases from 83 to 86 and the main acceptor site increases from 77 to 82	Neutral	The donor and acceptor sites is not recognized	2
c.622+103C>G	Neutral	Neutral	Neutral	The main donor site is not recognized	1
c.633A>G (p.(R211R))	Neutral	Score for the main donor site increases from 92 to 94	Neutral	The main donor site is not recognized and the acceptor decrease	2
c.637C>A (p.(R213R))	Neutral	Score for the main acceptor site decreases from 20 to 18	Neutral	Score for donor site increases and a new acceptor site is created	2
c.654T>A (p.(Y218*))	Neutral	Score for the main donor site increases from 92 to 94 and the main acceptor site decreases from 20 to 18	Neutral	Score for the main acceptor site decrease	2
c.790G>A (p.(D264N))	Neutral	Score for the main donor site decreases from 94 to 92	Neutral	The main donor site is not recognized	2
c.835G>T (p.(V278V))	Neutral	Neutral	Neutral	Score for donor site decreases and the acceptor site increase	1
c.853-22T>C	Neutral	Score for the main donor site decreases from 87 to 86	Neutral	Neutral	1
c.968+117G>A *BMPR2*	Neutral	Neutral	Neutral	The donor and acceptor sites is not recognized	1
c.968-124_968-122delTCT	Neutral	Neutral	Neutral	Neutral	0
c.893G>A (p.(W298*))	Neutral	Score for the main donor and acceptor site decreases	The WT consensus sequence is not recognized	The main donor site increase and a new acceptor site in created	2
c.981T>C (p.(P327P))	The WT consensus sequence is not recognized	Score for the main donor site decreases from 100 to 99	Neutral	A new donor site is created	2
c.1021G>A (p.(V341M))	Neutral	Neutral	The WT consensus sequence is not recognized	The main donor site is not recognized	2
c.1414-84C>T	Neutral	Neutral	Neutral	Score for the main acceptor site increases	1

Table 3. Cont.

Sequence variants	NNSplice	NetGene2	Splice View	HSF Human	Score
c.1467G>A (p.(E489E))	Neutral	Score for the main donor site increases from 89 to 93	Neutral	A new acceptor site is created	2
c.2034G>A (p.(K678K))	Neutral	Neutral	Neutral	The main donor site is not recognized	1
c.2324G>A (p.(S775N))	Neutral	Neutral	Neutral	The main donor site is not recognized	1
c.2811G>A (p.(R937R))	Neutral	Neutral	Neutral	The main donor site is not recognized	1

These results are considered positive if the score is equal or greater than two.
doi:10.1371/journal.pone.0100261.t003

sPaP (systolic pulmonary pressure), PVR (pulmonary vascular resistence), CI (cardiac index), 6MWT (6 minute walking test) and type of PAH (IPAH vs APAH). Variables were categorized according to the best cut off point by ROC curve.

The association of genotype with clinical and hemodynamics parameters showed statistically significant differences in mPaP (p = 0.043) and PVR (p = 0.043). Patients carrying a mutation had a higher value for these two parameters than non-carriers. In opposition, patients carrying a mutation had a significantly lower CI (p = 0.04) and 6MWT (p = 0.02). These results are shown in table 1. We did not found significant differences between gender for the presence of mutations (p = 0.216), mean age of onset of first symptoms (p = 0.437) and sPaP (p = 0.448). Pathological mutations

were seen in 10 patients with IPAH and 10 patients with associated PAH without statistical differences (p = 0,222). Clinical and hemodynamic parameters did not show any significant difference between associated and idiopathic PAH.

The mean follow-up period was 14 months. Three patients died during this time (2 APAH, 1 IPAH), so it was not possible to compare groups. Two of the three deceased patients present two pathogenic mutations in *BMPR2* gene. The other patient was carrier of a pathogenic mutation, (p.(A162P)) in *BMPR2* gene and showed several polymorphisms in *ACVRL1* (c.1047+31C>A, c.1186A>G (p.(T396A)), c.1502+7A>G) and *KCNA5* (c.1842+508A>T) genes.

Table 4. Results from four different bioinformatic programs used to predict the effect on the splicing process in *ACVRL1* gene (NNSplice, NetGene2, Splice View and HSF Human).

Sequence variants	NNSplice	NetGene2	Splice View	HSF Human	Score
c.24A>T (p.(K8N))	Score for the main acceptor site increases from 66 to 76	Neutral	Neutral	The main donor and acceptor sites are not recognized	2
c.176A>T (p.(E59V))	Neutral	Neutral	Neutral	The main donor site is not recognized and a new acceptor site is created	0
c.313+11C>T	Neutral	Neutral	Neutral	Score for acceptor site decreases	1
c.313+20C>A	Neutral	Neutral	Neutral	Score for acceptor site increase	1
c.476A>T (p.(E159V))	The WT consensus sequence is not recognized	The WT consensus sequence is not recognized	Neutral	The main donor site is not recognized and acceptor site increase	0
c.478delT (p.(S160Pfs*5))	Neutral	Neutral	Neutral	The main donor site is not recognized	1
c.673A>T (p.(S225C))	Score for the main donor site increases from 95 to 99	Score for the main donor site increases from 39 to 55	The WT consensus sequence is not recognized	The main donor site is not recognized and a new acceptor site is created	2
c.1047+31C>A ACVRL1	The WT consensus sequence is not recognized	The WT consensus sequence is not recognized	Neutral	The main donor site is not recognized	1
c.1186A>G (p.(T396A))	The WT consensus sequence is not recognized	Neutral	Neutral	Score for the main donor site increases	0
c.1246+41G>C	The WT consensus sequence is not recognized	Neutral	Neutral	The main acceptor site is not recognized	0
c.1502+7A>G	Neutral	Score for the main donor site decreases from 83 to 70	The WT consensus sequence is not recognized	Neutral	1

These results are considered positive if the score is equal or greater than two.

Table 5. Results from four different bioinformatic programs used to predict the effect on the splicing process in *KCNA5* gene (NNSplice, NetGene2, Splice View and HSF Human).

Sequence variants	NNSplice	NetGene2	Splice View	HSF Human	Score
c.125T>A (p.(L42H))	The WT consensus sequence is not recognized	The WT consensus sequence is not recognized	The WT consensus sequence is not recognized	The WT consensus sequence is not recognized	0
c.253C>A (p.(L85M))	The WT consensus sequence is not recognized	The WT consensus sequence is not recognized	The WT consensus sequence is not recognized	The WT consensus sequence is not recognized	0
c.340A>C (p.(T114P))	The WT consensus sequence is not recognized	The WT consensus sequence is not recognized	The WT consensus sequence is not recognized	The WT consensus sequence is not recognized	0
c.385C>G (p.(L119V))	The WT consensus sequence is not recognized	The WT consensus sequence is not recognized	The WT consensus sequence is not recognized	Neutral	0
c.477G>C (p.(L159L))	The WT consensus sequence is not recognized	The WT consensus sequence is not recognized	The WT consensus sequence is not recognized	Score for the main acceptor site increase	1
c.509C>G (p.(P170R))	The WT consensus sequence is not recognized	The WT consensus sequence is not recognized	The WT consensus sequence is not recognized	The WT consensus sequence is not recognized	0
c.551G>C (p.(R184P))	The WT consensus sequence is not recognized	The WT consensus sequence is not recognized	The WT consensus sequence is not recognized	The WT consensus sequence is not recognized	0
c.622G>T (p.(E208*))	The WT consensus sequence is not recognized	The WT consensus sequence is not recognized	The WT consensus sequence is not recognized	The main donor site is not recognized and acceptor site increase	1
c.1733G>A (p.(R577K))	The WT consensus sequence is not recognized	The WT consensus sequence is not recognized	The WT consensus sequence is not recognized	The WT consensus sequence is not recognized	0
c.1842+22T>G	The WT consensus sequence is not recognized	The WT consensus sequence is not recognized	The WT consensus sequence is not recognized	The WT consensus sequence is not recognized	0
c.1842+52A>T	The WT consensus sequence is not recognized	The WT consensus sequence is not recognized	The WT consensus sequence is not recognized	The WT consensus sequence is not recognized	0
c.1842+508A>T	The WT consensus sequence is not recognized	The WT consensus sequence is not recognized	The WT consensus sequence is not recognized	The WT consensus sequence is not recognized	0

These results are considered positive if the score is equal or greater than two.

Discussion

This study was designed to establish the prevalence of mutations found in certain genes potentially involved in the pathogenesis of PAH. We detected 53 different nucleotide changes in *BMPR2*, *ACVRL1* and *KCNA5* genes in 40 out of 41 PAH patients. Twenty two of these mutations (found in 51% of patients) were considered pathogenic according to the *in silico* analysis that was performed with several programs to reach a high reliability [21].

The mutational frequency for *BMPR2* gene in sporadic PAH range from 10–20%, as referred in previous studies [22,23,24].However, we found that 50% of our IPAH patients had a pathogenic mutation in *BMPR2* gene, higher than expected and corresponding to the highest value described until now. The percentage of mutations found in APAH was 36%, which is lower but also significantly elevated. Consider the suggestion made by Pfarr *et al* [25] that as soon a genetic defect had been identified in PAH patients they must be classified as familial PAH, it could be interesting to perform segregation analysis in order to confirm the familial nature of the disease in these families.

We identified two hot spots for mutations in exon 3 and exon 6 for *BMPR2* gene. These exons are located in a very important area rich in cysteine residues and therefore any mutation here could affect the catalytic ability of the BMPs, the ligand of *BMPR2*, disrupting the Smad signaling pathway [2,23,26,27,28]. These mutations may introduce subtle changes in the structure of the protein and might interfere with the downstream signaling of the BMP pathway [29]. It has been hypothesized that an imbalance of increased TGF-β levels and decreased BMP signals induced by *BMPR2* mutations leads to PAH [30]. Exon 6 is located in the N-terminus of a serine-threonine kinase domain which is formed by conserved subdomains that includes exons 6 to 11 of the gene. This region, responsible for binding adenosine triphosphate (ATP), is characterized by distinctive patterns of conserved residues. Mutations located here could produce heterogeneous defects for signaling activity by binding preventing of ATP and altering the functionality of the protein. We also detected several mutations in the C-terminus region for this serine-threonine kinase domain, which is involved in substrate recognition and initiation of the phosphorylation relay. In addition, one missense mutation and one synonymous change, which seems to alter the splicing process

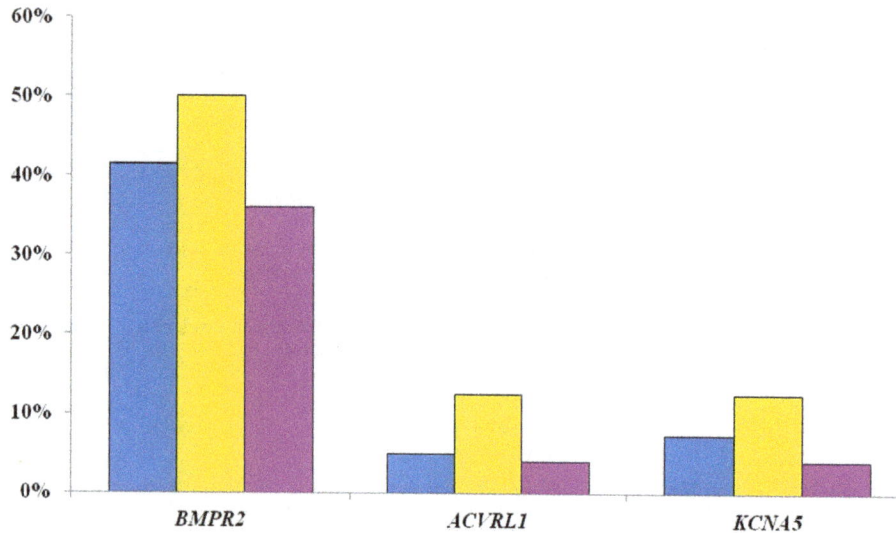

Figure 2. Frequency of pathological mutations found in our patients (blue all patients, yellow IPAH, purple APAH). *BMPR2* showed the greatest number of mutations.

according to *in silico* analysis, were identified in exon 8.Finally, we found the synonymous mutation p.(E489E) in exon 11, which is predicted to produce alterations at splicing level. An invariant arginine at position 491 in the protein is located around this point, which is essential for signaling [31], thereby making this area of special interest.

Synonymous mutations have always been considered safe, but they could cause serious physiological effects as they can interfere in the splicing accuracy, translation fidelity, mRNA structure and protein folding. Even, these mutations may decrease the half-life of mRNA, leading to a downregulation of the protein expression [32]. Different synonymous mutations, both new and already described, were seen in 46% of our patients and the 62.5% of these synonymous mutations are considered pathogenic and were not found in controls. It could be interesting to analyze synonymous mutations and intronic deletions [23] with a functional approach since no studies have been performed for these changes.

Regarding to the *ACVRL1* gene, several mutations have usually been described associated with HHT. Girerd *et al* describe a mutational frequency for this gene of 2.3% in IPAH patients from the French PAH Network, lower than 12.5% found in our patients [33]. Probably the small size of our series may explain these differences. When we compared the data for IPAH in this paper against our results, we found a higher mutational rate for *BMPR2* and *ACVRL1* genes (59% vs 16.6%), finding only one mutation (p.(S160P)fs*5) in *ACVRL1* in one APAH patient. Selva-O'Call-

aghan *et al*, who studied mutational load for *ACVRL1* gene in APAH to connective tissue disease patients [34], did not found any mutation. These findings suggest that *ACVRL1* gene do not have a significant role in APAH patients.

The p.(S225C) mutation is located in exon 6 of *ACVRL1* gene and it is placed in the serine-threonine kinase domain. Mutations in this region, a conserved serine–threonine kinase domain, have been associated with a higher risk of PAH in childhood and could affect the downstream SMAD signaling pathway as *BMPR2* [35,36]. The novel missense mutation, p.(T396A) was detected in 8 patients and does not appear in the control group. Functional studies from Abdalla et al [36] demonstrated that mutations located in this highly conserved protein domain may cause protein misfolding [36,37] and intracellular degradation, explaining the lack of surface expression of mutant proteins [36]. Although it has been classified as nonpathogenic, it would be interesting to determine its functionality.

Few mutations have been described in highly conserved aminoacid residues of the *KCNA5* gene in PAH patients [38]. Several *KCNA5* gene mutations have been involved in atrial fibrillation, a common cardiac arrhythmia, in 1.95% of patients with absence of known predisposing factors [39]. We detect pathological mutations in this gene in 7.3% of total patients. For IPAH patients this value raises to 12.5%, but only one mutation was identified in one APAH patient.

Table 6. List of patients with several pathogenic mutations in the studied genes.

Patient	BMPR2	ACVRL1	KCNA5	PAH Type
14.09	c.251G>T (p.(C84F)), c.259C>T (p.(H87Y))[a], c.981T>C (p.(P327P)) [a]	–	–	Associated
14.17	c.530+37C>G [a]	–	c.551G>C (p.(R184P))	Idiopathic
17.01	c.893G>A (p.(W298*))	c.24A>T (p.(K8N)) [a]	–	Idiopathic
PO.15	c.229A>T (p.(I77L))[a], c.633A>G (p.(R211R)) [a]	–	–	Idiopathic
PO.16	c.327G>C (p.(Q109Q)) [a], c.1021G>A (p.(V341M))	–	–	Associated

[a]These mutationsare considered pathogenic because they could produce alterations in the splicing process, according to *in silico* analysis.

The p.(P170R), p.(R184P) and p.(E208*) mutations in *KCNA5* gene are located within the T1 domain, which is highly conserved. The T1 domain is largely responsible for tetramerization and governs channel interaction by cytoplasmic regulatory subunits KVα and KVβ. Mutations located in this region have been shown to disrupt both KVα-KVβ with deleterious consequences on channel gating, protein expression [40] or cause both hyperpolarizing and depolarizing shifts on the activation relationship [41,42]. T1 domain has also been associated with other aspects of channel function as the interaction with S1 domain or the influence in gating properties and voltage sensitivity of KV channels. Furthermore, the p.(E208*) mutation is close to S1 domain and potentially can disrupt the creating side portals between the T1 domain and the pore. Even mutations that have been identify as no harmful for the protein and did not appear in controls, as p.(L42H), p.(T114P) and p.(R577K) could introduce subtle changes in the structure of the protein and might interfere with the proper operation of the Kv1.5 channels, since they are located between the 5′UTR region of the gene and heteromerization domain, where the association between different proteins occurs [38].

We found statistical differences for mPaP, PVR, CI and 6MWT when compared hemodynamics and clinical parameters between patients with and without pathogenic mutations. Patients who harbor mutations show higher values for mPaP and PVR. Conversely, values for CI and 6MWT were significantly smaller. These results seem to show that patients with mutations have a more severe disease and perhaps worse prognosis. Otherwise,Pfarr *et al* found significant differences only for a low PVR value [25]. On the other hand, no differences in these parameters were seen according to PAH type. Liu D *et al* have described that gender influences the phenotype in PAH patients with *BMPR2* mutations, being more severe in males, but we did not confirm this fact in our results [43]. Previous studies indicate that PAH patients carrying a mutation have an onset approximately 10 years earlier than non-carriers [31], but our results did not confirm this finding. The vast majority of these variations are private, so it makes very difficult to establish a correlation between the phenotype and one particular mutation. For this reason, genotype-phenotype correlation is made according to all mutations found in a group of patients.

We described for the first time 5 patients with multiple mutations, three of them with two or more mutations in *BMPR2* gene. Two patients, both with IPAH, were carriers of mutations in two genes, *BMPR2* and *KCNA5* genes in one case and *BMPR2* and *ACVRL1* genes in the other one. This genetic heterogeneity reinforces the complex pathogenicity of this disease, with several ways of actuation. The molecular mechanisms of PAH are not clearly understood but multiple factors are involved in the development of this disease and several genes could be mutated, so it is not surprising that one patient may require mutations in several genes to develop PAH. The small number of patients with various mutations does not allow comparisons, but 3 of these 5 patients had a younger age at diagnosis and 2 of them died during follow-up which may suggest a worse prognosis.

Obviously, the main limitation of our study is the small number of patients, although the low incidence of PAH and some cases that did not consent the inclusion in this study, did not allow us to have a larger series. The comprehensive study carried out and complete follow-up of all cases add value to our results.

In summary, we present a series of patients with idiopathic and associated PAH with a high percentage of mutations in *BMPR2* and lower in *ACVRL1* and *KCNA5* genes, some of them not previously described, showing some clinical and hemodynamic differences which suggest that the presence of these mutations may be associated with more severe disease. There is no doubt that other genes are involved in the pathogenesis of PAH and will be important to know the role they play in the development of this disease. Perhaps the presence of more than one mutation increases the risk of develop it. As in other pathologies with genetic basis, PAH may be caused by a total mutational load of the genes involved in. This genetic heterogeneity, when known, may allow us to establish a correlation with the severity and course of the disease. The more we known about the pathways involved the best we can design the treatment.

Acknowledgments

We are grateful to the patients who participated in our research and we thank the physicians who participated in the collection of patients and data.

Author Contributions

Conceived and designed the experiments: GP AB DV. Performed the experiments: GP DV. Analyzed the data: GP AB CV DV. Contributed reagents/materials/analysis tools: GP AB CV JMC DV. Wrote the paper: GP AB DV. Clinical data: AB CV JMC.

References

1. Johnson JA, Vnencak-Jones CL, Cogan JD, Loyd JE, West J (2009) Copy-number variation in BMPR2 is not associated with the pathogenesis of pulmonary arterial hypertension. Med Gen 10: 58–60.

2. Machado RD, Eickelberg O, Elliott G, Geraci MW, Hanaoka M, et al. (2009) Genetics and Genomics of Pulmonary Arterial Hypertension. J Am Coll Cardiol 54: 1, Suppl S.

3. Peacock AJ, Murphy NF, McMurray JJV, Caballero L, Stewart S (2007) An epidemiological study of pulmonary arterial hypertension. Eur Respir J 30: 104–109.

4. Ulrich S, Szamalek-Hoegel J, Hersberger M, Fischler M, Solera-García J, et al. (2010) Sequence Variants in BMPR2 and Genes Involved in the Serotonin and Nitric Oxide Pathways in Idiopathic Pulmonary Arterial Hypertension and Chronic Thromboembolic Pulmonary Hypertension: Relation to Clinical Parameters and Comparison with Left Heart Disease. Respiration 79: 279–287.

5. Sanchez O, Marié E, Lerolle U, Wermert D, Israël-Biel D, et al. (2010) Pulmonary arterial hypertension in women. Rev Mal Respir 27: e79–e87.

6. Austin ED, Phillips JA, Cogan JD, Hamid R, Yu C, et al. (2009) Truncating and missense BMPR2 mutations differentially affect the severity of heritable pulmonary arterial hypertension. Respir Res 10: 87–96.

7. Davies RJ, Morrell NW (2008) Molecular mechanisms of Pulmonary Arterial Hypertension: Morphogenetic protein type II receptor. Chest 134: 1271–1277.

8. Morrell NW (2010) Genetics of pulmonary arterial hypertension: do the molecular findings have translational value?. f1000 Biology Reports 2: 22–24.

9. O'Callaghan AS, Balada E, Serrano-Acedo S, Simeon-Aznar CP, Ordi-Ros J (2007) Mutations of activin-receptor-like kinase 1 (ALK-1) are not found in patients with pulmonary hypertension and underlying connective tissue disease. Clin Rheumatol 26: 947–949.

10. Upton PD, Davies RJ, Trembath RC, Morrell NW (2009) Bone Morphogenetic Protein (BMP) and Activin Type II Receptors Balance BMP9 Signals Mediated by Activin Receptor-like Kinase-1 in Human Pulmonary Artery Endothelial Cells. J Biol Chem 284: 15794–15804.

11. Garrido-Martin EM, Blanco FJ, Fernandez-L A, Langa C, Vary VP, et al. (2010) Characterization of the human Activin-A receptor type II-like kinase 1 (ACVRL1) promoter and its regulation by Sp1. BMC Molecular Biology 11: 51–73.

12. Wipff J, Dieudé P, Guedj M, Ruiz B, Riemekasten G, et al. (2010) Association of a KCNA5 Gene Polymorphism With Systemic Sclerosis–Associated Pulmonary Arterial Hypertension in the European Caucasian Population. Arthritis & Rheumatism 62: 3093–3100.

13. Burg ED, Remillard CV, Yuan JX (2008) Potassium channels in the regulation of pulmonary artery smooth muscle cell proliferation and apoptosis: pharmacotherapeutic implications. Br J Pharmacol 153: S99–S111.

14. Galié N, Hoeper MM, Humbert M, Torbicki A, Vachiery JL, et al. (2009) Guidelines for the diagnosis and treatment of pulmonary hypertension. Eur Heart J 30: 2493–537.

15. Deng Z, Morse JH, Slager SL, Cuervo N, Moore KJ, et al. (2000) Familial primary pulmonary hypertension (gene PPH1) is caused by mutations in the bone morphogenetic protein receptor-II gene. Am J Hum Genet 67: 737–44.
16. Berg JN, Gallione CJ, Stenzel TT, Johnson DW, Allen WP, et al. (2007) The Activin Receptor-Like Kinase 1 Gene: Genomic Structure and Mutations in Hereditary Hemorrhagic Telangiectasia Type 2. Am J Hum Genet 61: 60–67.
17. Yang T, Yang P, Roden DM, Darbar D (2010) A novel KCNA5 Mutation Implicates Tyrosine Kinase Signaling in Human Atrial Fibrillation. Heart Rhythm 7(9): 1246–1252.
18. Adzhubei I, Jordan DM, Sunyaev SR (2013) Predicting functional effect of human missense mutations using PolyPhen-2. Curr Protoc Hum Genet 7(7): 20.
19. Ferrer-Costa C, Orozco M, de la Cruz X (2004) Sequence-based prediction of pathological mutations. Proteins 57(4): 811–9.
20. Kumar P, Henikoff S, Ng PC (2009) Predicting the effects of coding non-synonymous variants on protein function using the SIFT algorithm. Nat Protoc 4(7): 1073–81.
21. Santos C, Peixoto A, Rocha P, Pinto P, Bizarro S, et al. (2014) Pathogenicity Evaluation of BRCA1 and BRCA2 Unclassified Variants Identified in Portuguese Breast/Ovarian Cancer Families. J Mol Diagn 16(3): 324–334.
22. Portillo K, Santos S, Madrigal I, Blanco I, Paré C, et al. (2010) Study of the BMPR2 gene in patients with pulmonary arterial hypertension. Arch Bronconeumol 46: 129–34.
23. Fessel JP, Loyd JE, Austin ED (2011) The genetics of pulmonary arterial hypertension in the post-BMPR2 era. Pulm Circ 1: 305–319.
24. Girerd B, Montani D, Eyries M, Yaici A, Sztrymf B, et al. (2010) Absence of influence of gender and BMPR2 mutation type on clinical phenotypes of pulmonary arterial hypertension. Respir Res 11: 73–80.
25. Pfarr N, Fischer C, Ehlken N, Becker-Grünig T, López-González V, et al. (2013) Hemodynamic and genetic analysis in children with idiopathic, heritable, and congenital heart disease associated pulmonary arterial hypertension. Respir Res 14: 3–12.
26. Elliot CG, Glissmeyer EW, Havlena GT, Carlquist J, McKinney JT, et al. (2006) Relationship of BMPR2 mutations to vasoreactivity in Pulmonary Arterial Hypertension. Circulation 113: 2509–2515.
27. Hamid R, Cogan JD, Hedges LK, Austin E, Phillips III JA, et al. (2009) Penetrance of Pulmonary Arterial Hypertension is modulated by the expression of normal BMPR2 allele. Hum Mutat 30(4): 649–654.
28. Majka S, Hagen M, Blackwell T, Harral J, Johnson JA, et al. (2011) Physiologic and molecular consequences of endothelial BMPR2 mutation. Respir Res 12: 84–96.
29. Pfarr N, Szamalek-Hoegel J, Fischer C, Hinderhofer K, Nagel C, et al. (2011) Hemodynamic and clinical onset in patients with hereditary pulmonary arterial hypertension and BMPR2 mutations. Respir Res 12: 99–109.
30. Chida A, Shintani M, Nakayama T, Furutani Y, Hayama E, et al. (2012) Missense Mutations of the BMPR1B (ALK6) Gene in Childhood Idiopathic Pulmonary Arterial Hypertension. Circ J 76(7): 1804–1811.
31. Machado RD, Aldred MA, James V, Harrison RE, Patel B, et al. (2006) Mutations of the TGF-b Type II Receptor BMPR2 in Pulmonary Arterial Hypertension. Hum Mutat 27(2): 121–132.
32. Czech A, Fedyunin I, Zhang G, Ignatova Z (2010) Silent mutations in sight: co-variations in tRNA abundance as a key to unravel consequences of silent mutations. Mol BioSyst 6: 1767–1772.
33. Girerd B, Montani D, Coulet F, Sztrymf B, Yaici A, et al. (2010) Clinical Outcomes of Pulmonary Arterial Hypertension in Patients Carrying an ACVRL1 (ALK1) Mutation. Am J Respir Crit Care Med 181: 851–861.
34. Selva-O'Callaghan A, Balada E, Serrano-Acedo S, Simeon-Aznar CP, Ordi-Ros J (2007) Mutations of activin-receptor-like kinase 1 (ALK-1) are not found in patients with pulmonary hypertension and underlying connective tissue disease. Clin Rheumatol 26: 947–949.
35. Fujiwara M, Yagi H, Matsuoka R, Akimoto K, Furutani M, et al. (2008) Implications of Mutations of Activin Receptor-Like Kinase 1 Gene (ALK1) in Addition to Bone Morphogenetic Protein Receptor II Gene (BMPR2) in Children With Pulmonary Arterial Hypertension. Circ J 72: 127–133.
36. Abdalla SA, Cymerman U, Johnson RM, Deber CM, Letarte M (2003) Disease-associated mutations in conserved residues of ALK-1 kinase domain. Eur J Hum Genet 11: 279–287.
37. Schulte C, Geisthoff U, Lux A, Kupkal S, Zenner HP, et al. (2005) High frequency of ENG and ALK1/ACVRL1 mutations in german HHT patients. Hum Mutat 25(6): 595–602.
38. Remillard CV, Tigno DD, Platoshyn O, Burg ED, Brevnova EE, et al. (2007) Function of Kv1.5 channels and genetic variations of KCNA5 in patients with idiopathic pulmonary arterial hypertension. Am J Physiol Cell Physiol 292: C1837–C1853.
39. Christophersen IE, Olesen MS, Liang B, Andersen MN, Larsen AP, et al. (2013) Genetic variation in KCNA5: impact on the atrial-specific potassium current IKur in patients with lone atrial fibrillation. Eur Heart J 34(20): 1517–25.
40. Burg ED, Platoshyn O, Tsigelny IF, Lozano-Ruiz B, Rana BK, et al. (2010) Tetramerization domain mutations in KCNA5 affect channel kinetics and cause abnormal trafficking patterns. Am J Physiol Cell Physiol 98(3): C496–509.
41. Kurata HT, Soon GS, Eldstrom JR, Lu GW, Steele DF, et al. (2002) Amino-terminal determinants of U-type inactivation of voltage-gated K+ channels. J Biol Chem 277(32): 29045–53.
42. Park WS, Firth AL, Han J, Ko EA (2010) Patho-, physiological roles of voltage-dependent K+ channels in pulmonary arterial smooth muscle cells. J. Smooth Muscle Res 46(2): 89–105.
43. Liu D, Wu WH, Mao YM, Yuan P, Zhang R, et al. (2012) BMPR2 mutations influence phenotype more obviously in male patients with pulmonary arterial hypertension. Circ Cardiovasc Genet 5(5): 511–8.

6

Exercise Training Improves Exercise Capacity and Quality of Life in Patients with Inoperable or Residual Chronic Thromboembolic Pulmonary Hypertension

Christian Nagel[1][9], Felix Prange[1][9], Stefan Guth[2][9], Jochen Herb[1], Nicola Ehlken[1], Christine Fischer[3], Frank Reichenberger[4], Stephan Rosenkranz[5], Hans-Juergen Seyfarth[6], Eckhard Mayer[2], Michael Halank[7][9], Ekkehard Grünig[1]*[9]

1 Centre for Pulmonary Hypertension, Thoraxclinic at University Hospital Heidelberg, Heidelberg, Germany, 2 Department of Thoracic Surgery, Kerckhoff-Klinik Bad Nauheim, Bad Nauheim, Germany, 3 Department of Human Genetics, University of Heidelberg, Heidelberg, Germany, 4 Department of Pneumology, University Gießen-Marburg, Gießen, Germany, 5 Department of Cardiology, University of Cologne, Cologne, Germany, 6 Department of Pneumology, University of Leipzig, Leipzig, Germany, 7 Department of Pneumology, University of Dresden, Dresden, Germany

Abstract

Background: Aim of this prospective study was to evaluate the effects of exercise training in patients with inoperable or residual chronic thromboembolic pulmonary hypertension (CTEPH).

Methods: Thirty-five consecutive patients with invasively confirmed inoperable or residual CTEPH (16 women;19 men; mean age 61±15 years, mean pulmonary artery pressure, 63±20 mmHg; primary inoperable n=33, persisting pulmonary hypertension after pulmonary endarterectomy n=2) on stable disease-targeted medication received exercise training in-hospital for 3 weeks and continued at home for 15 weeks. Medication remained unchanged during the study period. Efficacy parameters have been evaluated at baseline, after 3 and 15 weeks by blinded-observers. Survival rate has been evaluated in a follow-up period of median 36.4 months (interquartile range 26.6–46.6 months).

Results: All patients tolerated exercise training without severe adverse events. Patients significantly improved the mean distance walked in 6 minutes compared to baseline by 61±54 meters after 3 weeks (p<0.001) and by 71±70 meters after 15 weeks (p=0.001), as well as scores of quality-of-life questionnaire, peak oxygen consumption and maximal workload. NT-proBNP improved significantly after 3 weeks of exercise training (p=0.046). The 1-year survival rate was 97%, 2-year survival rate was 94% and the 3-year-survival 86% respectively.

Conclusion: Training as add-on to medical therapy may be effective in patients with CTEPH to improve work capacity, quality of life and further prognostic relevant parameters and possibly improves the 1-, 2- and 3-year survival rate. Further multicentric randomized controlled studies are needed to confirm these promising results.

Editor: Michael Lipinski, University of Virginia Health System, United States of America

Funding: The study was funded by a grant of the German patient organization Pulmonale Hypertonie e.V., Rheinstetten, Germany. The funders had no role in study design, data collection and analysis, decision to publish, or preparation of the manuscript.

Competing Interests: The authors have declared that no competing interests exist.

* E-mail: ekkehard.gruenig@thoraxklinik-heidelberg.de

[9] These authors contributed equally to this work.

Introduction

Chronic thromboembolic pulmonary hypertension (CTEPH) is a rare complication of acute pulmonary embolism due to unresolved emboli initiating remodeling of the non-obstructed pulmonary arteries leading to progressive increase in pulmonary vascular resistance (PVR) [1]. The incidence of CTEPH is not known, but recent studies suggest that 1–4.6% of patients develop the condition within 2 years after an episode of acute pulmonary embolism [2,3,4]. Pulmonary endarterectomy (PEA) with removal of the obstructive material is the only curative treatment and can

be performed in about 60% of patients [5]. However, about 40% of patients with CTEPH are not operable [5] and 16% to 32% of operated patients suffer from persistent or recurrent pulmonary hypertension (PH) [6]. Clinical presentation with right heart failure and histological damage of pulmonary arteries is similar in CTEPH and pulmonary arterial hypertension (PAH). Therefore, CTEPH patients may benefit from medical therapy that has been approved for PAH. Various uncontrolled clinical trials propound the hypothesis that prostanoids, endothelin receptor antagonists (ERAs) and phosphodiesterase type-5-inhibitors may improve hemodynamics and exercise capacity in patients with operable or inoperable CTEPH [7]. However, the only 2 controlled trials in CTEPH were inconclusive. Subgroup analysis of 57 patients with CTEPH of the Aerosolized Iloprost Randomization (AIR) study showed an improvement in quality of life but failed to prove a significant benefit on exercise capacity and hemodynamics [8]. The BENEFIT-study with Bosentan in CTEPH resulted in a significant improvement of pulmonary vascular resistance and Borg index but did not improve exercise capacity measured by 6-minute walking distance, WHO-functional class (WHO-FC) or time to clinical worsening [9]. Thus, until now beside lifelong anticoagulation no further medical therapy has been approved in Europe or USA for treatment in CTEPH [10,11]. Selected patients may benefit of PH-targeted drug therapy but cautious use is advised by current guidelines [10,11]. Preoperative treatment has been reported to have minimal effect on pre-PEA hemodynamics and no effect on post-PEA outcome [12], and may induce unnecessary delay to a potentially curative surgical intervention [12,13]. Although studies in CTEPH already showed an improvement of survival rate compared to earlier trials without optimized medical PH-targeted therapy [14] survival is still unsatisfying with 82–87%, 75–77% and 70–77% after 1, 2 and 3 years, respectively [15,16].

Therefore, patients with inoperable or residual CTEPH have a need for additional therapeutic tools addressing their exercise capacity, quality of life and survival. Exercise training has been a useful add-on therapy in other forms of PH [17,18]. The effect of exercise training in patients with inoperable or residual CTEPH has not yet been evaluated systematically. The objective of the present study was to evaluate safety and effectiveness of exercise training in patients with inoperable or residual CTEPH as add on to optimized medical PH-targeted therapy and to analyze long-term survival.

Methods

Study Population and Design

The protocol for this trial and supporting CONSORT checklist with flow-chart are available as supporting information; see Checklist S1, flow-chart Figure S1 and Protocol S1.

Our investigation included patients between 18 and 80 years with CTEPH and WHO-FC II–IV who received exercise and respiratory therapy as add-on to PH -targeted medication between June 2006 and October 2011. Patients had to be stable under optimized medical therapy including inhaled ERAs, inhaled or parenteral prostanoids, phosphodiesterase inhibitors, anticoagulants, diuretics, and supplemental oxygen for least 2 months before entering the study. According to current guidelines [11,12] all patients underwent a detailed clinical work up at the participating PH centers, including right heart catheterization, ventilation/perfusion lung scan, computed tomography angiography and pulmonary angiography to establish the diagnosis. The status "inoperable CTEPH" had been confirmed by experienced PEA-surgeons (SG, EM). All patients gave written informed consent for this study, which was approved by the Ethics Committee of the University of Heidelberg.

Outcome Measures

Efficacy parameters were assessed at baseline, week 3 and week 15 as described previously [17,18]. 6-minute-walking-distance (6MWD) was performed under standardized conditions [19]. Cardiopulmonary exercise testing and stress Doppler echocardiography were carried out during supine bicycle exercise as described previously [17]. Workload, heart rate, systolic pulmonary artery pressure (sPAP), systolic (RRsys) and diastolic

(RRdias) systemic blood pressures, ventilation (VE), oxygen uptake (VO_2), oxygen pulse (VO_2/heart rate), and carbon dioxide output (VCO_2) were evaluated continuously. V-slope method was used to detect the anaerobic threshold (AT). We analyzed gas exchange, Borg dyspnea index (with 6 representing no exertion and 20 maximal exertion) [20] and changes in WHO-FC after 3 and 15 weeks. Health related quality of life was measured by the Short Form Health Survey questionnaire (SF-36) [21] at baseline was compared to the results after 15 weeks. Serum N-terminal pro brain natriuretic peptide (NT-proBNP) was obtained at baseline and after 3 and 15 weeks. 6MWD, SF-36-questionnaire and NT-proBNP have been obtained and analyzed by investigators who have been blinded to clinical data of the patients.

Exercise Training Program

We designed a program for patients with PH with a minimum of 1.5 h/day exercise training as described earlier [17,18,22]. For the first 3 weeks the program took place in the Rehabilitation Clinic Koenigstuhl Heidelberg. The different parts of the program were interval bicycle ergometer training at low workloads, walking, respiratory training at 5 days/week and dumbbell-training of single muscle groups using low weights (500–1000 g). Patients continued training at home for at least 30 minutes/day at 5 days a week for 12 weeks. Additional to physical training patients received psychological support and performed mental training helping them to improve their perception of individual physical abilities and limits. During the study period the program was closely supervised by physicians specialized in rehabilitation medicine and PH-experts as described earlier [17,18,22]. Adverse events were recorded whenever they occurred. Oxygen saturation (sO2) and heart rate were monitored continuously throughout the training and used to adjust the training intensity. When patients' SO_2 passed below 90% during exercise they received supplemental oxygen (3–10 L/min) throughout the training. Before leaving the hospital after 3 weeks, patients were given an individualized training manual and a bicycle ergometer for use at home was ordered. Physiotherapists and physicians stayed in close contact to patients and supervised the planned training at home by phone call every 2–4 weeks. All patients were asked to keep close contact to physicians of the training program and to their general practitioners and specialized center.

Follow-up Assessment

In 2011 all participating patients were interviewed by telephone or at a control visit in the Thoraxklinik Heidelberg using a half-structured questionnaire. The patients were asked for present symptoms, WHO-FC, current medication, what kind of exercise training they pursued at home, for any adverse events of exercise training and any further cardiac events that might have occurred since last observation. If the index patient was deceased, date of death was recorded and their relatives and/or treating physicians were asked for the cause and circumstances of death.

Statistical Methods

The analyses were performed by a statistician (C.F.). Data are given as mean ± standard deviation and as median, 25% and 75% quantiles for more detailed description at baseline. Statistical tests shown in table 2 were performed without assuming normal distributions. The inner-group comparisons of baseline, weeks 3 and 15 for 6MWD, workload, Borg dyspnea index, parameters of gas exchange, PASP, systemic blood pressure, NT-proBNP, heart rate, summation and subscores of the SF-36 questionnaire were compared by Wilcoxon rank test. WHO-FC comparison at different time points was performed by McNemar-Bowden test.

All tests were two sided and p-values <0.05 were considered statistically significant. Bonferroni adjustment for multiple comparisons was performed for comparisons of the primary endpoints such as parameters of quality of life and 6-minute walking distances. In a previous study of 58 patients with pulmonary hypertension of other ethiology we showed an improvement in 6MWD of 84±49 meter. Under a conservative assumption of a difference of 40 meter and a standard deviation of 50 meter, taking multiple testing of 6MWD and 8 quality of life scales by Bonferroni adjustment into account, we calculated (t-test situation) that we would need 30 patients to detect the difference (if present) with a power of 90%. Furthermore, analysis of dropouts that did not attend the 15 week measurement was performed. All analyses were carried out with IBM SPSS V20 (IBM Corp. Armonk, NY, USA). For missing values we performed different imputation strategies and reported the values from the most strict one: 1. multiple imputation using the MCMC method as implemented in SPSS, 2. the last observation carried forward, 3. the baseline carried forward and a pessimistic imputation, in which 3 week 6MWD was imputed as 15 week measurement if it was lower than baseline, otherwise the baseline 6MWD. Kaplan-Meier estimates have been used for survival-analysis with 95% two-sided asymptotic confidence interval (CI). All treated patients were used for the survival analysis. Patients with deaths were counted as endpoints, survivors were regarded as censored.

Results

Study Population (Table 1)

We prospectively recruited 39 consecutive patients for this study, 2 had to be excluded due to a change in their PA-targeted medication 2–4 weeks before admission to the rehabilitation hospital, 2 patients had been misdiagnosed as CTEPH and turned out as PAH. Thus, the final study group consisted of 35 consecutive patients in our study group (16 women, 19 men): 33 patients with inoperable CTEPH (94%) and 2 patients with residual CTEPH after PEA (6%). Demographic data, diagnosis, functional class, hemodynamic values, lung function and medical therapy of the study population are summarized in table 1. At baseline 7 patients were in WHO-FC II (20%), 26 patients were classified in WHO-FC III (74%) and 2 in WHO-FC IV (6%). Combination therapies including 2 to 3 PAH-targeted agents were used in 46% of patients (Table 1).

Assessment of Training Effects

Training significantly improved the 6MWD from 408±108 meters by 61±54 meters after 3 weeks (p<0.001) and by 71±70 meters after 15 weeks (p=0.001) (Figure 1, Table 2). All patients except six improved in 6MWD (Figure 1). The patient with the highest decrease of 6MWD had experienced a syncope as described in the adverse events section and walked intentionally less after 3 and 15 weeks in order to avoid another syncope. Three of the 6 further "non-responders" deceased during follow-up (after 2, 2.2 and 2.8 years, respectively). In one of these patients other parameters of physical exercise capacity had improved during training. Two further patients improved in their 6MWD after 3 weeks but had a slight decrease compared to baseline after 15 weeks. All other patients improved in their 6MWD, most of them continued with exercise training at home.

Training also significantly improved quality of life parameters indicated by the SF-36 subscale scores for physical functioning (p=0.041) and vitality (p=0.03, Figure 2, Table 2). Using Bonferroni adjustment for 6MWD and quality of life scales improvement of 6 MWD remained statistically significant.

Mean peak oxygen consumption, peak oxygen consumption per kg body weight, workloads with an increase of maximal heart rate during cardiopulmonary exercise testing increased significantly from baseline to 3 weeks and to 15 weeks (Table 2). NT-proBNP plasma levels were significantly reduced after 3 weeks. The change in WHO-FC compared to baseline after 3 weeks and after 15 weeks was not significant (p=0.157 and p=0.157).

Missing Value Analysis

Thirteen patients (37%) did not attend the visit after 15 weeks (12 referred from other PH-centers than Heidelberg) mainly due to the long travel distance. They showed at baseline no significant differences for most parameters except maximal systolic and diastolic blood pressure. However, although statistically not significant, patients had a tendency of being older, having a higher BMI, lower 6MWD at baseline and after 3 weeks and lower improvement of 6MWD and slightly worse values for all quality of life scales in comparison to patients who completed all visits.

Results remained significant after imputation of missing values for the 6 MWD at 15 weeks using the rules described in the methods: a) the last observation carried forward method revealed an improvement of 60.2±62.5 Meters, p<0.001; b) the baseline carried forward revealed 42.6±62.5 meters, p<0.001; c) pessimistic imputation: improvement of 40.8±66.1 meters, p=0.001.

Adverse Events

During the 3 weeks in-hospital training 5 patients had an adverse event, in two cases (5.7%) it was related or possibly related to the training program. In one patient syncope occurred during the in-hospital rehabilitation after climbing three flights of stairs. Intensity of exercise training was reduced and the patient was able to continue the program without any further events. He was however concerned to get another syncope and walked intentionally less in the test of 6MWD after 3 and 15 weeks. The other patient had a herpes zoster infection 2 months after in-hospital training, which was possibly related to exercise training and was treated successfully by antiviral therapy and continued afterwards. In the other 3 patients adverse events had been respiratory infections, which were not related to the training itself. These patients had to interrupt the training program during the in-hospital rehabilitation and were treated successfully by antibiotic therapy. They continued with the training after recovery and showed an improvement in 6MWD and peak oxygen consumption after 15 weeks. All other patients (86%) tolerated exercise training well. There were no signs of clinical worsening of right heart failure during the in-hospital program. All patients reported that they had improved their awareness of their physical abilities and limitations.

Follow-up and Survival

Follow-up data were obtained after a median of 36.4 months (0.8 to 5.2 years after baseline/start of the in-hospital rehabilitation, interquartile range 26.6–46.6 months). During follow-up 6 patients died. Three due to CTEPH and right heart failure, one patient due to sudden cardiac death, one patient died due to lung cancer 4.2 years after baseline. In one further patient the cause of death remained unknown. The Kaplan-Meier overall-survival rate was 97% after 1-year, 94% after 2-years and 86% after 3 years (figure 3). We interviewed the 29 surviving patients for actual symptoms, worsening events and continuation of exercise training. Of the 29 patients assessed during follow-up, 23 (79%) had been continuing exercise training, 19 for more than 3 years after baseline. 20 of the 23 continued bicycle ergometer training, 13 dumbbell-training, 9 walking, 15 respiratory training and 17

Table 1. Baseline Characteristics.

				median	Q25	Q75
Patients [n]		35				
Gender [male/female]	19	/	16			
Age [years]	61	±	15	64	53	71
Height [cm]	170.5	±	10	170	161	178
Weight [kg]	78	±	13	78	70	86
WHO functional Class – No. [%]						
II	7		20%			
III	26		74%			
IV	2		6%			
6MWD [meters]	408	±	108	420	336	489
Cardiac Catheterization						
mPAP [mmHg]	48	±	16	50	35	57
PVR [dyn×sec×cm^{-5}]	784	±	399	701	497	945
RA pressure [mmHg]	7.2	±	4.8	7.0	3	10.5
SaO$_2$ [%]	91.4	±	3.1	91	90	93.9
PCWP [mmHg]	9.3	±	4.3	8.5	7	12
CI [L/min/m^2]	2.3	±	0.5	2.3	1.85	2.36
Echocardiography						
sPAP at rest, mmHg	64	±	20	60	50	80
sPAP during exercise, mmHg	94	±	25	95	75	110
RV area, cm^2	28.4	±	10.4	28.5	19	34
RA area, cm^2	26.0	±	8.5	26.5	18.5	33.5
TAPSE, cm	1.98	±	0.32	1.95	1.8	2.2
PAH-targeted medication						
Endothelin Receptor Antagonist	21		60%			
Phosphodiesterase-5-Inhibitor	21		60%			
Prostanoids inhaled	6		17%			
Prostanoids intravenous	1		3%			
Calcium Channel Blockers	2		6%			
Soluble guanyl cyclase Stimulator	2		6%			
Combination therapy						
Monotherapy	17		49%			
Dualtherapy	10		29%			
Tripletherapy	6		17%			

Values are given as mean±SD, median and 25 and 75% Quantile (Q25, Q75) or as n and %. mPAP = mean pulmonary arterial pressure, PVR = pulmonary vascular resistance, RA = right atrium, SaO$_2$ = oxygen saturation, PCWP = pulmonary capillary wedge pressure, CI = Cardiac Index, sPAP = systolic pulmonary arterial pressure, RV = right ventricle, TAPSE = tricuspid plane annular systolic excursion.

alternative training such as gymnastics. Nine patients combined two items, 5 patients three items and 5 patients four items. Four patients (14%) did not continue the training after the end of the study for the following reasons: one patient discontinued due to clinical worsening, two further patients mentioned lack of time, the fourth patient was mainly limited by musculoskeletal pain and did not see an improvement by exercise training.

Discussion

This is the first prospective clinical trial investigating short- and long-term effects of exercise training as add-on to PAH-targeted medication in patients with severe CTEPH. The results of the study suggest that training in pulmonary hypertension can significantly improve prognostic relevant parameters as exercise capacity and quality of life in this condition and has an excellent long-term survival of 97% after 1 year, 94% after 2 years and 86% after 3 years, respectively.

The results represent an important source of data on survival, exercise capacity and quality of life in patients with CTEPH treated with exercise and respiratory therapy. Mean 6MWD significantly improved by almost 20%, mean peak oxygen consumption by 16%, and mean maximal workload by 40% during 15 weeks of the training program. This had a significant impact on quality of life improving two of eight scores of the SF36 questionnaire. The positive effect of exercise training was also documented in a significant decrease (>20%) of mean NT-proBNP after 3 weeks. Overall compliance was excellent with a

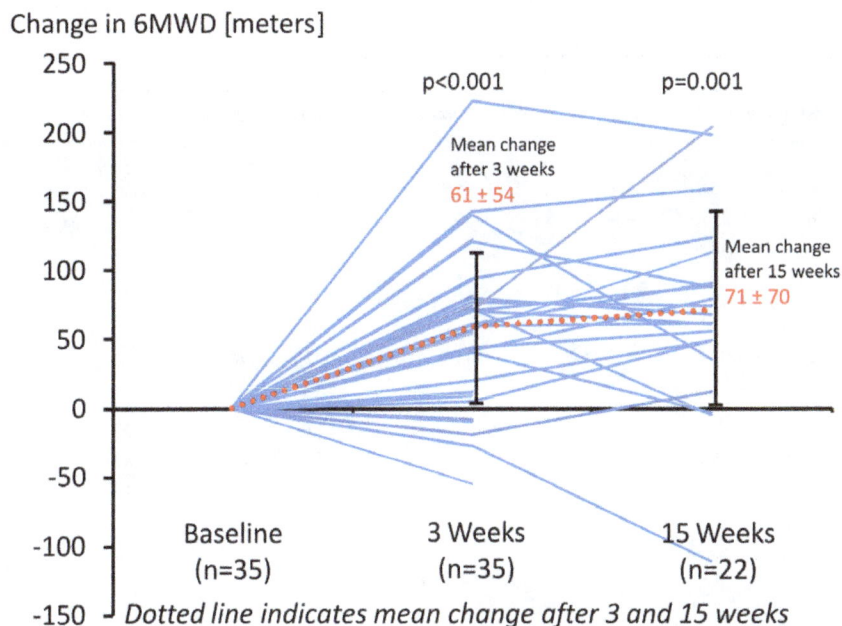

Figure 1. Individual changes in Six-Minute-Walking Distance (6MWD) after 3 and 15 weeks exercise training. With the use of Wilcoxon Rank Test according to baseline walking distance, p<0.001 was obtained for the comparison to baseline with weeks 3 (n = 35) and p = 0.001 with week 15 (n = 22). The dotted line indicates the mean change from baseline in 6MWD (61±54 meters and 71±70 meters).

continuation in 79% during the follow-up period of 36.5±17 months. However, these data must be confirmed in randomized, controlled studies. The results of this study are in line with previous studies of training in patients with other forms of PH/PAH [17,18,22,23,24]. These studies showed similar effects in patients with various forms of PH and right heart insufficiency in a randomized controlled study [17] and in single-arm, non-controlled designs [18,22,23]. However, in these studies only few patients with CTEPH had been included. Thus, there are almost no previous data on the effect of exercise training in patients with inoperable or residual CTEPH. The promising results of this study suggest that training may be an important add-on therapy in CTEPH regarding long-term survival, exercise capacity, quality of life and oxygen consumption.

Improvement in 6-Minute-walking-distance

The 6MWD has been used as primary end-point in many randomized controlled clinical trials in PAH [11] and correlated with mortality and prognostically relevant parameters [25]. In patients with medically treated inoperable CTEPH 6MWD was the only independent predictor of long-term survival [16,26]. Furthermore, 6MWD and NT-proBNP were independent predictors of perioperative mortality [27]. Pre-operative cut-off values for NT-proBNP of 1200 pg/ml and 345 m for 6MWD had both high negative predictive values for mortality [27].

Previous uncontrolled drug-trials with Riociguat [28] and Bosentan [29,30,31,32] in small cohorts of CTEPH-patients showed a significant increase in 6MWD, whereas in a randomized controlled trial Bosentan did not significantly improve 6MWD [10]. Therefore, a mean increase of 61 meters after 3 weeks and 71 meters after 15 weeks exercise and respiratory therapy is unexpectedly high. The absence of a non-trained "placebo" group may be considered a limitation of the study, with concern that some of the improvements were due to "placebo" effect, rather than efficacy of the training program. However, previously

reported placebo controlled PAH studies of Bosentan or other PAH-targeted drugs have not shown any clinically relevant improvements in placebo groups. In fact, they have generally shown a decline. Despite the limitations of this study the magnitude of the mean improvements from baseline in 6MWD and other parameters as quality of life makes the findings promising. Further randomized, controlled studies are warranted.

Survival of Patients with CTEPH after Training

The survival estimate of 97% after 1 year, 94% after 2 years and 86% after 3 years using exercise training as add-on to optimized PAH targeted medical treatment can be considered as a positive outcome in CTEPH. Despite optimized PAH-targeted therapy several studies report a lower 1 year (87%/82%), 2 year (77%/75%) and 3 year survival rate (77%/70%) [15,16]. One study showed a comparable 1 year survival rate of 96% [31].

The CTEPH-cohort assessed in this study has been severely affected with a mean 6MWD of 408±108 meters at baseline despite double or even triple PAH targeted therapy in 46% of patients and is therefore comparable to the cohorts described previously. However, we cannot exclude that we selected highly motivated and compliant patients with less outcome limitations. Nevertheless, exercise training may have improved survival by ameliorating prognostic relevant factors as quality of life and exercise capacity. Since maximal heart rate during cardiopulmonary exercise testing and peak oxygen consumption significantly improved, exercise training possibly improved right ventricular contractile reserve [18]. Similar effects of training have been seen in patients with IPAH and right heart failure [18,22].

Limitations

Limitations of our study include its relatively small sample size and lack of randomization. Because of this, there could be a referral bias that CTEPH patients who do well have been selected. Furthermore patients were well-aware of the assignment to a

Table 2. Efficacy parameters.

Characteristic	Baseline (n = 35)		3 weeks (n = 35)		p-value		15 weeks (n = 22)		p-value	
6MWD										
Walking distance [meters]	408	± 108	468	± 130			509	± 81		
mean change [meters]			60.5	± 54	<0.001	*	71	± 70	0.001	*
95% CI for the difference to baseline			41.3	– 79.8			39.2	– 102.9		
change: median Q25,Q75 [meters]			71.0	41.5	87.0		68.0	42.0	102.0	
Quality of life Questionnaire SF-36										
Physical functioning	36.2	± 20.4					40.9	± 27,4	0.041	#
Role-physical	33.9	± 36.8					40.9	± 44.0	0.67	
Bodily pain	70	± 28					73.2	± 30.8	0.367	
General health perception	40.9	± 16.6					44.7	± 15.3	0.777	
Vitality	46.4	± 16.6					51.1	± 18.1	0.03	#
Social functioning	62.9	± 31.9					67.9	± 29.4	0.114	
Role-emotional	54	± 47.5					60.8	± 45.7	0.177	
Mental Health	63.2	± 18.7					64.5	± 21.2	0.174	
Cardiopulmonary exercise testing										
peak VO$_2$/kg [mL/Min/kg]	12.1	± 1.7	13.4	± 3.7	0.003	*	14	± 2.9	0.017	#
peak VO$_2$ [mL/min]	933.2	± 335.3	1028.8	± 330.6	0.022	#	1111	± 304.2	0.014	#
EqCO$_2$ at AT [mL/min]	50	± 10.9	47.6	± 11.7	0.264		48	± 12.8	0.953	
VO$_2$ at AT [mL/min]	672.8	± 236.4	638	± 242.3	0.872		846.4	± 259.7	0.441	
O$_2$-pulse [(mL/min)/min-1]	8.2	± 2.7	8.8	± 2.9	0.345		8.8	± 3.1	0.185	
HR rest [min-1]	73.2	± 12	70.8	± 10.2	0.657		73.8	± 11.8	0.679	
HR max [min-1]	114.8	± 19.7	118.9	± 23.5	0.049	#	129.5	± 19.4	0.010	#
RR sys rest [mmHg]	117.6	± 15.5	118.4	± 13.4	0.989		112.8	± 30.3	0.852	
RR dia rest [mmHg]	77.5	± 11.3	76.8	± 9.1	0.266		78.3	± 9.9	0.924	
RR sys max [mmHg]	143.5	± 27.5	150.1	± 26	0.210		143.2	± 43.8	0.586	
RR dia max [mmHg]	85.4	± 15	83.1	± 20.4	0.653		89.6	± 13.6	0.811	
Oxygen saturation rest [%]	93	± 6.2	92.8	± 6.6	0.472		95.2	± 2.2	0.605	
Oxygen saturation max [%]	87.9	± 7.8	88.7	± 6.8	0.820		89.9	± 3.5	0.440	
sPAP rest [mmHg]	63.5	± 20.3	62.5	± 20.5	0.710		56.8	± 15.9	0.083	
sPAP max [mmHg]	94.1	± 25.2	91.9	± 32.9	0.458		94.1	± 27	0.243	
Workload max [Watt]	64.1	± 28	76.7	± 27.8	0.005	*	90	± 22	0.010	#
Borg Scale	14.9	± 2.3	15.6	± 2.2	0.071		16.2	± 1.6	0.015	#
Laboratory parameters										
NT-proBNP [pg/mL]	2334.5	± 2886.8	1715.9	± 2263.4	0.046	#	2500.6	± 2896.7	0.339	

Values are mean±SD, q25:25% quantile, q75:75% quantile, CI = 95% confidence interval 6MWD,
~p<0.08; #p<0.05; *p<0.01 in comparison to baseline we show Wilcoxon test p-values.
6-MWD = 6-minute walking distance, VO2/kg = max.oxygen consumption/kg, HR = heart rate, RR = Blood pressure.
sPAP = systolic Pulmonary arterial pressure.

training study, which may also have favored the results. The effects of exercise training after 15 weeks may be further biased due to the missing values of about 37% of patients who did not perform the last follow-up visit. However, the efficacy after 3 weeks exercise and respiratory therapy and the high proportion of patients who continued with the program suggest a positive effect in this cohort. The significant effect and high compliance of exercise training in inoperable CTEPH might also be due to the closely supervised in-hospital rehabilitation program, which probably cannot be simply translated to an out-patient program. This limits the application of this program in other countries which cannot provide in-hospital rehabilitation care. Therefore, further studies are necessary using ambulatory training programs.

It is a general issue of rehabilitation programs that the therapy cannot be performed in a blinded fashion and that a referral bias towards highly motivated patients with a better outcome may occur. Further studies are necessary to determine the effects of training programs on outcome in patients with pulmonary hypertension.

Conclusions

This is the first trial investigating exercise training in CTEPH as add-on to optimized medical therapy. The results indicate that exercise training is effective in CTEPH and may improve work capacity, quality of life and further prognostic relevant parameters. Exercise and respiratory therapy possibly improves survival rate.

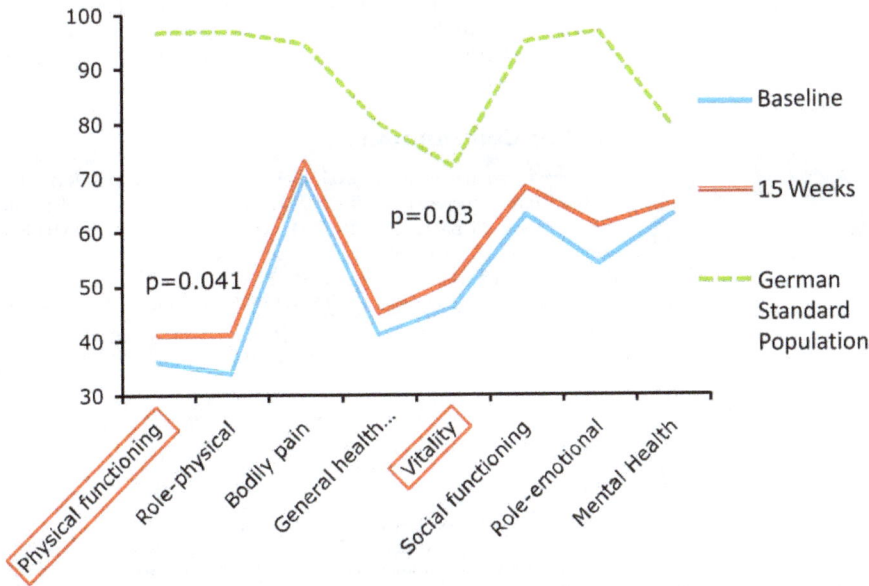

Figure 2. Mean SF-36 scores of Quality of life Subscales (SF-36 questionnaire) before and after Exercise Training. At baseline (straight line), mean SF-36 scores were significantly reduced in comparison to respective values of a normal population (dotted line). After 15 weeks (dashed line), the 2 subscales of the SF-36 questionnaire physical functioning and vitality improved significantly. P-values are indicated vs. baseline. No significant improvement was found for role emotional (ROLEM), role physical (ROLPH), general health (GH), social functioning (SF), mental health (MH), bodily pain (PAIN) after training. With Bonferroni adjustment, values of p<0.005 preserve statistical significance. At baseline data of 28 patients, after 15 weeks of 23 patients were available and included.

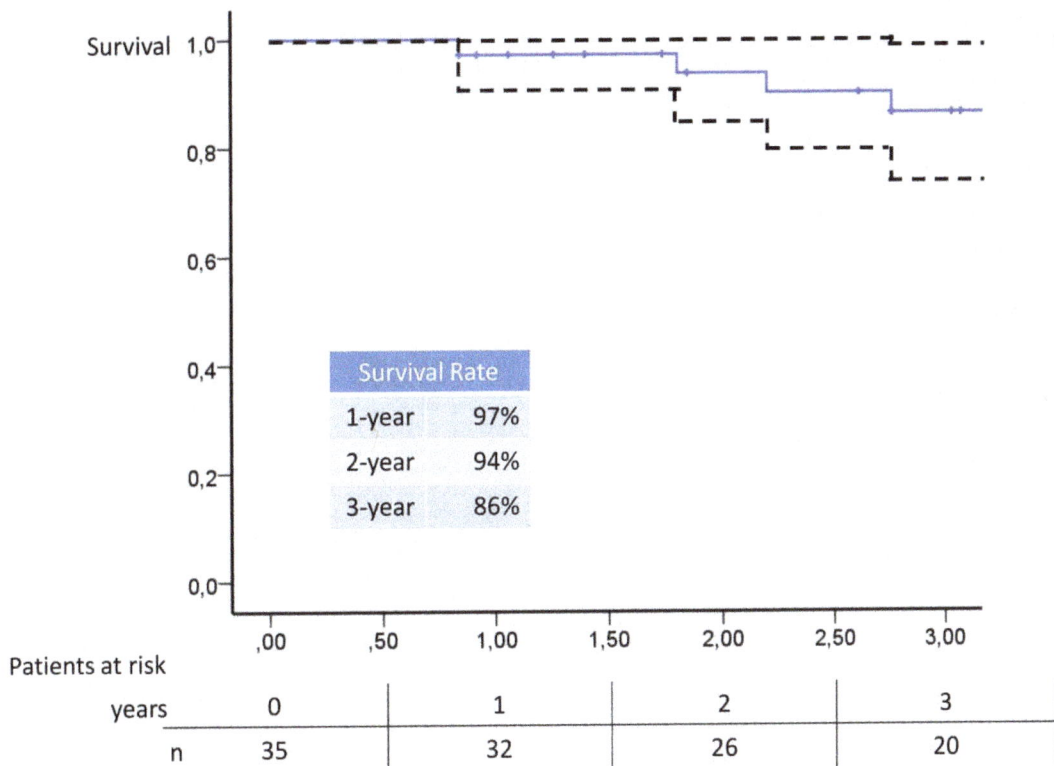

Figure 3. Survival by Kaplan Meier Analysis. Within a follow-up period of median 36.4 months (interquartile range 26.6–46.6 months) 6 patients deceased, 4 due to PH. One patient died due to lung cancer >4 years after baseline. In one patient cause of death remained unknown. The straight line indicates overall survival, with 97% after 1-year, 94% after 2-years and 86% after 3 years. The dashed line indicates 95% Confidence interval.

Further randomized studies are needed to confirm these promising results.

Supporting Information

Figure S1   CONSORT Flow-chart

Checklist S1   CONSORT Checklist

Protocol S1   Trial Protocol

Acknowledgments

We would like to thank all patients who participated, the self-help group pulmonary hypertension e.V., especially Bruno Kopp for their support. We are grateful and thank for the support of the clinic director Karl-Heinz Markmann and Dr. Nechwatal, all physicians, therapists, and physiotherapists of the Rehabilitation-Clinic Koenigstuhl Heidelberg, who took part in the rehabilitation program.

Author Contributions

Conceived and designed the experiments: CN EG NE SG EM MH. Performed the experiments: EG CN MH EM SG. Analyzed the data: CF NE FP. Wrote the paper: CN FP SG JH NE CF FR SR HJS EM MH EG. Directly involved in acquisition of data: FP JH. Principle investigators directly involved in data collection: SG EM FR SR HJS MH. Approved the final version of the paper: CN FP SG JH NE CF FR SR HJS EM MH EG.

References

1. Hoeper MM, Mayer E, Simonneau G, Rubin LJ (2006) Chronic thromboembolic pulmonary hypertension. Circulation 113: 2011–2020.
2. Pengo V, Lensing AW, Prins MH, Marchiori A, Davidson BL, et al. (2004) Incidence of chronic thromboembolic pulmonary hypertension after pulmonary embolism. N Engl J Med 350: 2257–2264.
3. Becattini C, Agnelli G, Pesavento R, Silingardi M, Poggio R, et al. (2006) Incidence of chronic thromboembolic pulmonary hypertension after a first episode of pulmonary embolism. Chest 130: 172–175.
4. Korkmaz A, Ozlu T, Ozsu S, Kazaz Z, Bulbul Y (2012) Long-Term Outcomes in Acute Pulmonary Thromboembolism: The Incidence of Chronic Thromboembolic Pulmonary Hypertension and Associated Risk Factors. Clin Appl Thromb Hemost.
5. Pepke-Zaba J, Delcroix M, Lang I, Mayer E, Jansa P, et al. (2011) Chronic thromboembolic pulmonary hypertension (CTEPH): results from an international prospective registry. Circulation 124: 1973–1981.
6. Freed DH, Thomson BM, Berman M, Tsui SS, Dunning J, et al. (2011) Survival after pulmonary thromboendarterectomy: effect of residual pulmonary hypertension. J Thorac Cardiovasc Surg 141: 383–387.
7. Lang IM (2009) Managing chronic thromboembolic pulmonary hypertension: pharmacological treatment options. Eur Respir Rev 18: 24–28.
8. Olschewski H, Simonneau G, Galie N, Higenbottam T, Naeije R, et al. (2002) Inhaled iloprost for severe pulmonary hypertension. The New England journal of medicine 347: 322–329.
9. Jais X, D'Armini AM, Jansa P, Torbicki A, Delcroix M, et al. (2008) Bosentan for treatment of inoperable chronic thromboembolic pulmonary hypertension: BENEFiT (Bosentan Effects in iNopErable Forms of chronIc Thromboembolic pulmonary hypertension), a randomized, placebo-controlled trial. J Am Coll Cardiol 52: 2127–2134.
10. Galie N, Hoeper MM, Humbert M, Torbicki A, Vachiery JL, et al. (2009) Guidelines for the diagnosis and treatment of pulmonary hypertension. Eur Respir J 34: 1219–1263.
11. Wilkens H, Lang I, Behr J, Berghaus T, Grohe C, et al. (2011) Chronic thromboembolic pulmonary hypertension (CTEPH): Updated Recommendations of the Cologne Consensus Conference 2011. Int J Cardiol 154 Suppl 1: S54–60.
12. Jensen KW, Kerr KM, Fedullo PF, Kim NH, Test VJ, et al. (2009) Pulmonary hypertensive medical therapy in chronic thromboembolic pulmonary hypertension before pulmonary thromboendarterectomy. Circulation 120: 1248–1254.
13. Mayer E, Jenkins D, Lindner J, D'Armini A, Kloek J, et al. (2011) Surgical management and outcome of patients with chronic thromboembolic pulmonary hypertension: results from an international prospective registry. J Thorac Cardiovasc Surg 141: 702–710.
14. Riedel M, Stanek V, Widimsky J, Prerovsky I (1982) Longterm follow-up of patients with pulmonary thromboembolism. Late prognosis and evolution of hemodynamic and respiratory data. Chest 81: 151–158.
15. Condliffe R, Kiely DG, Gibbs JS, Corris PA, Peacock AJ, et al. (2008) Improved outcomes in medically and surgically treated chronic thromboembolic pulmonary hypertension. Am J Respir Crit Care Med 177: 1122–1127.
16. Scholzel BE, Post MC, Thijs Plokker HW, Snijder RJ (2011) Clinical Worsening During Long-Term Follow-Up in Inoperable Chronic Thromboembolic Pulmonary Hypertension. Lung.
17. Mereles D, Ehlken N, Kreuscher S, Ghofrani S, Hoeper MM, et al. (2006) Exercise and respiratory training improve exercise capacity and quality of life in patients with severe chronic pulmonary hypertension. Circulation 114: 1482–1489.
18. Grünig E, Ehlken N, Ghofrani A, Staehler G, Meyer FJ, et al. (2011) Effect of Exercise and Respiratory Training on Clinical Progression and Survival in Patients with Severe Chronic Pulmonary Hypertension. Respiration 81: 394–401.
19. Guyatt GH, Pugsley SO, Sullivan MJ, Thompson PJ, Berman L, et al. (1984) Effect of encouragement on walking test performance. Thorax 39: 818–822.
20. Borg G (1982) Psychophysical bases of perceived exertion. Med Sci Sports Exerc: 377–381.
21. Ware J, Sherbourne C (1992) The MOS 36-Item Short-Form Health Survey (SF-36): I. Conceptual Framework and Item Selection. Medical Care 30: 473–483.
22. Grunig E, Lichtblau M, Ehlken N, Ghofrani HA, Reichenberger F, et al. (2012) Safety and Efficacy of Exercise Training in various forms of Pulmonary Hypertension. Eur Respir J.
23. de Man F, Handoko M, Groepenhoff H, van 't Hul A, Abbink J, et al. (2009) Effects of exercise training in patients with idiopathic pulmonary arterial hypertension. Eur Respir J 34: 669–675.
24. Handoko ML, de Man FS, Happé CM, Schalij I, Musters RJP, et al. (2009) Opposite Effects of Training in Rats With Stable and Progressive Pulmonary Hypertension. Circulation 120: 42–49.
25. Miyamoto S, Nagaya N, Satoh T, Kyotani S, Sakamaki F, et al. (2000) Clinical correlates and prognostic significance of six-minute walk test in patients with primary pulmonary hypertension. Comparison with cardiopulmonary exercise testing. Am J Respir Crit Care Med 161: 487–492.
26. Saouti N, de Man F, Westerhof N, Boonstra A, Twisk J, et al. (2009) Predictors of mortality in inoperable chronic thromboembolic pulmonary hypertension. Respir Med 103: 1013–1019.
27. Suntharalingam J, Goldsmith K, Toshner M, Doughty N, Sheares KK, et al. (2007) Role of NT-proBNP and 6MWD in chronic thromboembolic pulmonary hypertension. Respir Med 101: 2254–2262.
28. Ghofrani HA, Hoeper MM, Halank M, Meyer FJ, Staehler G, et al. (2010) Riociguat for chronic thromboembolic pulmonary hypertension and pulmonary arterial hypertension: a phase II study. Eur Respir J 36: 792–799.
29. Bonderman D, Nowotny R, Skoro-Sajer N, Jakowitsch J, Adlbrecht C, et al. (2005) Bosentan therapy for inoperable chronic thromboembolic pulmonary hypertension. Chest 128: 2599–2603.
30. Hoeper MM, Kramm T, Wilkens H, Schulze C, Schafers HJ, et al. (2005) Bosentan therapy for inoperable chronic thromboembolic pulmonary hypertension. Chest 128: 2363–2367.
31. Hughes RJ, Jais X, Bonderman D, Suntharalingam J, Humbert M, et al. (2006) The efficacy of bosentan in inoperable chronic thromboembolic pulmonary hypertension: a 1-year follow-up study. Eur Respir J 28: 138–143.
32. Ulrich S, Speich R, Domenighetti G, Geiser T, Aubert JD, et al. (2007) Bosentan therapy for chronic thromboembolic pulmonary hypertension. A national open label study assessing the effect of Bosentan on haemodynamics, exercise capacity, quality of life, safety and tolerability in patients with chronic thromboembolic pulmonary hypertension (BOCTEPH-Study). Swiss Med Wkly 137: 573–580.

7

Pulmonary Hypertension in Patients with Chronic Kidney Disease on Dialysis and without Dialysis: Results of the PEPPER-Study

Stefan Pabst[1⬥], **Christoph Hammerstingl**[1⬥], **Felix Hundt**[2⬥], **Thomas Gerhardt**[3], **Christian Grohé**[4], **Georg Nickenig**[1], **Rainer Woitas**[2], **Dirk Skowasch**[1]*

1 The Department of Internal Medicine II – Cardiology/Pneumology, University of Bonn, Bonn, Germany, **2** The Department of Internal Medicine I - Nephrology, University of Bonn, Bonn, Germany, **3** Praxis für Nieren- und Hochdruckkrankheiten Bonn, Bonn, Germany, **4** The Lungenklinik Berlin-Buch, Berlin, Germany

Abstract

Pulmonary hypertension (PH) is common in patients with dialysis-dependent chronic kidney disease and is an independent predictor of mortality. However, specific hemodynamics of the pulmonary circulation, changes induced by hemodialysis and characterization into pre- or postcapillary PH have not been evaluated in patients with chronic kidney disease. We assessed consecutive patients with end-stage chronic kidney disease in WHO FC≥II with dyspnea unexplained by other causes on hemodialysis (group 1, n = 31) or without dialysis (group 2, n = 31) using right heart catheterization (RHC). In group 1, RHC was performed before and after dialysis. In end-stage chronic kidney disease, prevalence of precapillary PH was 13% (4/31), and postcapillary PH was discovered in 65% (20/31). All four cases of precapillary PH were unmasked after dialysis. In group 2, two cases of precapillary PH were detected (6%), and postcapillary PH was diagnosed in 22 cases (71%). This is the first study examining a large cohort of patients with chronic kidney disease invasively by RHC for the prevalence of PH. The prevalence of precapillary PH was 13% in patients with end-stage kidney disease. That suggests careful screening for precapillary PH in this selected patient population. RHC should be performed after hemodialysis.

Editor: Jeremy Stuart Duffield, University of Washington, United States of America

Funding: The study was sponsored by Actelion Pharmaceuticals. The funder had no role in study design, data collection and analysis, decision to publish, or preparation of the manuscript.

Competing Interests: The authors have read the journal's policy and have the following conflicts: SP, CH, and DS received remuneration for lecturing and grants for travel expenses from Actelion Pharmaceuticals and GlaxoSmithKline. This does not alter the authors' adherence to all the PLoS ONE policies on sharing data and materials.

* E-mail: Dirk.Skowasch@ukb.uni-bonn.de

⬥ These authors contributed equally to this work.

Introduction

The prevalence of chronic kidney disease (CKD) in the developed world is 13% [1] and is recognized as a condition that elevates the risk of cardiovascular complications as well as kidney failure and other complications. End-stage kidney disease (ESKD) substantially increases the risk of death, cardiovascular disease, and use of specialized health care. In this context, pulmonary hypertension (PH) has been reported in patients with ESKD maintained on long-term hemodialysis. Based on echocardiographic studies, the prevalence of PH in these patient populations is estimated to be around 17–56% [2–7], and PH is an independent predictor of mortality in such patients [6,7]. However, these studies lack invasive hemodynamic data and thus cannot discriminate between pre- and postcapillary PH in unselected patients with or without symptoms.

PH is a hemodynamic and pathophysiological state found in a range of clinical conditions and is characterized by an increase in mean pulmonary arterial pressure (mPAP ≥25 mmHg); precapillary PH is defined by the additional criterion of a pulmonary arterial wedge pressure (PCWP) ≤15 mmHg [8]. The different forms of PH have been classified into five clinical groups with specific characteristics [8,9]. Group 1 consists of the major forms of pulmonary arterial hypertension (PAH: idiopathic, heritable and associated with connective tissue disease and congenital heart disease etc.). A diagnosis of PAH requires the exclusion of all other causes of PH, and specific treatments are available. Group 2 describes PH due to left heart disease including diastolic dysfunction, Group 3 PH due to lung diseases and/or hypoxia and Group 4 is chronic thromboembolic pulmonary hypertension (CTEPH). Group 5 consists of PH with unclear and/or multifactorial mechanisms including "chronic renal failure on dialysis" [8,9]. The pathogenesis of PAH is poorly understood, and the associated conditions that result in PAH are heterogenous and seemingly unrelated.

The purpose of the PEPPER-study ("prevalence of precapillary pulmonary arterial hypertension in patients with end-stage renal disease") was to assess the specific hemodynamics in CKD patients with otherwise unexplained dyspnea on hemodialysis and in those without dialysis, to elucidate possible risk factors contributing to PH, and to evaluate hemodynamic changes induced by hemodialysis – by use of right heart catheterization (RHC), the "gold standard" method for the diagnosis and characterization in pre- and postcapillary PH.

Methods

Patients

This was a prospective, single center study conducted at the University of Bonn, Germany. Local ethics committee approval was obtained prior to the inclusion of any patient in the study (Ethics committee, University of Bonn, Germany, 061/09) and the study was conducted according to the Declaration of Helsinki. Written informed consent was obtained from all participants involved in our study. Consecutive patients with severe CKD stage 4 or 5 [10] attending the clinic for regular treatment were assessed for enrollment suitability using defined inclusion and exclusion criteria. Within the one year ESKD patients with dialysis were recruited and compared to patients with CKD without dialysis. The study started in November 2009 and ended in October 2010 after 62 patients (31 patients in each group) were included. Detailed information is given in figure 1. Inclusion criteria were: adults ≥ 18 years old, stage 4 or 5 CKD (defined as serum creatinine ≥ 200 μmol/l [2.26 mg/dl] or glomerular filtration rate [GFR] ≤ 30 ml/min/1.73 m^2 assessed by MDRD4-formula [11,12] for a time span ≥ 1 year), on hemodialysis or without hemodialysis treatment, and in World Health Organization functional class (WHO FC) $\geq$II with dyspnea unexplained by other causes. Exclusion criteria were: uncontrolled arterial hypertension (defined as mean blood pressure before entry into the study $\geq 160/100$ mmHg), current malignant diseases, pregnancy, left ventricular ejection fraction (LVEF) $<50\%$, mitral or aortic regurgitation $>$grade 2, aortic or mitral surface <1.5 cm^2, myocarditis, endocarditis, pericarditis, severe anemia (hemoglobin concentration <10 g/dl), severe chronic obstructive pulmonary disease (COPD) defined by FEV$_1$ $<60\%$ predicted, lung fibrosis, and known PAH medication with prostanoids, endothelin receptor antagonists, or phosphodiesterase-5 inhibitors. The following assessments were undertaken in all patients: medical history (including exact data concerning immunosuppressive medication, other medication and duration of renal insufficiency before starting dialysis and the time under dialysis as well as the daily amount of residual diuresis); clinical examination, including height, (dry-)weight, blood pressure; standard 12-lead-electrocardiography (ECG); transthoracic echocardiography (TTE); lung function testing (bodyplethysmography); laboratory investigations including blood count, and potassium, sodium, aspartate aminotrasferase/alanine aminotransferase (AST/ALT), creatinine and urea levels.

Right heart catheterization

All patients underwent RHC. RHC in CKD patients on dialysis was performed before and after dialysis, if PH was confirmed with the first RHC. As shown in table 1 PH was defined as mean pulmonary arterial pressure (mPAP) ≥ 25 mmHg regardless of the pulmonary capillary wedge pressure (PCWP). If mPAP was ≥ 25 mmHg and PCWP was ≤ 15 mmHg, the diagnosis of precapillary PH was made. In case of precapillary PH, a complete work-up (including chest computertomography-scan, ventilation-perfusion-scan, sleep apnea screening, ultrasound of the liver and laboratory testing) was performed to verify or exclude PAH. Vasoreactivity testing (inhaled iloprost 5 μg; iNeb, Philips Healthcare, Eindhoven, Netherlands) was performed in case of precapillary PH/PAH. Positive vasoreactivity was defined as a decrease of mPAP ≥ 10 mmHg to reach ≤ 40 mmHg with a stable cardiac index (CI) [8]. Cardiac index was measured by direct Fick method.

Statistical analysis

The German version of SPSS V17.0 (IBM, Munich, Germany) was used as a database and for statistical analysis. Data are expressed as mean $\pm$ standard deviation and as a percentage for categorial parameters. Differences between groups were compared with Student's t-test and Mann-Witney-U test, as applicable. Chi-square test was used to estimate the occurrence of categorical variables. Two-tailed bivariate correlations were determined by the Pearson's coefficient. Statistical significance was set at p$<$0.05.

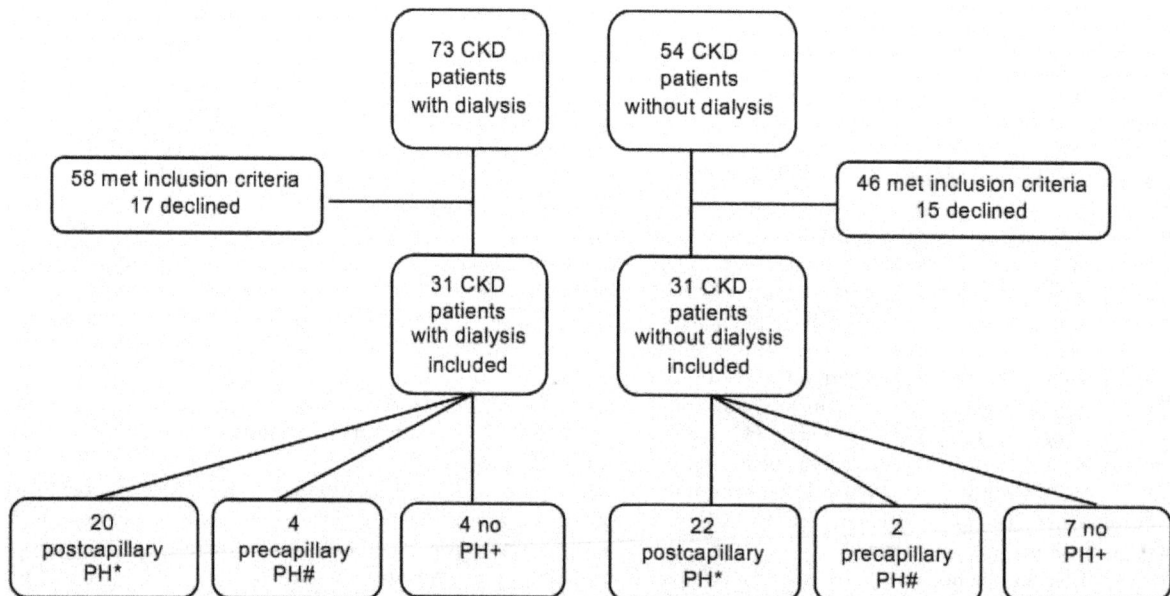

Figure 1. Enrolment of Patients. CKD: chronic kidney disease; Pulmonary hypertension (PH): mean pulmonary arterial pressure (mPAP) ≥ 25 mmHg; *postcapillary PH: mPAP ≥ 25 mmHg and pulmonary capillary wedge pressure (PCWP) ≥ 15 mmHg; #precapillary PH: mPAP ≥ 25 mmHg and PCWP <15 mmHg, +no PH: mPAP <25 mmHg.

Table 1. Distinction of PH, precapillary PH and postcapillary PH [8].

no PH	mPAP <25 mmHg
PH	mPAP ≥25 mmHg
precapillary PH	mPAP ≥25 mmHg and PCWP <15 mmHg
postcapillary PH	mPAP ≥25 mmHg and PCWP ≥15 mmHg

Results

Study population

From November 2009 to October 2010, consecutive patients with severe CKD stage 4 or 5 and in WHO FC ≥II with dyspnea unexplained by other causes were screened by transthoracic echocardiography (TTE) for study participation (Fig. 1).

In all, 62 patients met the inclusion criteria and agreed to participate in the study. The demographics and characteristics of the per-protocol population comprising 31 CKD patients on

Table 2. CHARACTERISTICS OF PEPPER PARTICIPANTS.

Characteristics	Dialysis patients	Patients with CKD (serum creatinine ≥200 µmol/l) without dialysis	p-value
	n = 31	n = 31	
Age at examination (yrs)	65.3±7.4	73.6±9.5	**<0.001**
Gender (% female)	35	48	0.303
BMI (kg/m²)	24.0±3.5 (post-dialysis)	26.8±5.17	**0.015**
GFR (re-expressed MDRD ml/min)	n.a.	21.94±4.37	n.a.
CKD cause			0.152
diabetes mellitus	10 (32%)	13 (42%)	0.430
arterial hypertension	4 (13%)	7 (23%)	0.319
Glomerulonephritis	3 (10%)	5 (16%)	0.449
ADPKD	4 (13%)	0 (0%)	**0.039**
others (including unclear)	10 (32%)	6 (19%)	0.246
Median time to enrollment (years)			
from first diagnosis of CKD	4.9±3.8	1.5±12.2	**<0.001**
from first dialysis	3.8±3.5	n.a.	n.a.
Comorbid conditions			
Cerebrovascular disease (CVD)	4 (13%)	8 (26%)	0.199
MI in medical history	4 (13%)	6 (19%)	0.490
CAD	10 (32%)	13 (42%)	0.430
PCI	8 (26%)	10 (32%)	0.258
CABG	2 (7%)	3 (10%)	0.416
Neoplasm in medical history	2 (7%)	0 (0%)	0.151
PAD	4 (13%)	4 (13%)	1.0
Atrial fibrillation	13 (42%)	19 (61%)	0.127
COPD (I–II)	9 (29%)	9 (29%)	1.0
Diabetes mellitus	12 (39%)	12 (39%)	1.0
Insulin use	8 (26%)	8 (26%)	1.0
Arterial hypertension	17 (55%)	19 (61%)	0.203
Smoking (actual and former)	19 (61%)	19 (61%)	1.0
Hyperlipidemia	23 (75%)	24 (77%)	0.767
Medication			
Beta blockade	21 (68%)	19 (61%)	0.596
Calcium channel blockade	11 (35%)	3 (10%)	**0.015**
ACE inhibitor	13 (42%)	13 (42%)	1.0
AT-1 blockade	4 (16%)	4 (13%)	1.0
Statin	23 (75%)	24 (77%)	0.767
Dyspnea WHO grade II/III/IV	22/7/2 (71%/23%/6%)	19/10/2 (61%/32%/7%)	0.586

BMI: body mass index; GFR: glomerular filtration rate; CKD: chronic kidney disease; ADPKD: autosomal dominant polycystic kidney disease; MI: myocardial infarction; CAD: coronary artery disease; PCI: percutaneous coronary intervention; CABG: coronary artery bypass graft; PAD: peripheral artery disease; COPD: chronic obstructive pulmonary disease; AT-1: angiotensin 1.

Table 3. HAEMODYNAMIC MEASUREMENTS IN TTE AND RHC.

	All dialysis patients	Dialysis patients with PH		p-value	CKD patients without dialysis	p-value	p-value	p-value
	before dialysis	before dialysis	after dialysis	dialysis before vs. dialysis after		dialysis before vs. no dialysis	patients with PH: dialysis before vs. no dialysis	patients with PH: dialysis after vs. no dialysis
	n=31	n=25	n=25		n=31			
TTE								
PAP systolic (mmHg)	43±16	44±16	37±13	**<0.001**	43±13	0.908	0.679	0.122
No. of patients PAP systolic ≥30 mmHg	22 (71%)	18 (72%)	15 (60%)	0.370	24 (77%)	0.562	0.642	0.159
LVEF (%)	59±12	61±12	60±11	0.870	56±6	0.170	0.057	0.121
Pericardial effusion	0	0	0	1.0	0	1.0	1.0	1.0
RHC								
PAP systolic (mmHg)	56±21	62±18	55±17	**<0.001**	52±15	0.324	**0.019**	0.456
PAP diastolic (mmHg)	27±13	30±11	26±10	**<0.001**	25±9	0.543	0.053	0.559
PAP mean (mmHg)	38±15	42±13	36±12	**<0.001**	35±11	0.315	**0.025**	0.573
PCWP (mmHg)	23±9	25±8	20±6	**<0.001**	22±8	0.917	0.263	0.255
PH	25 (81%)	25 (100%)	24 (96%)	0.327	24 (77%)	0.755	**0.011**	**0.048**
precapillary PH	0 (0%)	0 (0%)	4 (16%)	**0.043**	2 (6%)	0.151	0.196	0.251
postcapillary PH	25 (81%)	25 (100%)	20 (80%)	**0.012**	22 (71%)	0.374	**0.003**	0.438
RAP (mmHg)	14±8	13±9	13±9	1.0	13±6	0.788	0.167	0.167
PVR (dyn · sec · cm^{-5})	345±360	403±378	400±398	0.716	325±340	0.828	0.422	0.451
CI (l/min/m^2)	2.43±0.79	2.28±0.65	2.28±0.76	0.700	1.94±0.53	**0.005**	**0.033**	**0.028**
TPG (mmHg)	15±10	18±10	17±11	0.142	12±9	0.227	0.057	0.079

CI: cardiac index; CKD: chronic kidney disease: serum creatinine ≥200 µmol/l; LVEF: left ventricular ejection fraction; PAP: pulmonary artery pressure; PCWP: pulmonary capillary wedge pressure; PH: pulmonary hypertension (PAP mean ≥25 mmHg); PVR: pulmonary vascular resistance; RAP: right arterial pressure; RHC: right heart catheterization; TPG: transpulmonary gradient; TTE: transthoracic echocardiography.

Table 4. CHARACTERIZATION OF PATIENTS WITH PRECAPILLARY PH.

Patient	Dialysis/Non-Dialysis	Gender	Age	PAPmean (mmHg)	PCWP (mmHg)	TPG (mmHg)	CI (l/min/m²)	PVR (dyn · sec · cm⁻⁵)	RAP (mmHg)	putative cause for precapillary PH
1	Dialysis	m	75	40	12	28	1.3	861	6	dialysis
2	Dialysis	m	79	32	14	18	2.8	282	11	severe sleep apnea
3	Dialysis	f	70	30	12	18	1.9	497	11	dialysis
4	Dialysis	m	58	56	13	33	0.9	1911	20	dialysis
5	Non-Dialysis	f	58	29	12	17	1.8	400	6	COPD GOLD II
6	Non-Dialysis	m	74	41	13	28	2.8	373	7	COPD GOLD II

Haemodynamic data are from post-dialysis (in dialysis patients).
m: male; f: female; COPD: chronic obstructive pulmonary disease; GOLD stages: global initiative for chronic obstructive lung disease.

chronic hemodialysis treatment (group 1) and 31 patients with CKD (group 2) not on dialysis are presented in Table 2. We observed significant differences in age (the mean age of the dialysis cohort was 8 years lower than the nondialysis group), body mass index (BMI was lower in the dialysis group), median time to enrollment after manifestation of CKD (4.9 years in the dialysis group vs. 1.5 years in the non-dialysis group), and use of calcium channel blockers (increased in the dialysis group).

Right heart catheterization

All 62 patients underwent RHC; data are given in Table 3.

In group 1, RHC was performed before and after dialysis, if mPAP was ≥ 25 mmHg before dialysis (n = 25). If mPAP was determined as <25 mmHg by RHC before dialysis, PH/PAH was excluded, and patients did not undergo a second RHC (n = 6). PH was observed in 25/31 (81%) patients in the dialysis group (before dialysis) versus 22/31 (71%) in the nondialysis cohort. After dialysis in group 1, prevalence of PH was 24/31 (77%, 20/31 postcapillary PH, 4/31 precapillary PH). There was a significant decrease of mPAP and PCWP after dialysis (mPAP from 62 ± 18 to 55 ± 17 mmHg; and PCWP from 25 ± 8 to 20 ± 6 mmHg). All four cases of precapillary PH were identified only by the RHC performed after dialysis treatment; none of the four patients was vasoreactive to inhaled iloprost.

In nondialysis patients (group 2), postcapillary PH was diagnosed in 22/31 cases (71%); precapillary PH without vasoreactivity was found in 2/31 cases (6%). Hemodynamic data were similar to the dialysis group (Table 3); only the higher CI in the dialysis group reached significance.

Prevalence of precapillary and postcapillary PH

The clinical and hemodynamic profiles of the patients with precapillary PH are displayed in Table 4. Further diagnostic workup according to clinical guidelines [8], including chest CT-scan, ventilation-perfusion-scan, sleep apnea screening, ultrasound of the liver and laboratory testing, confirmed precapillary PH due to hemodialysis (Dana Point Group 5 [9]) in three patients, and excluded PAH and diagnosed PH due to lung diseases and/or hypoxia in three further cases (Dana Point Group 3 [9]; two patients with mild PH and COPD, one patient with mild PH and sleep disordered breathing). In a total of 3/31 CKD patients on dialysis precapillary PH that was not explained by the PH workup (i.e. Dana Point group 1 or 5) was diagnosed, whereas precapillary PH (Dana Point group 1 or 5) was not found in nondialysis CKD patients. Thus, prevalence of precapillary PH (Dana Point group 1 or 5) was 10% in CKD patients on dialysis. There were no further clinically remarkable differences between the patients with precapillary compared to postcapillary PH or between patients with or without PH.

Discussion

We present the results of the first prospective study evaluating the prevalence of precapillary PH by use of RHC in a large cohort of patients with CKD on dialysis or without dialysis. In this symptomatic cohort with dyspnea WHO FC $\geq$ II, the prevalence of precapillary PH (Dana Point group 1 or 5) was found to be 10% in the examined CKD patients requiring renal replacement therapy, whereas no cases of precapillary PH were detected in nondialysis CKD patients. In contrast, the prevalence of PH in CKD patients on or without dialysis was similar (77 vs. 71%, respectively) and considerably higher than previously reported (56 vs. 39% [3]; 44 vs. 32% [6]). The reason for the higher prevalence in our study could be due to the high risk nature of our cohort which included only patients with dyspnea in WHO FC $\geq$II, whereas other studies also included asymptomatic patients [2–7]. Another strength of our study is the use of invasive methodology (RHC), considered a requirement and the "gold standard" for the differential diagnosis between pre- and postcapillary PH and assessment of hemodymic impairment [8], for all study participants. Previous studies used only echocardiographic estimation of systolic PAP for PH diagnosis [2–7].

Since the prevalence of precapillary PH in our participants dramatically exceeds the prevalence of PAH in the general population of 15–50 per million adult population [8,10], end-stage kidney disease or dialysis itself may be a trigger for the development of precapillary PH in a predisposed patient, analogous to connective tissue disease, HIV, or portal hypertension. Hormonal and metabolic disturbances associated with CKD requiring dialysis might lead to pulmonary vascular constriction [8]. There are several pathogenetic mechanisms which may contribute to the development of precapillary PH in patients undergoing long-term dialysis, including impaired endothelial function [13], decreased bioavailability of nitric oxide (NO) [14,15], and increased levels of endothelin (ET)-1 [16–19]. PAP may also be increased by high cardiac output resulting from the arteriovenous access and/or concomitant renal anemia, as well as from fluid overload [9,20,21]. In addition, diastolic and systolic left heart dysfunctions are frequent in this setting [9] as also indicated by the high rate of postcapillary PH in this study. Due to the fact that we have excluded patients with reduced left ventricular ejection fraction the main diagnosis in our cohort probably is diastolic dysfunction.

In some patients, it may be difficult to distinguish between a diagnosis of precapillary PH and heart failure with preserved ejection fraction/diastolic dysfunction. In the present study, in CKD patients on dialysis, precapillary PH initially masked by fluid overload was unmasked by dialysis in 4/25 cases of primarily postcapillary PH. However, one may argue the opposite i.e. masking of postcapillary PH by fluid withdrawal. In particular, exercise hemodynamics or volume challenge have been proposed as means of identifying LV dysfunction, but these diagnostic tools require further standardization and can often not be applied to dialysis patients [8]. Even so, an elevated transpulmonary pressure gradient (TPG; mPAP minus PCWP) >12 mmHg is suggestive of intrinsic changes in the pulmonary circulation overriding the passive increase in PCWP. As demonstrated in Table 3, mPAP as well as PCWP were elevated before dialysis compared with afterwards, whereas TPG did not differ significantly. Moreover, in all CKD-precapillary-PH patients the stable "out-of-proportion" TPG suggests a precapillary component in addition to the fluid overload before dialysis. Therefore the elevated TPG might point towards CKD- precapillary-PH already at the time before hemodialysis. However, we propose that RHC should be performed after dialysis to unmask precapillary PH. The Dana Point classification assigns PH in patients with CKD to Group 5, i.e. all of the patients in the present study primarily belong into this group [8,9]. However, based on the present post-dialysis hemodynamics, a re-grouping of some CKD patients with precapillary PH into Group 1 at least is to be discussed in upcoming guidelines. Certainly there is need for more data, i.e. if histopathological changes of the here-described cohort are similar to those patients in Dana Point group 1 (PAH). We explicitly do not want to encourage CKD patients with a precapillary PH to be treated with specific PAH drugs, as there is no knowledge about the efficacy of those therapies in this cohort.

There are notable limitations of this single-center study. Each patient was only measured once invasively. Especially in the hemodialysis cohort it would be possible that RHC would have led to different results over the time caused by different fluid overload/dry weight. However, we think that our invasive approach is new and more catheterizations cannot be enforced in this patients' cohort. We did not obtain data measuring extracellular fluid (ECF). Another limitation is the measurement of CI by direct Fick method. Due to arteriovenous fistula, the product of the Fick formula and therefore CI and PVR might be changed. However, there is no influence on PAP and PCWP.

Treatment regimens were not assessed. Therefore, the question how best to treat patients with CKD and PH/PAH remains unresolved. Although information on specific PAH treatment or clinical outcome would be of interest, it would necessitate a controlled, prospective study analyzing clinical end points with specific PAH treatment and requiring a follow-up period of several years and the recruitment of a large patient cohort. With the exception of isolated case reports [22], the efficacy of current medical therapeutics for PAH such as prostanoids, endothelin receptor antagonists and phosphodiesterase-5 inhibitors have not been studied in CKD patients.

In conclusion, this study provides evidence that precapillary PH is a common co-morbidity in CKD patients on dialysis. End-stage kidney disease and/or hemodialysis rather than the renal insufficiency itself seems to be the main determining risk factor for developing precapillary PH. Diagnostic RHC should be performed after dialysis to diferentiate precapillary from postcapillary PH.

Acknowledgments

The authors thank Simone Krämer for excellent technical assistance.

Author Contributions

Conceived and designed the experiments: SP CG RW DS. Performed the experiments: SP FH RW DS. Analyzed the data: SP CH FH TG RW DS. Wrote the paper: SP CH FH TG CG GN RW DS.

References

1. Coresh J, Selvin E, Stevens LA, Manzi J, Kusek JW, et al. (2007) Prevalence of chronic kidney disease in the United States. JAMA 298: 2038–2047.

2. Yigla M, Nakhoul F, Sabag A, Tov N, Gorevich B, et al. (2003) Pulmonary hypertension in patients with end-stage renal disease. Chest 123: 1577–1582.

3. Havlucu Y, Kursat S, Ekmekci C, Celik P, Serter S, et al. (2007) Pulmonary hypertension in patients with chronic renal failure. Respiration 74: 503–510.

4. Bozbas SS, Akcay S, Altin C, Bozbas H, Karacaglar E, et al. (2009) Pulmonary hypertension in patients with end-stage renal disease undergoing renal transplantation. Transplant Proc 41: 2753–2756.

5. Ramasubbu K, Deswal A, Herdejurgen C, Aguilar D, Frost AE () A prospective echocardiographic evaluation of pulmonary hypertension in chronic hemodialysis patients in the United States: prevalence and clinical significance. Int J Gen Med 2010;3: 279–286.

6. Abdelwhab S, Elshinnawy S () Pulmonary hypertension in chronic renal failure patients. Am J Nephrol 2008;28: 990–997.

7. Yigla M, Fruchter O, Aharonson D, Yanay N, Reisner SA, et al. (2009) Pulmonary hypertension is an independent predictor of mortality in hemodialysis patients. Kidney Int 75: 969–975.

8. Task Force for Diagnosis and Treatment of Pulmonary Hypertension of European Society of Cardiology (ESC); European Respiratory Society (ERS); International Society of Heart and Lung Transplantation (ISHLT), Galié N, Hoeper MM, Humbert M, Torbicki A, et al. (2009) Guidelines for the diagnosis and treatment of pulmonary hypertension. Eur Respir J 34: 1219–1263.

9. Simonneau G, Robbins IM, Beghetti M, Channick RN, Delcroix M, et al. (2009) Updated clinical classification of pulmonary hypertension. J Am Coll Cardiol 54(1 Suppl): S43–S54.

10. Humbert M, Sitbon O, Chaouat A, Bertocchi M, Habib G, et al. (2006) Pulmonary arterial hypertension in France: results from a national registry. Am J Respir Crit Care Med 173: 1023–1030.

11. National Kidney Foundation. K/DOQI Clinical Practice Guidelines for Chronic Kidney Disease: Evaluation, Classification and Stratification (2002) Am J Kidney Dis 39(suppl. 1): S1–S266.

12. Levey AS, Bosch JP, Lewis JB, Greene T, Rogers N, et al. (1999) A more accurate method to estimate glomerular filtration rate from serum creatinine: a new prediction equation. Modification of Diet in Renal Disease Study Group. Ann Intern Med 130: 461–470.

13. Thambyrajah J, Landray MJ, McGlynn FJ, Jones HJ, Wheeler DC, et al. (2000) Abnormalities of endothelial function in patients with pre-dialysis renal failure. Heart 83: 205–209.

14. Arese M, Strasly M, Ruva C, Costamagna C, Ghigo D, et al. (1995) Regulation of nitric oxide synthesis in uraemia. Nephrol Dial Transplant 10: 1386–1397.

15. Aznar-Salatti J, Escolar G, Cases A, Gómez-Ortiz G, Anton P, et al. (1995) Uraemic medium causes endothelial cell dysfunction characterized by an alteration of the properties of its subendothelial matrix. Nephrol Dial Transplant 10: 2199–2204.

16. Stefanidis I, Wurth P, Mertens PR, Ikonomov V, Philippidis G, et al. (2004) Plasma endothelin-1 in hemodialysis treatment - the influence of hypertension. J Cardiovasc Pharmacol 44 Suppl 1: S43–S48.

17. Odetti P, Monacelli F, Storace D, Robaudo C, Rossi S, et al. (2006) Correlation between pentosidine and endothelin-1 in subjects undergoing chronic hemodialysis. Horm Metab Res 38: 817–820.

18. Tomić M, Galesić K, Markota I (2008) Endothelin-1 and nitric oxide in patients on chronic hemodialysis. Ren Fail 30: 836–842.

19. El-Shafey EM, El-Nagar GF, Selim MF, El-Sorogy HA, Sabry AA (2008) Is there a role for endothelin-1 in the hemodynamic changes during hemodialysis? Clin Exp Nephrol 12: 370–375.

20. Nakhoul F, Yigla M, Gilman R, Reisner SA, Abassi Z (2005) The pathogenesis of pulmonary hypertension in haemodialysis patients via arterio-venous access. Nephrol Dial Transplant 20: 1686–1692.

21. Unal A, Tasdemir K, Oymak S, Duran M, Kocyigit I, et al. (2010) The long-term effects of arteriovenous fistula creation on the development of pulmonary hypertension in hemodialysis patients. Hemodial Int 14: 398–402.

22. Liefeldt L, van Giersbergen PLM, Dingemanse J, Rudolph B, Walde T, et al. (2004) Treatment of secondary pulmonary hypertension with Bosentan and its pharmacokinetic monitoring in ESRD. Am J Kidney Dis 43: 923–926.

8

Lack of Bcr and Abr Promotes Hypoxia-Induced Pulmonary Hypertension in Mice

Min Yu[1,9,¤], Dapeng Gong[1,9], Min Lim[2], Anna Arutyunyan[1], John Groffen[1,2], Nora Heisterkamp[1,2]*

1 Section of Molecular Carcinogenesis, Division of Hematology/Oncology, and The Saban Research Institute of Children's Hospital, Los Angeles, California, United States of America, **2** Departments of Pediatrics and Pathology, Keck School of Medicine, University of Southern California, Los Angeles, California, United States of America

Abstract

Background: Bcr and Abr are GTPase activating proteins that specifically downregulate activity of the small GTPase Rac in restricted cell types *in vivo*. Rac1 is expressed in smooth muscle cells, a critical cell type involved in the pathogenesis of pulmonary hypertension. The molecular mechanisms that underlie hypoxia-associated pulmonary hypertension are not well-defined.

Methodology/Principal Findings: *Bcr* and *abr* null mutant mice were compared to wild type controls for the development of pulmonary hypertension after exposure to hypoxia. Also, pulmonary arterial smooth muscle cells from those mice were cultured in hypoxia and examined for proliferation, p38 activation and IL-6 production. Mice lacking Bcr or Abr exposed to hypoxia developed increased right ventricular pressure, hypertrophy and pulmonary vascular remodeling. Perivascular leukocyte infiltration in the lungs was increased, and under hypoxia *bcr*−/− and *abr*−/− macrophages generated more reactive oxygen species. Consistent with a contribution of inflammation and oxidative stress in pulmonary hypertension-associated vascular damage, Bcr and Abr-deficient animals showed elevated endothelial leakage after hypoxia exposure. Hypoxia-treated pulmonary arterial smooth muscle cells from Bcr- or Abr-deficient mice also proliferated faster than those of wild type mice. Moreover, activated Rac1, phosphorylated p38 and interleukin 6 were increased in these cells in the absence of Bcr or Abr. Inhibition of Rac1 activation with Z62954982, a novel Rac inhibitor, decreased proliferation, p38 phosphorylation and IL-6 levels in pulmonary arterial smooth muscle cells exposed to hypoxia.

Conclusions: Bcr and Abr play a critical role in down-regulating hypoxia-induced pulmonary hypertension by deactivating Rac1 and, through this, reducing both oxidative stress generated by leukocytes as well as p38 phosphorylation, IL-6 production and proliferation of pulmonary arterial smooth muscle cells.

Editor: James West, Vanderbilt University Medical Center, United States of America

Funding: This work was supported by a Children's Hospital Los Angeles Research Career Development award to MY and the National Institutes of Health (HL071945) to JG. The funders had no role in study design, data collection and analysis, decision to publish, or preparation of the manuscript.

Competing Interests: The authors have declared that no competing interests exist.

* E-mail: heisterk@hsc.usc.edu

9 These authors contributed equally to this work.

¤ Current address: Department of Anesthesiology, Jiangsu Province Hospital, Nanjing Medical University, Nanjing, China

Introduction

BCR (breakpoint cluster region) was originally identified as a gene involved in the development of Ph-chromosome-positive leukemias [1]. The normal Bcr protein of around 160-kDa contains multiple domains. One of these has an enzymatic function that is shared with Abr, a related protein encoded by a separate gene. The function of this domain has been relatively well characterized *in vivo*. It interacts with the small GTPase Rac when Rac is in its active GTP-bound conformation [2,3]. The interaction of Bcr and Abr with RacGTP results in the conversion of bound GTP to GDP and the inactivation of Rac. Thus Bcr and Abr belong to the class of GTPase activating proteins (GAPs), of which around 70 have been identified for Rho family members [4]. Although many of these GAPs are expressed in a cell-specific or developmentally-restricted fashion, both Abr and Bcr are expressed in many cell types in an overlapping pattern.

There are only three Rac proteins, that regulate a diversity of biological functions. The expression of Rac2 and Rac3 is relatively restricted, whereas that of Rac1 is ubiquitous. Specificity of Rac function is regulated through a tightly controlled cycle of activation and deactivation that is mediated by upstream activators, the guanine nucleotide exchange factors (GEFs), and through deactivation by the GAPs [5,6].

Mice lacking Bcr or Abr are phenotypically normal and fertile. However, when they are examined in more detail under conditions that generate pathology, significant differences with control wild type (WT) animals can be measured in specific functions. We found that ablation of Bcr and Abr results in abnormal reactivity of the innate immune system, and mice without both Abr and Bcr function also exhibit neuronal defects and inner ear developmental abnormalities [7–11].

Rac1 is also expressed in smooth muscle cells, which contribute to the pathology of pulmonary hypertension (PH), a life-threatening disorder [12]. Pulmonary vascular remodeling is a critical pathological feature of PH, and this is associated with the dysfunction and uncontrolled proliferation of the pulmonary arterial vascular smooth muscle cells (PASMCs) in the vascular wall. This in turn leads to increased thickening and muscularization of the small pulmonary arteries [13,14]. We therefore considered the possibility that Abr and Bcr could regulate Rac activity in this cell type and through this mechanism affect the pathology of hypoxia-generated pulmonary hypertension. Using mice deficient in Abr or Bcr function, we here demonstrate for the first time that endogenous Rac1 activity is elevated by hypoxia-induced PH and that this is controlled by Bcr and Abr.

Results

Increased Hypoxia-induced Pulmonary Hypertension (PH) and Right Ventricle Hypertrophy in bcr−/− or abr−/− Mice

To examine the impact of chronic hypoxia on pulmonary hemodynamics in mice lacking Abr or Bcr, we measured right ventricular systolic pressure (RVSP). As illustrated in Figure 1A, the RVSP of bcr−/− or abr−/− mice was similar to that of wt mice in normoxia. After 3 weeks of exposure to hypoxia, all three genotypes developed pulmonary hypertension, with a significant increase in RVSP, compared with their littermates in normoxia. In the hypoxic bcr−/− or abr−/− mice, the RVSP was significantly higher than that in the hypoxic wild type (wt) mice (Figure 1A).

We next calculated the ratio of RV to LV+S weight, to assess the impact of changes of pulmonary pressure on cardiac mass (Figure 1B). There was no significant difference in (RV/LV+S) between normoxic bcr−/−, abr−/− and wt mice. Consistent with the RVSP, hypoxia increased the value of (RV/LV+S) in all mice, indicating the development of right ventricular hypertrophy. Compared with the hypoxic wt mice, the (RV/LV+S) value of hypoxic bcr−/− or abr−/− mice was higher, implying that the right ventricular hypertrophy was greater in these mice.

Enhanced Hypoxia-induced Pulmonary Vascular Remodeling in bcr−/− or abr−/− Mice

To investigate the pathologic changes in hypoxia-induced PH, we performed histological analysis on the lungs of these animals. In normoxia, the percent wall thickness was similar for the bcr−/−, abr−/− and wt mice. However, bcr−/− and abr−/− mice exposed to hypoxia showed significantly greater increase in the wall thickness and larger percent wall thickness, compared with the wt mice (Figure 2A and B). Immunostaining with α-SMA antibodies on lung specimens from the mice showed, as expected, that hypoxia-challenged mice showed pulmonary vascular remodeling, characterized by increased areas of α-SMA–immunoreactive PASMCs in the pulmonary arteries. After chronic hypoxia exposure, the bcr−/− and abr−/− mice developed visibly more severe vascular remodeling, with greater areas of α-SMA–positive cells in remodeled arteries than the wt mice (Figure 2C and D).

Contribution of Inflammation to Hypoxia-generated Pulmonary Pathology in bcr−/− and abr−/− Mice

Inflammation and oxidative stress are thought to contribute to the pathology of PAH [15,16]. Since Abr and Bcr negatively regulate Rac in innate immune cells [8], we quantitated the numbers of perivascular leukocytes in H&E stained lung sections. Interestingly, pulmonary extravasation of leukocytes under hypoxia was significantly increased in the mice lacking Abr or Bcr function as compared to wt mice (Figure 3A). To examine if

reactive oxygen species (ROS) production could contribute to the exacerbated pathology in hypoxia-treated bcr−/− and abr−/− animals, we exposed macrophages from these mice to hypoxia and normoxia, and compared ROS production in their innate immune cells. We found that lack of these GAPs for Rac resulted in significantly increased ROS production under hypoxic conditions (Figure 3B). Excess ROS production by inflammatory cells can result in collateral damage to surrounding tissues including the endothelium. To address whether loss of Abr or Bcr function results in vascular injury, we exposed mice to hypoxia and then measured pulmonary endothelial dysfunction using Evans blue. Figure 3C shows that chronic hypoxia promoted loss of endothelial barrier function and, moreover, mice lacking Abr or Bcr were clearly more severely affected.

The VEGFR inhibitor SU5416 can cause emphysema in rodents and, when combined with chronic hypoxia, generates PAH [17,18]. Pathological features of combined treatment with SU5416 and chronic hypoxia include increased endothelial cell proliferation and moderately increased emphysema compared to mice exposed to hypoxia alone [19]. However, mice and rats with PAH induced by hypoxia alone did not show increased proliferation of pulmonary artery endothelial cells [20]. We therefore examined lungs of mice lacking Abr or Bcr for signs of emphysema. No obvious differences in airway hypertrophy between genotypes exposed to hypoxia were noted (Figure S1A). The mean linear intercept and average alveolar area in bcr−/− and abr−/− mice was increased upon chronic hypoxia exposure, but this was not significantly different from that of mice at normoxia, or of wt mice at hypoxia (Figure S1B, C).

Proliferation of bcr−/− and abr−/− PASMCs is Stimulated by Hypoxia

The progress of pulmonary vascular remodeling not only involves endothelial dysfunction, but also adventitial fibroblast growth, matrix deposition, acquisition of new mural cells and PASMCs proliferation [21]. These result in the narrowing of the lumen and decreased compliance of the small pulmonary arteries, constituted mainly by PASMCs [22,23]. To examine if Bcr and Abr are expressed in PASMCs, we performed Western Blot analysis. As shown in Figure 4A, both are expressed in this cell type. To explore the underlying mechanism of the enhanced pulmonary vascular remodeling in bcr−/− and abr−/− mice, we investigated the in vitro proliferation of PASMCs from these animals. As shown in Figure 4B, PASMCs from the different genotypes had similar proliferation in normoxia. The proliferation of all PASMCs increased under hypoxic conditions; furthermore, the proliferation of bcr−/− or abr−/− PASMCs was significantly higher than that of the wt cells.

We also investigated the effect of a novel Rac inhibitor, Z62954982, on the proliferation of the PASMCs. This compound has been shown to inhibit Rac but not RhoA or CDC42 activation in SMC [24]. Interestingly, Z62954982 clearly suppressed the proliferation of hypoxia-treated PASMCs, reducing it to that measured for normoxia. Flow cytometry cell cycle analysis confirmed that the hypoxic condition induced an increase in the PASMC proliferation as quantified by the proliferation index, which was more significantly elevated in PASMCs that lacked Bcr or Abr, and could be decreased by Z62954982 (Figure 4C).

Deficiency of Bcr or Abr Enhances Rac Activity during Hypoxia

Because Abr and Bcr can regulate all three Racs we used quantitative real-time PCR to investigate which Racs are

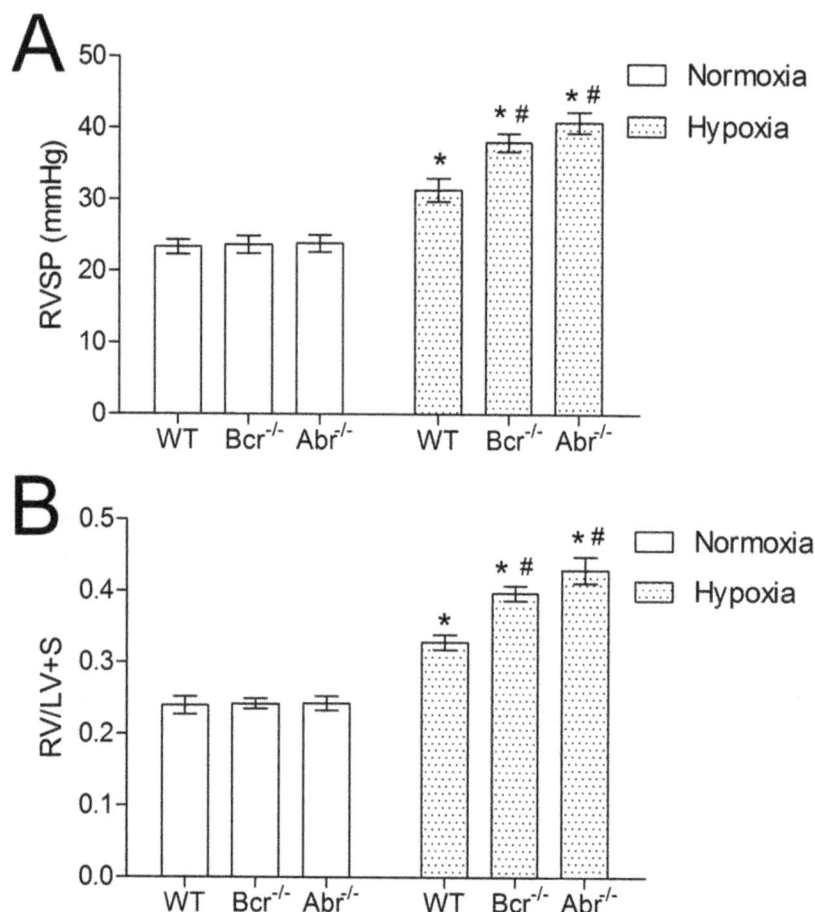

Figure 1. Hypoxia-treated *bcr−/−* **and** *abr−/−* **mice have higher RVSP and more severe right ventricular hypertrophy. A,** RVSP from *bcr−/−*, *abr−/−* and *wt* mice with exposure to normoxia or hypoxia. **B,** Ratio of RV/LV+S calculated using the weight of RV, LV+S from the hearts of normoxic and hypoxic *bcr−/−*, *abr−/−* and *wt* mice. *p<0.05 compared to the values of mice with the same genotype at normoxia. # p<0.05 when compared to *wt* mice in the same exposure condition. Bars represent mean ±SD; n =6 mice per group.

expressed in PASMCs. As shown in Figure 5A and 5B, *rac1* is highly expressed, *rac2* mRNA can not be detected, and *rac3* expression is very low in this cell type.

Regulation of Rac expression levels can be one mechanism to control the effect of Rac, but it is generally accepted that the most important mode of regulation is on its GTP- or GDP-bound state. In macrophages, astroglia and neutrophils, loss of Abr and Bcr function leads to increased levels of activated Rac [7–9,11]. Therefore, we examined the activation state of Rac1 protein in lungs from normoxic and hypoxic mice and in PASMCs. As shown in Figure 5C, the baseline levels of GTP-Rac1 (active Rac1) were similar in the lungs of normoxic *bcr−/−*, *abr−/−* and *wt* mice. Hypoxia increased the level of GTP-Rac1 in all lung samples. Interestingly, the level of GTP-Rac1 was higher in the lungs from hypoxic Bcr−/− or Abr−/− mice than in those of the WT mice (Figure 5C and D). In PASMCs, a similar basal level of GTP-Rac1 in different genotypes in normoxia was measured (Figure 5E, left 3 lanes). Hypoxia increased the levels GTP-Rac1 in PASMCs and this was higher in *bcr−/−* or *abr−/−* PASMCs than *wt* controls (Figure 5E, 5F). We also measured active Rac in hypoxia-treated PASMCs exposed to the Rac inhibitor Z62954982, and found that it significantly inhibited activation of Rac1.

To investigate the possible application of this compound *in vivo*, we treated *abr−/−* mice with intraperitoneal injections of 10 mg/kg, every second day for the duration of the hypoxia exposure. Analysis of RV/LV+S revealed that the right ventricle hypertrophy index was decreased in Z62954982-treated *abr−/−* mice under hypoxia but this was not statistically significant. The trend was more obvious in an experiment in which 20 mg/kg/d was used (p = 0.096) (Figure S2A). There was no evidence for hepatic toxicity (10 mg/kg, Figure S3A) or myelosuppression at 20 mg/kg (Figure S3B). Lung lysates isolated 60 minutes after application of the final lower dose of Z62954982 showed that Rac activation was inhibited at least temporarily in this target tissue (Figure S2B, C).

Lack of Bcr or Abr Promotes Phosphorylation of p38 MAPK and Increased IL-6 in Hypoxia

Among the various intracellular pathways that can be activated by Rac, the p38 MAPK pathway was reported to be specially relevant to the pathological changes that occur in pulmonary hypertension [25–28]. Also, p38 activation was found to be associated with increased IL-6 production [29–37]. To investigate whether the p38 kinase pathway and concomitant IL-6 production are involved in the Bcr or Abr deficiency-promoted pulmonary hypertension, activation of the p38 pathway in the lungs and IL-6 levels in the serum and lungs of these mice were assessed. Under

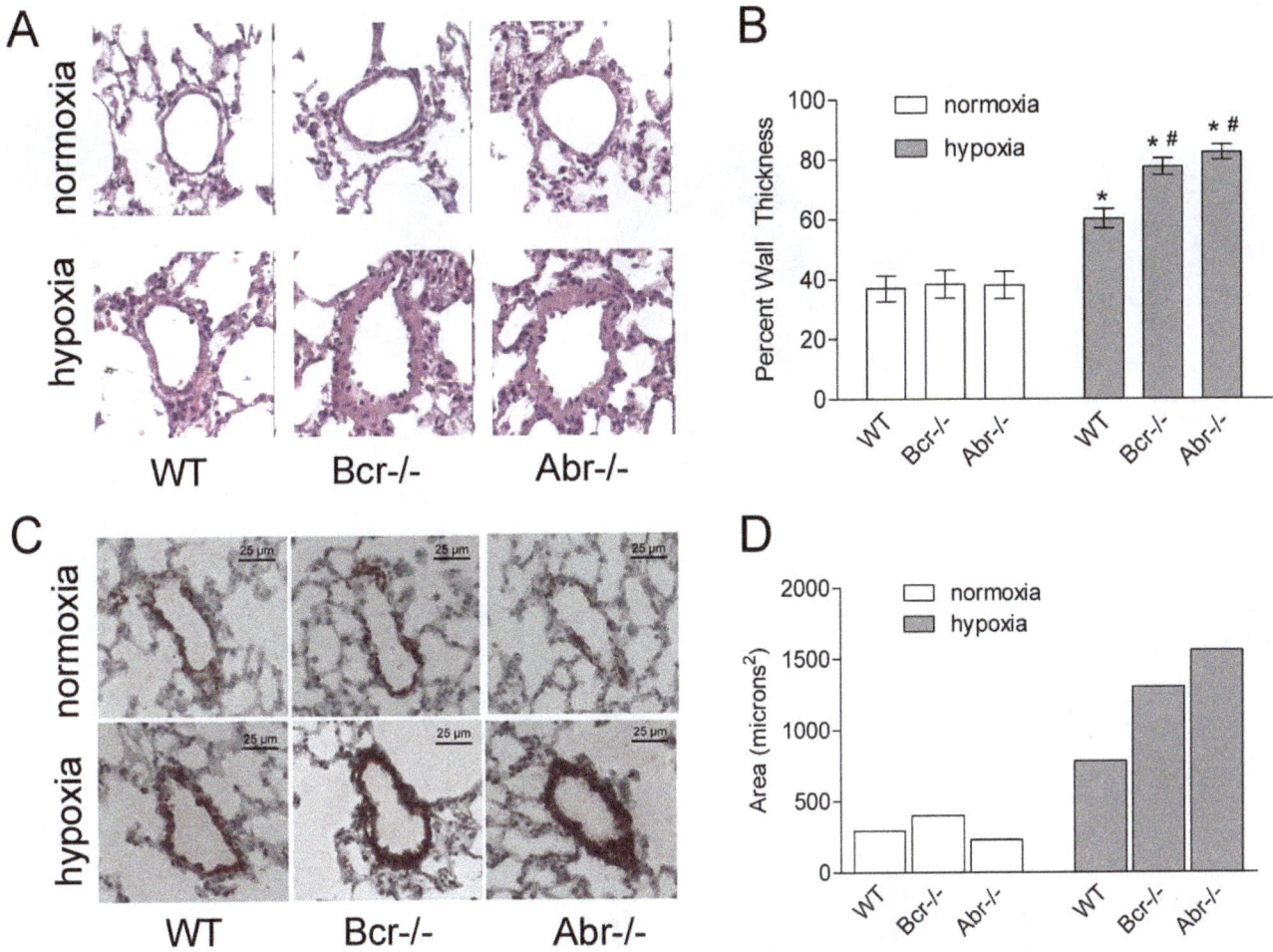

Figure 2. Hypoxia-induced pulmonary vascular remodeling in *bcr−/−* **and** *abr−/−* **mice. A,** Hematoxylin and eosin staining on representative lung specimens from *bcr−/−*, *abr−/−* and *wt* mice under normoxia or hypoxia. Note that the walls of the pulmonary arteries of the *bcr−/−* and *abr−/−* mice are remarkably thicker than those of the *wt* mice after hypoxia. Magnification, 200×. **B,** Quantification of changes in the pulmonary artery walls. Percent wall thickness was determined on H&E stained sections as described in Methods on nine vessels of comparable size per mouse, with 6 mice per genotype per condition. *p<0.05 compared with the same genotype at normoxia. # p<0.05 compared with WT mice in the same exposure condition. Bars, mean ± SD. **C,** Immunostaining with α-SMA antibodies on pulmonary vessels from representative normoxia or hypoxia-treated mice. **D,** Quantification of areas for α-SMA-positive cells. Areas of α-SMA-positive cells were calculated using ImageJ software as described in the Materials and Methods.

conditions of normoxia, the phosphorylation of p38 was minimal (Figure 6A, B) and IL-6 levels were low in serum and in lungs (Figure 6C, D). Exposure to hypoxia remarkably elevated the levels of p-p38 in lungs and this was increased significantly more in *bcr−/−* or *abr−/−* mice than in the *wt* mice (Figure 6A, B). This was accompanied by a significantly larger increase in IL-6 levels in lung and serum in the null mutant mice (Figure 6C, D).

We also evaluated p38 activation and IL-6 production in the PASMCs. When present at normoxia, PASMC had very low levels of p-p38 and produced little IL-6, but after hypoxia exposure this was significantly increased (Figure 6E–G), especially in *bcr−/−* or *abr−/−* PASMCs. To explore whether the Rac activation was correlated with the p38 MAPK phosphorylation and IL-6 production, we assessed p-p38 and IL-6 production in PASMCs treated with the Rac inhibitor Z62954982. Our results show that Z62954982 decreased both phosphorylation of p38 as well as secreted IL-6 in PASMCs in response to hypoxia (Figure 6E–G).

Discussion

Pulmonary hypertension is a devastating disease with poor prognosis. Because no validated therapy has been reported that can prevent it or affect its development [12,38], the identification of potential targets for treatment remains a crucial first step.

A number of studies indirectly suggest that Rac may play a role in PH and form such a potential target [39–42], but the possible contribution of endogenous Rac protein to PH has not been adequately examined. Firstly, since there are three distinct Rac proteins, Rac1, Rac2 and Rac3, there is a controversy regarding which of these are expressed in PASMCs, a critical cell type involved in the pathogenesis of PH. Although Rac2 is regarded as an isoform that is only expressed in hematopoietic cells, Rac2 was reported to also be present in aortic smooth muscle cells [43,44]. However Rac2 expression in PASMCs had not been reported. In the current study, using quantitative real-time RT/PCR, PASMCs cultured in standard culture medium [45] were found to contain virtually no *rac2* mRNA. Our results additionally showed low *rac3*

A

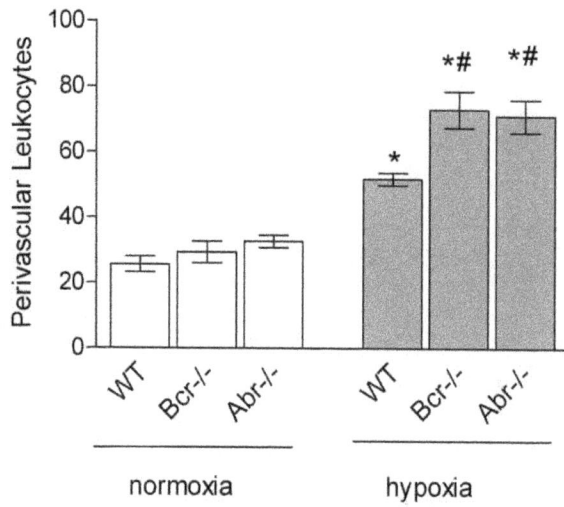

B

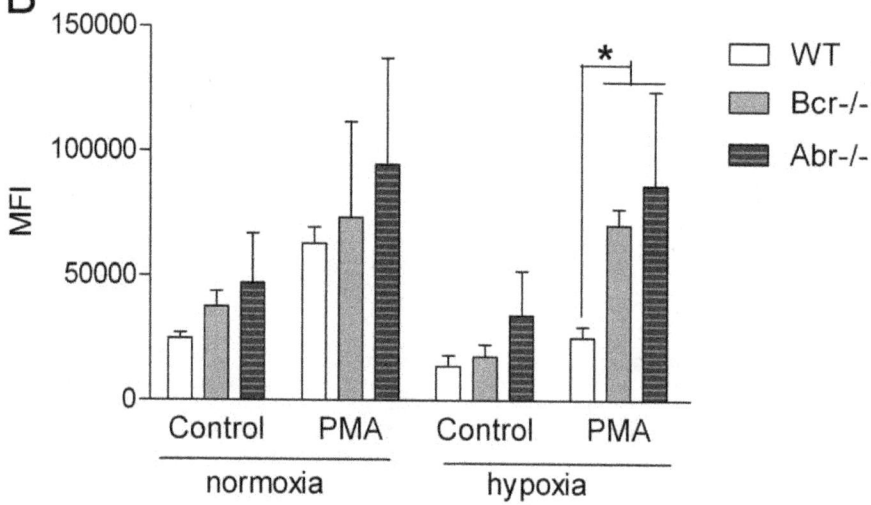

C

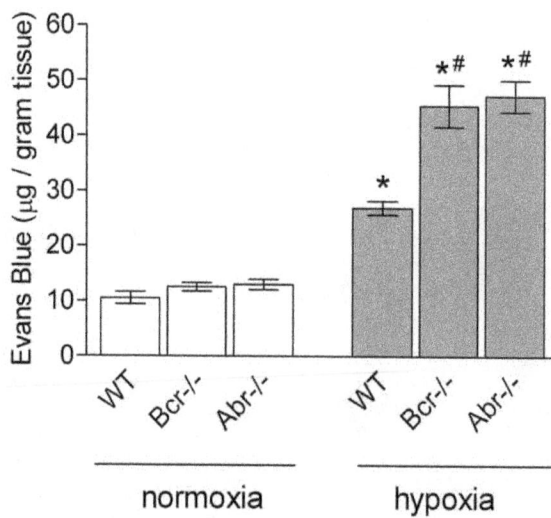

Figure 3. Lack of Abr and Bcr function exacerbates hypoxia-induced leukocyte involvement in PH. A, Numbers of perivascular leukocytes surrounding terminal arterioles. Data are expressed as total leukocyte counts per high-power field (200× amplification). Bars, mean±SEM. n = 3/group. **B,** Peritoneal-elicited macrophages exposed to normoxia or hypoxia for 24 hours activated with 1 μM PMA. ROS production was measured by FACS 1 hr later. Controls, cells without PMA activation. Bars, mean±SEM. n = 5 mice/group. *, p<0.05. MFI, mean fluorescent intensity. **C,** Vascular leakage. Evans blue was injected when mice had been exposed to normoxia or hypoxia for 3 weeks. Bars, mean±SEM. n=3–4 mice/group. A and C, *p<0.05 comparison between animals of the same genotype at normoxia. #p<0.05 compared to WT mice exposed to the same condition.

and high *rac1* mRNA levels in PASMC, indicating that Rac1 is likely to be the most important Rac for this cell type.

Secondly, previous reports that suggest Rac1 regulates processes relevant to pulmonary hypertension based their conclusions on the detection of increased levels of total Rac1 protein using Western blotting, or on the overexpression of constitutively active V12Rac or dominant negative N17Rac in PASMCs [40,46]. Although the latter studies obviously are important, under physiological conditions Rac proteins are never permanently frozen into a GTP- or GDP-bound state, but instead participate in a cycle of activation and deactivation. Also, in our study, no evidence was found for increased total Rac1 protein levels upon exposure of mouse lungs or PASMC to hypoxia (Figure 5E). Therefore, we here analyzed the levels of endogenously activated, GTP-bound Rac1 as a physiologically relevant readout for the putative involvement of Rac in PH.

We were able to detect not only the activation of endogenous Rac1 in the lungs in a mouse model of PH, but we also found enhanced hypoxia-induced activation of pulmonary Rac1 in mice deficient of Bcr or Abr. Consistent with the *in vivo* results, we confirmed that Rac1 becomes activated in PASMCs that are subjected to hypoxia. Moreover, the hypoxia-induced activation of Rac1 was significantly more notable in PASMCs lacking Bcr or Abr. We conclude that Bcr and Abr are very important components of a regulatory pathway that connects PH caused by hypoxia to Rac activation and the proliferation of PASMC. Our data also connect Bcr and Abr to the pathology of PH in a different cell type, namely by suppression of excessive ROS production in macrophages exposed to hypoxia.

The activation of Rac1 in PASMC can lead to a number of essential signaling events. The phosphorylation of p38 has been reported as a critical factor in the development of pulmonary hypertension [47,48]. Our results also showed for the first time that the suppression of endogenous Rac1 activation with the Rac inhibitor Z62954982 led to inhibition of phosphorylation of p38 in hypoxic PASMCs. This result is consistent with a previous study which reported that knock-down of Rac1 with siRNA suppresses the phosphorylation of p38 in aortic smooth muscle cells exposed to cyclic strain [49].

Of the various cytokines that are generated downstream of the phosphorylation and activation of the p38 pathway, IL-6 was recently highlighted because of its important role in pulmonary vascular remodeling and pulmonary hypertension [29,30,32]. In agreement with previous reports, our study showed increased IL-6 in mouse serum and lung homogenates in hypoxia-induced PH. We also observed further elevated IL-6 in hypoxic Bcr- or Abr-deficient mice. IL-6 can be secreted by vascular smooth muscle cells, and can also promote their growth [36,50]. Moreover, hypoxia is a factor that induces transcription and translation of IL-6 in human PASMCs [51]. Our results are consistent with these reports. We confirmed that hypoxia can increase IL-6 levels in the culture supernatant of PASMCs. Interestingly, we showed that decreasing activated Rac1 levels with Z62954982 can decrease IL-6 produced by hypoxia-exposed PASMC, suggesting that IL-6 is regulated by Rac1 activation, and is possibly related with phosphorylation of p38.

Figure 7 summarizes our data that link Abr and Bcr to the Rac cycle and downstream events in hypoxia-treated PASMCs. Which GEF is upstream of Rac in promoting PASMC proliferation, and how that GEF is activated in PH, is currently unknown. We noted that different GEFs for Rac including *DOCK1, TIAM1, TRIO, VAV1, VAV2* are highly expressed both in human control lung as well as PH RNA samples (GSE15197) This does not support the possibility that the GEFs are regulated at the level of gene transcription. Instead, we suggest that the GEF may be activated through tyrosine phosphorylation. In particular, PDGF-R signaling is known to play a role in pulmonary hypertension [52]. Since hypoxia induces increased *PDGF-BB* mRNA in human primary VSMCs, which also express the PDGF-R, paracrine signaling may contribute to VSMC cell proliferation under hypoxic conditions [53]. PDGF signaling in VSMC also generates reactive oxygen species, leading to the activation of the Src and Abl tyrosine kinases and promoting growth of these cells [54]. In fibroblasts, Abl is needed for the PDGF-R signaling that leads to Rac activation and mitogenesis [55]. Dock1 (DOCK180), a GEF for Rac, becomes tyrosine phosphorylated by Src downstream of PDGFRα activation in glioblastoma cells [56]. Thus, we speculate that one mechanism through which hypoxia could result in Rac activation is by paracrine PDGF-R signaling, that in turn leads to ROS production, Src/Abl activation and tyrosine phosphorylation/activation of a GEF for Rac. This mechanism would be consistent with the activity of the Abl and PDGF-R inhibitor Imatinib currently in clinical trials for PAH.

There are very few small molecule inhibitors available that decrease levels of activated Rac [24]. Z62954982 is a new compound that was identified through pharmacophore virtual screening, with the commonly used Rac inhibitor NSC23766 as reference compound [24]. Z62954982 does not inhibit Rac directly, but interferes with the interaction of Rac with a GEF, which activates Rac by catalyzing the exchange of the GDP bound to it for GTP. Considering the fact that there are 69 GEFs in mammals that act on various GTPases with a probable tissue specific pattern of expression [57], the targets of such inhibitors of the GEF-Rac interaction are not well-defined and need to be empirically discovered.

Z62954982 was tested in human vascular smooth muscle cells, in which it interfered with the binding of Rac1 to Tiam1 and was more efficient in reducing Rac1-GTP levels than the chemically unrelated Rac inhibitor NSC23766 [24]. However, Z62954982 has not been used in animals. In our experiments, we measured reduction in levels of activated Rac and found evidence for a beneficial effect on the pathology of hypoxia-induced PH in mice. The relatively moderate extent of this effect could be caused by, for example, a rapid clearance of the drug, and further pharmacokinetic and pharmacodynamic studies will be needed to determine the utility of this particular chemical compound for treatment of PAH.

Our results do establish that lack of Abr and Bcr function, resulting in elevated levels of activated Rac, affects macrophages and PASMC, two distinct cell types that are involved in the pathology of PH. Thus treatment with Rac inhibitors remains a viable approach to suppress hypoxia-induced pulmonary hyper-

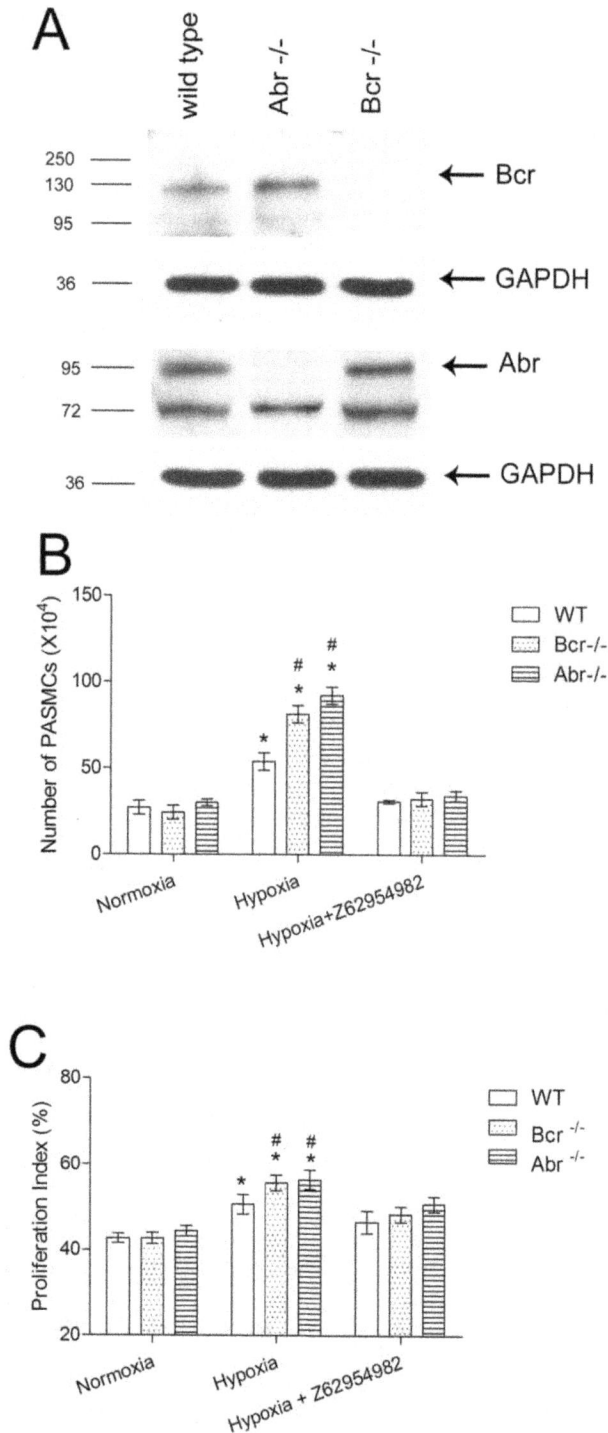

based on 10,000 PASMCs per sample, 3 samples per genotype per condition. * p<0.05 compared with the outcomes from the same genotype PASMCs in normoxia. # p<0.05 compared with *wt* PASMCs exposed to the same condition. Bars are shown as mean ±SD of triplicate wells.

tension, in particular if a combination of GEF inhibitors, or a single Rac inhibitor can be identified that would target Rac activation in PASMC as well as in innate immune cells.

Materials and Methods

Ethics Statement

Animal experiments were approved by the Children's Hospital Los Angeles Institutional Animal Care and Use Committee, and were conducted in compliance with the NIH guide for the Care and Use of Laboratory Animals.

Animals and Chronic Hypoxia Model

Bcr−/− and *abr−/−* mice were generated as previously reported [9,11] and were on an f6 FVB/J inbred genetic background.

Male *bcr−/−*, *abr−/−* and *wt* mice (8 to 10-week-old littermates) were exposed to hypoxia (10% O_2) or normoxia (21% O_2) for 3 weeks. For *in vivo* Rac1 inhibitor treatment experiments, Z62954982 was administered intraperitoneally (i.p.) at 10 mg/kg every other day or 20 mg/kg daily. Control mice were injected with the same volume of vehicle (DMSO : corn oil = 1: 9). During and at the end of the treatment, we monitored normoxia-exposed vehicle and Z62954982-treated wild type mice for possible obvious signs of toxicity of the drug. However there was no evidence for toxicity. Numbers of myeloid cells in the bone marrows were comparable and kidney (not shown) and liver appeared normal in both groups (Figure S3).

Mice were anesthetized with intraperitoneal ketamine hydrochloride (60 mg/kg) and xylazine (8 mg/kg). A catheter connected to a pressure transducer was inserted into the right ventricle (RV) through the right jugular vein. Right ventricular systolic pressure (RVSP) was measured by BP-1 (World Precision Instruments, FL, USA). The mice were then sacrificed with CO_2. The serum, hearts and lungs were immediately collected.

Pathology and Image Analysis

Percent wall thickness was calculated based on the analysis of the arterial area of pulmonary terminal arterioles, according to the following formula: wall thickness (%) = (area$_{ext}$−area$_{int}$)/area$_{ext}$×100 (area$_{ext}$ is the area bounded by external wall of the vessel, and area$_{int}$ is the area bounded by internal wall of the vessel). Nine vessels of comparable size (25–100 μm) per mouse were measured (6 mice per group). In total, 324 vessels were included. PASMCs were detected by immunohistochemistry with a mouse monoclonal antibody to α-smooth muscle actin (α-SMA; 1:1000, Sigma).

For assessment of right ventricle hypertrophy, right ventricles (RV), left ventricles and septae (LV+S) were isolated and weighed. The ratio of the weight of RV to LV+S (RV/LV+S) was analyzed as an index of right ventricle hypertrophy (RVH).

For examination of the lungs, the right primary bronchi of the lungs were ligated. The left lobes were inflated through the trachea with 10% formalin at a perfusion pressure of 20 cm H_2O. Excised inflated lung tissue was fixed in 10% formalin, processed and embedded with paraffin. Hematoxylin and eosin staining was performed on 5 μm sections. The images of the pulmonary terminal arterioles were captured with a Zeiss microscope digital

Figure 4. *Bcr−/−* **and** *abr−/−* **PASMC show increased proliferation when exposed to hypoxia** *in vitro.* **A,** Western blot analysis on PASMC lysates from *wt, bcr−/−* or *abr−/−* mice with anti-Bcr N20 antibodies or Abr antiserum. GAPDH, loading control. **B,** Third passage primary PASMC isolated from the intrapulmonary arteries of 5 different mice per genotype (1×10⁴ cells/well) were synchronized by serum free medium for 24 hrs, then cultured in medium with 10% FBS for 5 days, after which cells were counted. The Rac inhibitor Z62954982 was added to the indicated samples. * p<0.05 compared with the outcomes from the same genotype PASMCs in normoxia. # p<0.05 compared with *wt* PASMCs exposed to the same condition. Bars, mean ±SD of triplicate wells. **C,** Proliferation index of *wt, bcr−/−* and *abr−/−* PASMCs was calculated as described in Methods. Flow cytometry analysis was done

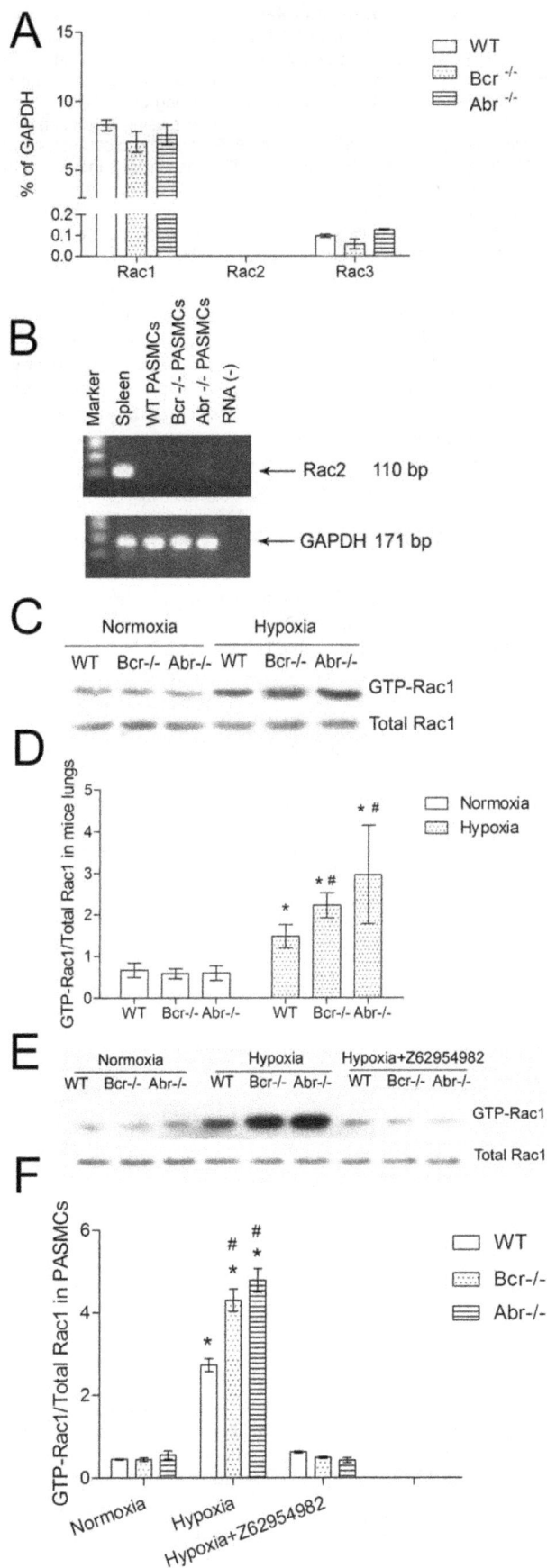

Figure 5. Loss of Bcr or Abr promotes hypoxia-induced Rac1 activation *in vitro* and *in vivo*. A, Real-time RT-PCR analysis for quantification of *rac1*, *rac2* and *rac3* mRNA in PASMCs. **B,** Representative gel electrophoresis of RT-PCR products showing absence of *rac2* in PASMCs. Samples loaded are indicated above the lanes; spleen, positive control; RNA (−), no RNA, negative control. **C–F,** Assay for Rac1 activation. **C–D,** Analysis of activation of Rac1 *in vivo* in the lungs of *bcr−/−*, *abr−/−* and *wt* mice after normoxia or hypoxia exposure. **E–F,** Analysis of Rac1 activation in PASMC under normoxia or hypoxia. **C** and **E,** representative Western blots; **D** and **F,** quantification. Three independent samples of each genotype were tested and the entire experiment was repeated independently. To quantitate results, Western blots were scanned and the ratio of GTP-Rac/total Rac was determined (panels **D, F**). * p<0.05 when compared with the results of the same genotype under normoxia. # p<0.05 when compared with WT exposed to the same condition.

camera. The arterial areas were analyzed with ImageJ 1.41 software (NIH, Bethesda, MD) for percentage wall thickness.

For immunohistochemistry, lung sections (5 μm) were deparaffinized. Vascular smooth muscle cells were detected by immunohistochemistry with a mouse monoclonal antibody to SMA, using a LAB-SA detection system (Invitrogen). Areas of cells positive for anti-SMA staining were quantified using ImageJ software (NIH). Briefly, contour plots were drawn around the α-SMA-stained cells. Images were then converted to grayscale format. A threshold was set for α-SMA-positive staining. Within the contour plots, pixels with intensities above the threshold were quantified and converted to areas using the scale bar on the image.

Measurement of the Mean Linear Intercept

For each image, 4 areas of interest, free of airways and blood vessels, were randomly picked for measuring the Mean Linear Intercept (MLI). A grid (5×5 with 20 μm between lines) was superimposed over the area of interest. The number of times (intercepts) that the alveoli intercepted the grid lines was counted. The MLI was calculated by multiplying the length of the lines and the number of lines per area, then dividing by the total number of intercepts [58].

The average alveolar area was quantified with Fiji ImageJ software [59]. The images were first processed with a median filter (radius 2.0 pixels), color deconvolution with an H&E 2 matrix, and an unsharp mask (radius 20 pixels, weight 0.9) on the H&E image. Default auto-thresholding and a binary fill-holes function were next applied. The area of all objects was measured with the Analyze Particles function, excluding objects with areas <60 μm². Objects representing trachea and blood vessels were manually excluded from the analysis. Data represent >100 measurements per genotype per condition.

Measurement of ROS Production in Macrophages

Mice were injected intraperitoneally with 4 ml of 4% thioglycollate medium. 4 days after the injection, macrophages were harvested from peritoneal cavities. Macrophages in complete RPMI-1640 medium (10% FBS) were exposed to normoxia or hypoxia for 24 hours. Cells were then treated with PBS (control cells for basal ROS production) or activated with PMA (1 μM) for 1 hr. Measurement of ROS production was performed using a CellROX Deep Red Reagent kit (Life Technologies, CA) according to the manufacturer's protocol. Data were collected using an Accuri flow cytometer (BD Biosciences).

Evans Blue Vascular Leakage Assay

Mice subjected to hypoxia for 3 weeks were injected with Evans blue (30 mg/kg body weight) via the tail vein. 20 min after the

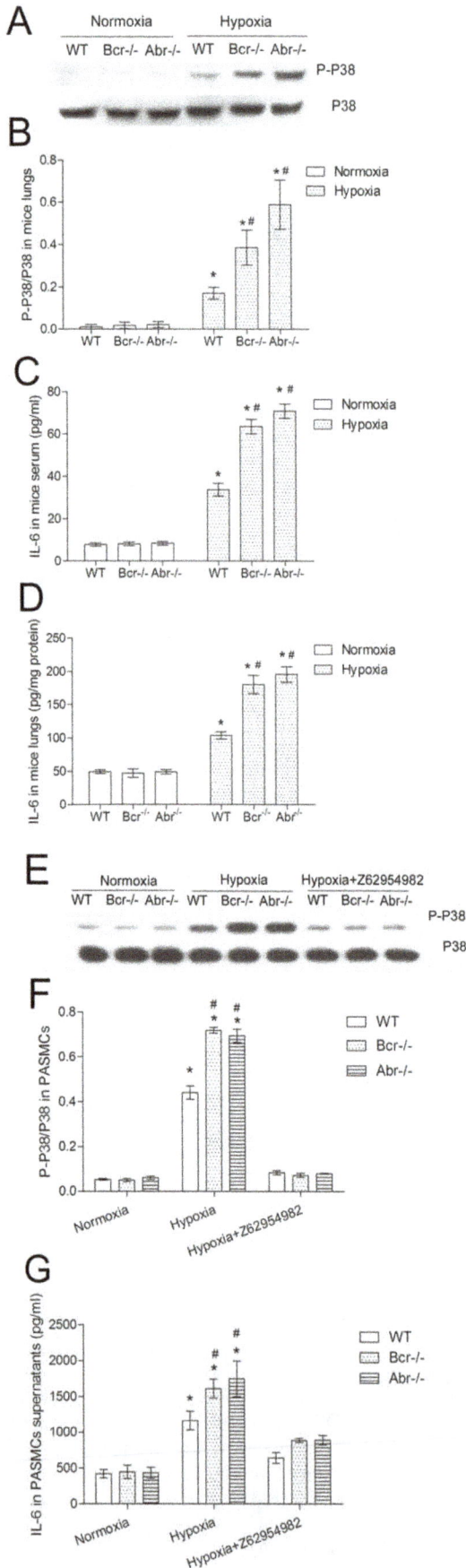

Figure 6. Enhanced phosphorylation of p38 and IL-6 production *in vivo* **and in null mutant PASMC. A,** Representative image of Western blots analyzing the phosphorylation of p38 in the lungs from *bcr−/−*, *abr−/−* and *wt* mice. **B,** Quantification of results for lungs from 6 mice/group. **C–D,** IL-6 was measured using an ELISA in serum (**C**) and lungs (**D**) of *bcr−/−*, *abr−/−* and *wt* mice using 6 independent samples per genotype per condition. **E–F,** Western blot analysis of PASMC for p-p38 (**E**) and quantification (**F**) of results of 3 independent samples of PASMCs/group. **G,** IL-6 in PASMC supernatants after normoxia or hypoxia exposure. *p<0.05 compared with the values from the same genotype, or PASMCs in normoxia. #p<0.05 when compared with WT exposed to the same condition.

injection, animals were sacrificed and perfused with PBS through the right ventricle. The vena cava was cut to drain blood and PBS, thus allowing PBS to pass through the pulmonary and systemic circulation to flush out blood. After perfusion, lungs were harvested, blotted on gauze and weighted. Lungs were then placed in 1 ml of formamide and incubated at 56°C for 24 h for the extraction of Evans blue. The concentration of Evans blue was measured at OD620 and calculated against a standard curve.

Pulmonary Arterial Smooth Muscle Cells Isolation and Culture

PASMCs were isolated from the intrapulmonary arteries of male *bcr−/−*, *abr−/−* and *wt* FVB/J mice as previously described [60]. In brief, mice were euthanized by CO_2. The thorax and abdomen were rinsed with 70% ethanol. The intrapulmonary arteries were dissected with sterile scissors and forceps under microscope. The adventitia and intima were removed from the arteries. The arteries was cut into 1–2 mm long pieces and incubated with 1.5 mg/ml type II collagenase (Sigma) for 4–6 hours at 37°C with gentle shaking. After two washes with culture medium (DMEM with 10% fetal bovine serum, 1% penicillin/streptomycin, 1% glutamine; Invitrogen), PASMCs were collected

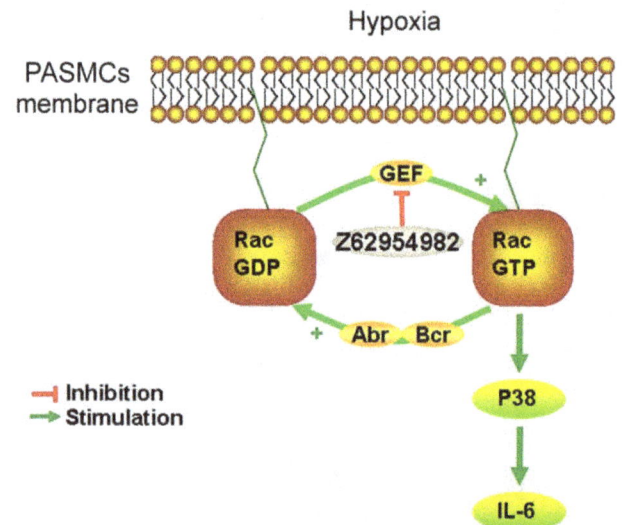

Figure 7. Schematic representation of the signal transduction pathways affected in PASMC lacking Abr and Bcr. Hypoxia directly or indirectly activates a G-nucleotide exchange factor (GEF) for Rac, resulting in elevated levels of GTP-bound Rac. In the absence of Bcr or Abr, Rac is not downregulated to its inactive GDP-bound form and this causes prolonged activation of p38 MAPK and production of IL-6. The inhibitor Z62954982 prevents the generation of the GTP-bound Rac that switches these pathways on, by interfering with the binding of Rac to the GEF that is chronically switched on in hypoxia.

and cultured at $37°C$ in 95% air/5% CO_2. The PASMC phenotype was confirmed by morphological features and immunostaining for SMA.

In vitro Cell Proliferation Assay and Flow Cytometric Cell Cycle Analysis

PASMCs (3rd passage) from male $bcr-/-$, $abr-/-$ and wt FVB/J mice were seeded in 6-well plates (1×10^4 cells/well) and cultured in serum-free medium for 24 hrs. Effective cell synchronization was confirmed by flow cytometry analysis. Triplicate wells of cells were then exposed to normoxia or hypoxia (5% O_2), with or without 25 µmol/L of the Rac inhibitor Z62954982 (ZINC08010136; Enamine Ltd, Cincinnati, USA). Z62954982 was made as a concentrated stock solution in DMSO (dimethyl sulfoxide). The final concentration of DMSO in the culture medium was 0.1%; control wells were treated with 0.1% DMSO only. Z62954982 did not have cytotoxic effects, since viability of the drug-treated PASMCs was around 95%, comparable with that of PASMCs treated with 0.1% DMSO. Medium was refreshed every 2 days. After 5 days, the supernatants were collected for measurement of IL-6. Cells were trypsinized and counted. PASMCs were then fixed with 70% ethanol and incubated with staining solution (20 µg/ml propidium iodide, 0.2 mg/ml DNase-free RNase, 0.01% Triton-100 in PBS). Cell cycle was analyzed using a flow cytometer (Accuri Cytometers). The proliferation index of the PASMCs was calculated as: $(S+G_2/M)/(G_0/G_1 + S + G_2/M) \times 100\%$. G_0/G_1, S, G_2/M represents the percentage of the cells in G_0/G_1, S, G_2/M phase, respectively.

Quantitative Real-time PCR

For the isolation of RNA and protein, 3rd passage PASMCs from Bcr$-/-$, Abr$-/-$ and WT mice were plated in 10 cm culture dishes (3×10^4/dish). Cells were treated either with DMSO or with Z62954982 (25 µmol/L, dissolved in DMSO, Enamine Ltd) in an incubator with normoxia or hypoxia (5% O_2) for 5 days. Medium was refreshed every other day. Fresh Z62954982 was added along with the change of medium for the Z62954982 treatment cells. On day 5, cells were harvested, washed 3 times with PBS, harvested by scraping and processed for RNA (RNA mini kit, Qiagen) or for protein isolation in MLB (see below). 2 µg of RNA was converted to cDNA. The primer pairs used for amplification were:

rac1, 5'- TGGCGAAAGAGATCGGTGCTGT-3' (sense), 5'-TTCTTGACAGGAGGGGGACAGAGA-3' (antisense); rac2, 5'-ACCTCCTAGCCACTCCATACCACT-3' (sense), 5'-CACCACACACTTGATGGCCTGCAT-3' (antisense); rac3, 5'-TGAGAATGTCCGTGCCAAGTGGT-3' (sense), 5'-CCGCAGCCGTTCAATCGTATCCTT-3' (antisense); Glyceraldehyde 3-phosphate dehydrogenase (gapdh), 5'-ACCCAGAAGACTGTGGATGG-3' (sense), 5'-CACCACACACTTGATGGCCTGCAT-3' (antisense).

Amplification reactions were performed with SYBR Green (Invitrogen) in an ABI Prism 7700 thermal cycler sequence detection system (Perkin-Elmer, CA). To confirm specificity of amplification, the PCR products from each primer pair were subjected to a melting curve analysis and electrophoresis on 2% agarose gels. The relative mRNA levels of target genes to that of gapdh were calculated.

Antibodies, Western Blotting

Rac activation assays were carried out as described previously [7]. Briefly, right lobes of the lungs from normoxia or hypoxia treated mice were isolated, washed 3 times with TBS, and

homogenized with Mg^{2+} lysis/wash buffer (MLB, 25 mmol/L Tris, pH 7.5, 150 mmol/L NaCl, 1% Igepal CA-630, 10 mmol/L $MgCl_2$, 1 mmol/L EDTA, 10% glycerol, 10 µg/ml leupeptin, 10 µg/ml aprotinin, 1 mmol/L sodium pervanadate, 1 mmol/L phenylmethylsulfonyl fluoride) on ice. These lysates were used for standard Western blotting and Rac activation assays. Lung lysates (in total, samples from 6 mice per genotype per condition) and PASMCs lysates in MLB (from triplicate wells and two independent experiments) were incubated with recombinant Pak1-GST PBD precoupled with glutathione-agarose beads at $4°C$ with rotation for 1 hour. Beads were washed 3 times with MLB and resuspended in SDS-sample buffer. Lysates to measure total Rac1 were collected before performing the Rac activation assay. Immunoblotting was performed with anti-Rac1 antibodies (1:1000, Cytoskeleton). Anti p38 and p-p38 antibodies (1:500) were from Cell Signaling. Abr antiserum (1:200) has been previously described. [8] Bcr (N-20; 1:500) antibodies were from Santa Cruz and GAPDH antibodies (1:5000) from Millipore. Anti-phosphotyrosine antibodies were obtained from BD Biosciences. Western blot results were quantified using Un-Scan-It software (Silk Scientific, Orem, UT) and analyzed as the ratio of phosphorylated p38 MAPK to total p38 MAPK or of GTP-bound Rac1 to total Rac. Western blot analysis was done with Abr antiserum (1:200) [8] and Bcr (N-20)(1:500, Santa Cruz) or GAPDH antibodies (1:5000, Millipore).

ELISA

The IL-6 levels in the serum and lungs of mice and PASMCs supernatants were measured by Enzyme-Linked Immunosorbent Assay (ELISA) according to the manufacturer's instructions (eBioscience).

Statistical Analysis

Statistical analysis was performed with SPSS 13.0 software (Chicago, USA). Data are expressed as mean $\pm$SD. One way-ANOVA was used to compare the differences between groups, followed by the Student-Newman-Keuls post-hoc analysis. Statistical significance was considered when $p < 0.05$.

Supporting Information

Figure S1 Emphysema and airway remodeling in normoxia- and hypoxia-exposed mice. A, Representative H&E stained lung sections of the indicated genotypes showing alveoli and bronchiolar walls. Bars, 25 µm. **B-C,** Quantification of **B,** mean linear intercept (MLI), and **C,** alveolar area. n.s., not significant.

Figure S2 Treatment of hypoxia- and normoxia-exposed mice with Z62954982. A, Right ventricle hypertrophy assessed by ratio of (RV/LV+S) from the hearts of normoxic and hypoxic wt and $abr-/-$ mice treated with Z62954982 at 10 mg/kg every other day or at 20 mg/kg daily for 3 wks. Control mice were administered i.p. with equal amount of vehicle. Bars, mean$\pm$SEM. n = 3–4 mice/group. *, $p < 0.05$, data were analyzed by one way ANOVA. **B–C,** Western blot analysis of representative samples (**B**) and quantification (**C**) of activated Rac1 in mice treated with 10 mg/kg Z62954982. n = 3 samples/group. Lysates were generated 1 hr after injection of the drug.

Figure S3 Lack of toxicity of Z62954982. A, representative H&E-stained liver sections of the indicated mice treated with 10 mg/kg every second day. **B,** analysis of total bone marrow cellularity and myeloid cell percentages of mice exposed to hypoxia and treated every day with 20 mg/kg drug or with vehicle. *$p<0.05$, n = 3 mice/group.

Acknowledgments

We thank Donna Foster for excellent care of the mice. Monica Wong and Sun Ju Yi are acknowledged for instruction on the RVSP measurements and the Rac activation assays, respectively. Dr. Bellusci kindly provided access to the hypoxia chamber and gas modulator. We thank Esteban Fernandez of the Imaging Core of the Saban Research Institute, Children's Hospital Los Angeles for help with quantification of the mean linear intercept, the alveolar size and of areas of α-SMA-positive cells. We thank Dr. Stefan M. Lee, who generously allowed us to use the BP-1 machine for invasive BP measurements.

Author Contributions

Conceived and designed the experiments: MY DG ML AA JG NH. Performed the experiments: MY DG ML AA. Analyzed the data: MY DG AA JG NH. Wrote the paper: MY DG AA JG NH.

References

1. Heisterkamp N, Stam K, Groffen J, de Klein A, Grosveld G (1985) Structural organization of the bcr gene and its role in the Ph' translocation. Nature 315: 758–761.

2. Chuang TH, Xu X, Kaartinen V, Heisterkamp N, Groffen J, et al. (1995) Abr and Bcr are multifunctional regulators of the Rho GTP-binding protein family. Proc Natl Acad Sci U S A 92: 10282–10286.

3. Diekmann D, Brill S, Garrett MD, Totty N, Hsuan J, et al. (1991) Bcr encodes a GTPase-activating protein for p21rac. Nature 351: 400–402.

4. Bernards A, Settleman J (2004) GAP control: regulating the regulators of small GTPases. Trends Cell Biol 14: 377–385.

5. Heasman SJ, Ridley AJ (2008) Mammalian Rho GTPases: new insights into their functions from in vivo studies. Nat Rev Mol Cell Biol 9: 690–701.

6. Van Aelst L, DSouza-Schorey C (1997) Rho GTPases and signaling networks. Genes Dev 11: 2295–2322.

7. Cho YJ, Cunnick JM, Yi SJ, Kaartinen V, Groffen J, et al. (2007) Abr and Bcr, two homologous Rac GTPase-activating proteins, control multiple cellular functions of murine macrophages. Mol Cell Biol 27: 899–911.

8. Cunnick JM, Schmidhuber S, Chen G, Yu M, Yi SJ, et al. (2009) Bcr and Abr cooperate in negatively regulating acute inflammatory responses. Mol Cell Biol 29: 5742–5750.

9. Kaartinen V, Gonzalez-Gomez I, Voncken JW, Haataja L, Faure E, et al. (2001) Abnormal function of astroglia lacking Abr and Bcr RacGAPs. Development 128: 4217–4227.

10. Oh D, Han S, Seo J, Lee JR, Choi J, et al. (2010) Regulation of synaptic Rac1 activity, long-term potentiation maintenance, and learning and memory by BCR and ABR Rac GTPase-activating proteins. J Neurosci 30: 14134–14144.

11. Voncken JW, van Schaick H, Kaartinen V, Deemer K, Coates T, et al. (1995) Increased neutrophil respiratory burst in bcr-null mutants. Cell 80: 719–728.

12. Macchia A, Marchioli R, Marfisi R, Scarano M, Levantesi G, et al. (2007) A meta-analysis of trials of pulmonary hypertension: a clinical condition looking for drugs and research methodology. Am Heart J 153: 1037–1047.

13. Janssens SP, Thompson BT, Spence CR, Hales CA (1991) Polycythemia and vascular remodeling in chronic hypoxic pulmonary hypertension in guinea pigs. J Appl Physiol 71: 2218–2223.

14. Rabinovitch M, Gamble W, Nadas AS, Miettinen OS, Reid L (1979) Rat pulmonary circulation after chronic hypoxia: hemodynamic and structural features. Am J Physiol 236: H818–827.

15. Crosswhite P, Sun Z (2010) Nitric oxide, oxidative stress and inflammation in pulmonary arterial hypertension. J Hypertens 28: 201–212.

16. Price LC, Wort SJ, Perros F, Dorfmuller P, Huertas A, et al. (2012) Inflammation in pulmonary arterial hypertension. Chest 141: 210–221.

17. Sakao S, Tatsumi K (2011) The effects of antiangiogenic compound SU5416 in a rat model of pulmonary arterial hypertension. Respiration 81: 253–261.

18. Tuder RM, Zhen L, Cho CY, Taraseviciene-Stewart L, Kasahara Y, et al. (2003) Oxidative stress and apoptosis interact and cause emphysema due to vascular endothelial growth factor receptor blockade. Am J Respir Cell Mol Biol 29: 88–97.

19. Ciuclan L, Bonneau O, Hussey M, Duggan N, Holmes AM, et al. (2011) A novel murine model of severe pulmonary arterial hypertension. Am J Respir Crit Care Med 184: 1171–1182.

20. Yu L, Hales CA (2011) Hypoxia does neither stimulate pulmonary artery endothelial cell proliferation in mice and rats with pulmonary hypertension and vascular remodeling nor in human pulmonary artery endothelial cells. J Vasc Res 48: 465–475.

21. Stenmark KR, Fagan KA, Frid MG (2006) Hypoxia-induced pulmonary vascular remodeling: cellular and molecular mechanisms. Circ Res 99: 675–691.

22. Humbert M, Morrell NW, Archer SL, Stenmark KR, MacLean MR, et al. (2004) Cellular and molecular pathobiology of pulmonary arterial hypertension. J Am Coll Cardiol 43: 13S–24S.

23. Stenmark KR, Mecham RP (1997) Cellular and molecular mechanisms of pulmonary vascular remodeling. Annu Rev Physiol 59: 89–144.

24. Ferri N, Corsini A, Bottino P, Clerici F, Contini A (2009) Virtual screening approach for the identification of new Rac1 inhibitors. J Med Chem 52: 4087–4090.

25. Das M, Bouchey DM, Moore MJ, Hopkins DC, Nemenoff RA, et al. (2001) Hypoxia-induced proliferative response of vascular adventitial fibroblasts is dependent on g protein-mediated activation of mitogen-activated protein kinases. J Biol Chem 276: 15631–15640.

26. Karakiulakis G, Papakonstantinou E, Aletras AJ, Tamm M, Roth M (2007) Cell type-specific effect of hypoxia and platelet-derived growth factor-BB on extracellular matrix turnover and its consequences for lung remodeling. J Biol Chem 282: 908–915.

27. Lu J, Shimpo H, Shimamoto A, Chong AJ, Hampton CR, et al. (2004) Specific inhibition of p38 mitogen-activated protein kinase with FR167653 attenuates vascular proliferation in monocrotaline-induced pulmonary hypertension in rats. J Thorac Cardiovasc Surg 128: 850–859.

28. Sodhi CP, Phadke SA, Batlle D, Sahai A (2001) Hypoxia stimulates osteopontin expression and proliferation of cultured vascular smooth muscle cells: potentiation by high glucose. Diabetes 50: 1482–1490.

29. Hattori Y, Suzuki M, Hattori S, Kasai K (2002) Vascular smooth muscle cell activation by glycated albumin (Amadori adducts). Hypertension 39: 22–28.

30. Tokunou T, Ichiki T, Takeda K, Funakoshi Y, Iino N, et al. (2001) Thrombin induces interleukin-6 expression through the cAMP response element in vascular smooth muscle cells. Arterioscler Thromb Vasc Biol 21: 1759–1763.

31. Lee JC, Kumar S, Griswold DE, Underwood DC, Votta BJ, et al. (2000) Inhibition of p38 MAP kinase as a therapeutic strategy. Immunopharmacology 47: 185–201.

32. Sano M, Fukuda K, Sato T, Kawaguchi H, Suematsu M, et al. (2001) ERK and p38 MAPK, but not NF-kappaB, are critically involved in reactive oxygen species-mediated induction of IL-6 by angiotensin II in cardiac fibroblasts. Circ Res 89: 661–669.

33. Selimovic N, Bergh CH, Andersson B, Sakiniene E, Carlsten H, et al. (2009) Growth factors and interleukin-6 across the lung circulation in pulmonary hypertension. Eur Respir J 34: 662–668.

34. Humbert M, Monti G, Brenot F, Sitbon O, Portier A, et al. (1995) Increased interleukin-1 and interleukin-6 serum concentrations in severe primary pulmonary hypertension. Am J Respir Crit Care Med 151: 1628–1631.

35. Steiner MK, Syrkina OL, Kolliputi N, Mark EJ, Hales CA, et al. (2009) Interleukin-6 overexpression induces pulmonary hypertension. Circ Res 104: 236–244, 228p following 244.

36. Berk BC (2001) Vascular smooth muscle growth: autocrine growth mechanisms. Physiol Rev 81: 999–1030.

37. Soon E, Holmes AM, Treacy CM, Doughty NJ, Southgate L, et al. (2010) Elevated levels of inflammatory cytokines predict survival in idiopathic and familial pulmonary arterial hypertension. Circulation 122: 920–927.

38. Galie N, Manes A, Negro L, Palazzini M, Bacchi-Reggiani ML, et al. (2009) A meta-analysis of randomized controlled trials in pulmonary arterial hypertension. Eur Heart J 30: 394–403.

39. Diebold I, Petry A, Djordjevic T, Belaiba RS, Fineman J, et al. (2010) Reciprocal regulation of Rac1 and PAK-1 by HIF-1alpha: a positive-feedback loop promoting pulmonary vascular remodeling. Antioxid Redox Signal 13: 399–412.

40. Grobe AC, Wells SM, Benavidez E, Oishi P, Azakie A, et al. (2006) Increased oxidative stress in lambs with increased pulmonary blood flow and pulmonary hypertension: role of NADPH oxidase and endothelial NO synthase. Am J Physiol Lung Cell Mol Physiol 290: L1069–1077.

41. Teng RJ, Eis A, Bakhutashvili I, Arul N, Konduri GG (2009) Increased superoxide production contributes to the impaired angiogenesis of fetal pulmonary arteries with in utero pulmonary hypertension. Am J Physiol Lung Cell Mol Physiol 297: L184–195.

42. Diebold I, Djordjevic T, Hess J, Gorlach A (2008) Rac-1 promotes pulmonary artery smooth muscle cell proliferation by upregulation of plasminogen activator inhibitor-1: role of NFkappaB-dependent hypoxia-inducible factor-1alpha transcription. Thromb Haemost 100: 1021–1028.

43. Tian Y, Autieri MV (2007) Cytokine expression and AIF-1-mediated activation of Rac2 in vascular smooth muscle cells: a role for Rac2 in VSMC activation. Am J Physiol Cell Physiol 292: C841–849.

44. Patterson C, Ruef J, Madamanchi NR, Barry-Lane P, Hu Z, et al. (1999) Stimulation of a vascular smooth muscle cell NAD(P)H oxidase by thrombin. Evidence that p47(phox) may participate in forming this oxidase in vitro and in vivo. J Biol Chem 274: 19814–19822.

45. Davie N, Haleen SJ, Upton PD, Polak JM, Yacoub MH, et al. (2002) ET(A) and ET(B) receptors modulate the proliferation of human pulmonary artery smooth muscle cells. Am J Respir Crit Care Med 165: 398–405.

46. Liu JQ, Zelko IN, Erbynn EM, Sham JS, Folz RJ (2006) Hypoxic pulmonary hypertension: role of superoxide and NADPH oxidase (gp91phox). Am J Physiol Lung Cell Mol Physiol 290: L2–10.

47. Hirota K, Semenza GL (2001) Rac1 activity is required for the activation of hypoxia-inducible factor 1. J Biol Chem 276: 21166–21172.

48. Carlin CM, Peacock AJ, Welsh DJ (2007) Fluvastatin inhibits hypoxic proliferation and p38 MAPK activity in pulmonary artery fibroblasts. Am J Respir Cell Mol Biol 37: 447–456.

49. Qi YX, Qu MJ, Yan ZQ, Zhao D, Jiang XH, et al. (2010) Cyclic strain modulates migration and proliferation of vascular smooth muscle cells via Rho-GDIalpha, Rac1, and p38 pathway. J Cell Biochem 109: 906–914.

50. Ikeda U, Ikeda M, Oohara T, Oguchi A, Kamitani T, et al. (1991) Interleukin 6 stimulates growth of vascular smooth muscle cells in a PDGF-dependent manner. Am J Physiol 260: H1713–1717.

51. Tamm M, Bihl M, Eickelberg O, Stulz P, Perruchoud AP, et al. (1998) Hypoxia-induced interleukin-6 and interleukin-8 production is mediated by platelet-activating factor and platelet-derived growth factor in primary human lung cells. Am J Respir Cell Mol Biol 19: 653–661.

52. Grimminger F, Schermuly RT (2010) PDGF receptor and its antagonists: role in treatment of PAH. Adv Exp Med Biol 661: 435–446.

53. Chanakira A, Dutta R, Charboneau R, Barke R, Santilli SM, et al. (2011) Hypoxia differentially regulates arterial and venous smooth muscle cell proliferation via PDGFR-beta and VEGFR-2 expression. Am J Physiol Heart Circ Physiol 302: H1173–1184.

54. Clempus RE, Griendling KK (2006) Reactive oxygen species signaling in vascular smooth muscle cells. Cardiovasc Res 71: 216–225.

55. Boureux A, Furstoss O, Simon V, Roche S (2005) Abl tyrosine kinase regulates a Rac/JNK and a Rac/Nox pathway for DNA synthesis and Myc expression induced by growth factors. J Cell Sci 118: 3717–3726.

56. Feng H, Hu B, Liu KW, Li Y, Lu X, et al. (2011) Activation of Rac1 by Src-dependent phosphorylation of Dock180(Y1811) mediates PDGFRalpha-stimulated glioma tumorigenesis in mice and humans. J Clin Invest 121: 4670–4684.

57. Meller N, Merlot S, Guda C (2005) CZH proteins: a new family of Rho-GEFs. J Cell Sci 118: 4937–4946.

58. Dunnill MS (1962) Quantitative methods in the study of pulmonary pathology. Thorax 17: 320–328.

59. Schindelin J, Arganda-Carreras I, Frise E, Kaynig V, Longair M, et al. (2012) Fiji: an open-source platform for biological-image analysis. Nat Methods 9: 676–682.

60. Morrell NW, Upton PD, Kotecha S, Huntley A, Yacoub MH, et al. (1999) Angiotensin II activates MAPK and stimulates growth of human pulmonary artery smooth muscle via AT1 receptors. Am J Physiol 277: L440–448.

9

Xanthine Oxidase-Derived ROS Upregulate Egr-1 via ERK1/2 in PA Smooth Muscle Cells; Model to Test Impact of Extracellular ROS in Chronic Hypoxia

Tanya Hartney[1,9], Rahul Birari[1,9], Sujatha Venkataraman[1], Leah Villegas[1,2], Maylyn Martinez[1], Stephen M. Black[3], Kurt R. Stenmark[1,2], Eva Nozik-Grayck[1,2]*

1 Department of Pediatrics, University of Colorado Denver, Aurora, Colorado, United States of America, 2 Cardiovascular Pulmonary Research Laboratory, University of Colorado Denver, Aurora, Colorado, United States of America, 3 Georgia Health Sciences University, Augusta, Georgia, United States of America

Abstract

Exposure of newborn calves to chronic hypoxia causes pulmonary artery (PA) hypertension and remodeling. Previous studies showed that the redox-sensitive transcription factor, early growth response-1 (Egr-1), is upregulated in the PA of chronically hypoxic calves and regulates cell proliferation. Furthermore, we established in mice a correlation between hypoxic induction of Egr-1 and reduced activity of extracellular superoxide dismutase (EC-SOD), an antioxidant that scavenges extracellular superoxide. We now hypothesize that loss of EC-SOD in chronically hypoxic calves leads to extracellular superoxide-mediated upregulation of Egr-1. To validate our hypothesis and identify the signaling pathways involved, we utilized PA tissue from normoxic and chronically hypoxic calves and cultured calf and human PA smooth muscle cells (PASMC). Total SOD activity was low in the PA tissue, and only the extracellular SOD component decreased with hypoxia. PA tissue of hypoxic calves showed increased oxidative stress and increased Egr-1 mRNA. To mimic the in vivo hypoxia-induced extracellular oxidant imbalance, cultured calf PASMC were treated with xanthine oxidase (XO), which generates extracellular superoxide and hydrogen peroxide. We found that 1) XO increased Egr-1 mRNA and protein, 2) XO induced the phosphorylation of ERK1/2 and, 3) pretreatment with an ERK1/2 inhibitor prevented induction of Egr-1 by XO. siRNA knock-down of EC-SOD in human PASMC also upregulated Egr-1 mRNA and protein, activated ERK1/2, and enhanced SMC proliferation and reduced apoptosis. We conclude that an oxidant/antioxidant imbalance arising from loss of EC-SOD in the PA with chronic hypoxia induces Egr-1 via activation of ERK1/2 and contributes to pulmonary vascular remodeling.

Editor: Rory Edward Morty, University of Giessen Lung Center, Germany

Funding: This work was supported by National Institutes of Health grants 5RO1-HL086680-04 (EN-G) and 5PO1-HL014985-37 (KS) and March of Dimes research grant #6-FY06-316 (EN-G). The funders had no role in the study design, data collection and analysis, decision to publish or preparation of the manuscript.

Competing Interests: The authors have declared that no competing interests exist.

* E-mail: Eva.Grayck@ucdenver.edu

9 These authors contributed equally to this work.

Introduction

Infants, children and adults with chronic lung diseases complicated by alveolar hypoxia are at risk for developing pulmonary hypertension, which is associated with a high morbidity and mortality [1]. Exposure of animals to chronic hypoxia is a well-established and useful model to interrogate the mechanisms that may contribute to human disease. Accumulating evidence indicates that reactive oxygen species including superoxide $(O_2^{·-})$ are important in the pathogenesis of pulmonary hypertension, including chronic hypoxia-induced pulmonary hypertension [2,3]. There are a number of known sources of $O_2^{·-}$ in the pulmonary artery including NADPH oxidase, the mitochondrial electron transport chain, uncoupled endothelial nitric oxide synthase and xanthine oxidase (XO) that have been implicated in generation of $O_2^{·-}$ in response to hypoxia [3,4]. There is accumulating evidence that $O_2^{·-}$ generated specifically in the extracellular compartment contributes to the development of pulmonary hypertension. The antioxidant enzyme which defends against extracellular $O_2^{·-}$, extracellular superoxide dismutase (EC-SOD or SOD3), is highly expressed in the pulmonary circulation,

and its level of expression may modulate the development of pulmonary hypertension. Lung EC-SOD expression and activity decreases in rodent models associated with oxidative stress, including hypoxia and bleomycin-induced lung injury, as well as in the bronchus of humans with end-stage idiopathic pulmonary arterial hypertension [5–9]. Furthermore, enhancing lung EC-SOD activity either in genetically engineered mice or with adenoviral gene delivery protects against pulmonary hypertension and pulmonary vascular remodeling due to monocrotaline, bleomycin, or chronic hypoxia [10–12]. Overexpression of EC-SOD protects by limiting fibrosis and inflammation and prevents the upregulation of key genes involved in these processes. Among many redox-regulated genes, the transcription factor, early growth response-1 (Egr-1) is of interest because we and others have shown it increases in the lung and pulmonary vascular cells early in response to hypoxia and activates a number of downstream targets critical to proliferation, fibrosis and inflammation [10,11,13–19]. Therefore, Egr-1 can play a critical role in pulmonary vascular remodeling though its regulation in pulmonary hypertension by ROS is not clearly understood.

The contribution of EC-SOD to the pathogenesis of neonatal pulmonary hypertension has not been substantially investigated. Broadly it has been recognized that the neonatal lung is susceptible to oxidative stress due to the developmental regulation of antioxidant defenses [20]. The neonatal calf is particularly susceptible to hypoxia-induced pulmonary hypertension, with severe inflammation, pulmonary vascular remodeling and pulmonary hypertension, and Egr-1 is increased in the pulmonary artery in the chronically hypoxic neonatal calf [19]. The calf model is a useful model not only because of the severe pathology similar to human disease, but also because of the availability of primary pulmonary artery cells from the neonatal calf to test mechanisms responsible for the pathogenesis of pulmonary hypertension. We hypothesized that loss of EC-SOD specifically within the pulmonary artery of the newborn calf in response to hypoxia leads to extracellular superoxide-mediated upregulation of Egr-1. We utilized PA tissue isolated from normoxic and chronically hypoxic calves along with cultured calf to test this hypothesis and investigate the signaling pathway involved in the ROS modulation of Egr-1. In addition, we also knocked-down EC-SOD in human PASMC to directly test the contribution of EC-SOD to Egr-1 expression as well as SMC proliferative ability.

Methods

Animal Model and Tissue Harvesting

This study was carried out in strict accordance with the recommendations in the Guide for the Care and Use of Laboratory Animals of the National Institutes of Health. All animal studies were approved by the Institutional Animal Use and Care Committees (Colorado State University School of Veterinary Medicine, Fort Collins, CO (Protocol 10-1927A) or University of Colorado School of Medicine, Aurora, CO (Protocol # 71108(03)1E). Chronic exposure to hypoxia is a well-established model of pulmonary hypertension, characterized by elevated pulmonary artery pressures and pulmonary artery remodeling. In this study, 1-day-old male Holstein calves (Laluna Dairy Farm, Fort Collins) were placed in a hypobaric hypoxia chamber at P_B 445 mm Hg (simulating 15,000 ft or 12% FIO_2) for 14 days along with age-matched calves maintained in ambient Denver altitude (P_B 640 mm Hg). Tissue from chronically hypoxic calves was harvested within the chamber under hypobaric hypoxic conditions while tissue from normoxic calves was obtained in normobaric atmosphere. Calves were euthanized with an overdose of pentobarbital sodium (160 mg/kg body weight) and lung tissue and intraparenchymal proximal pulmonary artery tissue containing all three layers of the vessel wall were rapidly dissected and flash frozen. Another pulmonary artery segment was placed in cold media for preparation of primary vascular cell lines. Tissue was flash frozen for analysis.

Cell Culture model

To test how extracellular $O_2^{.-}$ generated in the pulmonary artery wall can upregulate the redox sensitive transcription factor, Egr-1, experiments were done with smooth muscle cells (SMC) isolated from the pulmonary artery of normoxic or chronically hypoxic calves using an explant technique as previously described [21]. This cell type was selected as a key cell type implicated in the pathogenesis of pulmonary hypertension that also expresses Egr-1 [19,22]. Cells were grown in DMEM with 10% bovine calf serum (Gemini, West Sacramento, CA) and supplemented with Cellgro 1% NEAA (Mediatech, Inc, Manassas, VA), 4 mM Cellgro L-Glutamine (Mediatech, Inc) and Cellgro pen-strep (100 I.U/mL pen and 100 µg/mL strep, Mediatech, Inc) and maintained in

humidified incubator at 5% CO_2 and 37°C. Cells were used between passages 4 and 8. The cell culture data, unless specified otherwise in a particular experiment, is derived from three separate wells or plates of cells derived from a single chronically hypoxic calf and performed on a single day to control for day-to-day variability and enable comparisons between experimental groups. The experiments were repeated on at least 3 different days with cells from at least 3 different calves to ensure reproducibility. The qPCR was also performed in triplicate for each cell isolation. Human PASMC purchased from Lonza were grown in designated SMC media (Clonetics LONZA smBm media cat no: CC3181).

Treatment groups

Cells were treated with XO because it is an enzyme known to be upregulated in the pulmonary circulation in models of pulmonary hypertension and it is a reproducible method to generate extracellular $O_2^{.-}$ in order to study the impact of $O_2^{.-}$ released in this particular cell compartment. Cells were treated with XO dissolved in phosphate buffered saline (PBS) (Sigma, St Louis, MO) and hypoxanthine (HX) (Sigma) dissolved in 0.1 M sodium hydroxide (NaOH). The optimal dose of XO and HX was established with a dose and time response curve. Based on pilot results, all remaining studies were carried out using cells treated for 1 hour with 8 mU/mL XO and 0.5 mM HX (XO/HX). Control cells for XO/HX treatment received the vehicles alone (PBS and 0.1 M NaOH). For studies with extracellular antioxidant treatments, cells were pretreated for 30 minutes with 500 U/mL SOD (Sigma) and/or catalase 600 U/mL (Boehringer Mannheim, Mannheim, Germany). Catalase was first dialyzed against PBS for 24 hours in PBS and activity determined as previously described [23]. Catalase was stored at −20°C until used. For MAPK inhibitor studies, cells were pretreated for 30 minutes with the ERK1/2 Inhibitor PD98059 (10 µM, Cell Signaling Danvers, MA) followed by the 1 hour treatment with XO. One series of PASMC were exposed in sealed humidified gas chambers to 21% or 1% oxygen tension with 5% CO_2 and balanced N_2 for 4 and 24 hours, as previously described, to evaluate the relative impact of hypoxia on Egr-1 expression and extracellular $O_2^{.-}$ release compared to XO/HX-treated cells [10–12]. An additional series of cells were treated for 2 hours with low dose (0.25 µM) or high dose (250 µM) antimycin A, an inhibitor of the mitochondrial electron transport chain, to generate endogenous $O_2^{.-}$. Antimycin A was dissolved in DMSO and the appropriate vehicle was used for control conditions.

siRNA transfection

An siRNA targeting EC-SOD and a non-targeting siRNA were transfected into human PASMC (Lonza Walkersville, Walkersville, MD) using the siPORT NeoFX transfection reagent (Ambion). Cells ($12×10^5$) in a 6-well plate, were transfected with a final concentration of 5 nM of non-targeting (negative control, siNEG)) or siRNA targeting EC-SOD, (siEC-SOD). The manufacturer's suggested protocol of a reverse transfection was followed. Transfected cells were then harvested after 48 h for mRNA or protein analysis. After every transfection, the EC-SOD knockdown was confirmed by qPCR.

mRNA isolation from calf PA and cultured cells

For pulmonary artery segments, the fibrous tissue was first pulverized using a mortar and pestle on liquid nitrogen to facilitate homogenization. Cells, $4×10^4$ per well, were seeded in a 6 well plate (Corning, Lowell MA) and allowed to grow for 48 hours prior to treatment. RNA was isolated from tissue using TRIzol (Invitrogen, Carlsbad, CA) and from cells using the RNeasy Plus kit (Qiagen, Germantown, MD) according to manufacturers' instructions. The concentration and purity of each total RNA sample was determined by the NanoDrop® ND-1000 spectrophotometer (NanoDrop, Wilmington, DE). The integrity of total RNA samples was examined by 2100 Bioanalyzer and the RNA 6000 Nano Kit (Agilent Technologies).

mRNA analysis by real time RT-PCR (qPCR)

RNA (1 μg per reaction) was reverse transcribed with the Maxima First Strand cDNA synthesis kit (Fermentas International Inc, Glen Burnie, MD). PCR was performed on the MyiQ Detection System (Bio-Rad, Hercules, CA) with the RT^2 Real-Time SYBR Green/Fluorescein PCR master mix (SABiosciences, Frederick, MD). Reactions were run in triplicate and results analyzed by the 2 (−delta delta CT) Method, normalizing the gene copy numbers to hypoxanthine-guanine phosphoribosyl-transferase (HPRT). Data are expressed in figures as either actual copies of Egr-1/HPRT or, to more easily visualize fold change in certain experiments, Egr-1/HPRT normalized to the mean expression of the control group. Primers for calf tissue were designed with NCBI Primer-BLAST software. Primers used were Egr-1 forward: CCTTCAG TACCCACCTCCTG Egr-1 reverse: AGGGCTTCTGATCTGGTGTG. HPRT forward: CCAAA-GATGGTCA AGGTTGC HPRT reverse: GGGCATATCC-CACAACAAAC. Human Egr-1 and GAPDH primers were purchased from SABiosciences. For human EC-SOD mRNA analysis, Taqman EC-SOD primers were purchased along with the corresponding GAPDH primers and qPCR performed with Taqman master mix according to instructions (Applied Biosciences).

Protein isolation

Pulverized lung or pulmonary artery tissue was homogenized in RIPA buffer (Sigma) containing protease (Sigma) and phosphatase (Thermo Scientific, Rockford, IL) inhibitors and centrifuged to remove cellular debris. For total cell lysates from cultured cells, 5.0×10^5 cells were seeded in 100 mm dishes (Corning) and allowed to grow for 48 hours prior to treatment. After appropriate treatment, media was removed and plates placed on ice, cells washed $2 \times$ PBS and then lysed in RIPA buffer (Sigma) containing protease (Sigma) and phosphatase (Thermo Scientific) inhibitors. Cells were scraped and placed in −80°C overnight followed by sonication and centrifugation at 4°C degrees to collect the supernatant. Protein concentration was determined using the Pierce 660 nm protein assay reagent (Thermo Scientific). Nuclear protein was extracted from calf PASMC (1×10^6 cells per condition) using NE-PER Nuclear and Cytoplasmic Extraction Reagents according to product instructions (Pierce Biotechnology, Rockford, IL).

Western blot analysis

For Western blot analysis with the phosphoERK1/2 and total ERK1/2 antibodies, 20 μg human or calf total PASMC protein was loaded on a 4–12% Bis-Tris Gel (Invitrogen, Carlsbad, CA) and protein separated by gel electrophoresis. Proteins were transferred to PDVF membranes using the semi-dry method (Invitrogen). Blots were blocked with 5% milk in Tris Buffered Saline with 0.05% Tween 20 (TBST) and probed with the primary monoclonal mouse phospho-p44/42 MAPK antibody (Cell Signaling, 1:1000) overnight at 4°C followed by an anti-mouse HRP-conjugated secondary antibody (Millepore, Billerica, MA). Blots were developed with Enhanced Chemiluminescence (ECL) plus (Thermo Scientific) and then stripped with Restore Plus Western Blot Stripping Buffer according to kit instructions

(Thermo Scientific) and reprobed with rabbit monoclonal Total ERK antibody (Cell Signaling, 1:1000), for normalization: Bands were quantified by densitometry and expressed as the ratio of phosphoERK/totalERK. Blots from human PASMC total cell lysates were also probed with polyclonal rabbit anti-Egr-1 (Cell Signaling, 1:500), cyclin D1 (Cell Signaling , 1:1,000) and ß-actin as a loading control. For calf PASMC, to reduce non-specific binding by the Egr-1 antibody, likely due to poor cross-reactivity with the anti-human Egr-1 antibody, 25 μg nuclear extracts were used instead for Western blot. Equal nuclear protein loading was confirmed by Ponceau S staining (Millipore). For the Western blot with protein from pulmonary artery or lung tissue, 20–100 mg of protein homogenate was loaded on the gel as well as 1 mg purified bovine EC-SOD protein as a positive control. The blot was probed overnight at 4°C with 1:1,000 rabbit anti-human EC-SOD ab in 5% milk, which recognizes bovine EC-SOD (purified EC-SOD and EC-SOD antibody kindly provided by Tim Oury, MD, PhD, University of Pittsburgh). Western blots for PA protein were also probed with antibodies against Cu,Zn SOD (Abcam, 1:2,000) Mn SOD (Millipore, 1:1,000), and ß-actin in protein homogenates from normoxic and chronically hypoxic calves.

Reactive oxygen species measurements

2,3-bis-(2-methoxy-4-nitro-5-sulfophenyl)-2H-tetrazolium-5-carboxanilide, disodium salt (XTT) (Sigma) was used to detect extracellular $O_2\cdot^-$ generated in response to XO/HX or hypoxia in cultured calf PASMC. SMC (3×10^4), were plated in triplicate in a 96 well plate in phenol free medium containing the supplements as described above. Cells were grown for 48 hours and prior to treatment, cells were washed with $1 \times$ PBS and replaced with fresh phenol-free medium. To measure the change in extracellular $O_2\cdot^-$ generated by XO/HX, XTT (100 μm) was added to the cells along with either XO/HX or vehicle. The change in absorbance at 470 nm was read by a Biorad 680 microplate reader (Biorad, Hercules, CA) at 1 hr following XO/HX. One set of cells were pre-treated for 30 minutes with 500 U/mL SOD (Sigma) prior to the addition of XO/HX. The experiment was repeated three times. Using the extinction coefficient of $21600 \ M^{-1} \ cm^{-1}$ (XTT), the superoxide flux was calculated and data expressed as rate of superoxide flux ($M \cdot s^{-1}$). Hydrogen peroxide was measured in calf PASMC treated with 1 hour of XO/HX using a fluorometric assay as described by Hyslop et al [24] and the rate of H_2O_2 production was expressed in $M \cdot s^{-1}$. Briefly, in this assay, cells are rinsed and incubated with phenol red-free buffer containing horseradish peroxidase (HRP, 1.6 mM), HEPES buffer, $NaHCO_3$ (60 mM) and para-hydroxyphenyl acetic acid (pHPA, 95 μg/mL) for two hours. The reaction of H_2O_2 with HRP forms compound I, which then oxidizes pHPA and results in the formation of a fluorescent dimer product detectable by a fluorometric plate reader (polarstar Omega, BMG Labtech) [24].

SOD Activity assay

Pulverized lung and pulmonary artery tissue (300 mg) were homogenized in 10 volumes of ice-cold buffer (50 mM potassium phosphate, pH 7.4, with 0.3 M KBr, 0.05 mM phenylmethylsul-fonyl flouride, and 3 mM diethylene-triaminepentaacetic acid) and centrifuged to remove cellular debris. For the pulmonary artery homogenates, EC-SOD was separated from intracellular SOD (Cu,Zn SOD and Mn SOD) using a concanavalin A column (Pierce,Rockford,Illinois) as previously described [25]. Briefly, pulmonary artery homogenates were applied to the column. Intracellular SODs were collected by washing the column with

5 mL of equilibration buffer (50 mM HEPES, pH 7.0 with 0.25 M NaCl). The EC-SOD fraction was eluted with 3 mL 50 mM HEPES, pH 7.0 with 0.25 M NaCl with 1 M alpha-methylmannoside, final pH 5. The EC-SOD fraction was concentrated 10-fold by centrifuging with a centriprep concentrator (Amicon-ultracel-10K, Millipore) at 4°C for 60 minutes. EC-SOD and intracellular SOD separation was confirmed by Western blot, as described above, and activity levels were measured using the SOD assay kit-WST (Dojindo Molecular Technologies, Maryland, USA). This kit utilizes a water-soluble tetrazolium salt, WST-1 [2-(4-iodophenyl)-3-(4-nitrophenyl)-5-(2,4-disulfo-phenyl)-2H-tetrazolium, monosodium salt], to produce a water-soluble formazan dye upon reduction with a superoxide anion, detectable by a colorimetric assay. A standard curve was linear between SOD concentrations of 0.1 to 5 U/mL. SOD activity data were expressed as units of SOD activity per gram of tissue.

GSH/GSSG assay

The GSH/GSSG ratio was measured as a marker of oxidative stress in PA tissue following chronic hypoxia as previously described [26,27]. Briefly, cow PA tissue (50 mg) was homogenized in MES (Morpholino ethanesulfonic acid) (2:1, w/v) at 4°C and centrifuged at 12,000 g. Total glutathione was determined after reducing GSSG to GSH with glutathione reductase by the method of Anderson [26]. GSSG alone was determined by incubating the sample with 2-vinyl pyridine to eliminate the GSH. The glutathione concentrations were normalized to the protein content in the sample as assayed by the Pierce 660 nm protein assay reagent (Thermo Scientific) and the ratio of GSH/GSSG was calculated.

Cell Proliferation and Apoptosis Assays

These assays were carried out using human PASMC. Cell proliferation was measured by MTS assay using CellTiter 96 AQueous One Solution (Promega, Madison, WI). Twenty-dour hours after transfection with siRNA, ~2000 cells were plated in a 96-well plate and twenty microliters of 3-(4,5-dimethylthiazol-2-yl)-5-(3-carboxymethoxyphenyl)-2-(4-sulfophenyl)-2H-tetrazolium inner salt (MTS) was added to the wells on consecutive dates. MTS is bio-reduced by cells into a colored formazan product that reduces absorbance at 490 nm. Plates were read at 24 and 48 hours using a BioTek *MODEL* plate reader (Winooski, VT) two hours after MTS reagent was added. Apoptosis was assayed forty-eight hours after siRNA transfection. Phosphatidylserine externalization (a marker of early apoptosis) was analyzed using the Guava Nexin reagent. Cells were counted following staining with Guava ViaCount reagent (Millipore, Billerica, MA) and the amount of apoptosis determined using Guava Nexin reagent (Millipore). Samples were run on a Guava EasyCyte Plus flow cytometer (Millipore). Experiments were done in triplicate.

Statistical Analysis

Data are expressed as means ± SE. Unpaired t-test analysis or one-way Anova with Bonferroni post-hoc analysis was performed using Prism software (GraphPad, San Diego, CA, USA). Statistical significance was defined as $p<0.05$.

Results

A. From experiments with *in vivo* tissue samples

Chronic hypoxia decreases EC-SOD activity in the pulmonary artery of the neonatal calf. We speculated that chronic hypoxia would lead to a loss of EC-SOD activity in the pulmonary artery of the chronically hypoxic neonatal calf, similar to our observation in the lungs of weanling mice exposed to hypoxia [10]. We separated the intracellular SODs from extracellular SOD in bovine pulmonary artery homogenates using a concavalin A column and measured the activity in each fraction. Extracellular SOD activity in the pulmonary artery was decreased by 36% following 14 days of chronic hypoxia compared to normoxic sample (**Figure 1A**). In contrast, the intracellular SOD activity levels increased 7.6-fold (**Figure 1B**). Furthermore, while extracellular SOD comprised 60% of total SOD activity under normoxic conditions, it only accounted for 7.5% of total SOD activity by the end of the hypoxic exposure (**Figure 1C**). We performed Western blot analysis on the two fractions of SOD to confirm that the Cu,Zn SOD (SOD1) and Mn SOD (SOD2) were only detectable in the intracellular fraction (IC-SOD), while EC-SOD (SOD3) was almost exclusively bound to the concavalin A column based on its glycosylated state, and eluted in the extracellular SOD fraction. (**Figure 1D**) Further, we performed several comparison measurements of SOD activity and EC-SOD expression in the mouse and calf lung tissue to corroborate the low enzymatic defenses against extracellular $O_2{}^{.-}$ measured in the neonatal calf. We observed the total SOD activity was significantly lower in two week old calf lungs compared with immature (four week old) mouse lungs (**Figure S1A**). Furthermore, when we performed Western blot analysis using 25–100 μg protein prepared from peripheral calf lung or pulmonary arteries, we were unable to detect any signal with an EC-SOD antibody. We have previously observed that EC-SOD is easily detectable in 25 μg mouse lung, and we used 1 μg purified bovine EC-SOD (kindly provided by Dr. Tim Oury, University of Pittsburgh.) as a positive control (**Figure S1B**). Therefore, any small change in SOD activity level in calf is crucial as it is more prone to oxidative stress. Despite the increase in intracellular SOD, there was no significant change in Cu,Zn or Mn SOD protein expression (**Figure S1C**). As there was a significant decrease in EC-SOD in calf PA after chronic hypoxia, we carried out further experiments with calf PA to study the role of ECSOD and the impact of chronic hypoxia.

Oxidative stress is increased in the pulmonary artery of chronically hypoxic neonatal calves. Since EC-SOD activity is markedly decreased in the tissues of chronic hypoxic calves, it could trigger oxidative stress. Oxidative stress in the pulmonary artery was evaluated by determining the ratio of reduced to oxidized glutathione (GSH/GSSG) in the calf PA following 2 weeks of hypoxia. During periods of increased oxidative stress, GSSG will accumulate and the ratio of GSH to GSSG will decrease. Therefore, the determination of the GSH/GSSG ratio is a general indicator of oxidative stress in cells and tissues. We observed that the ratio of GSH/GSSG in calf PA decreased by 50% with hypoxia (**Figure 2**). The ratio was low in calf PA compared to our previously published findings in the mouse lung [10].

The redox sensitive transcription factor, Egr-1, is increased in the pulmonary artery of the chronically hypoxic neonatal calf. We have previously reported that the level of EC-SOD activity in the lung modulates the hypoxic upregulation of Egr-1 in mice [10]. In addition, it has previously been reported that Egr-1 is highly expressed in the pulmonary artery adventitia of chronically hypoxic calves and Egr-1 contributes to hypoxia-induced cyclin D1 expression and fibroblast proliferation [10]. To confirm the vascular changes in Egr-1, we compared the mRNA expression of Egr-1 in lung and intraparenchymal proximal pulmonary artery of chronically hypoxic calves compared to age-matched normoxic calves. We found that Egr-1 mRNA expression did not increase in the lung

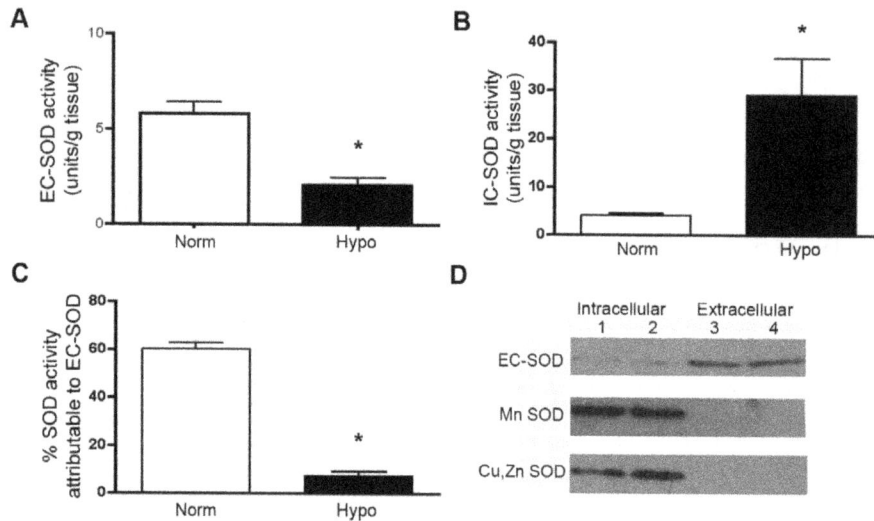

Figure 1. EC-SOD is decreased in the pulmonary artery in response to chronic hypoxia. In pulmonary artery tissue homogenates from two-week old chronically hypoxic (Hypo) and age-matched normoxic (Norm) control calves, extracellular SOD was separated from intracellular SODs (Cu,Zn SOD or SOD1 and Mn SOD or SOD2) using a concavalin A sepharose column, based on EC-SOD's predominantly glycosylated state that enables it to bind to the column and thus separate intracellular SODs (nonbound) from extracellular SOD (bound, then eluted) fraction. SOD activity was measured in each fraction using the SOD assay kit-WST. **A.** EC-SOD activity. **B.** Intracellular SOD (IC-SOD) activity. **C.** The percent of total SOD activity attributable to EC-SOD. Data expressed as mean ± SEM. *p<0.05 vs. Norm; n = 5. **D.** Western blot analysis of Cu,Zn SOD, Mn SOD and EC-SOD in the intracellular and extracellular fractions to confirm adequate separation of IC-SOD from EC-SOD. Lane 1 and 2 are the intracellular fractions from the two normoxic calves and the corresponding extracellular fraction is shown in Lanes 3 and 4.

tissue (data not shown) but was increased by 2 fold in the pulmonary artery of chronically hypoxic calves (**Figure 3**).

B. From *in vitro* experiments with calf PASMC cells

Extracellular reactive oxygen species upregulate Egr-1 in pulmonary artery smooth muscle cells (PASMC). To evaluate whether the increased Egr-1 expression detected in the pulmonary artery of chronically hypoxic calves could be directly mediated by extracellular ROS, we performed a series of experiments in SMC treated with XO+HX as an exogenous source of ROS. A dose response curve with a concentration of XO between 1–16 mU/mL and a time course between 30 minutes to 4 hours was initially performed to select the experimental

conditions (**Figure S2**). Based on these pilot studies, we selected one hour incubation with 8 mU/mL XO and 0.5 mM HX for subsequent experiments. This experimental condition significantly increased Egr-1 mRNA expression in SMC (**Figure 4A**).

XO generates extracellular $O_2^{\cdot-}$, which rapidly dismutates to H_2O_2, though XO can also generate H_2O_2 directly, depending on conditions such as pH or oxygen concentration [28–30]. In our experimental conditions, we detected an increase in extracellular $O_2^{\cdot-}$ flux when cells were treated with XO/HX for 1 hour, as shown by the SOD-inhibitable reduction of XTT, which specifically reflects extracellular $O_2^{\cdot-}$ generation (**Figure 4B**). H_2O_2 production was also significantly elevated following a 1 hour treatment with XO/HX while H_2O_2 was below the level of

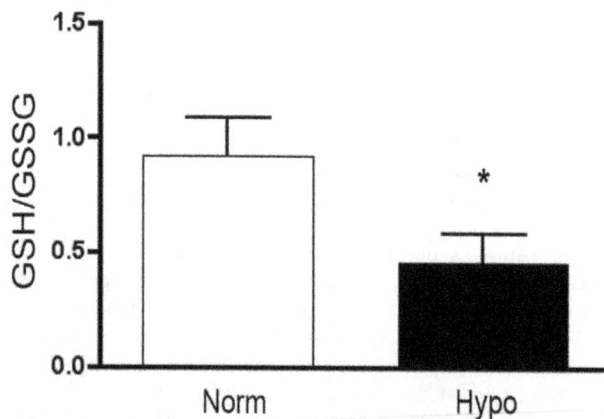

Figure 2. The GSH/GSSG ratio is decreased in the pulmonary artery of the chronic hypoxic calf (Hypo) compared to the normoxic control calf (Norm). A. GSH and total glutathione levels were measured and data expressed as the ratio of GSH to GSSG. Data expressed as mean ± SEM. *p<0.05 vs. Norm; n = 4.

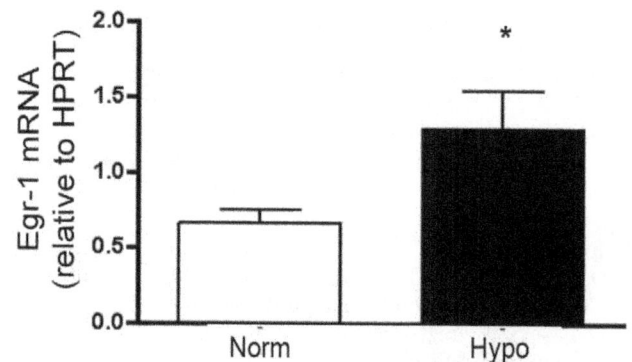

Figure 3. The redox-sensitive transcription factor Egr-1 is increased in the pulmonary artery of chronically hypoxic calves (Hypo) compared to age-matched normoxic control calves (Norm). Egr-1 mRNA expression was measured by qPCR in the pulmonary artery of 2 week old chronically hypoxic calves compared to age-matched normoxic control calves . Data are expressed as copies of Egr-1 per copy HPRT, mean ± SEM. *p<0.05 vs. Norm; n = 4–5.

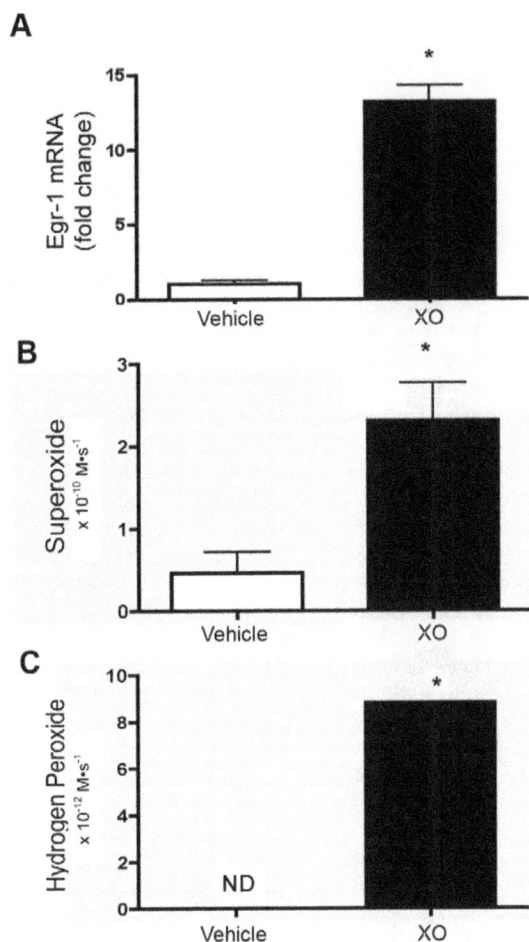

Figure 4. Xanthine oxidase upregulates Egr-1 in calf pulmonary artery smooth muscle cells. (**A**) Egr-1 mRNA expression was measured by qPCR in PASMC exposed to xanthine oxidase (XO- 8 mU/mL) and hypoxanthine (0.5 mM) at 37°C for 1 hour (XO). Data are expressed as fold change in Egr-1/HPRT relative to vehicle treated cells and presented as mean ± SEM. *p<0.05 vs. vehicle treated cells. **B.** Extracellular $O_2^{\cdot-}$ was measured by the SOD-inhibitable reduction of XTT in XO+hypoxanthine-treated (XO), and vehicle-treated smooth muscle cells with and without SOD (500 U/mL). 20,000 cells were treated in a final volume of 150 μL and exposed to XTT for 1 hour at 37°C and pH 7.4. An extinction coefficient of 21600 M^{-1} cm^{-1} (XTT) was used to calculate $O_2^{\cdot-}$ flux and data expressed in $M{\cdot}s^{-1}$. *p<0.05 vs. vehicle-treated cells, n=3. **C.** H_2O_2 was measured with a standard fluorometric assay utilizing in which H_2O_2 reacts with HRP to forms compound I, which subsequently oxidizes pHPA to its dimer form which can be detected on a fluorometer. Experiments were performed with 30,000 cells per well and a final volume of 150 μL for 2 hours at 37°C and pH 7.4 and H_2O_2 flux expressed in $M{\cdot}s^{-1}$. *p<0.05 vs. vehicle-treated cells, n=3. Data expressed as mean ± SEM.

detection in vehicle-treated cells, though the rate of accumulation of H_2O_2 was lower than the production of $O_2^{\cdot-}$ indicating that extracellular H_2O_2 was being rapidly removed by the cells, likely through GSH (**Figure 4C**). Compared to PASMC treated with XO/HX, exposure of cells to hypoxia produced a significantly smaller rise in Egr-1 mRNA (**Figure 5A**) as well as less extracellular $O_2^{\cdot-}$ production (**Figure 5B**). Low dose antimycin A, at a dose known to generate endogenous ROS due to inhibition of complex III of the mitochondrial electron transport chain, did not upregulate Egr-1, though high dose antimycin A did result in an increase in Egr-1 mRNA (**Figure 5C**).

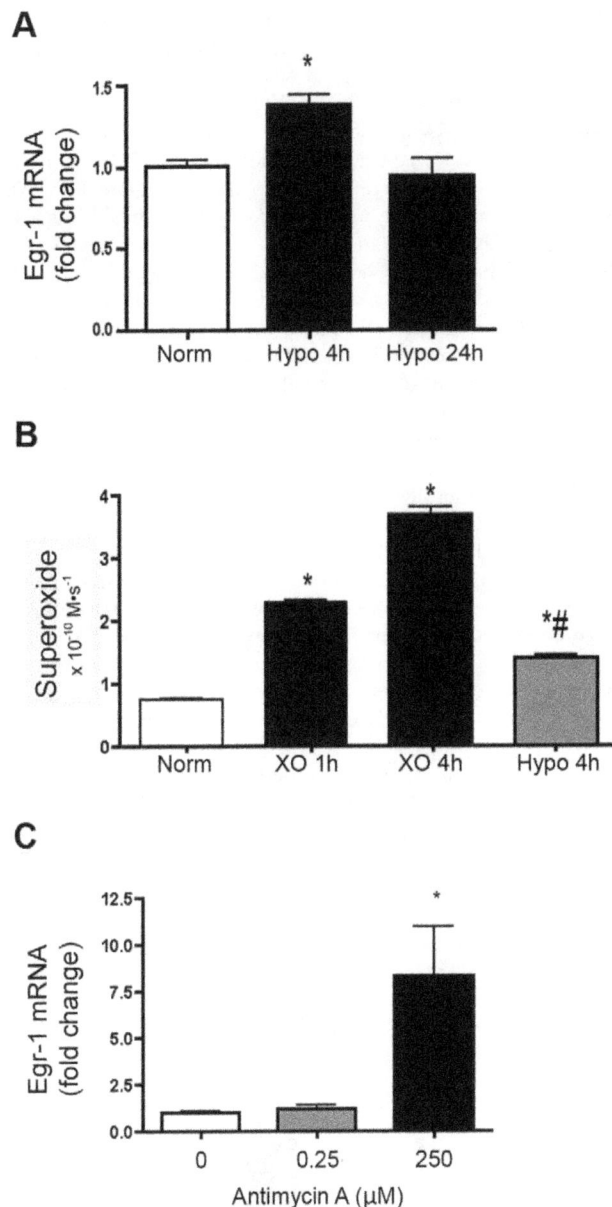

Figure 5. Exposure of calf PASMC to hypoxia resulted in less induction of Egr-1 and less extracellular superoxide generation than XO. A. Egr-1 mRNA expression in calf PASMC exposed in sealed humidified gas chambers with 21% or 1% O_2 plus 5% CO_2 and balanced N_2 at 37°C for 4 and 24 hours and shown compared to XO/HX treatment for 1 hour (XO). **B.** Extracellular $O_2^{\cdot-}$ production in PASMC exposed to XO/HX (XO) or hypoxia as described above. 20,000 cells treated in a final volume of 150 μL were exposed to XO/HX (XO) for 1 or 4 hours or hypoxia for 4 hours at 37°C and pH 7.4 in the presence of XTT. An extinction coefficient of 21600 M^{-1} cm^{-1} was used to calculate $O_2^{\cdot-}$ flux (M-s^{-1}). **C.** Egr-1 mRNA expression in calf PASMC exposed to antimycin A to increase endogenous ROS generated in the mitochondria. 20,000 cells were exposed to 0.25 μM or 250 μM antimycin A for 2 hours at 37°C. All data expressed as mean ± SEM. *p<0.05 vs. vehicle-treated cells, n=3.

Xanthine oxidase-derived extracellular reactive oxygen species upregulated Egr-1 via the activation of ERK1/2 in pulmonary artery smooth muscle cells. MAPK/ERK signaling pathways have been shown to regulate Egr-1, and many MAPK enzymes are redox sensitive. To determine if extracellular $O_2{}^{\cdot-}$, or H_2O_2 arising from the dismutation of $O_2{}^{\cdot-}$, induced the upregulation of Egr-1 via MAPK, we first evaluated whether XO/HX treatment resulted in phosphorylation of ERK1/2. Treatment with XO/HX led to phosphorylation of ERK1/2 (**Figure 6A**) in PASMC. Pretreatment with the ERK1/2 inhibitor, PD98059 (10 μM) attenuated the XO/HX-mediated upregulation of Egr-1, as measured by qPCR (**Figure 6B**). We also detected an increase in Egr-1 protein levels in the nuclear protein of cells exposed to XO/HX that was blocked by the PD98059. (**Figure 7B**). The combined pretreatment of cells with SOD and catalase reversed both XO/HX-mediated ERK1/2 phosphorylation (**Figure 6C**) as well as upregulation of Egr-1 mRNA and protein (**Figure 6D and 7B**). Catalase also significantly attenuated the upregulation of Egr-1 by XO/HX, while pretreatment with SOD alone did not prevent the upregulation of Egr-1 (**Figure S3**). These data cumulatively demonstrate a loss of EC-SOD and increased oxidative stress in the PA of chronically hypoxic calves and define a role for extracellular ROS in the upregulation of Egr-1 via the activation of EKR1/2 signaling in the pulmonary circulation.

Xanthine oxidase treatment of PASMC isolated from chronically hypoxic calves with lower PA EC-SOD activity augmented the upregulation of Egr-1 mRNA and protein. Upon completing studies that tested the impact of extracellular $O_2{}^{\cdot-}$ on Egr-1 expression, we performed a final series of experiments in PASMC isolated from normoxic and chronically hypoxic calves and in human PASMC following siRNA silencing of EC-SOD. These experiments were designed to confirm the impact of the level of EC-SOD expression on Egr-1 expression in the *in vitro* model and tested the impact of EC-SOD activity on SMC growth characteristics. The PASMCs isolated from chronically hypoxic calves showed a more significant increase in Egr-1 mRNA in response to XO/HX (**Figure 7A**) compared to cells isolated from normoxic calves. PASMC from three normoxic calves and three hypoxic calves were simultaneously passaged and treated with XO/HX to minimize experimental variability. Cells from both normoxic and hypoxic calves increased nuclear Egr-1

protein expression following XO/HX, with a higher signal detectable in cells isolated from a chronically hypoxic calf compared to cells isolated from a normoxic calf. Pretreatment with SOD+catalase or ERK inhibition attenuated the increase in XO/HX induced Egr-1 protein expression (**Figure 7B**). Equal loading in the nuclear extracts was confirmed via Ponceau S stain (**Figure S4**).

C. From *in vitro* experiments with human PASMC cells

EC-SOD silencing in human PASMC by siRNA transfection augmented Egr-1 mRNA and protein expression. We then performed additional experiments with human PASMC to confirm the impact of EC-SOD on Egr-1 expression. We selected human PASMC because these cells express high levels of EC-SOD at baseline, thus knock-down of EC-SOD would have a more significant impact than in the calf cells with low EC-SOD expression levels at baseline. Human PASMC were transfected with human EC-SOD siRNA (siEC-SOD) or the negative control siRNA vector (siNEG), and EC-SOD mRNA and protein was measured. We first confirmed that we significantly knocked down EC-SOD mRNA (**Figure 8A**) and protein (**Figure 8C**) in human PASMC with siRNA treatment. Knock down of EC-SOD in human PASMC increased Egr-1 mRNA and protein, as measured by qPCR and Western blotting respectively. (**Figure 8B and 8C**) Since activated ERK1/2 is implicated in Egr-1 expression, and Egr-1 can promote cell proliferation by increasing cyclin D1, we measured phosphorylated and total ERK1/2 as well as cyclin D1 protein expression. Knock down of EC-SOD resulted in increased phosphorylated ERK1/2/total ERK1/2 and increased cyclin D1 protein levels (**Figure 8C**).

EC-SOD silencing in hPASMC by siRNA transfection led to increased cell proliferation and attenuated cell apoptosis. Pulmonary vascular cells isolated from humans with PAH or animals with experimental PH exhibit increased cell proliferation and decreased cell apoptosis. To evaluate the impact of EC-SOD on PASMC growth characteristics, we

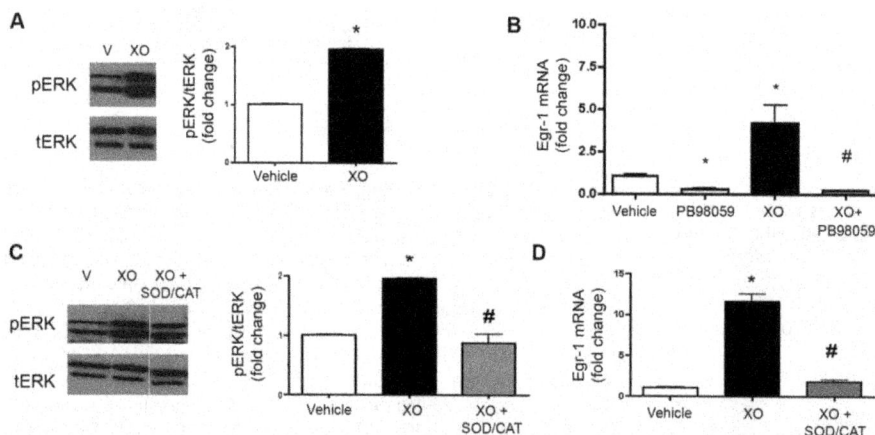

Figure 6. ROS derived from xanthine oxidase increase Egr-1 expression through ERK1/2 signaling. Calf PASMC were treated with XO (8 mU/mL) and hypoxanthine (0.5 mM) for 1 hour (XO) and protein was isolated for Western blot analysis. **A.** Blots were probed with antibodies against phosphorylated ERK1/2 (pERK) and total ERK1/2 (tERK) Each panel shows representative lanes from a single immunoblot as well as the densitometry data representing the ratio of the phosphorylated to total ERK1/2. **B.** Calf PASMC were pretreated with the MAPK/ERK1/2 inhibitor PD98059 (10 μM) for 30 min followed by either XO/HX (XO) or vehicle control. mRNA was isolated and analyzed by qPCR for Egr-1 expression relative to HPRT. **C.** Calf PASMC were pretreated with CuZn SOD (500 U/mL) and catalase (600 U/mL) for 30 minutes prior to XO (8 mU/mL) and hypoxanthine (0.5 mM). Total protein was subjected to Western blot analysis for phosphorylated ERK1/2 (pERK) and total ERK1/2 (tERK). The band intensities were quantified by densitometry and normalized to that of vehicle. **D.** PASMC were pretreated with CuZn SOD (500 U/mL) and catalase (600 U/mL) for 30 minutes prior to XO (8 mU/mL) and hypoxanthine (0.5 mM). mRNA was isolated and analyzed by qPCR for Egr-1 expression relative to HPRT. All data expressed as mean ± SEM. *p<0.05 vs. vehicle treated cells; #p<0.05 vs. 1 hour XO-treated cells; n=3.

A

B

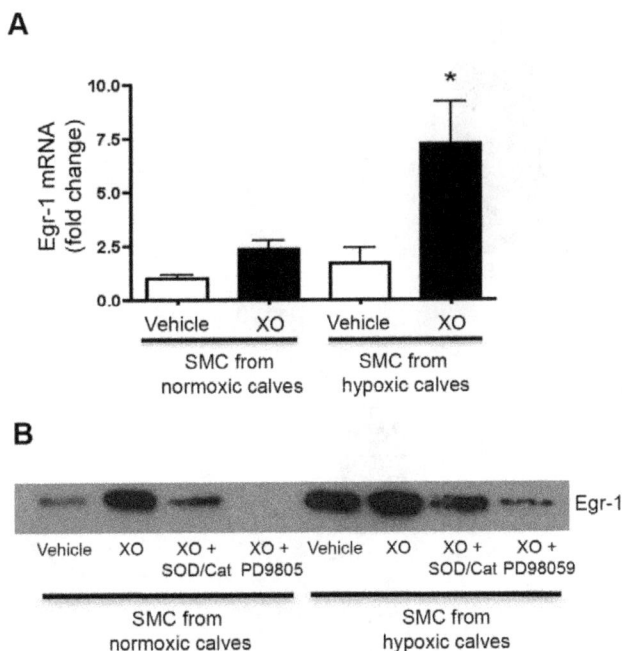

Figure 7. PASMC isolated from chronically hypoxic calves had a more marked upregulation of Egr-1 in response to xanthine oxidase compared to cells isolated from normoxic calves. A. PASMC isolated from three chronically hypoxic calves and three normoxic age-matched control calves were treated simultaneously with xanthine oxidase (8 mU/mL) and hypoxanthine (0.5 mM) at 37°C for 1 hour (XO). Egr-1 mRNA expression was measured by qPCR and expressed as fold change in Egr-1/HPRT relative to the vehicle-treated PASMC isolated from normoxic calves. Data are presented as mean ± SEM. *$p<0.05$ vs. vehicle treated cells. **B.** For protein analysis, PASMC (1×10^6 cells per plate) isolated from a chronically hypoxic calf and a normoxic age-matched control calf were treated simultaneously with xanthine oxidase (8 mU/mL) and hypoxanthine (0.5 mM) at 37°C for 1 hour (XO) with and without a 30 minute pretreatment with either Cu,Zn SOD (500 U/mL) and catalase (600 U/mL) or with the MAPK/ERK1/2 inhibitor PD98059 (10 µM). Nuclear protein was isolated using Thermo-Scientific NE-PER Nuclear and Cytoplasmic Extraction Reagents, and 25 µg was loaded on a gel for Western blot analysis with the Egr-1 antibody (1:1,000). Ponceau S staining was performed on the gel to confirm protein equal loading. (see Figure S4).

measured cell proliferation and apoptotic index following knock down of EC-SOD. After siRNA treatment to knock down EC-SOD, there was significant increase in cell proliferation (**Figure 8D**). We then measured the apoptotic status of cells after knock down of EC-SOD by flow cytometry. As shown in **Figure 8E**, inhibition of EC-SOD led to a significant decrease in the cell apoptotic index. These indicate that depletion of EC-SOD in human PASMC results in increased cell survival and proliferation.

Discussion

Understanding the molecular mechanism that induces pulmonary hypertension in neonates is important for the development of improved therapeutics. In this current study, we used the chronically hypoxic calf model of pulmonary hypertension to evaluate the activity of EC-SOD in a severe neonatal disease model and to better understand the role for extracellular $O_2{}^{\cdot-}$ in the upregulation of Egr-1, a redox sensitive transcription factor implicated in vascular remodeling. We tested the hypothesis that

loss of EC-SOD in chronically hypoxic calves leads to extracellular $O_2{}^{\cdot-}$-mediated upregulation of Egr-1 via activation of MAPK pathways. We tested tissue from chronically hypoxic calves to demonstrate the decrease in EC-SOD in the pulmonary artery *in vivo* and then treated isolated pulmonary vascular smooth muscle cells with xanthine oxidase to show that ROS generated outside the cell could upregulate Egr-1 via activation of MAPK/ ERK1/2. We used human PASMC following siRNA knock-down of EC-SOD to confirm the impact of EC-SOD expression on Egr-1 expression and SMC proliferative ability. Our data provide new insight into the importance and targets of EC-SOD and extracellular $O_2{}^{\cdot-}$ in chronic hypoxic pulmonary hypertension.

We previously reported that EC-SOD activity is impaired following exposure to chronic hypoxia, and overexpression of lung EC-SOD in two murine models of pulmonary hypertension protected against pulmonary vascular remodeling and prevented the early upregulation of the redox sensitive transcription factor, Egr-1 [10,11]. In this study, we report that total SOD activity levels in the calf lung and pulmonary artery were very low compared to the mouse lung, and extracellular SOD activity decreased in the pulmonary artery of calves exposed to 2 weeks of chronic hypoxia. The low SOD activity level measured in the calf pulmonary artery tissue was also substantially less than published activity levels reported for baboon and human pulmonary artery; though we report, similar to the baboon and human, that EC-SOD activity accounted for the majority of the total SOD activity in the pulmonary artery under normal conditions [31]. The low activity levels of total SOD may be in part due to the young age of the calves, as lung antioxidant defenses are known to be low early in life and increase in the perinatal period to prepare for the relative hyperoxia of room-air breathing. Consistent with this, we previously reported in the developing rabbit that EC-SOD activity in the lung increased during the first month of life [25]. Several pieces of data support the premise that the low SOD activity is associated with an increase in oxidative stress in the pulmonary artery of the chronically hypoxic calf. The ratio of GSH/GSSG was low in the calf pulmonary artery and decreased further with hypoxia. This result is similar to our published observation in mice in which the GSH/GSSG ratio decreased by 50% in response to hypoxia [10]. In chronic hypoxic mice, where we were able to examine a time-course, we had reported an early increase in EC-SOD expression and activity, which may reflect an adaptive response to combat increased oxidant stress [22]. Interestingly, in this study, we measured an increase in intracellular SOD (IC-SOD) activity in the calf PA at 2 weeks of hypoxia. This may also be adaptive in response to increased intracellular oxidative stress. It is possible that intracellular SOD activity would decrease over time, as we observed in the lung of chronically hypoxic mice over a 5 week period, but the large animal models are limited by cost and the longer exposures were not feasible. The loss of EC-SOD activity was even more pronounced when considered as the percentage of total SOD activity, decreasing its contribution to total SOD activity from 60% to less than 10%. We speculate that an increased susceptibility to oxidative stress due to the low total SOD activity along with a further loss of extracellular EC-SOD could contribute to the significant remodeling in the medial and adventitial layer of the pulmonary arteries observed in the neonatal calf compared to the modest vascular remodeling characteristic of chronically hypoxic mice [19,32–35].

To test the impact of extracellular $O_2{}^{\cdot-}$ on Egr-1 expression in PASMC, we treated cells with XO, as an enzymatic source of $O_2{}^{\cdot-}$. This exogenous model has potential relevance to the *in vivo* setting, as XO is upregulated in the hypoxic pulmonary circulation and can contribute to pulmonary hypertension [4,36–38]. A key

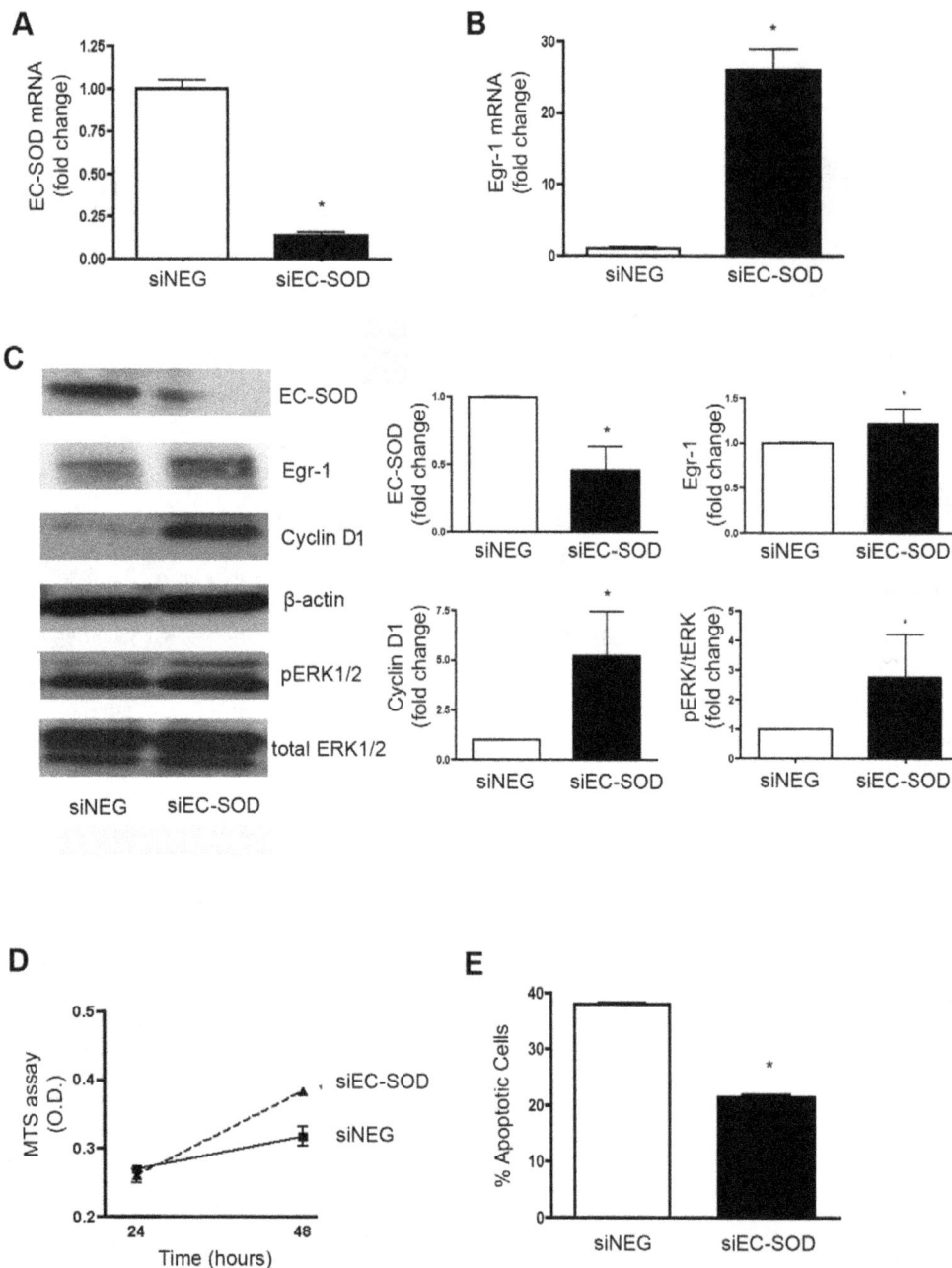

Figure 8. siRNA-mediated knock down of EC-SOD in human pulmonary artery smooth muscle cells increased Egr-1 mRNA and protein and promoted a pro-proliferative and anti-apoptotic phenotype. Human PASMC were transfected with human EC-SOD siRNA (siEC-SOD) or the negative control siRNA vector (siNEG) and experiments were performed 48 hours later. **A.** EC-SOD mRNA expression expressed relative to GAPDH to test the extent of knock-down of EC-SOD with siRNA. **B.** Fold change in Egr-1 mRNA expression expressed relative to GAPDH in human PASMC treated with siEC-SOD compared to cells treated with siNEG. Data are presented as mean ± SEM. *p<0.05 vs. siNEG. **C.** Western blot analysis in total cell lysates from human PASMC treated with siEC-SOD or siNEG. The blots were probed sequentially with the human EC-SOD antibody (1:1,000), Egr-1 antibody (1:500) cyclin D1 and ß-actin (1:1,000) to confirm equal protein loading. Blots were also probed with the phosphorylated ERK1/2 and total ERK1/2 antibodies (1:1,000). Densitometry shows fold change in EC-SOD, Egr-1 or cyclin D1 relative to ß-actin and fold change in phosphorylated relative to total ERK1/2 (n=2). **D.** Cell proliferation measured by MTS assay. Experiments were done in triplicate. *p<0.05 vs. siNEG. Solid line (■): siNEG; dashed line (▲): siEC-SOD *p<0.05 vs. siNEG **E**. Apoptosis was assayed using the Guava Nexin kit (Guava Technologies) according to the manufacturer's protocol. Fluorescence emission for Annexin V staining and 7-AAD was measured by flow cytometry. Experiments were done in triplicate. *p<0.05 vs. siNEG.

finding in the cell culture experiments was that exogenous generation of extracellular O_2^{-} by XO in smooth muscle cells strongly upregulated Egr-1 mRNA and protein expression. Furthermore, cells isolated from chronically hypoxic calves had

a more marked response to XO than cells isolated from normoxic calves. Since the SMC are a major source of vascular EC-SOD and we detected less EC-SOD in the pulmonary artery of chronically hypoxic calves, we speculate that the loss of EC-SOD in these cells contributed to the enhanced upregulation of Egr-1 in response to XO. This was supported by our finding in human PASMC in which knock-down of EC-SOD increased Egr-1 mRNA and protein. In the bovine cell culture model, pretreatment with both SOD and catalase was required to fully block the XO-induced signal. This indicates that H_2O_2, which also will increase with XO treatment due to the rapid dismutation of $O_2^{\cdot-}$ or its direct generation of H_2O_2, was capable of inducing Egr-1 expression in this system. In contrast, in the human cells, knocked down of EC-SOD expression was sufficient to increase Egr-1, consistent with our previous observation in the mouse model, that overexpression of EC-SOD in the lung blunted the hypoxic induction of Egr-1 expression[10]. These data demonstrate that we can use XO as a model to test how extracellular ROS can regulate Egr-1 mRNA expression; however, we must also consider the impact of exogenous vs. endogenous sources of ROS and the model when we interpret the data. Our data support the conclusion that extracellular $O_2^{\cdot-}$ may upregulate Egr-1 directly or following its dismutation to H_2O_2. Consistent with our cell culture findings, one published study reported that the exogenous administration of H_2O_2 in cardiac cells also increased Egr-1 mRNA and protein expression [39]. In our study when SOD+catalase was compared to catalase pretreatment alone, there is a small difference, suggesting that $O_2^{\cdot-}$ may have an effect independent of its dismutation to H_2O_2. It is also possible that EC-SOD modulates Egr-1 expression by regulating NO bioavailability. This mechanism was not tested in this study. Overall, these data indicate that while the bovine cell culture experiments do not fully mimic the *in vivo* setting, extracellular $O_2^{\cdot-}$, either directly or indirectly following its dismutation to H_2O_2, can upregulate Egr-1 in smooth muscle cell, and provides an opportunity to further understand how $O_2^{\cdot-}$ can regulate the redox sensitive transcription factor, Egr-1.

Published studies have shown enhanced induction of Egr-1 with hypoxia [10,14–19], For example, fetal bovine pulmonary artery fibroblasts exhibited an increase in Egr-1 mRNA by Northern blot analysis following four hours of 3% oxygen [18]. However, we observed that exposure of PASMCs to hypoxia (1% for 1–4 hours), in addition to generating lower concentrations of extracellular $O_2^{\cdot-}$ than XO, also had a much smaller impact on Egr-1 mRNA expression. This demonstrates that hypoxic induction of Egr-1 is specific to tissue or cell types, particularly given the known heterogeneity in cells within the vessel wall. The response can also vary with the hypoxic condition and the extent of hypoxic exposure. We speculate that an important source of extracellular ROS in the pulmonary circulation is that generated by recruited or resident inflammatory cells in response to hypoxia. Thus, a short bolus exposure to hypoxia in a single vascular cell type does not mimic the in vivo model system. While we focused in this study on the impact of extracellular $O_2^{\cdot-}$ on Egr-1 regulation, our data with antimycin A suggest that under certain conditions, intracellular ROS production can also modulate the expression of this transcription factor. Further studies will dissect the origin and sources of extracellular ROS, distinct from cytosolic or mitochondrial sources, in the lung and pulmonary circulation in response to hypoxia. Since the use of hypoxia in cultured vascular cells was limited by the low levels of extracellular $O_2^{\cdot-}$ generated and a minimal impact on Egr-1 regulation, we selected XO treatment as a model to test whether extracellular $O_2^{\cdot-}$ upregulated Egr-1 via the activation of MAPK pathways.

There is extensive data implicating the MAPK/ERK1/2 pathway in the regulation of Egr-1 and in the pathogenesis of chronic hypoxic pulmonary hypertension [1,17,18,39–41]. Furthermore, it is well-established that reactive oxygen species can activate MAPK through its phosphorylation [42]. These two observations formed the basis of our decision to test whether ROS generated outside the cell upregulated Egr-1 via MAPK. We found that extracellular ROS, generated by XO, phosphorylated ERK1/2, while inhibition of the ERK1/2 pathway prevented the upregulation of Egr-1. This identifies the importance of MAPK/ERK pathway in the redox regulation of Egr-1 in neonatal PASMC. A recent study showed that an increased extracellular oxidation in vascular smooth muscle cells activated the EGFR membrane receptor, leading to phosphorylation of ERK1/2 and activation of downstream transcription factors [43]. Our work thus provides a basis for future studies to better understand how the activity of EC-SOD may regulate extracellular redox state and further dissect its targets leading to ERK1/2 phosphorylation and regulation of Egr-1. Accordingly, targeting Egr-1 regulation may represent a novel therapeutic strategy to prevent PA remodeling.

The regulation of Egr-1 has been implicated in vascular remodeling in a number of models including the calf model of chronic hypoxic pulmonary hypertension. For example, upregulation of Egr-1 contributes to cyclin D1 expression and hypoxia-induced cell proliferation in fetal lung fibroblasts and stimulates insulin-like growth factor-1 receptor, resulting in vascular remodeling of vein grafts [44]. In addition, a pro-proliferative and anti-apoptotic phenotype has been attributed to SMC in pulmonary hypertension. Consistent with these studies, we were also able to show that knock-down of EC-SOD in human PASMC upregulated cyclin D1 and ERK1/2 activation, augmented proliferation and blunted apoptosis, providing direct evidence for EC-SOD in regulating PASMC phenotype.

In summary, we report that the neonatal calf has low SOD activity levels in the pulmonary artery and EC-SOD activity decreases further in the calf with pulmonary hypertension secondary to chronic hypoxia. The loss of EC-SOD is associated with an increase in Egr-1 mRNA in the pulmonary artery. We thus tested the impact of extracellular $O_2^{\cdot-}$ and its product, H_2O_2, on Egr-1 expression in vascular smooth muscle and found that exogenous production of these ROS, via xanthine oxidase, upregulated Egr-1. Hypoxia itself had a minimal effect on either Egr-1 expression or $O_2^{\cdot-}$ production. Extracellular ROS together with activation of ERK1/2 by phosphorylation regulated the increase in Egr-1. Therefore, targeting Egr-1 by controlling extracellular ROS generation and thereby balancing the cellular redox status could be a potential therapeutic pathway for pulmonary artery remodeling. Our data provided new insight into the role of extracellular $O_2^{\cdot-}$ and EC-SOD in the pathogenesis of pulmonary hypertension.

Supporting Information

Figure S1 Total SOD activity is less in the calf lung compared to the mouse lung. A. Total lung SOD, measured with an SOD activity kit (Dojindo Molecular Technologies) and expressed as units of SOD activity per gram tissue (U/g tissue), compared the activity in control two week old calves to immature control four week old mice. *p<0.05; n = 5. **B.** Western blot analysis of calf lung protein (25 µg) and purified bovine EC-SOD (1 µg) with a rabbit polyclonal EC-SOD antibody quantified. **C.** Representative Western blot of total PA homogenates for Cu,Zn SOD and Mn SOD with densitometry normalized to ß-actin, n = 5–6. p = 0.07 between groups for both blots.

Figure S2 Dose response curve and time course for xanthine oxidase on Egr-1 mRNA expression. A. Calf PASMC were treated with 0, 1, 4, 8 and 16 mU/mL xanthine oxidase+0.5 mM hypoxanthine for 1 hour and Egr-1 mRNA expression was determined by qPCR. Experiment was performed in triplicate and data expressed as Egr-1/HPRT relative to control cells. *p<0.05 vs control. **B.** Calf PASMC were treated with 8 mU/mL xanthine oxidase+0.5 mM hypoxanthine for 0.5, 1, 2 and 4 hours and Egr-1 mRNA expression was determined by qPCR. Experiment was performed in triplicate and data expressed as Egr-1/HPRT relative to vehicle-treated control cells. *p<0.05 vs control.

Figure S3 Combined treatment with SOD and CAT significantly inhibited XO induced Egr-1 expression. PASMC were pretreated with SOD (500 U/mL), Cat (600 U/mL) or combined SOD+CAT for 30 minutes prior to xanthine oxidase (8 mU/mL) and hypoxanthine (0.5 mM) to evaluate the contribution of superoxide and hydrogen peroxide to Egr-1 upregulation. mRNA was isolated analyzed by real-time RT-PCR for Egr-1 and HPRT expression. *p<0.05 vs. Vehicle and #p<0.05 vs. XO+SOD treatment.

Figure S4 Ponceau S stain of the blot presented in Figure 7 to demonstrate equal protein loading. The membrane shown in Figure 7B was stained with Ponceau S to confirm equal nuclear protein loading.

Author Contributions

Conceived and designed the experiments: EN-G. Performed the experiments: TH RB SV MM LV. Analyzed the data: EN-G TH RB SV SB KS. Contributed reagents/materials/analysis tools: EN-G KS. Wrote the paper: EN-G TH SV LV. Assisted with editing: SV SB KS RB MM.

References

1. Stenmark KR, Fagan KA, Frid MG (2006) Hypoxia-induced pulmonary vascular remodeling: cellular and molecular mechanisms. Circ Res 99: 675–691.
2. Nozik-Grayck E, Huang YC, Carraway MS, Piantadosi CA (2003) Bicarbonate-dependent superoxide release and pulmonary artery tone. Am J Physiol Heart Circ Physiol 285: H2327–2335.
3. Liu JQ, Zelko IN, Erbynn EM, Sham JS, Folz RJ (2006) Hypoxic pulmonary hypertension: role of superoxide and NADPH oxidase (gp91phox). Am J Physiol Lung Cell Mol Physiol 290: L2–10.
4. Jankov RP, Kantores C, Pan J, Belik J (2008) Contribution of xanthine oxidase-derived superoxide to chronic hypoxic pulmonary hypertension in neonatal rats. Am J Physiol Lung Cell Mol Physiol 294: L233–245.
5. Fattman CL, Chu CT, Kulich SM, Enghild JJ, Oury TD (2001) Altered expression of extracellular superoxide dismutase in mouse lung after bleomycin treatment. Free Radic Biol Med 31: 1198–1207.
6. Oury TD, Schaefer LM, Fattman CL, Choi A, Weck KE, et al. (2002) Depletion of pulmonary EC-SOD after exposure to hyperoxia. Am J Physiol Lung Cell Mol Physiol 283: L777–784.
7. Giles BL, Suliman H, Mamo LB, Piantadosi CA, Oury TD, et al. (2002) Prenatal hypoxia decreases lung extracellular superoxide dismutase expression and activity. Am J Physiol Lung Cell Mol Physiol 283: L549–554.
8. Tan RJ, Fattman CL, Watkins SC, Oury TD (2004) Redistribution of pulmonary EC-SOD after exposure to asbestos. J Appl Physiol 97: 2006–2013.
9. Mamo LB, Suliman HB, Giles B-L, Auten RL, Piantadosi CA, et al. (2004) Discordant extracellular superoxide dismutase expression and activity in neonatal hyperoxic lung. Am J Respir Crit Care Med 170: 313–318.
10. Nozik-Grayck E, Suliman HB, Majka S, Albietz J, Van Rheen Z, et al. (2008) Lung EC-SOD overexpression attenuates hypoxic induction of Egr-1 and chronic hypoxic pulmonary vascular remodeling. Am J Physiol Lung Cell Mol Physiol 295: L422–430.
11. Van Rheen Z, Fattman C, Domarski S, Majka S, Klemm D, et al. (2010) Lung EC-SOD Overexpression Lessens Bleomycin-Induced Pulmonary Hypertension and Vascular Remodeling. Am J Respir Cell Mol Biol doi:10.1165/rcmb.2010-0065OC.
12. Kamezaki F, Tasaki H, Yamashita K, Tsutsui M, Koide S, et al. (2008) Gene transfer of extracellular superoxide dismutase ameliorates pulmonary hypertension in rats. Am J Respir Crit Care Med 177: 219–226.
13. Khachigian LM (2006) Early growth response-1 in cardiovascular pathobiology. Circ Res 98: 186–191.
14. Yan SF, Mackman N, Kisiel W, Stern DM, Pinsky DJ (1999) Hypoxia/Hypoxemia-Induced activation of the procoagulant pathways and the pathogenesis of ischemia-associated thrombosis. Arterioscler Thromb Vasc Biol 19: 2029–2035.
15. Yan SF, Lu J, Zou YS, Soh-Won J, Cohen DM, et al. (1999) Hypoxia-associated induction of early growth response-1 gene expression. J Biol Chem 274: 15030–15040.
16. Yan SF, Lu J, Xu L, Zou YS, Tongers J, et al. (2000) Pulmonary expression of early growth response-1: biphasic time course and effect of oxygen concentration. J Appl Physiol 88: 2303–2309.
17. Jin N, Hatton N, Swartz DR, Xia X, Harrington MA, et al. (2000) Hypoxia activates jun-N-terminal kinase, extracellular signal-regulated protein kinase, and p38 kinase in pulmonary arteries. Am J Respir Cell Mol Biol 23: 593–601.
18. Gerasimovskaya EV, Ahmad S, White CW, Jones PL, Carpenter TC, et al. (2002) Extracellular ATP is an autocrine/paracrine regulator of hypoxia-induced adventitial fibroblast growth. Signaling through extracellular signal-regulated kinase-1/2 and the Egr-1 transcription factor. J Biol Chem 277: 44638–44650.
19. Banks MF, Gerasimovskaya EV, Tucker DA, Frid MG, Carpenter TC, et al. (2005) Egr-1 antisense oligonucleotides inhibit hypoxia-induced proliferation of pulmonary artery adventitial fibroblasts. J Appl Physiol 98: 732–738.
20. Sharma S, Grobe AC, Wiseman DA, Kumar S, Englaish M, et al. (2007) Lung Antioxidant Enzymes are Regulated by Development and Increased Pulmonary Blood Flow. Am J Physiol Lung Cell Mol Physiol.
21. Frid MG, Aldashev AA, Dempsey EC, Stenmark KR (1997) Smooth muscle cells isolated from discrete compartments of the mature vascular media exhibit unique phenotypes and distinct growth capabilities. Circ Res 81: 940–952.
22. Yu HW, Liu QF, Liu GN (2011) Positive regulation of the Egr-1/osteopontin positive feedback loop in rat vascular smooth muscle cells by TGF-beta, ERK, JNK, and p38 MAPK signaling. Biochem Biophys Res Commun 396: 451–456.
23. Beers RF, Sizer IW (1952) A spectrophotometric method for measuring the breakdown of hydrogen peroxide by catalase. J Biol Chem 195: 133–140.
24. Hyslop PA, Sklar LA (1984) A quantitative fluorimetric assay for the determination of oxidant production by polymorphonuclear leukocytes: its use in the simultaneous fluorimetric assay of cellular activation processes. Anal Biochem 141: 280–286.
25. Nozik-Grayck E, Dieterle CS, Piantadosi CA, Enghild JJ, Oury TD (2000) Secretion of extracellular superoxide dismutase in neonatal lungs. Am J Physiol Lung Cell Mol Physiol 279: L977–984.
26. Anderson M (1985) Handbook of Methods for Oxygen Radical Research: Boca Raton, Fla, USA: CRC Press.
27. Griffith O (1980) Determination of glutathione and glutathione disulfide using glutathione reductase and 2-vinylpyridine. Analytical Biochemistry 106: 207–212.
28. Fridovich I (1970) Quantitative aspects of the production of superoxide anion radical by milk xanthine oxidase. J Biol Chem 245: 4053–4057.
29. Buettner GR, Ng CF, Wang M, Rodgers VG, Schafer FQ (2006) A new paradigm: manganese superoxide dismutase influences the production of H2O2 in cells and thereby their biological state. Free Radic Biol Med 41: 1338–1350.
30. Kelley EE, Khoo NK, Hundley NJ, Malik UZ, Freeman BA, et al. (2010) Hydrogen peroxide is the major oxidant product of xanthine oxidase. Free Radic Biol Med 48: 493–498.
31. Oury TD, Day BJ, Crapo JD (1996) Extracellular superoxide dismutase in vessels and airways of humans and baboons. Free Radic Biol Med 20: 957–965.
32. Stenmark KR, Meyrick B, Galie N, Mooi WJ, McMurtry IF (2009) Animal models of pulmonary arterial hypertension: the hope for etiological discovery and pharmacological cure. Am J Physiol Lung Cell Mol Physiol 297: L1013–1032.
33. Hassoun PM, Mouthon L, Barbera JA, Eddahibi S, Flores SC, et al. (2009) Inflammation, growth factors, and pulmonary vascular remodeling. J Am Coll Cardiol 54: S10–19.
34. Frid MG, Li M, Gnanasekharan M, Burke DL, Fragoso M, et al. (2009) Sustained hypoxia leads to the emergence of cells with enhanced growth, migratory, and promitogenic potentials within the distal pulmonary artery wall. Am J Physiol Lung Cell Mol Physiol 297: L1059–1072.
35. Li M, Scott DE, Shandas R, Stenmark KR, Tan W (2009) High pulsatility flow induces adhesion molecule and cytokine mRNA expression in distal pulmonary artery endothelial cells. Ann Biomed Eng 37: 1082–1092.
36. Durmowicz AG, Frid MG, Wohrley JD, Stenmark KR (1996) Expression and localization of tropoelastin mRNA in the developing bovine pulmonary artery is dependent on vascular cell phenotype. Am J Respir Cell Mol Biol 14: 569–576.
37. Hoshikawa Y, Ono S, Suzuki S, Tanita T, Chida M, et al. (2001) Generation of oxidative stress contributes to the development of pulmonary hypertension induced by hypoxia. J Appl Physiol 90: 1299–1306.
38. Kelley EE, Hock T, Khoo NK, Richardson GR, Johnson KK, et al. (2006) Moderate hypoxia induces xanthine oxidoreductase activity in arterial endothelial cells. Free Radic Biol Med 40: 952–959.
39. Aggeli IKS, Beis I, Gaitanaki C (2010) ERKs and JNKs mediate hydrogen peroxide-induced Egr-1 expression and nuclear accumulation in H9c2 cells. Physiol Res 59: 443–454.

40. Das M, Burns N, Wilson SJ, Zawada WM, Stenmark KR (2008) Hypoxia exposure induces the emergence of fibroblasts lacking replication repressor signals of PKCzeta in the pulmonary artery adventitia. Cardiovascular research 78: 440–448.

41. Li C-J, Ning W, Matthay MA, Feghali-Bostwick CA, Choi AMK (2007) MAPK pathway mediates EGR-1-HSP70-dependent cigarette smoke-induced chemokine production. Am J Physiol Lung Cell Mol Physiol 292: L1297–1303.

42. Hasan RN, Schafer AI (2008) Hemin Upregulates Egr-1 Expression in Vascular Smooth Muscle Cells via ROS ERK-1/2 Elk-1 and NF-{kappa}B. Circ Res 102: 42–50.

43. Stanic B, Katsuyama M, Miller FJ, Jr. (2010) An oxidized extracellular oxidation-reduction state increases Nox1 expression and proliferation in vascular smooth muscle cells via epidermal growth factor receptor activation. Arterioscler Thromb Vasc Biol 30: 2234–2241.

44. Wu X, Cheng J, Li P, Yang M, Qiu S, et al. (2010) Mechano-sensitive transcriptional factor Egr-1 regulates insulin-like growth factor-1 receptor expression and contributes to neointima formation in vein grafts. Arterioscler Thromb Vasc Biol 30: 471–476.

10

Risk Factors for Death in 632 Patients with Sickle Cell Disease in the United States and United Kingdom

Mark T. Gladwin[1,2]*, Robyn J. Barst[3], J. Simon R. Gibbs[4], Mariana Hildesheim[1,2], Vandana Sachdev[5], Mehdi Nouraie[6], Kathryn L. Hassell[7], Jane A. Little[8], Dean E. Schraufnagel[9], Lakshmanan Krishnamurti[1,10], Enrico Novelli[1], Reda E. Girgis[11], Claudia R. Morris[12], Erika Berman Rosenzweig[3], David B. Badesch[7], Sophie Lanzkron[11], Oswaldo L. Castro[6], James G. Taylor VI[5], Jonathan C. Goldsmith[13], Gregory J. Kato[5], Victor R. Gordeuk[9], Roberto F. Machado[9], on behalf of the walk-PHaSST Investigators and Patients

1 Vascular Medicine Institute, University of Pittsburgh, Pittsburgh, Pennsylvania, United States of America, 2 Division of Pulmonary Allergy and Critical Care Medicine, University of Pittsburgh Medical Center, Pittsburgh, Pennsylvania, United States of America, 3 Columbia University, New York, New York, United States of America, 4 National Heart & Lung Institute, Imperial College London, London, United Kingdom, 5 Cardiovascular Branch, NHLBI, Bethesda, Maryland, United States of America, 6 Howard University, Washington, DC, United States of America, 7 University of Colorado HSC, Denver, Colorado, United States of America, 8 Case Western Reserve University, Cleveland, Ohio, United States of America, 9 University of Illinois, Chicago, Illinois, United States of America, 10 Children's Hospital of Pittsburgh, Pittsburgh, Pennsylvania, United States of America, 11 Johns Hopkins University, Baltimore, Maryland, United States of America, 12 Emory University School of Medicine, Atlanta, Georgia, United States of America, 13 National Heart Lung and Blood Institute/NIH, Bethesda, Maryland, United States of America

Abstract

Background: The role of pulmonary hypertension as a cause of mortality in sickle cell disease (SCD) is controversial.

Methods and Results: We evaluated the relationship between an elevated estimated pulmonary artery systolic pressure and mortality in patients with SCD. We followed patients from the walk-PHaSST screening cohort for a median of 29 months. A tricuspid regurgitation velocity (TRV)$\geq$3.0 m/s cuttof, which has a 67–75% positive predictive value for mean pulmonary artery pressure $\geq$25 mm Hg was used. Among 572 subjects, 11.2% had TRV$\geq$3.0 m/sec. Among 582 with a measured NT-proBNP, 24.1% had values $\geq$160 pg/mL. Of 22 deaths during follow-up, 50% had a TRV$\geq$3.0 m/sec. At 24 months the cumulative survival was 83% with TRV$\geq$3.0 m/sec and 98% with TRV<3.0 m/sec (p<0.0001). The hazard ratios for death were 11.1 (95% CI 4.1–30.1; p<0.0001) for TRV$\geq$3.0 m/sec, 4.6 (1.8–11.3; p = 0.001) for NT-proBNP$\geq$160 pg/mL, and 14.9 (5.5–39.9; p<0.0001) for both TRV$\geq$3.0 m/sec and NT-proBNP$\geq$160 pg/mL. Age >47 years, male gender, chronic transfusions, WHO class III–IV, increased hemolytic markers, ferritin and creatinine were also associated with increased risk of death.

Conclusions: A TRV$\geq$3.0 m/sec occurs in approximately 10% of individuals and has the highest risk for death of any measured variable.

The study is registered in ClinicalTrials.gov with identifier: NCT00492531

Editor: James West, Vanderbilt University Medical Center, United States of America

Funding: This project has been founded with federal funds from the National Heart, Lung, and Blood Institute, National Institutes of Health, Department of Health and Human Services, under contract HHSN268200617182C. NHLBI was involved in the design and conduct of the original study and their staff had input in the writing of the manuscript.

Competing Interests: The following authors have no conflicts to report: Castro, Girgis, Goldsmith, Hildesheim, Kato, Krishnamurti, Little, Machado, Nouraie, and Sachdev. Badesch has received honoraria for service on steering committees or advisory boards (or as a consultant) to the following companies working in the area of pulmonary hypertension: Actelion/CoTherix, Gilead, Pfizer, Mondo-Biotech/Mondogen, United Therapeutics/Lung Rx, GlaxoSmithKline, Lilly/ICOS, Bayer, Ikaria, and Arena. He has received grant support for clinical studies from GlaxoSmithKline, Actelion/CoTHerix, Gilead, Pfizer, United Therapeutics/Lung Rx, Lilly/ICOS, Bayer, and Novartis. He provided information pertinent to a legal matter for Actelion. Barst has received honoraria for consulting for: Actelion, Eli Lilly, Gilead, Ikaria, Novartis, Pfizer, VentriPoint, and owns stock/stock options in VentriPoint. Gibbs serves on advisory boards and/or performs consultancy work for Actelion, Bayer, Gilead, GSK, Novartis, Pfizer, and United Therapeutics. Mark Gladwin receives grant support from the NIH, Bayer Corporation, and Gilead Sciences. He is listed as a co-inventor on a US government patent for the use of nitrate salts and is a co-author on patent applications related to treating hemolysis. He also performs consulting for Bayer Corp and serves in an advisory capacity for Aires Pharmaceuticals. The Vascular Medicine Institute is funded by the Institute for Transfusion Medicine and the Hemophilia Center of Western Pennsylvania. Victor Gordeuk serves as a consultant for AesRx Pharmaceutical Company regarding developing a drug for sickle cell disease. He has also received an honorarium from AesRx and provided a testimonial review during a legal case involving sickle cell disease. Hassell has received research support for a multicenter study from Glycomimetics, Inc and Emmaus, Inc. and served on the advisory board for ApoPharma; AGA, Inc. Lanzkron serves on the scientific advisory board of Hemaquest. She also receives K award funding from the NHLBI K23HL083089. Morris is the inventor or co-inventor of patent applications owned by Children's Hospital & Research Center Oakland (CHRCO) involving biomarkers and therapies that target arginine dysregulation, and has received royalties from IP licensed from CHRCO to NourishLife for a nutritional supplement that targets oxidative stress. Novelli receives research funding from the American Society of Hematology Scholar Award and the Gilead Sciences Research Award. Berman Rosenzweig has received honoraria for consultation with Actelion, Gilead, and United Therapeutics in the past 2 years. She has received research funding from Actelion, Gilead, United Therapeutics, GSK, Eli Lily, Bayer, and Novartis in the past 2 years. Schraufnagel, MD serves on the Board of Directors for the International Union Against Tuberculosis and Lung Disease; Union North America. This does not alter the authors' adherence to PLOS ONE policies on sharing data and materials.

* Email: gladwinmt@upmc.edu

Introduction

As patients with sickle cell disease age, repetitive cycles of end-organ ischemia-reperfusion injury caused by vaso-occlusive events and intravascular hemolysis and anemia lead to end organ injury and failure [1,2]. The development of pulmonary vascular disease and renal failure are particularly ominous. A series of studies using Doppler-echocardiography to estimate pulmonary artery systolic pressure has suggested that even mild elevations in estimated pulmonary pressures are associated with a significant increase in the risk of death [3–5]. Three clinical cohort studies have been recently published defining pulmonary hypertension (PH) by the gold standard, right heart catheterization [6–8]. These studies reported a prevalence of PH of 6–10.5% and in all cases the patients with PH exhibited an increased risk for early death. Despite the consistent findings of these echocardiographic cohort studies, and more recent right heart catheterization studies, the importance of PH as both a common complication observed in the adult sickle cell population and an attributable risk factor for death has been questioned in editorial forums [9,10].

In the current study we estimate the prevalence of Doppler-echocardiography defined PH and the impact on survival in the largest screening cohort of patients with sickle cell disease, the Treatment of Pulmonary Hypertension and Sickle Cell Disease

Table 1. Characteristics of Patients in Screening Cohort.

	Total	Median(IQR)[1]
Demographics, Genotype, and Vital Status		
Age, years	632	37 (26–47)
Male, N(%)	632	294 (46.5)
SS Genotype, N(%)	632	466 (73.7)
Deaths, N(%)	632	22 (3.5)
Follow-up time, months	632	29.0 (25.1–33.4)
Clinical and Echocardiographic Measures		
Hydroxyurea, current use, N(%)	632	238 (37.7)
Chronic Transfusions, N(%)	627	76 (12.1)
O2 Sat, %	625	97 (95–99)
Systolic Blood Pressure, mm Hg	628	118 (109–129)
Diastolic Blood Pressure, mm Hg	628	69 (62–75)
Six Minute Walk Distance, m	618	436 (378–500)
TRV, m/sec	572	2.5 (2.3–2.7)
Laboratory Measures		
BNP, pg/mL	582	67.9 (29.0–155.0)
Ferritin, ng/mL	576	228.8 (93.2–520.8)
Fetal Hemoglobin, %	566	4.8 (1.5–10.6)
Hemolytic Component, relative unit	546	0.09 (−1.20–1.29)
Absolute Reticulocyte Count, $\times 10^6/\mu L$	594	217.6 (139.0–320.1)
Reticulocytes, %	587	7.7 (4.2–11.8)
Hemoglobin, g/dL	615	9.2 (8.0–10.7)
Hematocrit, %	616	26.8 (22.9–31.0)
MCHC, g/dL	612	34.6 (33.6–35.7)
MCV, μm^3	614	89.2 (81.6–98.1)
Platelets, $\times 10^3/\mu L$	614	341 (262–430)
RBC, $\times 10^6/\mu L$	615	2.95 (2.41–3.67)
WBC, $\times 10^3/\mu L$	615	9.2 (7.0–11.9)
Albumin, g/dL	615	4.2 (3.9–4.4)
Alkaline Phosphatase, U/L	615	86 (67–118)
ALT, U/L	619	22 (16–32)
AST, U/L	604	39 (27–54)
BUN, mg/dL	616	10.0 (7.0–28.0)
Creatinine, mg/dL	620	0.7 (0.6–0.9)
LDH, IU/L	584	367 (250–555)
Total Bilirubin, mg/dL	618	2.3 (1.4–3.6)

[1]Unless otherwise indicated.

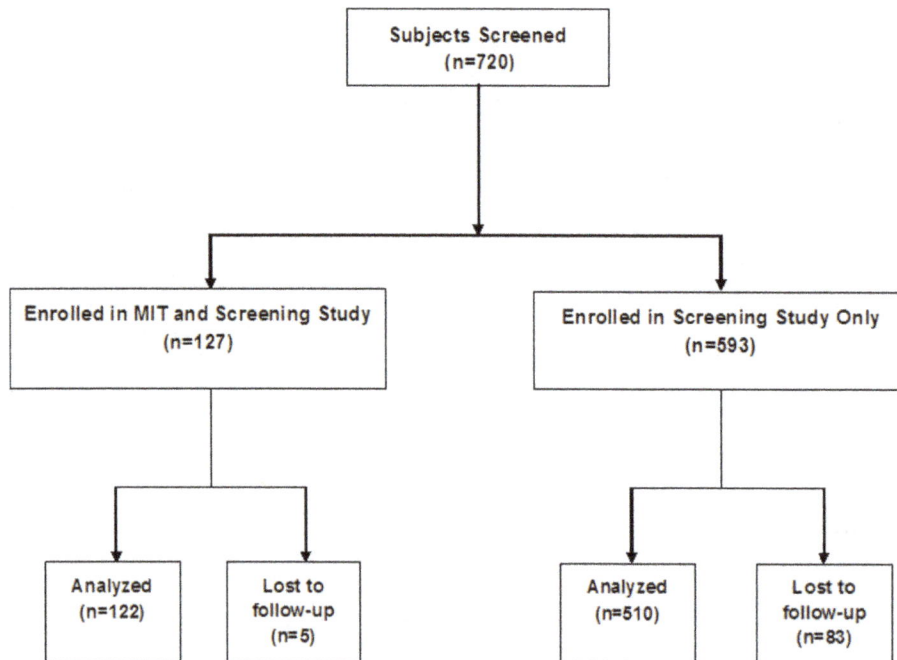

Figure 1. Study Flowchart.

with Sildenafil Therapy (walk-PHaSST) study [11,12]. This was designed both as a screening study to assemble a large cohort of patients with sickle cell disease and as an intervention trial to examine the effects of sildenafil therapy on PH. In addition to identifying the PH subjects eligible for the Main Intervention Trial (MIT), the screening study collected extensive data on demographic, medical history, physical examination, laboratory, and echocardiographic characteristics, and resulted in a large, multi-

center cohort of over 600 patients with sickle cell disease. An observational follow-up study of screening study participants was also implemented as part of the original protocol, during which data on clinical outcomes, including deaths, were collected prospectively during a follow-up period of approximately two years. In this report, we present the results from this observational follow-up and an examination of mortality in the walk-PHaSST screening cohort and its association with various patient characteristics.

For our analysis of prevalence and hazards ratios for death we chose a conservative value for the tricuspid regurgitation velocity of ≥ 3.0 m/sec. This value had a 67% positive predictive value for PH measured by right heart catheterization (defined by a mean pulmonary artery pressure of ≥ 25 mm Hg) in the French screening study published by Parent and colleagues [6], and had a 77% positive predictive value for PH in the NIH-pulmonary hypertension screening study [8]. This TRV value provides a more conservative population estimate of Doppler-defined PH prevalence and impact on mortality than a cut-off value of 2.5 m/sec. We recognize that the gold-standard for PH diagnosis is a right heart catheterization, but this was not considered feasible for the large number of patients enrolled in this NIH funded trial.

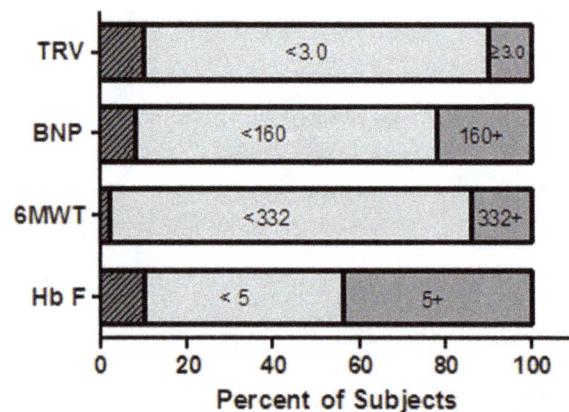

Figure 2. Prevalence of TRV, BNP, Six Minute Walk Distance, and Fetal Hemoglobin. The screening study patient population consisted of 671 patients with sickle cell anemia, 632 of whom were followed for mortality over a median of 29 months. Ten percent (n = 64) had TRV measurements of 3.0 m/sec or higher and 80% (n = 508) had measurements less than 3.0 m/sec. TRV measurements were not available for 10% (n = 60) of the patient population (diagonal stripes). Twenty-two percent of patients (n = 140) had BNP measurements of 160 pg/mL or higher. Fourteen percent (n = 85) had six minute walk distances less than 332 meters, and 46% (n = 289) had fetal hemoglobin levels less than 5%.

Methods

Study Design and Selection of Subjects

The protocol for this trial and supporting CONSORT checklist are available as supporting information; see Checklist S1 and Protocol S1. The study population and design have been described in detail elsewhere [11,12]. In brief, we analyzed all members of the screening cohort for whom follow-up data were available. Local institutional review boards or ethics committees (University of Pittsburgh, Columbia University, National Heart & Lung Institute, Imperial College London, Howard University, University of Colorado, Denver, University of Illinois Chicago, Johns Hopkins University, National Heart Lung and Blood Institute/

Table 2. Cox Proportional Hazards Regression Analysis of Mortality for Demographic, Clinical, and Laboratory Characteristics.

Characteristic	Category	Total	Deaths	Hazard Ratio (95% CI)[1]	p
Age, years	----	632	22	2.02 (1.1–3.8)	0.032
Gender	F	338	7	1.0	
	M	294	15	2.48 (1.0–6.1)	0.048
Genotype	SS	446	17	1.0	
	SC	166	5	0.83 (0.3–2.2)	0.71
Hydroxyurea use	none/past	394	11	1.0	
	current	238	11	1.64 (0.7–3.8)	0.25
Chronic Transfusions	no	551	15	1.0	
	yes	76	6	3.00 (1.2–7.7)	0.023
Moderate/Severe Pain episodes in past year	0–2	209	7	1.0	
	>2	420	14	1.02 (0.4–2.5)	0.96
Systolic BP, mm Hg	----	628	21	1.62 (0.93–2.8)	0.086
TRV, m/sec	<3.0	508	10	1.0	
	3.0+	64	11	9.55 (4.1–22.5)	<0.001
BNP, pg/mL[2]	---	582	19	2.56 (1.8–3.6)	<0.001
BNP, pg/mL	<160	442	8	1.0	
	≥160	140	11	4.55 (1.8–11.3)	0.001
Hemolytic Component, relative unit	<1.28	412	9	1.0	
	≥1.28	134	10	3.43 (1.4–8.4)	0.007
Lactate dehydrogenase, IU/L[3]	----	584	19	1.68 (1.1–2.6)	0.021
Aspartate aminotransferase, IU/L[3]	----	604	21	1.91 (1.3–2.7)	<0.001
Reticulocytes, %[2]	----	585	20	1.07 (0.6–2.0)	0.83
Total bilirubin, mg/dL[2]	----	618	21	1.15 (0.7–2.0)	0.63
Six-Minute Walk, m	≥332	533	19	1.0	
	<332	85	3	1.01 (0.3–3.4)	0.99
NYHA/WHO Class	I	439	11	1.0	
	II	141	7	1.96 (0.8–5.1)	0.17
	III,IV	35	4	4.52 (1.4–14.3)	0.010
Hemoglobin, g/dL	----	615	21	0.72 (0.4–1.4)	0.31
White blood cell count, ×10³/μL[2]	----	615	21	1.55 (0.8–2.9)	0.175
Absolute neutrophil count[2]	----	605	21	1.34 (0.8–2.3)	0.28
Platelets, ×10³/μL[2]	----	614	21	0.65 (0.4–1.0)	0.050
Hemoglobin F, %[2]	----	537	16	0.72 (0.3–1.5)	0.39
BUN, mg/dL[2]	----	616	20	1.24 (0.7–2.3)	0.49
Creatinine, mg/dL[2]	----	620	21	1.74 (1.4–2.2)	<0.001
Albumin, g/dL	----	615	20	0.60 (0.4–0.8)	0.002
Alkaline phosphatase, U/L[2]	----	615	21	1.88 (1.2–3.0)	0.009
Alanine aminotransferase, U/L[2]	----	619	21	1.68 (1.1–2.6)	0.023
Ferritin, ng/mL[2]	----	576	21	2.58 (1.5–4.4)	<0.001

[1]Hazard ratios presented for 75th relative to the 25th percentile, unless otherwise indicated. All results are unadjusted.
[2]Transformed using the log or square root function.
[3]Adjusted for site-specific differences in normal ranges.

NIH) approved the protocol and written informed consent was obtained (ClinicalTrials.gov identifier NCT00492531). Written informed consent was obtained from patients or their guardians in the case of minors. Overall, we recruited 720 subjects age 12 and over at steady state from nine different study sites in the United States and one site in the United Kingdom. Of these, 632 (94.2%) were followed for mortality and were included in our analysis; over a median of 29 months, we observed 22 deaths. Deaths were reported by study site coordinators and verified by review of medical records, contact with next-of-kin, and/or death certificates when available.

A

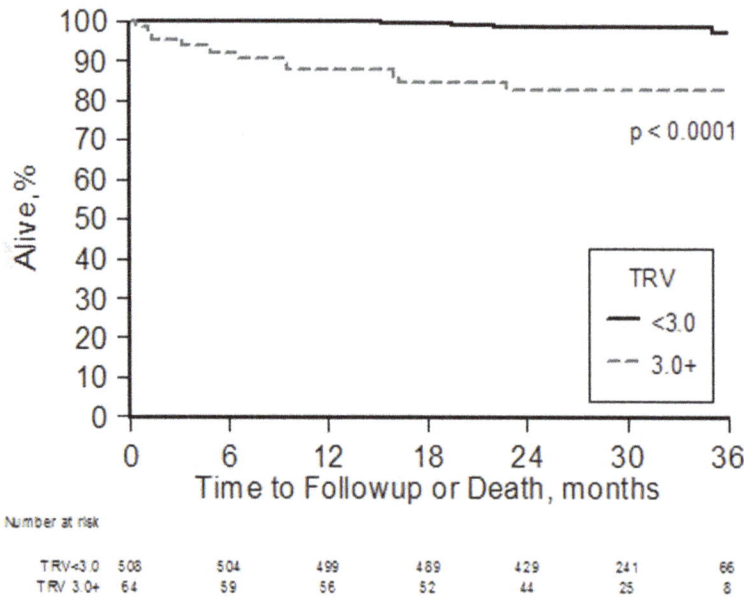

B

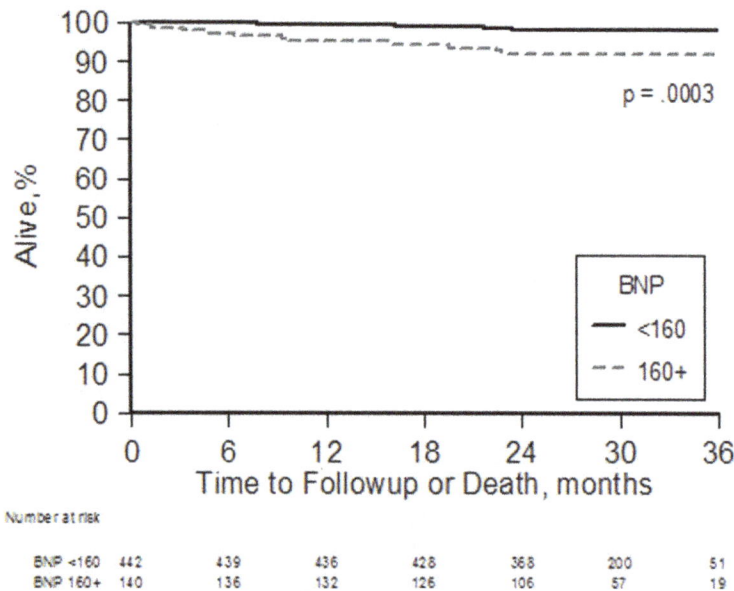

Figure 3. Kaplan-Meier Analysis of Survival Time by TRV and BNP. Longer survival times were observed for a) subjects with TRV less than 3.0 m/sec (p<0.0001) and b) for subjects with BNP levels less than 160 pg/mL (p = 0.0003).

Evaluation of Subjects

All screening study subjects were evaluated by histories of clinical events and lifetime treatments, physical examination, laboratory screening, transthoracic Doppler echocardiography, and the six-minute walk test. Routine laboratory tests (complete blood count, serum chemistry profile, and lactate dehydrogenase) from samples taken at the subject's screening visit were performed in the local laboratories of the participating institutions. Echocardiography was performed at the participating institutions and read centrally in the NHLBI echocardiography core laboratory. Percentage of hemoglobin F was measured by high-performance liquid chromatography (HPLC) (Ultra Resolution System, Trinity

Biotech). Alpha-thalassemia was detected by molecular methodology based on polymerase chain reaction at the University of Pittsburgh. Serum N-terminal pro-brain natriuretic peptide (NT-pro BNP) concentration was measured by a sandwich immunoassay using polyclonal antibodies that recognize epitopes located in the N-terminal segment (1–76) of pro-BNP (1–108) (Elecsys analyser; Roche Diagnostics, Mannheim, Germany), as previously described [13]. Ferritin was measured with an enzyme immunoassay (Ramco Laboratories Inc, Stafford, TX; reference range, 20–300 ng/mL).

Table 3. Multivariate Cox Proportional Hazards Regression Analysis of Mortality.

Risk Factor	Category	N at Risk (deaths)	Hazard Ratio (95% CI)[1]	p
TRV, m/sec	<3.0	445 (10)	1.0	
	3.0+	57 (10)	4.12 (1.4–11.8)	0.008
Ferritin, ng/mL	---	502 (20)	1.80 (1.0–3.1)	0.038
Aspartate aminotransferase, U/L	---	502 (20)	1.85 (1.0–3.5	0.062
Creatinine, mg/dL and BNP, pg/mL[2]	0	339 (8)	1.0	
(# of risk factors)	1	104 (2)	0.53 (0.1–2.5)	0.43
	2	59 (10)	2.73 (0.9–8.4)	0.079

[1]HR is presented for 75th relative to the 25th percentile, calculated as $e^{coefficient \times (75th\ percentile - 25th\ percentile)}$, for each variable listed in the table, unless otherwise indicated. Values shown are adjusted for all other variables in the model.
[2]HR is given for the combined influence of creatinine and BNP on mortality as defined by the creatinine levels >0.9 or BNP levels ≥160, or both, relative to creatinine ≤ 0.9 and BNP<160.

Statistical Analysis

Patient characteristics are presented as median and interquartile range (IQR) or number and percentage of participants with a given characteristic. TRV was categorized into two groups, ≥ 3.0 m/sec and below 3.0 m/sec, based on now established high PPV of this cut-off for PH defined by right heart catheterization; NT-proBNP was categorized into two groups based on a cut-off value of 160 pg/mL. A hemolytic component variable was derived using principal component analysis from four markers of hemolysis (lactate dehydrogenase, aspartate aminotransferase, total bilirubin, and reticulocyte percent), as described elsewhere [14], and divided into two groups based on the 75th percentile. Composite variables combining correlated risk factors were derived to minimize the effects on risk estimates of entering collinear variables simultaneously into statistical models. Associations of patient characteristics with mortality were assessed using Cox proportional hazards regression analysis, Kaplan-Meier survival curves, and the log-rank test for differences across groups. Continuous variables were log-transformed as necessary to normalize skewed distributions. Patients were censored at the point of their last contact with study staff if they did not have an event. Time to event or censoring was measured from the date of entry into the screening study. Regression coefficients were tested for significant differences from zero by the Wald test. The proportional hazards assumption was evaluated by testing the significance of each variable entered into the model as a time dependent covariate. For the final model, variables were entered in a stepwise approach if they had a significant univariate association with mortality. All statistical analyses were performed using PROC MEANS in SAS, version 9.1 (SAS Institute, Inc., Cary, NC) and STCOX and STS GRAPH in Stata, version 11.1 (Statacorp, LP, College Station, TX).

Results

Characteristics of the walk-PHaSST Screening Cohort

Demographic, clinical, laboratory, and echocardiographic characteristics of the screening cohort are shown in **Table 1 and Figure 1**. Of the 632 participants, 47% were male and 74% were homozygous for the hemoglobin S mutation. Study participants ranged in age from 12 to 84 years, and the median age was 37 years. A total of 22 deaths were observed during a median follow-up time of 29 months.

The prevalence of characteristics that are generally thought to be markers of poor relative health in patients with sickle cell disease is shown in **Figure 2**. Sixty-four patients (10.1%) had TRV measurements of 3.0 m/sec or higher, and140 (22.2%) had NT proBNP measurements at least as high as 160 pg/mL, a previously validated cut-off value associated with both PH and mortality in patients with sickle cell disease [15,16]. Thirty-nine (6.2%) patients had both TRV≥3.0 m/sec and NT-proBNP≥ 160 pg/mL. Walk distances of less than 332 meters were observed in 85 (13.5%) patients, and fetal hemoglobin levels less than 5% were observed in 289 (45.7%) patients.

Table 4. Cox Proportional Hazards Regression Analysis of Mortality for Composite of TRV and BNP.

Risk Factor	Category	N at Risk (deaths)	Hazard Ratio (95% CI)[1]	p
Unadjusted TRV/BNP Composite[1]	0	381 (7)	1.0	
(# of risk factors)	1	105 (3)	1.56 (0.4–6.0)	0.52
	2	39 (9)	14.86 (5.5–39.9)	<0.001
Adjusted TRV/BNP Composite[1,2]	0	366 (7)	1.0	
(# of risk factors)	1	96 (3)	1.44 (0.4–5.6)	0.60
	2	36 (9)	11.10 (4.0–30.8)	<0.001
Ferritin, ng/mL[3]	---		2.15 (1.2–3.8)	0.008

[1]HR is given for the combined influence of TRV and BNP on mortality as defined by TRV levels ≥3.0 or BNP levels ≥160, or both, relative to TRV<3.0 and BNP<160.
[2]Adjusted for ferritin.
[3]HR presented for 75th relative to the 25th percentile, calculated as $e^{coefficient \times (75th\ percentile - 25th\ percentile)}$, and adjusted for TRV/BNP composite.

Univariate Associations with Mortality

Patient characteristics and their associations with mortality were analyzed with Cox proportional hazards regression analysis (**Table 2**). In this study, an increased risk of death was observed for both age and gender, with males at two and a half times the risk of dying relative to females (p = 0.05), and patients older than 47 years at twice the risk of dying compared with patients less than 26 years (p = 0.03). Associations with mortality were also observed for chronic transfusions (p = 0.02) and a NYHA/WHO class value or III or IV (p = 0.01). Variables not associated with mortality included current hydroxyurea use, SC genotype, self-reported history of painful episodes, and six-minute walk distance.

We also observed associations with mortality for two separate biomarkers of pulmonary hypertension, TRV and NT-proBNP, both of which were identified as risk factors for death in other cohorts [3–5,13]. At 24 months the cumulative survival was 83% for patients with TRV measurements of 3.0 m/sec or greater and 98% for patients below 3.0 m/sec (p<0.0001; **Figure 3a**). Similarly, the cumulative survival was lower for patients with NT-proBNP levels of 160 pg/mL or higher compared with levels less than 160 pg/mL, although the magnitude of the difference was not as large (92% for NT-proBNP≥160 vs. 98% for NT-proBNP<160, log-rank p = 0.0003; **Figure 3b**). The unadjusted hazard ratios for death were 11.14 (95% CI 4.1–30.1; p<0.0001) for patients with TRV≥3.0 m/sec relative to TRV<2.7 m/sec and 4.55 (95% CI 1.8–11.3; p = 0.001) for patients with NT-proBNP≥160 pg/mL relative to NT-proBNP levels < 160 (**Table 2**). For log-transformed NT-proBNP, the risk ratio for death was 2.56 (95% CI 1.8–3.6; p<0.0001) for NT-proBNP levels in the 75th percentile relative to NT-proBNP levels in the 25th percentile (**Table 2**).

Other variables associated with mortality in our cohort included the calculated hemolytic component and two of the variables from which it was calculated, aspartate aminotransferase (AST) and lactate dehydrogenase, as well as ferritin and creatinine. Patients with a hemolytic component value at least as large as 1.28, the 75th percentile in this dataset, were at more than three times the risk of dying relative to those patients with smaller values (HR = 3.43, 95% CI 1.4–8.4; p = 0.007) (**Table 2**).

Multivariate Associations with Mortality

In stepwise multiple proportional hazards regression analysis, the magnitude of the association between TRV and mortality was decreased but still significant after adjustment for ferritin, AST, creatinine and NT-proBNP (HR 4.27, 95%CI 1.3–14.1; p = 0.04; **Table 3**). Comparing the 75th with the 25th percentiles of log-transformed values, ferritin (HR 1.80, 95% CI 1.0–3.1; p = 0.04) was also associated with mortality after adjustment for all other variables in the model. AST was associated with mortality in the multivariate model at the $\alpha = 0.10$ level (HR 1.84; 95%CI 0.95–3.5; p = 0.07), as were creatinine and NT-proBNP, which were entered into the model as a composite variables due to their high pairwise correlation (Pearson r = 0.48, p<0.0001). Patients who had both a high creatinine and a high NT-proBNP were at almost 3 times the risk of dying compared with patients with lower levels (HR 2.71, 95% CI 0.9–6.2; p = 0.08).

The results from an analysis of TRV as a composite variable combined with NT-proBNP are presented in **Table 4**. For patients with both high TRV (≥3.0 m/sec) and high NT-proBNP (≥160 pg/mL), the unadjusted hazard ratio was 14.86 (95% CI 5.5–39.9; p<0.0001) and 11.10 (95% CI 4.0–30.8; p<0.0001) after adjustment for ferritin. Adjustment for AST and creatinine had little effect on the significance of the association between the

combined TRV and NT-proBNP variable and mortality and were not included in the model.

Discussion

Here we show that amongst a large multinational cohort of patients with SCD, a TRV≥3.0 m/sec is common and has the highest risk for death of any measured variable. This risk is higher when an elevated TRV is combined with an elevated NT-proBNP level confirming the value of these measurements as risk stratification screening tools in patients with SCD.

An estimate based on a Doppler-echocardiographic measured TRV value ≥3.0 m/sec suggests that 11.2% of the SCD population screened are at high risk of having PH. This result is consistent with the recently published analysis of the NIH-Pulmonary Hypertension Screening Study, which reported 84 right heart catheterizations in 531 SCD subjects and a PH prevalence of 10.4% [8]. It is also consistent with a PH prevalence of 10% reported by Fonseca et al. in the evaluation of a smaller Brazilian cohort [7]. These numbers are higher than the 6% prevalence observed by Parent and colleagues, however they excluded 10% of their patient population from screening, those with elevated international normalized prothrombin time ratio > 1.7, estimated creatinine clearance <30 mL per minute and forced expiratory vital capacity <70% predicted [6]. Because hepatic dysfunction, renal insufficiency and low total lung capacity are associated with PH in the sickle cell disease population [3,17], they likely excluded a group with a much higher prevalence of PH. This would be expected to reduce prevalence estimates.

This study identified a number of risk factors for early death previously described in the Cooperative Study of Sickle Cell Disease (CSSCD) such as age and male gender [18]. It also confirmed risks associated with elevated TRV, elevated NT-proBNP, increasing creatinine, intensity of hemolytic anemia, and ferritin. Additionally, the New York Heart Functional Classification and number of red blood cell units transfused were also found to be associated with higher risk of death in univariate analysis. In multivariate analysis TRV, ferrritin, AST, and creatinine or NT-pro-BNP remained independent predictors of mortality. Of all the measured parameters the TRV carried the highest hazards ratio for early death, associated with a 10-fold increased risk. This was even more significant when combined with a high NT-proBNP (14-fold increased risk of death), potentially reflecting PH with right heart failure.

There are a number of major limitations to this study. Most patients with an elevated TRV did not have a right heart catheterization to confirm the diagnosis of PH. For these estimates we refer to the recent RHC studies and published operating characteristics for this test at this threshold value. The causes of death are largely unknown as there were no autopsies available and the trial was not funded to establish the definitive cause of death for all patients. In the recent analysis of the NIH-PH cohort, death certificates were available for 15 out of 23 (65%) subjects with PH and 80% of these subjects were reported to have had right heart failure or sudden cardiac death stated as a cause of death [8]. In addition, we cannot estimate the percentage of patients with an elevated TRV that had pulmonary arterial hypertension (PAH) or pulmonary venous (or post-capillary) hypertension (PVH). According to the NIH cohort [8] study 5.8% of the entire cohort had PAH and in the Fonseca study 3.75% had PAH [7]; based on these data it is likely that half of the patients with PH would have PAH and half PVH. It is notable in the Mehari study that even patients diagnosed with PVH had elevated transpulmonary gradients and the pulmonary vascular resistance and transpulmonary gradients predicted risk of death, while the pulmonary capillary wedge pressure did not [8,19]. These data suggest that pulmonary vascular disease is central to the mechanism of disease and death observed in the current study.

Recent editorials have suggested that PH is rare in patients with sickle cell disease and not a cause of death "per se" in this patient population [9,10]. To our knowledge, scleroderma, with a prevalence of 7–11% and portopulmonary hypertension (1–6% prevalence) are the only diseases with a prevalence of PAH that is comparable to sickle cell disease. Based on this accepted high prevalence, all patients with scleroderma and patients with portal hypertension being evaluated for liver transplantation are screened for the development of PH and referred to specialty care [20]. Similar to certain diseases associated with PAH, there have been no completed trials in patients with sickle cell disease with sufficient power to evaluate the efficacy of PAH targeted therapy. However, there are a number of interventions that would be expected to reduce morbidity and mortality in this population, including more aggressive hydroxyurea or transfusion therapy, iron chelation, supplemental oxygen and identification and treatment of thromboembolic disease and sleep disordered breathing. For these reasons, we suggest that screening for PH associated with sickle cell disease is helpful and would have a positive impact on the well-being of these patients.

Acknowledgments

This project has been funded with federal funds from the National Heart, Lung, and Blood Institute, National Institutes of Health, Department of Health and Human Services, under contract HHSN268200617182C. The views expressed by the authors in this article are theirs and do not represent the views of the government.

Author Contributions

Performed the experiments: RJB JSRG VS MN KLH JAL DES LK EN REG CRM EBR DBB SL OLC JGT JCG GJK VRG. Analyzed the data: MTG RFM MH. Contributed reagents/materials/analysis tools: MTG RFM MH RJB JSRG VS MN KLH JAL DES LK EN REG CRM EBR DBB SL OLC JGT JCG GJK VRG. Wrote the manuscript: MTG MH RFM. Edited the manuscript: RJB JSRG VS MN KLH JAL DES LK EN REG CRM EBR DBB SL OLC JGT JCG GJK VRG.

References

1. Gladwin MT, Vichinsky E (2008) Pulmonary complications of sickle cell disease. N Engl J Med 359: 2254–2265.
2. Rees DC, Williams TN, Gladwin MT (2010) Sickle-cell disease. Lancet 376: 2018–2031.
3. Gladwin MT, Sachdev V, Jison ML, Shizukuda Y, Plehn JF, et al. (2004) Pulmonary hypertension as a risk factor for death in patients with sickle cell disease. N Engl J Med 350: 886–895.
4. Ataga KI, Moore CG, Jones S, Olajide O, Strayhorn D, et al. (2006) Pulmonary hypertension in patients with sickle cell disease: a longitudinal study. Br J Haematol 134: 109–115.
5. De Castro LM, Jonassaint JC, Graham FL, Ashley-Koch A, Telen MJ (2008) Pulmonary hypertension associated with sickle cell disease: clinical and laboratory endpoints and disease outcomes. Am J Hematol 83: 19–25.
6. Parent F, Bachir D, Inamo J, Lionnet F, Driss F, et al. (2011) A hemodynamic study of pulmonary hypertension in sickle cell disease. N Engl J Med 365: 44–53.
7. Fonseca GH, Souza R, Salemi VM, Jardim CV, Gualandro SF (2012) Pulmonary hypertension diagnosed by right heart catheterization in sickle cell disease. Eur Respir J.
8. Mehari A, Gladwin MT, Tian X, Machado RF, Kato GJ (2012) Mortality in adults with sickle cell disease and pulmonary hypertension. JAMA : the journal of the American Medical Association 307: 1254–1256.
9. Nathan DG (2011) Guilt by association. Blood 118: 3758–3759.
10. Simonneau G, Parent F (2012) Pulmonary hypertension in patients with sickle cell disease: not so frequent but so different. Eur Respir J 39: 3–4.
11. Nouraie M, Lee JS, Zhang Y, Kanias T, Zhao X, et al. (2012) The relationship between the severity of hemolysis, clinical manifestations and risk of death in 415 patients with sickle cell anemia in the US and Europe. Haematologica.
12. Sachdev V, Kato GJ, Gibbs JS, Barst RJ, Machado RF, et al. (2011) Echocardiographic Markers of Elevated Pulmonary Pressure and Left Ventricular Diastolic Dysfunction Are Associated With Exercise Intolerance in Adults and Adolescents With Homozygous Sickle Cell Anemia in the United States and United Kingdom. Circulation 124: 1452–1460.
13. Machado RF, Hildesheim M, Mendelsohn L, Kato GJ, Gladwin MT (2009) NT-Pro Brain Natriuretic Peptide Levels and the Risk of Stroke and Death in the Cooperative Study of Sickle Cell Disease. Blood 114: 1541.
14. Minniti CP, Sable C, Campbell A, Rana S, Ensing G, et al. (2009) Elevated tricuspid regurgitant jet velocity in children and adolescents with sickle cell disease: association with hemolysis and hemoglobin oxygen desaturation. Haematologica 94: 340–347.
15. Machado RF, Anthi A, Steinberg MH, Bonds D, Sachdev V, et al. (2006) N-terminal pro-brain natriuretic peptide levels and risk of death in sickle cell disease. JAMA : the journal of the American Medical Association 296: 310–318.
16. Machado RF, Hildesheim M, Mendelsohn L, Remaley AT, Kato GJ, et al. (2011) NT-pro brain natriuretic peptide levels and the risk of death in the cooperative study of sickle cell disease. Br J Haematol 154: 512–520.
17. Anthi A, Machado RF, Jison ML, Taveira-Dasilva AM, Rubin IJ, et al. (2007) Hemodynamic and functional assessment of patients with sickle cell disease and pulmonary hypertension. Am J Respir Crit Care Med 175: 1272–1279.
18. Platt OS, Brambilla DJ, Rosse WF, Milner PF, Castro O, et al. (1994) Mortality in sickle cell disease. Life expectancy and risk factors for early death [see comments]. N Engl J Med 330: 1639–1644.
19. Mehari A, Alam S, Tian X, Cuttica MJ, Barnett CF, et al. (2013) Hemodynamic Predictors of Mortality in Adults with Sickle Cell Disease. American journal of respiratory and critical care medicine.
20. McLaughlin VV, Archer SL, Badesch DB, Barst RJ, Farber HW, et al. (2009) ACCF/AHA 2009 expert consensus document on pulmonary hypertension: a report of the American College of Cardiology Foundation Task Force on Expert Consensus Documents and the American Heart Association: developed in collaboration with the American College of Chest Physicians, American Thoracic Society, Inc., and the Pulmonary Hypertension Association. Circulation 119: 2250–2294.

11

Megakaryocytic Leukemia 1 (MKL1) Regulates Hypoxia Induced Pulmonary Hypertension in Rats

Zhibin Yuan[1,2,3], Jian Chen[1,2,3], Dewei Chen[1,2,3], Gang Xu[1,2,3], Minjie Xia[4], Yong Xu[4]*, Yuqi Gao[1,2,3]*

1 Department of Pathophysiology and High Altitude Physiology, College of High Altitude Military Medicine, Third Military Medical University, Chongqing, China, 2 Key Laboratory of High Altitude Medicine, Ministry of Education, Third Military Medical University, Chongqing, China, 3 Key Laboratory of High Altitude Medicine, PLA, Third Military Medical University, Chongqing, China, 4 Key Laboratory of Cardiovascular Disease, Department of Pathophysiology, Nanjing Medical University, Nanjing, Jiangsu, China

Abstract

Hypoxia induced pulmonary hypertension (HPH) represents a complex pathology that involves active vascular remodeling, loss of vascular tone, enhanced pulmonary inflammation, and increased deposition of extracellular matrix proteins. Megakaryocytic leukemia 1 (MKL1) is a transcriptional regulator known to influence cellular response to stress signals in the vasculature. We report here that in response to chronic hypobaric hypoxia, MKL1 expression was up-regulated in the lungs in rats. Short hairpin RNA (shRNA) mediated depletion of MKL1 significantly ameliorated the elevation of pulmonary arterial pressure *in vivo* with a marked alleviation of vascular remodeling. MKL1 silencing also restored the expression of NO, a key vasoactive molecule necessary for the maintenance of vascular tone. In addition, hypoxia induced pulmonary inflammation was dampened in the absence of MKL1 as evidenced by normalized levels of pro-inflammatory cytokines and chemokines as well as reduced infiltration of pro-inflammatory immune cells in the lungs. Of note, MKL1 knockdown attenuated fibrogenesis in the lungs as indicated by picrosirius red staining. Finally, we demonstrate that MKL1 mediated transcriptional activation of type I collagen genes in smooth muscle cells under hypoxic conditions. In conclusion, we data highlight a previously unidentified role for MKL1 in the pathogenesis of HPH and as such lay down groundwork for future investigation and drug development.

Editor: Rory Edward Morty, University of Giessen Lung Center, Germany

Funding: This study was supported, in part, by the National Basic Science Research "973" Program of China (2012CB518201, 2012CB517503), the Program for New Century Excellent Talents in University of China (NCET-11-0991), Natural Science Foundation of China (81100041, 31270805), Natural Science Foundation of Jiangsu Province (BK2012043), the Ministry of Education (212059), and the Postdoctoral Research Grant of China (20100471771). The funders had no role in study design, data collection and analysis, decision to publish, or preparation of the manuscript.

Competing Interests: The authors have declared that no competing interests exist.

* E-mail: gyq@mail.tmmu.edu.cn (YQG); yxu2005@gmail.com (YX)

Introduction

Hypoxia induced pulmonary hypertension (HPH) is a debilitating disease that will eventually lead to right ventricular failure [1]. HPH represents a complicated pathophysiological process that includes a series of interconnected events. Although the precise mechanism underlying the pathogenesis of HPH is largely unknown, it is generally believed that active vascular remodeling as a result of smooth muscle cell proliferation, increased pulmonary inflammation due to leukocyte adhesion and aggregation, disruption of vascular tone, and accelerated fibrogenesis all play a critical role. Importantly, the gene expression profile within the lungs is altered significantly in response to hypoxic stress [2]. For instance, it has been documented that accompanying pulmonary inflammatory response, the production and release of a number of cytokines, including IL-6 and TNF-α, are markedly up-regulated [3,4]. Another exemplary alteration of gene expression taking place in the lungs is the induction of extracellular matrix (ECM) proteins such as type I collagen in smooth muscle cells [5,6]. How these diverse transcriptional events are coordinated remains obscure.

Megakaryocytic leukemia 1 (MKL1), also termed myocardin-related transcription factor A (MRTF-A), belongs a family of transcriptional regulators initially reported to be involved in the phenotypic modulation of smooth muscle cells [7,8]. Several recent investigations have strongly indicated that MKL1 may function as a stress protein orchestrating cellular response to a range of extrinsic and intrinsic insults. It has been demonstrated the MKL1 participates in ischemia induced cardiac remodeling by regulating type I collagen transcription in fibroblast cells [9]. Meanwhile, MKL1 has shown to mediate the hypertrophic response in mice by activating the transcription of brain natriuretic peptide (BNP) gene [10]. Recently, Fang et al have reported that MKL1 mediates the deleterious effects of oxLDL, a major risk factor for atherosclerosis, by up-regulating intercellular adhesion molecule 1 (ICAM-1) transcription while simultaneously down-regulating NO synthase (eNOS) transcription in vascular endothelial cells [11]. In light of these findings, we hypothesized that MKL1 might be a key player in the pathogenesis of HPH. Our data as presented here suggest that MKL1 expression is elevated in the lungs in rats with HPH and that MKL1 silencing ameliorates HPH. Therefore, targeting MKL1 may yield novel therapeutic solutions for the intervention of HPH in the future.

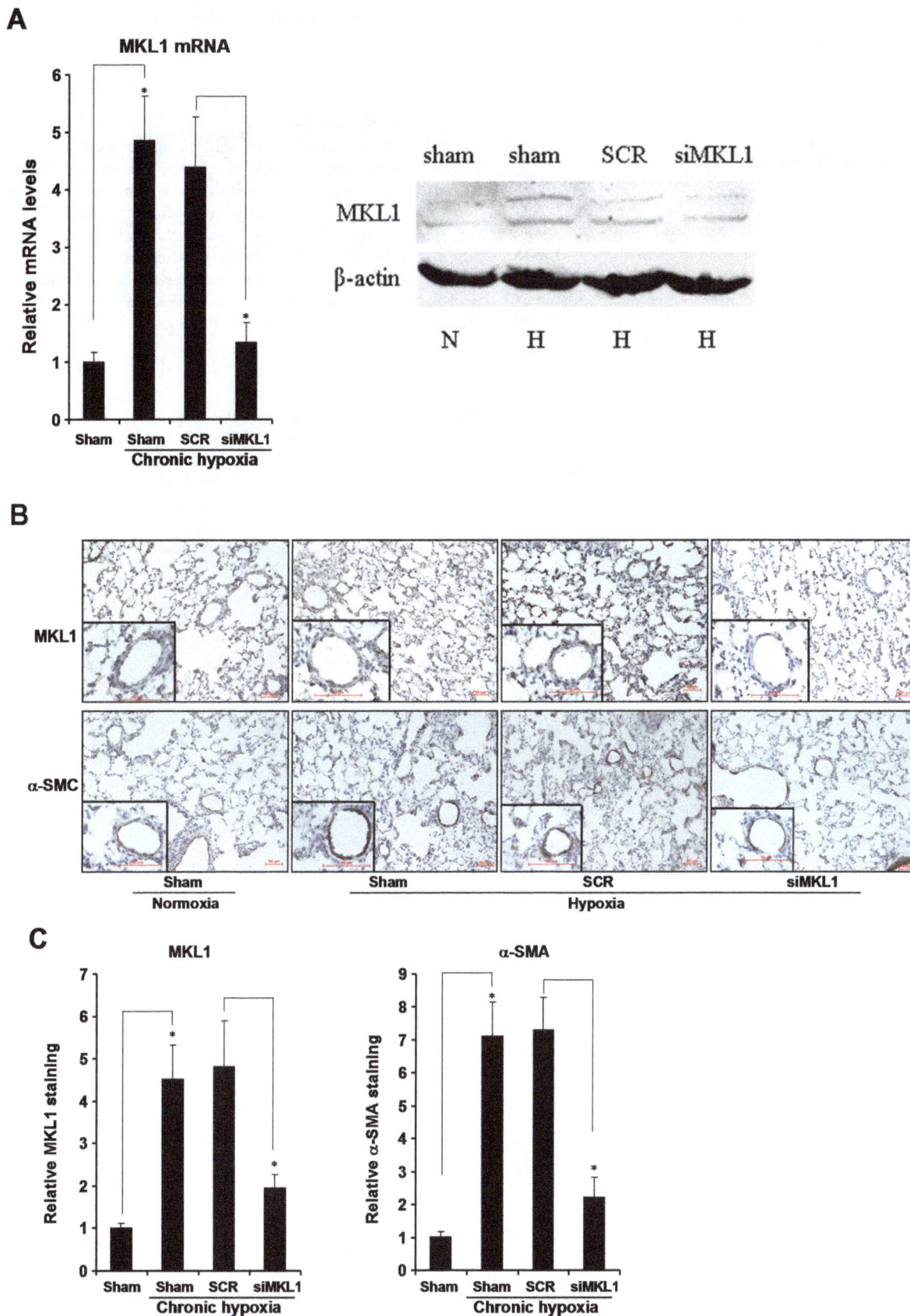

Figure 1. MKL1 expression is up-regulated in the lungs in rats with hypoxia-induced pulmonary hypertension. Sprague Dawley rats were injected with lentiviral particles carrying shRNA targeting MKL1 or random shRNA (SCR) and induced to develop HPH as described under *Methods*. (A) MKL1 mRNA and protein levels in pulmonary arteries were assessed by qPCR and Western blotting. (B) MKL1 and α-SMA levels in

pulmonary arteries were examined by immunohistochemistry. (**C**) Protein expression of MKL1 and α-SMA was quantified by Image Pro and expressed as relative staining compared to the control group set as 1. N = 10 rats for each group.

Materials and Methods

Cell culture, plasmids, and transfection

Rat vascular smooth muscle cells (A10) were cultured in DMEM as described previously [12]. Primary human pulmonary arterial smooth muscle cells (Lonza) were maintained SMBM supplemented with growth factors supplied by the vendor. Where indicated, hypoxia (1% O_2) was achieved by a mixture of ultra-high purity gases (5% CO_2, 10% H_2, 85% N_2) in a 37°C incubator (Thermo Fisher). MKL1 expression construct, shRNA plasmid targeting MKL1, *col1a2* promoter luciferase construct, and *col1a1* promoter luciferase construct have been described previously [11,13,14]. Small interfering RNA sequences for rat MKL1 were as follows: #1, CAGGUGAAUUACCCAAAGGUATT, and #2, UGGAGCUGGUGGAGAAGAATT. Transient transfections were performed with Lipofectamine 2000 (Invitrogen). Experiments were routinely performed in triplicate wells and repeated three times.

Animals and *in vivo* gene silencing

All animal experiment protocols were approved by the Committee on Ethical Practice of Animal Studies of the Third Military Medical University. Briefly, 8-week old male Sprague-Dawley rats were housed in a closed chamber with an ambient air pressure of 405.35 mmHg (approx. 0.53atm, or equivalent of 5000 m altitude, or equivalent of 11.2% O_2) for 4 weeks to induce pulmonary hypertension. shRNA targeting MKL1 (CATG-GAGCTGGTGGAGAAGAA) was cloned into a SuperSilencing lentiviral vector. At week 1 and week 3, these rodents were injected via sublingual vein purified lentivirus (1×10^8 viral particles/per injection). Detailed description for the measurement of hemodynamic parameters Key cardiac/pulmonary metrics can be found in the supplementary material.

Isolation of pulmonary arteries from SD rats

Isolation of pulmonary arteries was performed essentially as described before [15]. Briefly, the rats were anesthetized with amobarbital. The lungs were removed from the chest cavity and rinsed with washing buffer (138 mM NaCl, 4.7 mM KCl, 1.2 mM NH2PO4, 1.2 mM MgSO4, 1.8 mM CaCl2, 5 mM HEPES and 10 mM glucose). The superficial tissue and the bronchus artery were discarded with fine micro-scissors. The adventitia is carefully removed from isolated arteries under a dissection scope. Tertiary lobular branches (≤300 μm) were used for subsequent experiments.

Measurement of hemodynamics

Following the development of HPH, rats were anesthetized and the right internal jugular vein was dissected. A pulmonary artery catheter (PV 1, 0.28 mm diameter) was inserted through an introducer under pressure waveform monitoring and pulmonary arterial pressure was recorded. A PE-50 catheter was inserted into the left carotid artery with connection to a digital blood pressure analyzer (BPA, Micro-Med. Inc., Louisville, KY) for continuous recordings of systolic, diastolic and mean arterial blood pressures and heart rate.

Morphometric analysis

Wall thickness was measured with an ocular micrometer and expressed as the medial wall thickness (the distance between the internal and external lamina) divided by the diameter of the vessel (the distance between the external lamina). Muscularity was determined using α-SMA as a marker. Each vessel was categorized as fully muscular (>75% α-SMA staining), partially muscular (<75% α-SMA staining), or nonmuscular (no α-SMA staining), and values were expressed as the percentage of total vessels. Percent medial thickness was determined using Image J as previously described [16]. For each animal, at least 20 different fields and 100 different vessels (50–200 μM) were scored.

Protein extraction and Western blotting

For cells, lysates were obtained by re-suspending cell pellets in RIPA buffer (50 mM Tris pH 7.4, 150 mM NaCl, 1% Triton X-100) with freshly added protease inhibitor tablet (Roche). For tissues, lysates were obtained by homogenizing samples in lysis buffer (10 mM Tris pH 8.0, 130 mM NaCl, 1% Triton-X100). Western blot analyses were performed with anti-β-actin (Sigma; 1:5,000), anti-collagen type I (Rockland; 1:5,000), and anti-MKL1 (Santa Cruz; 1:1,000) antibodies.

Enzyme-linked immune absorbance assay (ELISA)

ELISA was performed using rat pulmonary artery homogenates to measure MCP-1/CCL2 (Pierce), RANTES/CCL5 (Invitrogen), IL-6, TNF-α, MIP-1/CCL4 (USCN Life Sciences), and TGF-β (R&D) as described previously [17].

RNA Isolation and Real-time PCR

RNA was extracted with the RNeasy RNA isolation kit (Qiagen) as described before [18,19]. Reverse transcriptase reactions were performed using a SuperScript First-strand Synthesis System (Invitrogen). Real-time PCR reactions were performed on an ABI Prism 7500 system. Primers are listed in Table S1.

Histology

Immunohistochemistry was performed as previously described [20]. Briefly, the sections were blocked with 10% normal goat serum for 1 hour at room temperature and then incubated with anti-MKL1 (Santa Cruz; 1:100), anti-sm-MHC (Sigma; 1:100), anti-α-SMA (Sigma; 1:100), anti-CD3 (BD Bioscience; 1:100), anti-CD45 (Abcam; 1:100), or anti-F4/80 (Abcam; 1:100) antibodies. Staining was visualized by incubation with an appropriate biotinylated 2° antibody and developed with a streptavidin-horseradish peroxidase kit (Pierce) for 20 min. Sections were counterstained with hematoxylin. Pictures were taken using an Olympus IX-70 microscope. Picrosirius red, Masson's trichrome (both from Sigma), and elastica von Gieson (Millipore) stainings were performed according to vendor's recommendations.

Immunofluorescence staining

The plastic-embedded sections were incubated with primary antibodies, anti-α-SMA and anti-Von Willebrand factor (both from Abcam), followed by incubation with rabbit secondary antibodies (Jackson ImmunoResearch). The nuclei were counter-stained with DAPI (Sigma).

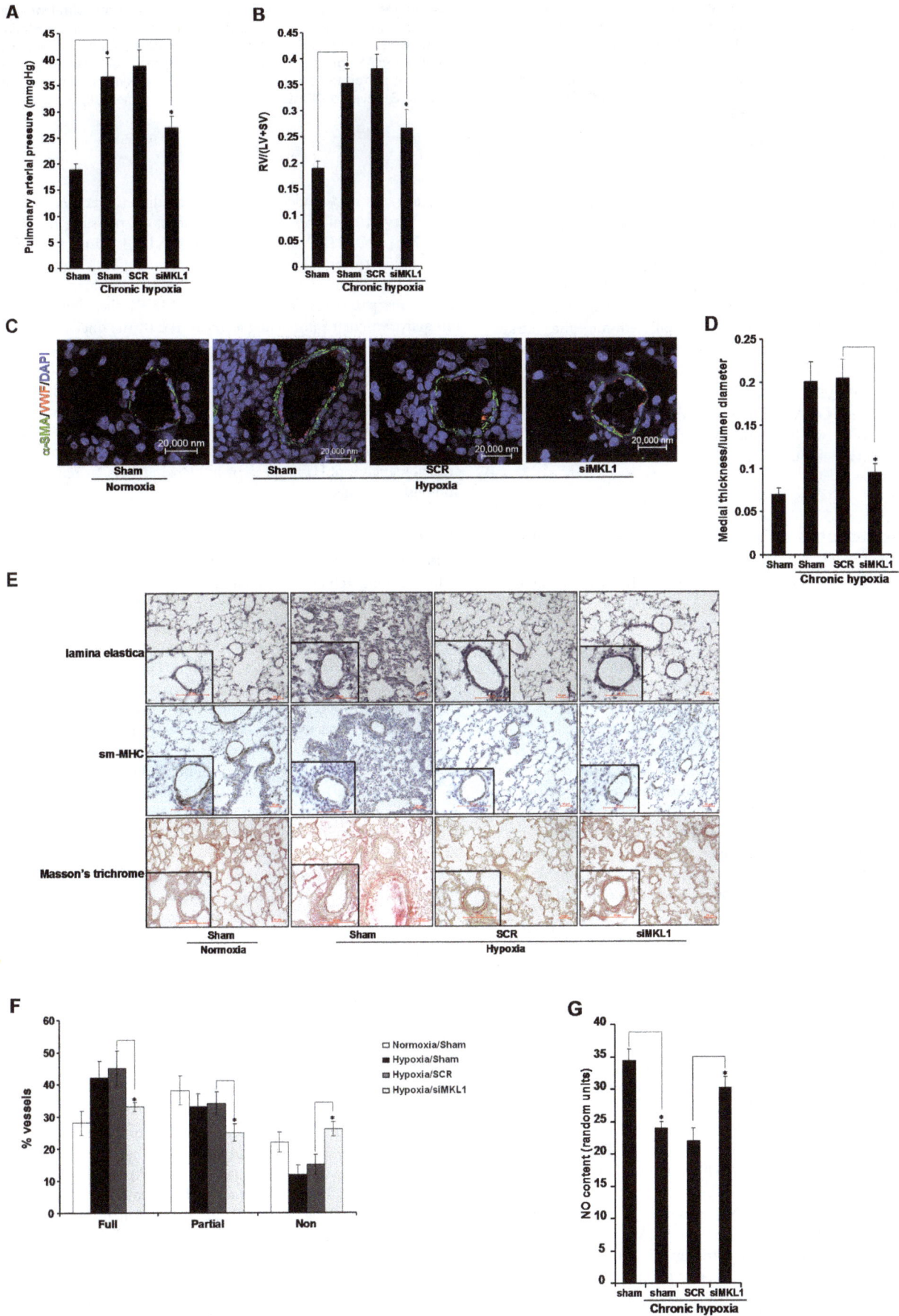

Figure 2. MKL1 silencing attenuates hypoxia-induced pulmonary hypertension in rats. Sprague Dawley rats were injected with lentiviral particles carrying shRNA targeting MKL1 or random shRNA (SCR) and induced to develop HPH as described under *Methods*. (**A**) Pulmonary arterial pressure was measured. N = 10 rats for each group (**B**) RV/(LV+SV) was measured to assess right ventricle hypertrophy. N = 10 rats for each group (**C, D**) Immunofluorescence staining was performed with anti-α-SMA (orange) and anti-VWF (green). Medial thickness and lumen diameter were measured by Image J. N = 10 rats for each group (**E, F**) Histochemical stainings were performed as described under Methods. Muscularization of pulmonary vessels was evaluated as described in Methods. N = 10 rats for each group (**G**) Levels of NO were evaluated by a commercially available kit as described under *Methods*. N = 5 rats for each group.

NO measurement

NO measurement has been described before [11]. Briefly, tissues were pre-heated to 95°C for 5 min to denature proteins and then homogenized in Kreb's solution (118 mM NaCl, 4.6 mM KCl, 27.2 mM NaHCO3, 1.2 mM MgSO4, 2.5 mM CaCl2, 1.2 mM KH2PO4, and 11.1 mM glucose) for 1 hour at 37°C. Afterwards, 100 μl supernatant was collected and the nitrate content was measured with a Griess reagent system (Promega).

Statistical Analysis

One-way ANOVA with post-hoc Scheffe analyses were performed using an SPSS package. p values smaller than .05 were considered statistically significant and designated *.

Results

MKL1 expression is up-regulated in pulmonary arteries by hypoxia in rats

We first evaluated the expression levels of MKL1 in the lungs of rats that had been allowed to develop HPH when housed in a hypoxic chamber for 4 weeks. Quantitative PCR (qPCR) assays revealed that mRNA level of MKL1 was significantly (by 486%) induced in pulmonary arteries rats with HPH as opposed to control rats; MKL1 protein level as examined by Western blotting was also increased in hypoxic rats (Fig. 1A). By comparison, MKL1 mRNA expression was only modestly up-regulated (by 203%) in aortic arteries (Fig. S1A). These data were corroborated by immunohistochemistry staining, which demonstrated that MKL1 was strongly stimulated in pulmonary arteries in rats in response to chronic hypoxia (Fig. 1B, 1C, S1B); there was a partial overlapping of MKL1 expression and α-SMA expression, indicating the presence of MKL1 in the vessel wall. We also probed the expression of MKL1 in cultured rat vascular smooth muscle cells (A10) and human primary pulmonary arterial smooth muscle cells (HPASMC) challenged with 1% O_2. Both mRNA and protein levels of MKL1 were increased by low oxygen tension (Fig. S1C, S1D). Together, our results indicate that MKL1 is activated in the lungs in response to hypoxic challenge *in vivo and in vitro*.

MKL1 silencing attenuates hypoxia-induced pulmonary hypertension in rats

Next, we assessed the possibility that MKL1 silencing might avert HPH in rats. To this end, we injected lentivirus carrying either shRNA targeting MKL1 (siMKL1) or random shRNA (SCR) into rats via the sublingual vein. As a result, MKL1 expression was suppressed in pulmonary arteries (Fig. 1A, 1B), but not in aortic arteries (Fig. S1A, S1B), at both mRNA and protein levels.

Depletion of MKL1 by shRNA resulted in a marked reduction of pulmonary arterial pressure (Fig. 2A) and significantly attenuated right ventricular hypertrophy (Fig. 2B), indicating that MKL1 indeed is required for the development of HPH *in vivo*. Meanwhile, neither systemic blood pressure nor heart rate was impacted by MKL1 knockdown (Fig. S2A, S2B). Of note, MKL1

silencing in rats under normoxic conditions did not alter pulmonary arterial pressure, or systemic blood pressure, or heart rate (Fig. S2C–S2E), suggesting that MKL1 is dispensable for maintaining cardiopulmonary function under physiological conditions. Expansion of the pulmonary vessel wall marks a critical step in the pathogenesis of HPH [21]. MKL1 silencing blocked this active vascular remodeling as measured by the thickness of the medial layer (Fig. 2C, 2D). MKL1 knockdown also alleviated muscularization of pulmonary vessels (Fig. 2E, 2F). Endothelium-derived NO serves as a key vasodilator that helps maintain the vascular tone [22]. As expected, NO levels were decreased in the lungs in HPH rats, but were normalized in the absence of MKL1 (Fig. 2G). Combined, these results suggest that MKL1 might be a critical regulator of HPH *in vivo* by influencing vascular remodeling and vascular tone.

MKL1 silencing attenuates hypoxia-induced pulmonary inflammation in rats

In the lungs challenged with hypoxia, there is an increased adhesion and aggregation of immune cells creating a pro-inflammatory milieu [23,24]. These immune cells, in turn, may secrete inflammatory mediators to promote the pathogenesis of HPH [25,26]. Indeed, production of both TNF-α and IL-6 were both increased in the lungs in HPH rats (Fig. 3A). MKL1 elimination, however, potently suppressed the synthesis of these cytokines. Chemokines, such as MCP-1/CCL2, MIP-1/CCL4, and RANTES/CCL5, are responsible for the recruitment of immune cells to the lung to initiate pro-inflammatory response [27]. As expected, all three chemokines were up-regulated by hypoxia in rats (Fig. 3B). On the other hand, MKL1 knockdown was able to neutralize the induction of CCL2 and CCL5, but no CCL4. We then directly assessed the effect of MKL1 silencing on the recruitment of immune cells to the lungs by immunohisto-chemistry. As shown in Fig. 3C, chronic hypoxia resulted in a significant increase in the number of macrophages (labeled by F4/80), leukocyte (labeled by CD45), and T lymphocyte (labeled by CD3) within the lungs. MKL1 loss-of-function abrogated the adhesion and aggregation of all three types of immune cells (Fig. 3D). Collectively, these results suggest that MKL1 may play a role in establishing and/or maintaining the pro-inflammatory microenvironment in the lungs in HPH rats.

MKL1 silencing attenuates hypoxia-induced pulmonary fibrogenesis in rats

At late stages of HPH, there is an increase in the production of extracellular matrix (ECM) proteins, collagen type I being the most prominent one, in the lungs leading to pulmonary fibrosis [28]. We first examined whether MKL1 could alter collagen deposition in the lungs in HPH rats. As shown in Fig. 4A and Fig. 4B, more collagen fibers were present in the lungs of HPH rats whereas MKL1 deletion caused a significant reduction of collagen secretion. By using qPCR, we confirmed that induction of a panel of fibrogenic genes under hypoxic conditions, including type I collagen (col1a1, col1a2), type III collagen (col1a3), fibronectin (fn)

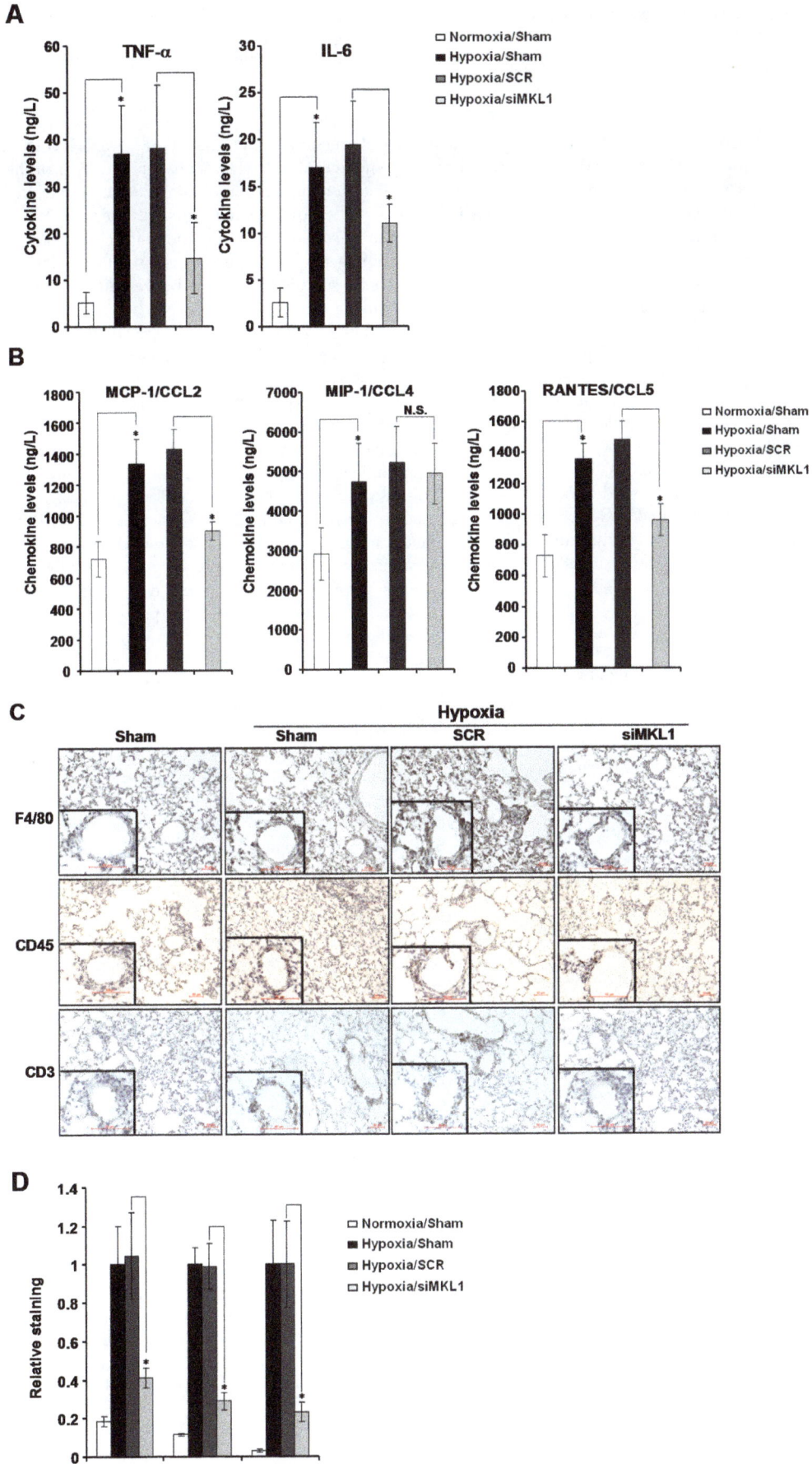

Figure 3. MKL1 silencing attenuates hypoxia-induced pulmonary inflammation in rats. Sprague Dawley rats were injected with lentiviral particles carrying shRNA targeting MKL1 or random shRNA (SCR) and induced to develop HPH as described under *Methods*. (**A, B**) Levels of cytokines and chemokines were assessed by ELISA. N = 5 rats for each group (**C, D**) Immunohistochemistry was performed with indicated antibodies as described under *Methods* and quantified by Image J. N = 5 rats for each group.

and transforming growth factor (tgf-b1), was all down-regulated in the absence of MKL1 in pulmonary arteries (Fig. 4C). MKL1 silencing also led to a decrease in protein expression of type I collagen (Fig. 4D). In accordance, MKL1 depletion prevented the accumulation of TGF-β proteins in the lungs (Fig. 4E).

Vascular smooth muscle cells (VSMC) are one of the major sources of ECM production in the lungs [5,6]. To further verify the role of MKL1 in hypoxia-induced collagen production, we transfected collagen type I gene promoter (col1a1 or col1a2) luciferase construct into cultured rat VSMC (A10). Hypoxia activated the transcription of type I collagen genes (Fig. 5A). Over-expression of MKL1 further potentiated the transcriptional activation of type I collagen genes. In contrast, knockdown of MKL1 by shRNA abolished the induction of collagen transcription by hypoxia (Fig. 5B). Finally, small interfering RNA (siRNA) mediated depletion of MKL1 prevented the increased synthesis of endogenous collagen type I mRNA in VSMC under hypoxic conditions (Fig. 5C, 5D). Taken together, MKL1 may participate in hypoxia-induced fibrogenesis in the lungs by transcriptionally activating collagen type I genes.

Discussion

Hypoxic pulmonary hypertension (HPH) is a devastating disease that eventually leads to right heart failure and death. Although there is a lack of unifying model for the pathogenesis of HPH, it is generally agreed that accumulation of pro-inflammatory mediators in the lungs and vascular remodeling as a result of extracellular matrix over-production likely provide two of the most important links [29]. Here we report that shRNA mediated silencing of MKL1, a multifaceted transcriptional modulator, effectively ameliorated HPH in rats by dampening pulmonary inflammation and normalizing collagen type I synthesis in smooth muscle cells.

Increased production and release of pro-inflammatory mediators have been observed in the plasma of patients with HPH [3,30,31]. Accumulation of pro-inflammatory mediators will injure vascular endothelium, promote the encroachment of medial smooth muscle cells to actively remodel pulmonary vasculature, and encourage the adhesion and aggregation of immune cells to the vessel wall, all of which cause irreparable damages and exacerbate HPH. At the transcriptional level, expression of these cytokines and chemokines depend on NF-κB, the master regulator of the innate immunity [32]. Indeed, it is well documented that hypoxia activates NF-κB to initiate and perpetuate a pro-inflammatory microenvironment in the context of pulmonary hypertension [33–35]. In the present study, we have found that when MKL1 was depleted by shRNA, levels of pro-inflammatory mediators were significantly down-regulated in the lungs of rats with HPH (Fig. 3A, 3B). In addition, recruitment of immune cells was greatly diminished (Fig. 3C, 3D). Our previous findings suggest that MKL1 directly interacts with NF-κB and potentiates NF-κB dependent transcription [11]. Therefore, it is possible that MKL1 may influence the synthesis of these cytokines and chemokines in a NF-κB dependent manner in immune cells. On the other hand, the interaction between immune cells and vascular endothelial cells that serves as a prerequisite for extravasation relies on the expression of a group of cell-cell adhesion molecules such as ICAM-1 and VCAM-1 [36,37]. MKL1 has been shown to

promote leukocyte adhesion by inducing ICAM-1 and VCAM-1 transcription in endothelial cells [11]. Thus, an equally plausible explanation for decreased infiltration of immune cells in the lungs following MKL1 knockdown would be that endothelial cells cannot produce sufficient amount of adhesion molecules to attract and sustain the interaction with immune cells. Future investigations employing tissue-specific MKL1 knockout animal models will be able to differentiate these two possibilities.

Another important finding presented here is that MKL1 silencing attenuated pulmonary fibrosis in rats with HPH (Fig. 4). In response to hypoxia, pulmonary vascular smooth muscle cells undergo several changes typical to HPH, including accelerated proliferation and migration and augmented ability to synthesize ECM proteins such collagen and fibronectin [38]. Collagen type I is the most prominent component of ECM in the lungs and pulmonary fibrosis as a result of enhanced collagen transcription is deemed a hallmark event in HPH [39]. We show here that MKL1 is both sufficient and necessary for hypoxia-induced collagen type I transactivation in smooth muscle cells (Fig. 5). Recently, two research groups have identified collagen type I as a direct transcriptional target for MKL1. Small et al propose that MKL1 is recruited to the collagen promoter by serum response factor (SRF) in cardiac fibroblast challenged with ischemia [9]. Luchsinger et al, in the meantime, suggest that Sp1 is responsible for bringing MKL1 to the collagen promoter to activate transcription in lung fibroblast [40]. Both SRF and Sp1 can be activated by hypoxia themselves and are known to mediate a range of cellular responses to hypoxia [41–43]. In light of our observation that MKL1 was up-regulated by hypoxia in the lungs (Fig. 1A, 1B), it is conceivable that a large transcriptional complex containing MKL1, SRF, and/or Sp1 could be assembled on the collagen promoter in response to hypoxia in smooth muscle cells. Alternatively, we have also observed that induction of TGF-β, a major pro-fibrogenic growth factor, was blunted in the absence of MKL1, suggesting that TGF-β might be a direct transcriptional target of MKL1. Of note, Parmacek and colleagues have recently discovered that MKL2, a closely related family member of MKL1, directly activates TGF-β transcription during vascular development [44]. Since TGF-β is responsible for the synthetic ability of smooth muscle cells, we propose that MKL1 may exert its pro-fibrogenic effect, at least in part, through activating TGF-β expression in the lungs. Still, another possibility is that the observed improvements of pulmonary function were a consequence of MKL1 blocking in the heart since Small et al have shown that MKL1 deficiency alleviates cardiac infarction [9]. In essence, systemic MKL1 expression on hemodynamics under chronic hypoxia cannot be excluded at this point. Tissue-specific deletion of MKL1 will likely shed more light on dissolving this issue in the future.

In conclusion, our data have suggested a potential role for MKL1 in the pathogenesis of HPH. In order for MKL1 to be targeted in the prevention and/or treatment of HPH, future research should scrutinize the role of MKL1 in more relevant animal models (e.g., Sugen-induced HPH) and probe the tissue-specific role of MKL1 in HPH.

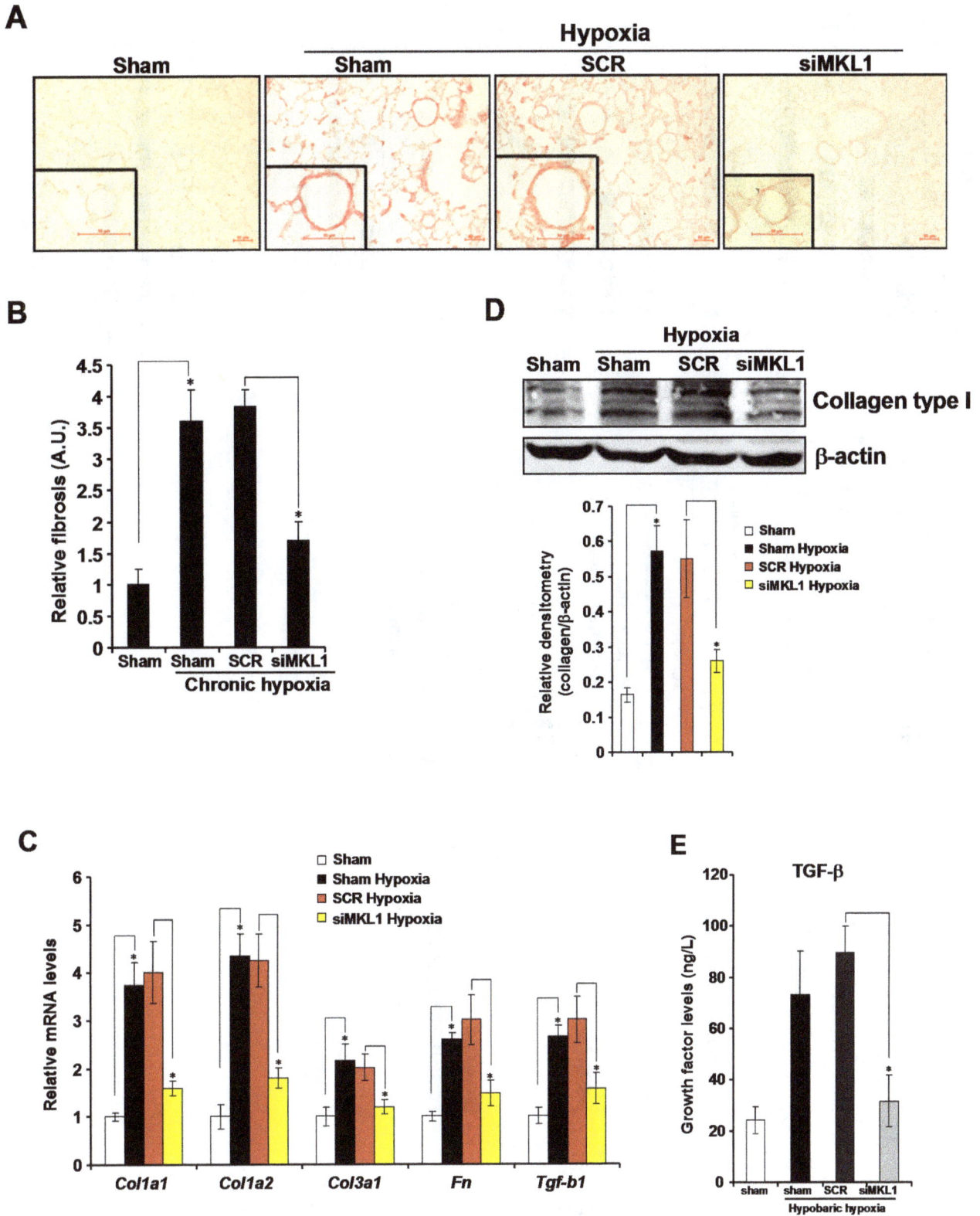

Figure 4. MKL1 silencing attenuates hypoxia-induced pulmonary fibrogenesis in rats. Sprague Dawley rats were injected with lentiviral particles carrying shRNA targeting MKL1 or random shRNA (SCR) and induced to develop HPH as described under *Methods*. (**A**) Picrosirius red staining was performed as described under *Methods*. (**B**) Positive staining was quantified by Image J and expressed as relative fibrosis compared to the control group. A. U., arbitrary unit (**C, D**) Expression of molecules involved in fibrogenesis in pulmonary arteries was measured by qPCR (C) and Western blotting (D). N = 5 rats for each group (**E**) Levels of TGF-β in pulmonary arteries were assessed by ELISA. N = 4 rats for each group.

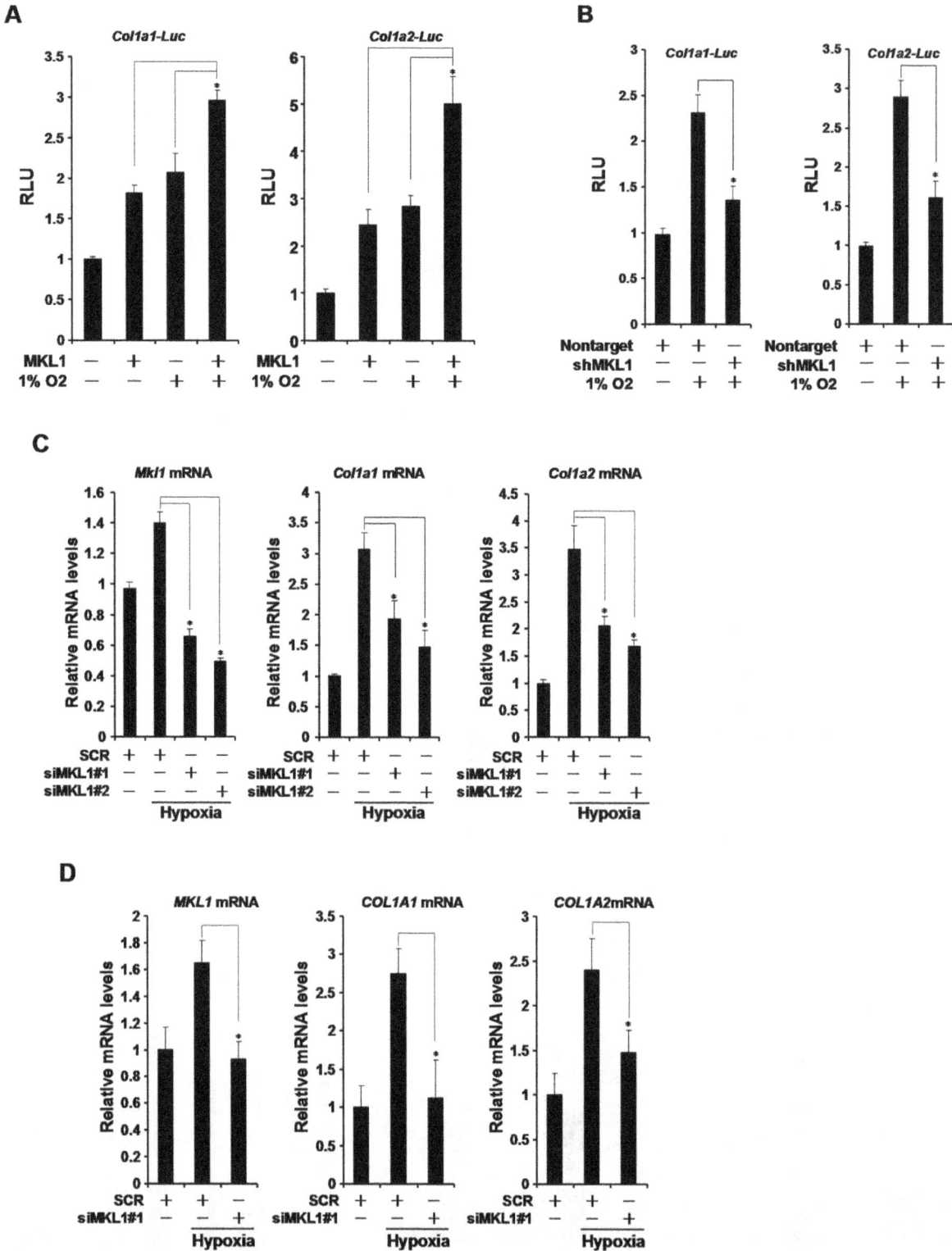

Figure 5. MKL1 regulates hypoxia-induced collagen transcription in smooth muscle cells. (**A**) Col1a1 or col1a2 promoter luciferase construct was transfected into A10 cells with MKL1 expression construct followed by exposure to 1% O_2 for 24 hours. Luciferase activities were expressed as relative luciferase unit (RLU). (**B**) Col1a1 or col1a2 promoter luciferase construct was transfected into A10 cells with shRNA plasmid targeting MKL1 or a control shRNA plasmid (nontarget) followed by exposure to 1% O_2 for 24 hours. Luciferase activities were expressed as RLU. (**C, D**) A10 (C) or primary human pulmonary arterial smooth muscle (D) cells were transfected with MKL1 specific or control siRNA (SCR) followed by exposure to 1% O_2 for 24 hours. Expression of collagen type I genes was measured by qPCR.

Supporting Information

Figure S1 (**A, B**) Sprague Dawley rats were injected with lentiviral particles carrying shRNA targeting MKL1 or random shRNA (SCR) and induced to develop HPH as described under *Methods*. MKL1 mRNA (A) and protein (B) levels in aortic arteries were assessed by qPCR and immunohistochemistry. N = 5 mice for each group (**C, D**) A10 cells (C) and HPASMCs (D) were exposed to 1% O_2 and harvested at indicated time points. mRNA and protein levels of MKL1 were measured by qPCR and Western.

Figure S2 (**A, B**) Sprague Dawley rats were injected with lentiviral particles carrying shRNA targeting MKL1 or random shRNA (SCR) and induced to develop HPH as described under *Methods*. Systemic blood pressure (A) and heart rate (B) were measured by using the PowerLab data acquisition system. N = 5 mice for each group (**C–E**) Sprague Dawley rats were injected with lentiviral particles carrying siMKL1 or SCR and maintained under normoxic conditions for 4 weeks. Pulmonary arterial pressure (C), systemic blood pressure (D), and heart rate (E) were recorded. N = 5 mice for each group

Table S1 Real-time quantitative PCR primers.

Acknowledgments

The authors wish to thank members of the Gao laboratory (Third Military Medical University) and the Xu laboratory (Nanjing Medical University) for technical assistance and helpful discussion during manuscript preparation. YX is a Fellow at the Collaborative Innovation Center for Cardiovascular Disease Translational Medicine.

Author Contributions

Conceived and designed the experiments: YX YQG ZBY JC GX DWC MJX. Performed the experiments: ZBY JC GX DWC MJX. Analyzed the data: ZBY JC GX DWC MJX. Wrote the paper: YX.

References

1. Stenmark KR, Fagan KA, Frid MG (2006) Hypoxia-induced pulmonary vascular remodeling: cellular and molecular mechanisms. Circ Res 99: 675–691.
2. Rabinovitch M (2008) Molecular pathogenesis of pulmonary arterial hypertension. J Clin Invest 118: 2372–2379.
3. Kubo K, Hanaoka M, Hayano T, Miyahara T, Hachiya T, et al. (1998) Inflammatory cytokines in BAL fluid and pulmonary hemodynamics in high-altitude pulmonary edema. Respiration Physiology 111: 301–310.
4. Tsai BM, Wang M, Pitcher JM, Meldrum KK, Meldrum DR (2004) Hypoxic pulmonary vasoconstriction and pulmonary artery tissue cytokine expression are mediated by protein kinase C. Am J Physiol Lung Cell Mol Physiol 287: L1215–1219.
5. Crouch EC, Parks WC, Rosenbaum JL, Chang D, Whitehouse L, et al. (1989) Regulation of collagen production by medial smooth muscle cells in hypoxic pulmonary hypertension. American Review of Respiratory Disease 140: 1045–1051.
6. Durmowicz AG, Parks WC, Hyde DM, Mecham RP, Stenmark KR (1994) Persistence, re-expression, and induction of pulmonary arterial fibronectin, tropoelastin, and type I procollagen mRNA expression in neonatal hypoxic pulmonary hypertension. Am J Pathol 145: 1411–1420.
7. Wang DZ, Li S, Hockemeyer D, Sutherland L, Wang Z, et al. (2002) Potentiation of serum response factor activity by a family of myocardin-related transcription factors. Proc Natl Acad Sci U S A 99: 14855–14860.
8. Cen B, Selvaraj A, Burgess RC, Hitzler JK, Ma Z, et al. (2003) Megakaryoblastic leukemia 1, a potent transcriptional coactivator for serum response factor (SRF), is required for serum induction of SRF target genes. Mol Cell Biol 23: 6597–6608.
9. Small EM, Thatcher JE, Sutherland LB, Kinoshita H, Gerard RD, et al. (2010) Myocardin-related transcription factor-a controls myofibroblast activation and fibrosis in response to myocardial infarction. Circ Res 107: 294–304.
10. Kuwahara K, Kinoshita H, Kuwabara Y, Nakagawa Y, Usami S, et al. (2010) Myocardin-related transcription factor A is a common mediator of mechanical stress- and neurohumoral stimulation-induced cardiac hypertrophic signaling leading to activation of brain natriuretic peptide gene expression. Mol Cell Biol 30: 4134–4148.
11. Fang F, Yang Y, Yuan Z, Gao Y, Zhou J, et al. (2011) Myocardin-related transcription factor A mediates OxLDL-induced endothelial injury. Circ Res 108: 797–807.
12. Xia J, Wu X, Yang Y, Zhao Y, Fang M, et al. (2012) SIRT1 deacetylates RFX5 and antagonizes repression of collagen type I (COL1A2) transcription in smooth muscle cells. Biochem Biophys Res Commun 428: 264–270.
13. Fang M, Kong X, Li P, Fang F, Wu X, et al. (2009) RFXB and its splice variant RFXBSV mediate the antagonism between IFNgamma and TGFbeta on COL1A2 transcription in vascular smooth muscle cells. Nucleic Acids Res 37: 4393–4406.
14. Lee SM, Vasishtha M, Prywes R (2010) Activation and repression of cellular immediate early genes by serum response factor cofactors. J Biol Chem 285: 22036–22049.
15. Ko EA, Song MY, Donthamsetty R, Makino A, Yuan JX (2010) Tension Measurement in Isolated Rat and Mouse Pulmonary Artery. Drug Discov Today Dis Models 7: 123–130.
16. Prie S, Leung TK, Cernacek P, Ryan JW, Dupuis J (1997) The orally active ET(A) receptor antagonist (+)-(S)-2-(4,6-dimethoxy-pyrimidin-2-yloxy)-3-methoxy-3,3-diphe nyl-propionic acid (LU 135252) prevents the development of pulmonary hypertension and endothelial metabolic dysfunction in monocrotaline-treated rats. J Pharmacol Exp Ther 282: 1312–1318.
17. Tian W, Xu H, Fang F, Chen Q, Xu Y, et al. (2012) Brahma related gene 1 (Brg1) bridges epigenetic regulation of pro-inflammatory cytokine production to steatohepatitis. Hepatology.
18. Kong X, Fang M, Fang F, Li P, Xu Y (2009) PPARgamma enhances IFNgamma-mediated transcription and rescues the TGFbeta antagonism by stimulating CIITA in vascular smooth muscle cells. J Mol Cell Cardiol 46: 748–757.
19. Kong X, Fang M, Li P, Fang F, Xu Y (2009) HDAC2 deacetylates class II transactivator and suppresses its activity in macrophages and smooth muscle cells. J Mol Cell Cardiol 46: 292–299.
20. Xu Y, Luchsinger L, Lucey EC, Smith BD (2011) The effect of class II transactivator mutations on bleomycin-induced lung inflammation and fibrosis. American Journal of Respiratory Cell and Molecular Biology 44: 898–905.
21. Zhao L, Mason NA, Morrell NW, Kojonazarov B, Sadykov A, et al. (2001) Sildenafil inhibits hypoxia-induced pulmonary hypertension. Circulation 104: 424–428.
22. Berkenbosch JW, Baribeau J, Perreault T (2000) Decreased synthesis and vasodilation to nitric oxide in piglets with hypoxia-induced pulmonary hypertension. Am J Physiol Lung Cell Mol Physiol 278: L276–283.
23. Vergadi E, Chang MS, Lee C, Liang OD, Liu X, et al. (2011) Early macrophage recruitment and alternative activation are critical for the later development of hypoxia-induced pulmonary hypertension. Circulation 123: 1986–1995.
24. Hanaoka M, Kubo K, Yamazaki Y, Miyahara T, Matsuzawa Y, et al. (1998) Association of high-altitude pulmonary edema with the major histocompatibility complex. Circulation 97: 1124–1128.
25. Steiner MK, Syrkina OL, Kolliputi N, Mark EJ, Hales CA, et al. (2009) Interleukin-6 overexpression induces pulmonary hypertension. Circ Res 104: 236–244, 228p following 244.
26. Chang SW (1994) TNF potentiates PAF-induced pulmonary vasoconstriction in the rat: role of neutrophils and thromboxane A2. J Appl Physiol 77: 2817–2826.
27. Stenmark KR, Davie NJ, Reeves JT, Frid MG (2005) Hypoxia, leukocytes, and the pulmonary circulation. J Appl Physiol 98: 715–721.
28. Poiani GJ, Wilson FJ, Fox JD, Sumka JM, Peng BW, et al. (1992) Liposome-entrapped antifibrotic agent prevents collagen accumulation in hypertensive pulmonary arteries of rats. Circ Res 70: 912–922.
29. Archer SL, Weir EK, Wilkins MR (2010) Basic science of pulmonary arterial hypertension for clinicians: new concepts and experimental therapies. Circulation 121: 2045–2066.
30. Chaouat A, Savale L, Chouaid C, Tu L, Sztrymf B, et al. (2009) Role for interleukin-6 in COPD-related pulmonary hypertension. Chest 136: 678–687.
31. Li M, Riddle SR, Frid MG, El Kasmi KC, McKinsey TA, et al. (2011) Emergence of fibroblasts with a proinflammatory epigenetically altered phenotype in severe hypoxic pulmonary hypertension. J Immunol 187: 2711–2722.
32. Oeckinghaus A, Hayden MS, Ghosh S (2011) Crosstalk in NF-kappaB signaling pathways. Nat Immunol 12: 695–708.
33. Ryan S, Taylor CT, McNicholas WT (2005) Selective activation of inflammatory pathways by intermittent hypoxia in obstructive sleep apnea syndrome. Circulation 112: 2660–2667.
34. BelAiba RS, Djordjevic T, Bonello S, Artunc F, Lang F, et al. (2006) The serum- and glucocorticoid-inducible kinase Sgk-1 is involved in pulmonary vascular remodeling: role in redox-sensitive regulation of tissue factor by thrombin. Circ Res 98: 828–836.

35. Raychaudhuri B, Dweik R, Connors MJ, Buhrow L, Malur A, et al. (1999) Nitric oxide blocks nuclear factor-kappaB activation in alveolar macrophages. American Journal of Respiratory Cell and Molecular Biology 21: 311–316.

36. Voraberger G, Schafer R, Stratowa C (1991) Cloning of the human gene for intercellular adhesion molecule 1 and analysis of its 5′-regulatory region. Induction by cytokines and phorbol ester. J Immunol 147: 2777–2786.

37. Cybulsky MI, Gimbrone MA, Jr. (1991) Endothelial expression of a mononuclear leukocyte adhesion molecule during atherogenesis. Science 251: 788–791.

38. Stenmark KR, Aldashev AA, Orton EC, Durmowicz AG, Badesch DB, et al. (1991) Cellular adaptation during chronic neonatal hypoxic pulmonary hypertension. Am J Physiol 261: 97–104.

39. Raiesdana A, Loscalzo J (2006) Pulmonary arterial hypertension. Annals of Medicine 38: 95–110.

40. Luchsinger LL, Patenaude CA, Smith BD, Layne MD (2011) Myocardin Related Transcription Factor-A Complexes Activate Type I Collagen Expression in Lung Fibroblasts. J Biol Chem.

41. Bell RD, Deane R, Chow N, Long X, Sagare A, et al. (2009) SRF and myocardin regulate LRP-mediated amyloid-beta clearance in brain vascular cells. Nat Cell Biol 11: 143–153.

42. Jeong JK, Park SY (2012) Transcriptional regulation of specific protein 1 (SP1) by hypoxia-inducible factor 1 alpha (HIF-1alpha) leads to PRNP expression and neuroprotection from toxic prion peptide. Biochem Biophys Res Commun 429: 93–98.

43. Koizume S, Ito S, Miyagi E, Hirahara F, Nakamura Y, et al. (2012) HIF2alpha-Sp1 interaction mediates a deacetylation-dependent FVII-gene activation under hypoxic conditions in ovarian cancer cells. Nucleic Acids Res 40: 5389–5401.

44. Li J, Bowens N, Cheng L, Zhu X, Chen M, et al. (2012) Myocardin-like protein 2 regulates TGFbeta signaling in embryonic stem cells and the developing vasculature. Development 139: 3531–3542.

12

Clinical Impact of Atrial Fibrillation in Patients with Pulmonary Hypertension

Dennis Rottlaender[1][*][◑], **Lukas J. Motloch**[1][◑], **Daniela Schmidt**[2], **Sara Reda**[1], **Robert Larbig**[1], **Martin Wolny**[3], **Daniel Dumitrescu**[2], **Stephan Rosenkranz**[2,3], **Erland Erdmann**[2], **Uta C. Hoppe**[1,2,3]

1 Department of Internal Medicine II, Paracelsus Medical University, Salzburg, Austria, 2 Department of Internal Medicine III, University of Cologne, Cologne, Germany, 3 Center of Molecular Medicine Cologne, University of Cologne, Cologne, Germany

Abstract

Background: Pulmonary hypertension (PH) is associated with progressive impairment of right ventricular function, reduced exercise capacity and a poor prognosis. Little is known about the prevalence, clinical manifestation and impact of atrial fibrillation (AF) on cardiac function in PH.

Methods: In a four year single-centre retrospective analysis 225 patients with confirmed PH of various origins were enrolled to investigate the prevalence of AF, and to assess the clinical manifestation, 6-minute walk distance, NT-proBNP levels, echocardiographic parameters and hemodynamics obtained by right heart catheterization in PH with AF.

Results: AF was prevalent in 31.1%. In patients with PH and AF, parameters of clinical deterioration (NYHA/WHO functional class, 6-minute walk distance, NT-proBNP levels) and renal function were significantly compromised compared to patients with PH and sinus rhythm (SR). In the total PH cohort and in PH not related to left heart disease occurrence of AF was associated with an increase of right atrial pressure (RAP) and right atrial dilatation. While no direct association was found between pulmonary artery pressure (PAP) and AF in these patients, right ventricular function was reduced in AF, indicating more advanced disease. In PH due to left heart failure the prevalence of AF was particularly high (57.7% vs. 23.1% in other forms of PH). In this subgroup, left atrial dilatation, increase of pulmonary capillary wedge pressure, PAP and RAP were more pronounced in AF than in SR, suggesting that more marked backward failure led to AF in this setting.

Conclusion: PH is associated with increased prevalence of AF. Occurrence of AF in PH indicates clinical deterioration and more advanced disease.

Editor: Denice Hodgson-Zingman, University of Iowa Carver College of Medicine, United States of America

Funding: The authors have no support or funding to report.

Competing Interests: The authors have declared that no competing interests exist.

* E-mail: dennis.rottlaender@uk-koeln.de

◑ These authors contributed equally to this work.

Introduction

Pulmonary hypertension (PH) – i.e. an elevated mean pulmonary artery pressure (PAP), ≥ 25 mmHg at rest – defines a group of diseases characterized by a progressive increase in pulmonary vascular resistance leading to right ventricular failure and premature death [1,2,3]. Based on the pathophysiological mechanisms and etiology, the current clinical classification distinguishes five groups of PH [4]. Left heart failure (HF) is one common cause of PH, representing group 2 of the Dana-Point classification. Left ventricular systolic dysfunction, diastolic dysfunction or valvular disease may all result in elevated PAP. In fact, PH is being found in more than 60% of patients with moderate or severe HF [5]. However, from a pathophysiological point of view and with regard to therapeutic options, PH due to left heart disease is clearly differentiated from pulmonary arterial hypertension (PAH) and has to be appreciated as a separate entity. At present, targeted PAH therapies are not recommended for this subgroup.

Atrial fibrillation (AF) is the most common chronic arrhythmia. Chronic left heart failure and AF often coexist. Both are responsible for increased mortality, more frequent hospitalizations, reduced exercise capacity, decreased quality of life and substantial health care expenditures [6]. In addition to merely having risk factors in common, AF and heart failure are believed to directly predispose to each other [7,8]. The risk of developing AF during long-term follow-up appears to be 5 to 10 times higher in patients with left heart failure than in healthy persons [9,10,11,12]. Some studies have shown that the onset of AF in these patients is associated with clinical and hemodynamic deterioration due to loss of atrial contractility, tachycardia, and lack of atrioventricular synchrony, as well as a worse long-term prognosis [13,14].

Although the association between AF and left heart failure is well documented, the predisposing factors for developing AF in this setting are not fully understood. Moreover, the prevalence of AF in PH with or without compromised right ventricular function has not been defined. Learning more about which types of patients with PH develop AF may yield important insights into the

Table 1. Patients' Characteristics.

Characteristic	PH-SR (n = 155) n	% or Mean ± SEM	PH-AF (n = 70) n	% or Mean ± SEM
Age	155	62.9±1.2	70	71.2±1.1
Male	58	37.4%	25	35.7%
Female	97	62.6%	45	64.3%
Mean heart rate (bpm)	155	79.5±1.3	70	74.6±1.9
**WHO group	PH subgroup**				
Pulmonary arterial hypertension	78	50.3%	32	45.7%
Idiopathic	31	20.0%	24	34.3%*
Heritable	2	1.3%	0	0%
Drug- and toxin-induced	4	2.6%	0	0%
Associated with				
Congenital heart disease	6	3.9%	3	4.3%
HIV infection	3	1.9%	0	0%
Connective tissue disease	32	20.6%	3	4.3%*
Portal hypertension	0	0%	2	2.9%
Veno-occlusive disease	0	0%	0	0%
Pulmonary hypertension due to left heart failure	22	14.2%	30	42.9%*
Systolic dysfunction	6	3.9%	10	14.3%*
Diastolic dysfunction	13	8.4%	17	24.3%*
Valvular disease	3	1.9%	3	4.3%
Pulmonary hypertension due to pulmonary disease	21	13.5%	5	7.1%
Chronic obstructive pulmonary disease	7	4.5%	3	4.3%
Interstitial lung disease	14	9.0%	2	2.9%
Chronic thromboembolic pulmonary hypertension	31	20.0%	2	2.9%*
Others	3	1.9%	1	1.4%
Medication				
Phosphodiesterase-5-inhibitor	51	32.9%	31	44.3%
Endothelin-1 antagonist	47	30.3%	15	21.4%
Prostacyclin	7	4.5%	3	4.3%
Calcium channel blockers	29	18.7%	17	24.3%
Betablocker	65	41.9%	51	72.9%*
Digitalis	8	5.2%	26	37.1%*
Amiodarone	1	0.6%	7	10.0%*
Sotalol	2	1.3%	1	1.4%
Diuretics	112	72.3%	65	92.9%*
Angiotensin receptor blockers/AT-1 antagonist	82	52.9%	42	60.0%
Cumarine	61	39.4%	55	78.6%*
Acetylsalicylic acid	49	31.6%	11	15.7%*
Clopidogrel	10	6.5%	4	5.7%
Statins	41	26.5%	27	38.6%
Nitrates	11	7.1%	3	4.3%
Concomitant disease				
Coronary artery disease	39	25.2%	19	27.1%
Myocardial infarction	9	5.8%	8	11.4%
Coronary artery bypass graft	5	3.2%	7	10.0%
Dilated cardiomyopathy	3	1.9%	7	10.0%*
Valvular disease	14	9.0%	20	28.6%*
Arterial hypertension	75	48.4%	45	64.3%*

Table 1. Cont.

Characteristic	PH-SR (n = 155)		PH-AF (n = 70)	
	n	% or Mean ± SEM	n	% or Mean ± SEM
Pulmonary disease	97	62.6%	27	38.6%*

*p<0.05 vs. PH-SR.

pathogenesis of AF in this condition, and importantly may help guide clinicians in the monitoring, evaluation, and management of these patients.

Methods

Study participants

The study was performed according to good clinical practice and in compliance with the Helsinki declaration. Individual patient were not identified. An individual written consent was obtained by every patient, which is usually performed due to quality management issues in our hospital. The study and study design was approved by the institutional review board. The study cohort comprised 225 consecutive patients with confirmed diagnosis of PH referred to a single-centre between October 01, 2006 and March 31, 2010. In all eligible patients, exact classification of PH into one of the five groups according to the Dana-Point classification was performed [4], and information about the clinical severity (NYHA/WHO functional class), medication, concomitant diseases, 6-minute walk distance and N-terminal pro-brain natriuretic peptide (NT-proBNP) levels were obtained from the University Patient Database. Furthermore, if available, echocardiography was analyzed. Patients were divided into two groups: 1. patients with PH and sinus rhythm (PH-SR) and 2. patients with PH and atrial fibrillation (PH-AF). Given distinct cardiac pathomechanisms, subgroup analysis was performed in patients with PH due to left heart failure (a. PH-HF SR and b. PH-HF AF) and PH due to any other cause (c. PH-nonHF SR and d. PH-nonHF AF).

Definition of prevalent AF

"Prevalent AF" was defined as the presence of AF on electrocardiogram during the index hospitalization and/or as indicated by a diagnosis found in medical records, the hospitalization database, or ambulatory visit databases. "Electrocardiographic AF" was defined as the presence of an irregular rhythm with fibrillatory waves and no defined P-waves [9]. Diagnoses were based on physician-assigned diagnoses in the medical records and/or the presence of corresponding ICD-9-CM codes for AF (427.31) in the hospital discharge or ambulatory visit clinical databases. Atrial fibrillation was sub-classified into paroxysmal AF or chronic AF (persistent or permanent) according to international guidelines.

Etiology and severity of PH

Patients were classified according to the Dana Point classification of PH, and clinical severity was assessed according to the WHO functional classes for PH [4]. In PH due to left heart failure with reduced ejection fraction, left ventricular ejection fraction was defined as lower than 40% (as assessed by echocardiography, biplane Simpson method in apical four chamber view). Heart failure with preserved ejection fraction was diagnosed following the consensus statement of the Association of the European

Society of Cardiology [15]. Valvular disease was defined as mitral and/or aortic stenosis or insufficiency or valve repair.

Six-minute walk testing

Patients were instructed to walk down a 100-foot corridor at their own pace, attempting to cover as much ground as possible. At the end of the six minute interval the total distance was determined. The test was performed by personnel that had been trained according to the current ATS consensus statement on six-minute walk testing [16]. Forty-two patients were excluded from testing due to disability of movement.

Clinical laboratory parameters

N-terminal pro-brain natriuretic peptide (NT-proBNP) was measured in every patient as a marker of heart failure known to correlate with survival and the severity of disease in both left and right heart failure. Additionally, renal function parameters, i.e. creatinine, urea nitrogen and estimated glomerular filtration rate (eGFR, using the MDRD equation [17]) were determined.

Echocardiography

All transthoracic echocardiographic studies were obtained by experienced investigators using a Philips iE 33 echocardiography system (Philips, Hamburg, Germany). Left atrial diameter (edge-to-edge method, parasternal view), right atrial area (measured at end-systole in the apical four chamber view), left ventricular ejection fraction (biplane Simpson method), Tricuspid Annular Plane Systolic Excursion (TAPSE) and pulmonary artery systolic pressure were recorded according to current recommendations [18]. Only complete datasets were included in the statistical analysis.

Right heart catheterization

Right heart catheterization was performed via the femoral vein using a balloon flotation catheter (PWP catheter, Medtronic, Minneapolis, USA). Fluoroscopic guidance was used to cannulate the pulmonary artery and obtain pulmonary capillary wedge position. Right heart catheterization studies were analyzed for systolic and mean pulmonary arterial pressure, pulmonary capillary wedge pressure (PCWP), right atrial pressure and pulmonary vascular resistance. Cardiac output was estimated using the Fick technique. Echocardiograms and right heart catheterization were performed at the same time.

Statistical analysis

Statistical analyses were performed using PASW statistics 18 software (SPSS, Chicago, USA). All variables were tested for normal distribution with the Kolmogorov-Smirnov test. The results are given as mean ± standard error of mean (SEM). All groups and subgroups were compared for PH classification, clinical manifestation, 6-minute-walk-testing, laboratory parameters, data of echocardiography and right heart catheterization.

Table 2. Effect of AF on NYHA class and renal function in PH.

NYHA classification	PH-SR n	PH-SR %	PH-AF n	PH-AF %
NYHA I	2	1.3%	0	0%[#]
NYHA II	52	33.5%	17	24.3%[#]
NYHA III	98	63.2%	51	72.9%[#]
NYHA IV	3	1.9%	2	2.9%[#]
Renal function				
CKD class I	31	20.0%	3	4.3%[#]
CKD class II	62	40.0%	23	32.9%[#]
CKD class III	55	35.5%	35	50.0%[#]
CKD class IV	6	3.9%	8	11.4%[#]
CKD class V	1	0.6%	1	1.4%[#]

CKD = Chronic kidney disease classification.
#p<0.05 vs. PH-SR.

Differences between groups and subgroups were evaluated by chi-square-testing for discrete variables and student-t test for continuous variables. For ordinal data Mann-Whitney-U test was used. A p<0.05 was considered as statistically significant.

Results

Baseline characteristics and prevalence of AF

A total of 225 patients with PH were analyzed in this retrospective study. Seventy patients (31.1%) of the total study cohort had evidence of AF. In patients with AF, 41.3% had paroxysmal AF, whereas 58.7% presented with chronic AF. The demographic variables of the individual groups with and without AF are shown in table 1. Patients in both groups were predominantly female. Mean age did not differ significantly between the PH-SR and PH-AF group.

When evaluating the relative percentage of the distinct etiologies of PH according to the Dana Point classification in the PH-AF group versus PH-SR group, we obtained no significant difference for PH due to pulmonary disease. However, PH due to left heart failure (PH-HF) was markedly more common in the PH-AF group (PH-AF 42.9% vs. PH-SR 14.2%, p<0.05). This observation was consistent for all causes of left heart failure, though for valvular disease the difference did not reach statistical significance most likely due to the limited number of patients in this subgroup (table 1). Notably, 57.7% of all patients with PH-HF presented with AF, compared to 23.1% in the PH-nonHF group. Conversely, the relative percentage of chronic thromboembolic pulmonary hypertension (CTEPH) was higher in the PH population with SR (PH-SR 20.0% vs. PH-AF 2.9%, p<0.05). While we observed a similar percentage of pulmonary arterial hypertension (PAH) per se in the PH-AF and PH-SR group (45.7% vs. 50.3%, n.s.), idiopathic PAH was more frequent in those with AF (PH-AF 34.3% vs. PH-SR 20.0%, p<0.05), reflecting an AF prevalence of 43.6% in this subpopulation.

A comparison of patients with paroxysmal (PH-AF paroxysmal) and chronic (PH-AF chronic) AF in PH revealed chronic AF to be associate with PH due to pulmonary disease (PH-AF paroxysmal 0% vs. PH-AF chronic 11.9%, p<0.05). Moreover, PH due to systolic dysfunction was associated with chronic AF, while diastolic dysfunction was related to paroxysmal AF (systolic dysfunction:

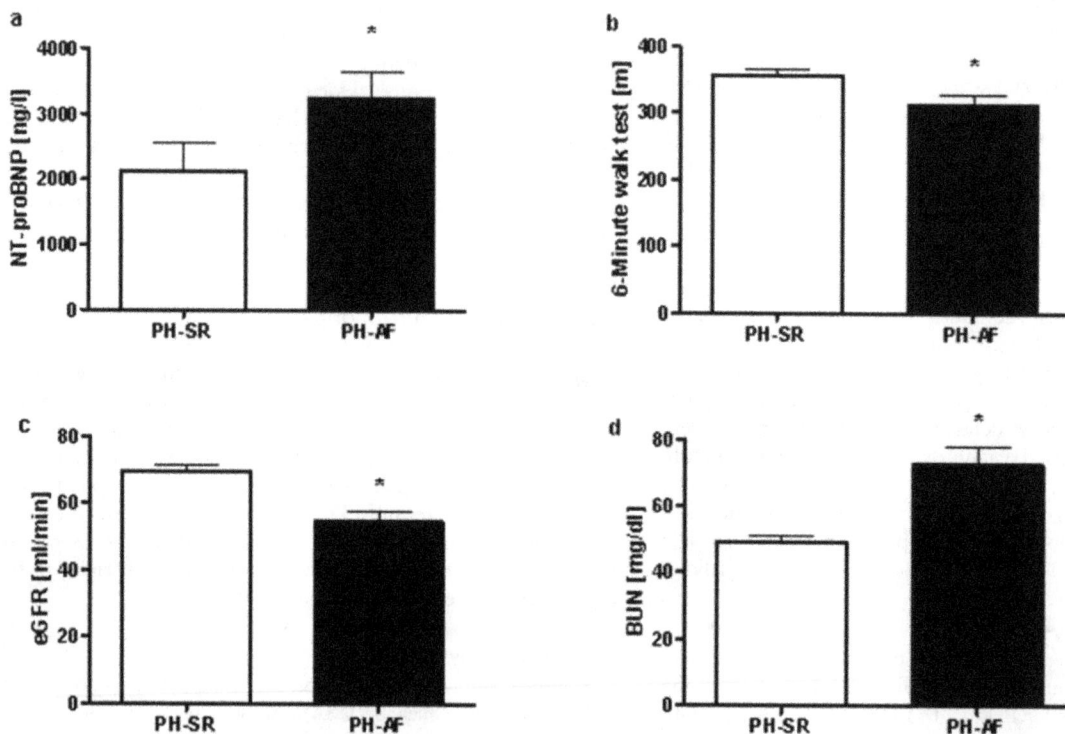

Figure 1. Laboratory parameters and exercise capacity in PH with and without AF. NT-pro-BNP, estimated glomerular filtration rate (eGFR), urea nitrogen (BUN) and 6-minute walk distance of patients with PH were compared in those with AF (PH-AF) and SR (PH-SR). * p<0.05. Error bars representing standard error of mean.

Table 3. Effect of AF on hemodynamic parameters in PH.

Echocardiography	n (PH-SR)	Mean ± SEM (PH-SR)	n (PH-AF)	Mean ± SEM (PH-AF)
Left atrial diameter [mm]	154	37.09±0.64	69	46.16±1.28*
Right atrial area [mm²]	154	23.15±0.62	69	28.59±1.19*
TAPSE [mm]	154	20.97±0.48	69	18.07±0.68*
Systolic pulmonary artery pressure [mmHg]	154	64.59±1.82	69	60.10±2.18
Left ventricular ejection fraction [%]	154	63.81±0.55	69	59.84±1.52*
Right heart catheterization				
Systolic pulmonary artery pressure [mmHg]	155	65.00±1.86	70	67.51±2.34
Mean pulmonary artery pressure [mmHg]	155	40.25±1.12	70	40.80±1.56
Mean right atrial pressure [mmHg]	135	9.4±0.43	61	12.85±0.86*
PCWP [mmHg]	155	11.96±0.38	70	16.50±0.90*
Pulmonary vascular resistance [Wood units]	146	7.29±0.42	66	6.45±0.54
Cardiac output [l/min]	127	4.36±0.12	47	3.91±0.16*

*$p < 0.05$ vs. PH-SR.

PH-AF paroxysmal 3.6% vs. PH-AF chronic 21.4%, $p < 0.05$; diastolic dysfunction: PH-AF paroxysmal 32.1% vs. PH-AF chronic 19.0%, $p < 0.05$).

Targeted therapy for PAH such as prostacyclin analogues, endothelin receptor antagonists and phosphodiesterase-5 inhibitors were equally prescribed in PAH patients with and without AF. Expectedly, treatment for AF, i.e. betablockers, digitalis, amiodarone and cumarine was more common in the PH-AF group. Notably, patients with PH-AF more often received diuretics indicating more advanced heart failure.

Clinical presentation of patients with AF in PH

Thus far, clinical manifestation of AF in PH has not been analyzed systematically. Therefore, we evaluated functional class, exercise capacity, and laboratory parameters indicative of hemodynamic status in this population. The clinical condition in patients with AF in PH was more severe than in patients without AF, as indicated by the NYHA/WHO functional class (table 2). Consistently, the 6-minute walk distance was significantly shorter in the PH-AF group (PH-SR vs. PH-AF: 355.55±9.86 m, n = 130 vs. 321.98±14.1 m, n = 53; $p < 0.05$, figure 1). Moreover, in patients with AF, the elevation of NT-proBNP serum levels was more pronounced (PH-SR vs. PH-AF: 2128.88±429.97 ng/l, n = 155 vs. 3252.79±401.76 ng/l, n = 70; $p < 0.05$, figure 1).

Given that renal failure was shown to correlate with reduced survival and clinical deterioration, standard parameters of renal function (creatinine, urea nitrogen, eGFR) and chronic renal failure classification were analyzed. As shown in figure 1, AF was associated with impaired renal function, reflected by a significant

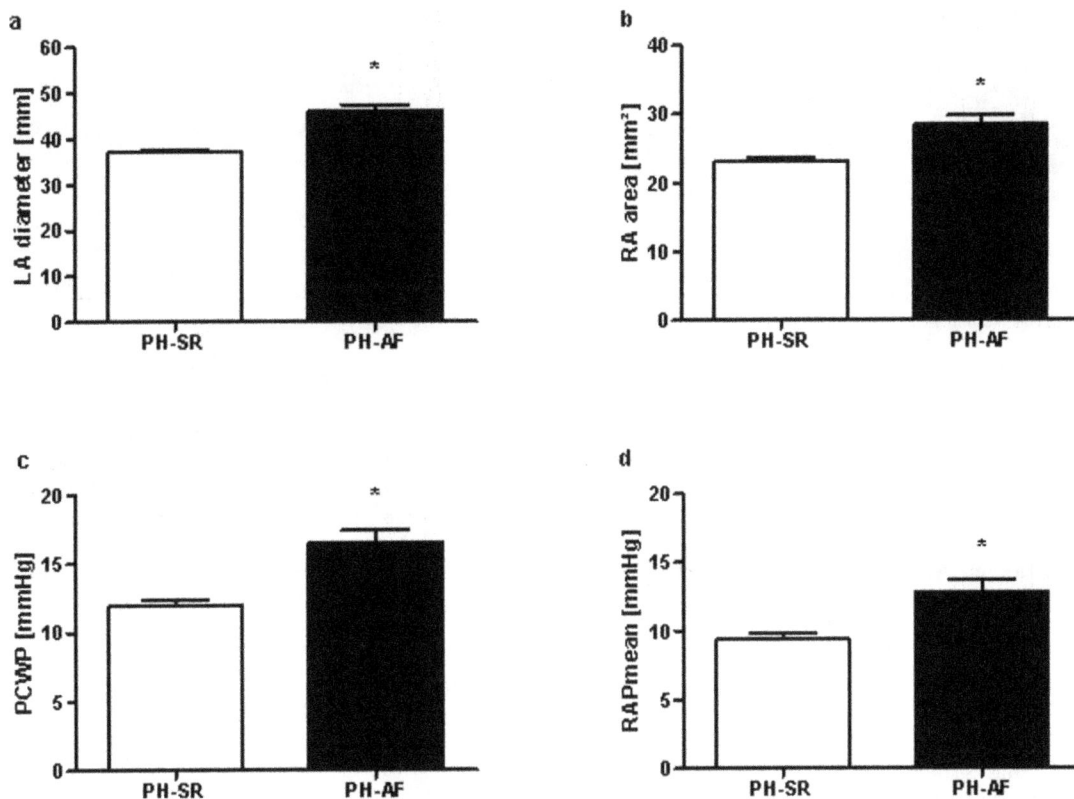

Figure 2. Hemodynamic parameters associated with AF in PH. Left atrial (LA) diameter and right atrial (RA) area were measured by echocardiography in PH-AF compared to PH-SR. PCWP and mean right atrial pressure (RAPmean) were obtained by right heart catheterization in the presence (PH-AF) or absence (PH-SR) of AF in patients with PH. * $p < 0.05$.

Table 4. Comparison of subgroups with SR vs. AF in PH not related to left heart disease (nonHF).

	PH-SR nonHF		PH-AF nonHF	
Echocardiography	n	% or Mean ± SEM	n	% or Mean ± SEM
Left atrial diameter [mm]	132	37.05±0.68	39	43.31±1.55*
Right atrial area [mm^2]	132	23.53±0.66	38	30.51±1.61*
TAPSE [mm]	132	20.74±0.52	38	18.35±0.87*
Systolic pulmonary artery pressure [mmHg]	132	66.67±1.98	39	65.72±3.15
Left ventricular ejection fraction [%]	132	64.52±0.43	40	64.30±1.16
Right heart catheterization				
Systolic pulmonary artery pressure [mmHg]	133	67.02±2.04	40	68.25±3.24
Mean pulmonary artery pressure [mmHg]	133	41.25±1.23	40	40.38±2.04
Mean right atrial pressure [mmHg]	115	8.93±0.45	36	11.03±0.63*
PCWP [mmHg]	133	10.86±0.30	40	12.35±0.63
Pulmonary vascular resistance [Wood units]	126	7.74±0.46	38	7.16±0.75
Cardiac output [l/min]	111	4.36±0.13	25	3.94±0.19
Laboratory parameters				
NT-proBNP [pg/l]	133	1738.86±212.05	40	3449.40±547.61*
Creatinine [mg/dl]	133	1.06±0.03	40	1.23±0.08*
Urea nitrogen [mg/dl]	133	48.23±2.10	40	64.40±5.39*
eGFR [ml/min//1.72 m^2]	133	70.78±2.34	40	58.18±3.51*
NYHA classification				
NYHA I	1	0.8%	0	0%#
NYHA II	51	38.3%	8	20.0%#
NYHA III	78	58.6%	31	77.5%#
NYHA IV	3	2.3%	1	2.5%#
6-minute walk test				
6-minute walk test [m]	113	364.67±10.51	31	303.87±17.36*
Renal function				
CKD class I	28	21.1%	2	5.0%#
CKD class II	56	42.1%	15	37.5%#
CKD class III	43	32.3%	20	50.0%#
CKD class IV	6	4.5%	3	7.5%#
CKD class V	0	0%	0	0%#

CKD = Chronic kidney disease classification, eGFR = estimated glomerular filtration rate.
*$p<0.05$ vs. PH-SR (student t-test).
#$p<0.05$ vs. PH-SR (Mann-Whitney test).

increase of creatinine and urea nitrogen in patients suffering from AF compared to those without AF (PH-SR vs. PH-AF: 1.07±0.03 mg/dl, n = 154 vs. 1.37±0.11 mg/dl, n = 73; 49.17±1.97 mg/dl, n = 154 vs. 72.61±5.44 mg/dl, n = 69; $p<0.05$), and a reduced eGFR (PH-SR vs. PH-AF: 69.68±2.11 ml/min, n = 154 vs. 54.96±2.65 ml/min, n = 69; $p<0.05$). Accordingly, patients with AF in PH were found to be in more severe stages of chronic renal failure (table 2).

Hemodynamic parameters in PH with AF

Cardiac function and hemodynamic data were evaluated by echocardiography and right heart catheterization (table 3). Expectedly, left atrial diameter was significantly larger, pulmonary capillary wedge pressure (PCWP) was higher (figure 2, table 3), and left ventricular ejection fraction was reduced in the PH-AF group, reflecting the marked fraction of PH due to left heart disease.

Notably, systolic and mean pulmonary artery pressures showed no differences in the PH-AF compared to the PH-SR group,

implicating that pulmonary artery pressure per se has no direct effect on the occurrence of AF or vice versa. However, we obtained a significant increase of the right atrial area and mean right atrial pressure in PH with versus without AF (figure 2, table 3). Moreover, right ventricular function assessed by TAPSE was significantly reduced in PH-AF. Consistently, cardiac output was lower in the PH-AF group compared to the PH-SR group (table 3).

A comparison of patients with paroxysmal (PH-AF paroxysmal) and chronic (PH-AF chronic) AF in PH indicated increased right atrial area and mean right atrial pressure in patients with chronic AF versus paroxysmal AF (PH-AF paroxysmal 25.04±1.46 mm^2 and 10.69±0.98 mmHg vs. PH-AF chronic 30.93±1.36 mm^2 and 14.91±1.03 mmHg, $p<0.05$).

AF in PH not related to left heart disease

Given the distinct pathopyhsiology of pre- versus postcapillary PH, in a subanalysis patients with PH due to left heart disease (PH-HF, group 2) were separated from patients with PH due to any

Table 5. Comparison of subgroups with SR vs. AF in PAH.

	PAH-SR		PAH-AF	
Echocardiography	n	% or Mean ± SEM	n	% or Mean ± SEM
Left atrial diameter [mm]	77	37.04±0.81	31	43.61±1.53*
Right atrial area [mm²]	77	22.92±0.87	31	31.33±1.49*
TAPSE [mm]	77	20.99±0.65	31	17.74±0.94*
Systolic pulmonary artery pressure [mmHg]	77	62.83±2.62	31	66.58±3.38
Left ventricular ejection fraction [%]	77	64.49±0.49	32	64.06±1.40
Right heart catheterization				
Systolic pulmonary artery pressure [mmHg]	78	65.27±2.31	32	70.03±3.83
Mean pulmonary artery pressure [mmHg]	78	41.22±1.73	32	41.47±2.45
Mean right atrial pressure [mmHg]	66	8.90±0.49	32	11.43±0.65*
PCWP [mmHg]	78	10.53±0.38	32	12.84±0.63
Pulmonary vascular resistance [Wood units]	74	7.49±0.60	32	7.58±0.87
Cardiac output [l/min]	66	4.41±0.19	21	3.98±0.26
Laboratory parameters				
NT-proBNP [pg/l]	78	1705.81±232.49	32	3529.84±537.77*
Creatinine [mg/dl]	78	1.06±0.04	32	1.38±0.09*
Urea nitrogen [mg/dl]	78	45.98±2.38	32	68.19±4.55*
eGFR [ml/min//1.72 m²]	78	73.76±3.47	32	59.09±3.09*
NYHA classification				
NYHA I	1	1.3%	0	0%#
NYHA II	35	44.9%	7	21.9%#
NYHA III	41	52.6%	24	75.0%#
NYHA IV	1	1.3%	1	3.1%#
6-minute walk test				
6-minute walk test [m]	66	384.21±11.67	26	311.35±18.04*
Renal function				
CKD class I	20	25.6%	2	6.3%#
CKD class II	30	38.5%	13	40.6%#
CKD class III	24	30.8%	15	46.9%#
CKD class IV	4	5.1%	2	6.3%#
CKD class V	0	0%	0	0%#

CKD = Chronic kidney disease classification, eGFR = estimated glomerular filtration rate.
*$p<0.05$ vs. PAH-SR (student t-test).
#$p<0.05$ vs. PAH-SR (Mann-Whitney test).

other cause (PH-nonHF, groups 1, 3, 4, or 5). In PH not related to left heart disease, AF was observed in 23.1% (table 4). In PAH (group 1) AF was found in 29.1% (table 5). AF was associated with clinical deterioration, as indicated by a higher NYHA/WHO functional class, shorter 6-minute walk distance, more severely elevated NT-proBNP serum levels and compromised renal function compared to patients in SR (table 4, table 5).

While consistent with the total PH cohort, no difference of systolic and mean pulmonary arterial pressures in the presence or absence of AF was obtained; increased right atrial pressure and size as well as reduced right ventricular function were the most obvious hemodynamic differences between prevalent AF versus no AF in PH-nonHF and PAH. As expected, left ventricular ejection fraction and PCWP were similar in both groups (table 4, table 5).

AF in left heart disease with PH

In patients with PH due to left heart disease, AF was prevalent in 57.7%. While AF in this cohort did not further diminish exercise capacity or NYHA/WHO functional class, we still observed higher NT-proBNP values and more severely compromised renal function in those patients with AF versus SR (table 6).

Left atrial size was significantly larger and PCWP tended to be higher in prevalent AF, although the latter did not reach statistical significance. Invasive measurements demonstrated increased systolic and mean pulmonary arterial and right atrial pressures associated with AF. Moreover, echocardiography indicated right heart impairment, i.e. increased right atrial area and suppressed TAPSE in the subgroup with prevalent AF (table 6).

Discussion

Atrial fibrillation affects 1–2% of the general population. The prevalence of AF increases with age, from 0.5% at 40–50 years, to 5–15% at 80 years [19]. Atrial fibrillation is highly prevalent among patients with left ventricular heart failure, and can lead to adverse consequences, including tachycardia-related cardiomyop-

Table 6. Comparison of subgroups with SR vs. AF in PH related to left heart disease (HF).

	PH-SR HF		PH-AF HF	
Echocardiography	n	% or Mean ± SEM	n	% or Mean ± SEM
Left atrial diameter [mm]	22	37.36±1.89	30	49.87±1.96*
Right atrial area [mm²]	22	20.87±1.65	30	26.17±1.69*
TAPSE [mm]	22	22.32±1.25	29	17.45±0.94*
Systolic pulmonary artery pressure [mmHg]	22	52.14±3.75	30	52.80±2.34
Left ventricular ejection fraction [%]	22	59.55±2.69	29	53.69±2.90
Right heart catheterization				
Systolic pulmonary artery pressure [mmHg]	22	52.86±3.29	30	64.10±3.36*
Mean pulmonary artery pressure [mmHg]	22	34.23±2.01	30	41.37±2.46*
Mean right atrial pressure [mmHg]	20	12.10±1.16	25	16.92±1.37*
PCWP [mmHg]	22	18.63±1.21	30	22.13±1.37
Pulmonary vascular resistance [Wood units]	20	4.48±0.77	28	5.50±0.77
Cardiac output [l/min]	16	4.33±0.26	22	3.89±0.28
Laboratory parameters				
NT-proBNP [pg/l]	22	1149.00±181.61	30	3257.30±568.65*
Creatinine [mg/dl]	21	1.11±0.06	29	1.58±0.25*
Urea nitrogen [mg/dl]	21	55.10±5.60	29	83.93±10.35*
eGFR [ml/min//1.72 m²]	21	62.71±4.27	29	50.52±3.97*
NYHA classification				
NYHA I	2	9.1%	0	0.0%
NYHA II	4	18.2%	11	36.7%
NYHA III	16	72.7%	19	63.3%
NYHA IV	0	0%	0	0%
6-minute walk test				
6-minute walk test [m]	17	294.88±24.29	22	333.41±23.99
Renal function				
CKD class I	3	13.6%	1	3.3%#
CKD class II	8	36.4%	8	26.7%#
CKD class III	10	45.5%	15	50.0%#
CKD class IV	0	0%	5	16.7%#
CKD class V	1	4.5%	1	3.3%#

CKD = Chronic kidney disease classification, eGFR = estimated glomerular filtration rate.
*p<0.05 vs. PH-SR (student t-test).
#p<0.05 vs. PH-SR (Mann-Whitney test).

athy, reduction in left ventricular preload attributable to disorganized atrial contractions, increased risk of systemic embolism, and overall poorer long-term outcome [20,21,22]. Supraventricular tachyarrhythmias occurred in patients with pulmonary hypertension with an annual incidence of 2.8%. Atrial flutter and atrial fibrillation were equally common and both arrhythmias led to acute clinical deterioration with signs of right heart failure, while only atrial fibrillation exerted an impact on mortality [23]. However, little is known about the total prevalence of AF in patients with PH and possible differences among distinct etiological groups of PH have not been defined. In the present cohort of patients with confirmed PH of various origins, we found that AF affected approximately one-third of patients. Thus, the prevalence of AF in PH is considerably higher than in the normal population at similar age [24]. This was also true for all PH subgroups except for patients with chronic thromboembolic pulmonary hypertension (CTEPH).

Particularly, more than half of the patients with PH related to left heart disease were affected by AF. Symptomatic heart failure has been reported in 30% of AF patients and AF is found in up to 30% of heart failure patients, depending on the underlying cause and severity of heart failure [9,19]. Pulmonary hypertension in heart failure is associated with a poor prognosis and an increased severity of disease [5]. Compared to the cited populations mentioned above we observed a significantly higher prevalence of AF in patients with left heart disease combined with PH (57.7%), supporting the notion that our patients suffered from more severe heart failure, which was also indicated by the high prevalence of patients with NYHA III and markedly elevated NT-proBNP levels. Moreover, these data suggest that more advanced heart failure leading to PH is a relevant risk factor for the development of AF. Given the retrospective design of our study, we may even have underestimated the true prevalence of AF in PH. Diagnosis of AF was made by carefully analyzing patient's history and standard electrocardiograms. Because of the lack of other means of rhythm monitoring (i.e. periodical Holter recordings, implanted event recorders), it is likely that some self-limiting silent AF episodes might have been missed.

When analyzing hemodynamic factors promoting AF in PH it seems plausible to separately evaluate patients with and without left heart disease. Previously, reduced left ventricular function, elevated end-diastolic left ventricular pressure and, thus, higher PCWP and larger left atrial diameter have been associated with an increased propensity of AF in left heart disease. Consistently, in the present study these parameters were more severely altered in prevalent AF than in patients with SR. Notably, in PH-HF with AF we observed increased pulmonary artery pressures in invasive measurements, which are more accurate than echocardiographic estimation [25], and signs of right heart impairment, indicating that AF in PH related to left heart disease was associated with more marked backward failure compared to SR.

Thus far, hemodynamic factors that might contribute to onset of AF in PH not related to left heart disease have not been evaluated. In the present analysis, elevated right atrial pressure and right atrial dilatation were the most prominent parameters associated with prevalent AF in PH-nonHF. While systolic and mean pulmonary pressures did not directly correlate with AF occurrence in nonHF patients, the severity of pulmonary hypertension might have been masked by impairment of right ventricular function, thus rather supporting the notion that AF is more common in more advanced PH. These results provide insight into the possible pathophysiology of AF in PH and indicate a different pathomechanism of AF induction in PH with versus without left heart disease. In the absence of left heart disease (i) left atrial pressure does not play a pathophysiological role and (ii) pulmonary artery pressure does not seem to provoke AF by itself, but an increase in right atrial pressure leading to right atrial dilatation seems to be responsible for onset of AF.

There is only limited data available regarding the clinical consequences of AF in patients with various forms of PH. Previous studies indicated that elevated heart rate might lead to increased mortality in patients suffering from PH. Notably, mean heart frequency in PH-AF was not significantly different compared to PH-SR in our population.

The influence of AF on clinical performance and cardiac function in PH has not been investigated yet. In our cohort patients with PH-AF demonstrated significant impairment in NYHA/WHO functional class and 6-minute walk distance compared to PH-SR. This clinical deterioration in the presence of AF was also evident by the higher prescription rate of diuretics. Elevation of NT-proBNP as a marker for heart failure and renal insufficiency have been implicated to correlate with prognosis and severity of disease in PH. In the present study these laboratory parameters were consistently increased in the total PH population and in all subgroups with prevalent AF compared to SR, further supporting the notion that AF in PH is associated with more advanced compromise of hemodynamic function.

Recently, renal failure, reduced 6-minute walk distance, elevated mean right atrial pressure, and increased brain natriuretic peptide have been suggested as independent predictors of mortality in PH. Therefore, it remains to be determined in a larger prospective study whether AF in PH is just a marker of more advanced disease, is an independent risk factor, and/or if cardioversion might improve symptoms, exercise capacity and possibly prognosis in this population.

Author Contributions

Conceived and designed the experiments: DR LJM S. Reda UCH. Performed the experiments: DR LJM S. Reda UCH DS DD. Analyzed the data: DR LJM S. Reda UCH EE S. Rosenkranz RL MW. Contributed reagents/materials/analysis tools: DR LJM S. Reda UCH S. Rosenkranz EE. Wrote the paper: DR LJM MW S. Reda UCH.

References

1. D'Alonzo GE, Barst RJ, Ayres SM, Bergofsky EH, Brundage BH, et al. (1991) Survival in patients with primary pulmonary hypertension. Results from a national prospective registry. Ann Intern Med 115: 343–349.
2. Runo JR, Loyd JE (2003) Primary pulmonary hypertension. Lancet 361: 1533–1544.
3. Humbert M, Morrell NW, Archer SL, Stenmark KR, MacLean MR, et al. (2004) Cellular and molecular pathobiology of pulmonary arterial hypertension. J Am Coll Cardiol 43: 13S–24S.
4. Simonneau G, Robbins IM, Beghetti M, Channick RN, Delcroix M, et al. (2009) Updated clinical classification of pulmonary hypertension. J Am Coll Cardiol 54: S43–54.
5. Ghio S, Gavazzi A, Campana C, Inserra C, Klersy C, et al. (2001) Independent and additive prognostic value of right ventricular systolic function and pulmonary artery pressure in patients with chronic heart failure. J Am Coll Cardiol 37: 183–188.
6. Maisel WH, Stevenson LW (2003) Atrial fibrillation in heart failure: epidemiology, pathophysiology, and rationale for therapy. Am J Cardiol 91: 2D–8D.
7. Shinebane JS, Wood MA, Jensen DN, Ellenbogen KA, Fitzpatrick AP, et al. (1997) Tachycardia-induzed cardiomyopathy: A review of animal models and clinical studies. J Am Coll Cardiol 29: 709–715.
8. Li D, Fareh S, Leung TK, Nattel S (1999) Promotion of atrial fibrillation by heart failure in dogs: atrial remodeling of a different sort. Circulation 100: 87–95.
9. Ruo B, Capra AM, Jensvold NG, Go AS (2004) Racial variation in the prevalence of atrial fibrillation among patients with heart failure: the Epidemiology, Practice, Outcomes, and Costs of Heart Failure (EPOCH) study. J Am Coll Cardiol 43: 429–435.
10. Hoppe UC, Casares JM, Eiskjaer H, Hagemann A, Cleland JG, et al. (2006) Effect of cardiac resynchronization on the incidence of atrial fibrillation in patients with severe heart failure. Circulation 114: 18–25.
11. Benjamin EJ, Levy D, Vaziri SM, D'Agostino RB, Belanger AJ, et al. (1994) Independent risk factors for atrial fibrillation in a population-based cohort: the Framingham Heart Study. JAMA 271: 840–844.
12. Crijns HJ, Tjeerdsma G, de Kam PJ, Boomsma F, van Gelder IC, et al. (2000) Prognostic value of the presence and development of atrial fibrillation in patients with advanced chronic heart failure. Eur Heart J 21: 1238–1245.
13. Swedberg K, Olsson LG, Charlesworth A, Cleland J, Hanrath P, et al. (2005) Prognostic relevance of atrial fibrillation in patients with chronic heart failure on long-term treatment with beta-blockers: results from COMET. Eur Heart J 26: 1303–1308.
14. Stevenson WG, Stevenson LW (1999) Atrial fibrillation in heart failure. N Engl J Med 341: 910–911.
15. Paulus WJ, Tschope C, Sanderson JE, Rusconi C, Flachskampf FA, et al. (2007) How to diagnose diastolic heart failure: a consensus statement on the diagnosis of heart failure with normal left ventricular ejection fraction by the Heart Failure and Echocardiography Associations of the European Society of Cardiology. Eur Heart J 28: 2539–2550.
16. Crapo RO, Casburi R, Coates AL, Enright PL, MacIntyre NR, et al. (2002) ATS statement: guidelines for the six-minute walk test. Am J Respir Crit Care Med 166: 111–117.
17. Levey AS, Bosch JP, Lewis JB, Greene T, Rogers N, et al. (1999) A more accurate method to estimate glomerular filtration rate from serum creatinine: a new prediction equation. Modification of Diet in Renal Disease Study Group. Ann Intern Med 130: 461–470.
18. Rudski LG, Lai WW, Afilalo J, Hua L, Handschumacher MD, et al. (2010) Guidelines for the echocardiographic assessment of the right heart in adults: a report from the American Society of Echocardiography endorsed by the European Association of Echocardiography, a registered branch of the European Society of Cardiology, and the Canadian Society of Echocardiography. J Am Soc Echocardiogr 23: 685–713; quiz 786-688.
19. Camm AJ, Kirchhof P, Lip GY, Schotten U, Savelieva I, et al. (2010) Guidelines for the management of atrial fibrillation: the Task Force for the Management of Atrial Fibrillation of the European Society of Cardiology (ESC). Eur Heart J 31: 2369–2429.
20. Dries DL, Exner DV, Gersh BJ, Domanski MJ, Waclawiw MA, et al. (1998) Atrial fibrillation is associated with an increased risk for mortality and heart failure progression in patients with asymptomatic and symptomatic left ventricular systolic dysfunction: a retrospective analysis of the SOLVD trials. Studies of Left Ventricular Dysfunction. J Am Coll Cardiol 32: 695–703.
21. Aronow WS, Ahn C, Kronzon I (2001) Prognosis of congestive heart failure after prior myocardial infarction in older persons with atrial fibrillation versus sinus rhythm. Am J Cardiol 87: 224–225, A228–229.

22. Pozzoli M, Cioffi G, Traversi E, Pinna GD, Cobelli F, et al. (1998) Predictors of primary atrial fibrillation and concomitant clinical and hemodynamic changes in patients with chronic heart failure: a prospective study in 344 patients with baseline sinus rhythm. J Am Coll Cardiol 32: 197–204.

23. Tongers J, Schwerdtfeger B, Klein G, Kempf T, Schaefer A, et al. (2007) Incidence and clinical relevance of supraventricular tachyarrhythmias in pulmonary hypertension. Am Heart J 153: 127–132.

24. Naccarelli GV, Varker H, Lin J, Schulman KL (2009) Increasing prevalence of atrial fibrillation and flutter in the United States. Am J Cardiol 104: 1534–1539.

25. Fisher MR, Forfia PR, Chamera E, Housten-Harris T, Champion HC, et al. (2009) Accuracy of Doppler echocardiography in the hemodynamic assessment of pulmonary hypertension. Am J Respir Crit Care Med 179: 615–621.

13

Stiffening-Induced High Pulsatility Flow Activates Endothelial Inflammation via a TLR2/NF-κB Pathway

Yan Tan[1,2¤a]**, Pi-Ou Tseng**[1]**, Daren Wang**[2]**, Hui Zhang**[2¤b]**, Kendall Hunter**[2]**, Jean Hertzberg**[1]**, Kurt R. Stenmark**[2]**, Wei Tan**[1]*

1 Department of Mechanical Engineering, University of Colorado at Boulder, Boulder, Colorado, United States of America, **2** Department of Pediatrics, University of Colorado at Denver, Aurora, Colorado, United States of America

Abstract

Stiffening of large arteries is increasingly used as an independent predictor of risk and therapeutic outcome for small artery dysfunction in many diseases including pulmonary hypertension. The molecular mechanisms mediating downstream vascular cell responses to large artery stiffening remain unclear. We hypothesize that high pulsatility flow, induced by large artery stiffening, causes inflammatory responses in downstream pulmonary artery endothelial cells (PAECs) through toll-like receptor (TLR) pathways. To recapitulate the stiffening effect of large pulmonary arteries that occurs in pulmonary hypertension, ultrathin silicone tubes of variable mechanical stiffness were formulated and were placed in a flow circulatory system. These tubes modulated the simulated cardiac output into pulsatile flows with different pulsatility indices, 0.5 (normal) or 1.5 (high). PAECs placed downstream of the tubes were evaluated for their expression of proinflammatory molecules (ICAM-1, VCAM-1, E-selectin and MCP-1), TLR receptors and intracellular NF-κB following flow exposure. Results showed that compared to flow with normal pulsatility, high pulsatility flow induced proinflammatory responses in PAECs, enhanced TLR2 expression but not TLR4, and caused NF-κB activation. Pharmacologic (OxPAPC) and siRNA inhibition of TLR2 attenuated high pulsatility flow-induced pro-inflammatory responses and NF-κB activation in PAECs. We also observed that PAECs isolated from small pulmonary arteries of hypertensive animals exhibiting proximal vascular stiffening demonstrated a durable ex-vivo proinflammatory phenotype (increased TLR2, TLR4 and MCP-1 expression). Intralobar PAECs isolated from vessels of IPAH patients also showed increased TLR2. In conclusion, this study demonstrates for the first time that TLR2/NF-κB signaling mediates endothelial inflammation under high pulsatility flow caused by upstream stiffening, but the role of TLR4 in flow pulsatility-mediated endothelial mechanotransduction remains unclear.

Editor: Joseph Najbauer, University of Pécs Medical School, Hungary

Funding: This study was funded in part by grants from the National Institutes of Health (NIH) (HL K25-097246 to W.T., HL-14985-36 to K.R.S.) and the American Heart Association (13GRNT16990019 to W.T.). The funders had no role in study design, data collection and analysis, decision to publish, or preparation of the manuscript.

Competing Interests: The authors have declared that no competing interests exist.

* Email: wei.tan-1@colorado.edu

¤a Current address: Department of Geriatrics, Nanfang Hospital, Guangdong, China
¤b Current address: Department of Pediatrics, Shengjing Hospital and China Medical University, Shenyang, China

Introduction

It is increasingly accepted that large artery stiffening, which commonly occurs with aging, hypertension, diabetes, etc., contributes to the microvascular abnormalities of the kidney, brain, and eyes that characterize these pathophysiologic conditions [1–5]. In pulmonary hypertension, a group of progressive and fatal diseases, it has also become evident that stiffening of large proximal pulmonary arteries occurs, often early, in the course of this spectrum of diseases that have been conventionally characterized by dysfunction and obliteration of small distal pulmonary arteries [6]. However, while both clinical and animal studies convincingly demonstrate an association between proximal artery stiffening and distal artery dysfunction, few studies have examined the underlying cellular and molecular mechanisms through which these pathologic features might be inherently linked.

Besides being a conduit between the heart and distal vasculature, elastic proximal arteries act as a cushion or hydraulic buffer transforming highly pulsatile flow into semi-steady flow through the arterioles [4]. Normally, the so-called arterial windkessel effect is efficiently performed such that the mean flow, which reflects the steady-state energy, is well maintained throughout the arterial tree, whereas flow pulsatility, which reflects the kinetic energy of flow, is reduced by the deformation of compliant proximal arteries [7,8]. Thus, flow pulsatility in distal arteries is usually low, due to kinetic energy dissipated by the proximal compliance. In the cases of aging and diabetes in the systemic circulation or various forms of pulmonary hypertension, stiff proximal arteries reduce their cushion function to modulate flow pulsation, extending high flow pulsatility into distal vessels where the pulse remnant might be reduced via smooth muscle contractility. Therefore, proximal stiffening may contribute to small artery abnormalities found in high flow, low impedance organs including the kidney, brain, eye, and lung [2,3,5]. It is thus clear that a better understanding of the contribution of pulsatility (the kinetic component) of unidirectional physiologic flow to molecular changes in the downstream vascular endothelium is necessary for a better understanding of the effects of artery stiffening on cardiovascular health.

The endothelium, uniquely situated at the interface between the blood and the vessel wall, is an efficient biological flow sensor that converts flow stresses to biochemical signals, which in turn modulate vascular tone, infiltration of inflammatory cells and other cell activities important in vascular remodeling [9–11]. Endothelial cells (ECs) not only sense the mean magnitude of flow shear stress, but also discriminate among distinct flow patterns [10]. While a majority of studies on EC mechano-transduction of flow involve turbulent or disturbed flows with low wall shear stress (≤ 2 dyne/cm^2) simulating atherosclerosis-related flow conditions [9–11], few systems exist to examine the impact of stiffening on EC physiology. We have previously established flow pulsatility, a stiffening-related flow parameter, as a determinant of pulmonary artery endothelial function [12]. In response to unidirectional high pulsatility flow (HPF) with the mean shear stress remaining at a physiological level (12 dyne/cm^2), ECs demonstrate pro-inflammatory and vasoconstrictive responses [12], though the mechanisms involved in the ECs' ability to sense and respond to pulse flow remained unclear. Growing evidence supports the role of TLRs, a family of integral membrane proteins, in the initiation and progression of vascular diseases that are associated with disturbed blood flow such as atherosclerosis. It was found that ECs are the first cells to display increased TLR expression in early lesions of atherosclerotic prone vessels [13]. It is also known that ECs normally express TLR4 and a very low level of TLR2, which is further reduced under physiological flow conditions [14]. The TLRs are essential factors not only in the innate immune response, functioning as the first line of defense against pathogens, but also in homeostasis mediating cell responses to stress and danger signals [13]. Upon activation, TLRs may activate several downstream signaling nuclear factors, thus leading to a local inflammatory response [15]. Though the key role that TLRs play in atherosclerosis is becoming recognized [16], few studies have examined possible roles of TLRs in other vascular diseases, particularly those absent of turbulent flow. We therefore sought to test the hypothesis that reduced upstream compliance in the large pulmonary arteries enhances high flow pulsatility in distal vessels which in turn induces endothelial inflammation via a TLR/NF-κB pathway. To address this hypothesis, we developed an *ex-vivo* model flow system to simulate the effects of stiffening of upstream arteries on the downstream endothelial function. In addition to the model system, we also determined whether TLR expression in small PAECs was increased with pulmonary hypertension in calves and humans whose large pulmonary arteries are characterized by significant stiffening [17,18].

Methods

Endothelial cell isolation and culture

Bovine PAECs were isolated from pulmonary arterial endothelium of normal (CO-ECs) and pulmonary hypertensive (PH-ECs) calves. The use of calves conforms to the Guide for the Care and Use of Laboratory Animals published by the United States National Institutes of Health, and was approved by the Institutional Animal Care Use Committee (IACUC) at the Colorado State University. Animals were euthanized using an overdose of pentobarbital as recommended by the Panel on Euthanasia of the American Veterinary Medical Association. The cell isolation of the endothelium from calf small arteries (after 4th generation) as intact monolayers, involved brief pretreatment with Dispase (Becton Dickinson Inc, Franklin Lakes, NJ) followed by a single scrape with a flexible plastic scraper. Cell monolayers were plated onto at least 10 culture dishes, either plastic or covered with 1% denatured type I collagen (gelatin) in complete D-Valine MEM medium (Sigma Inc, Saint Louis, MO) with 10% fetal bovine serum. Freshly separated cells were characterized for their expressions of MCP-1 and TLRs. Primary cultures were confirmed to be free of contamination with smooth muscle cells by thorough screening of at least 2 culture dishes using immunostaining for smooth muscle marker. For all the *in vitro* flow experiments, CO-ECs at passages 4–8 were used. There was little difference in TLR2 and TLR4 expression or their responsiveness to various stimuli between cells of different passages.

Preparation methods of silicone tubes as mechanical equivalents to pulmonary artery

To employ silicone tubes that simulate the buffering function of proximal elastic pulmonary arteries in normal and hypertensive conditions, we utilized silicone elastomers with various elastic moduli to form tubes, and placed them upstream to the flow chambers where PAECs were cultured (Figure 1A). Silicone elastomer base and curing agent (Sylgard184 elastomer kit, Dow Corning Inc, Midland, MI) were mixed at different ratios to obtain varied elastic moduli. To determine appropriate polymer compositions that simulate the compliance function of large pulmonary arteries, we studied how the ratio between the base solution and the crosslinker (curing agent) influences the elastic modulus of silicone elastomer. The tensile modulus of samples was measured with a tensile tester (Instron Inc, Norwood, MA). For this study, we used a base-to-crosslinker ratio of 36:1 for a "soft" tube and 10:1 for a "stiff" tube, which respectively simulate buffering function of normotensive and hypertensive proximal pulmonary arteries, while the thickness and length of both tubes were kept the same (~0.3 mm thick, 5 cm long). Fabrication of silicone tubes involves a repeated dip-cure process. Briefly, a stainless steel cannula (14 G) was briefly dipped into the silicone prepolymer mixture with a predetermined base-to-crosslinker ratio, and then placed into an oven set at 60°C for 4 h to cure the polymer coating on the cannula. This was followed by repeating the dipping process with the same silicone elastomer mixture and back to the oven for additional 4 h. The ultrathin silicone tube was then carefully removed from the stainless steel cannula. The resultant silicone tubes (cut into a length of 5 cm) exhibit appropriate distensibility and cushion function to mimic the flow buffering of normotensive and hypertensive pulmonary arteries, respectively.

Mechanical properties of silicone elastomers were characterized with tube compliance testing and stress-strain tensile testing. For tube compliance testing that reveals the pressure-diameter relationship, a tube was loaded onto a custom-made fixture through tube adapters, using suture threads to secure the tubes near the adapters on both ends. The tube was then connected to a flow network via pressure gauges (Living Systems Instrumentation, Burlington, VT) on both ends of the tube. The pressure in the tube was controlled using varying speed of a water pump, to obtain a steady pressure from 0 mmHg to 100 mmHg, with a gradual increment. At each pressure, images of the tube dilatation were taken using a Canon EOS 450D camera (Canon, Tokyo, Japan). These images were analyzed using a customized script in MatlabVR (MathWorks, Natick, MA) to obtain the tube diameter at each pressure point.

To measure the mechanical properties of human pulmonary arteries, we performed ultrasonic imaging to determine the pressure-diameter relationship *in vivo* and stress-strain tensile testing *in vitro* to measure the elastic moduli of pulmonary arteries in the circumferential direction. With informed consent and/or

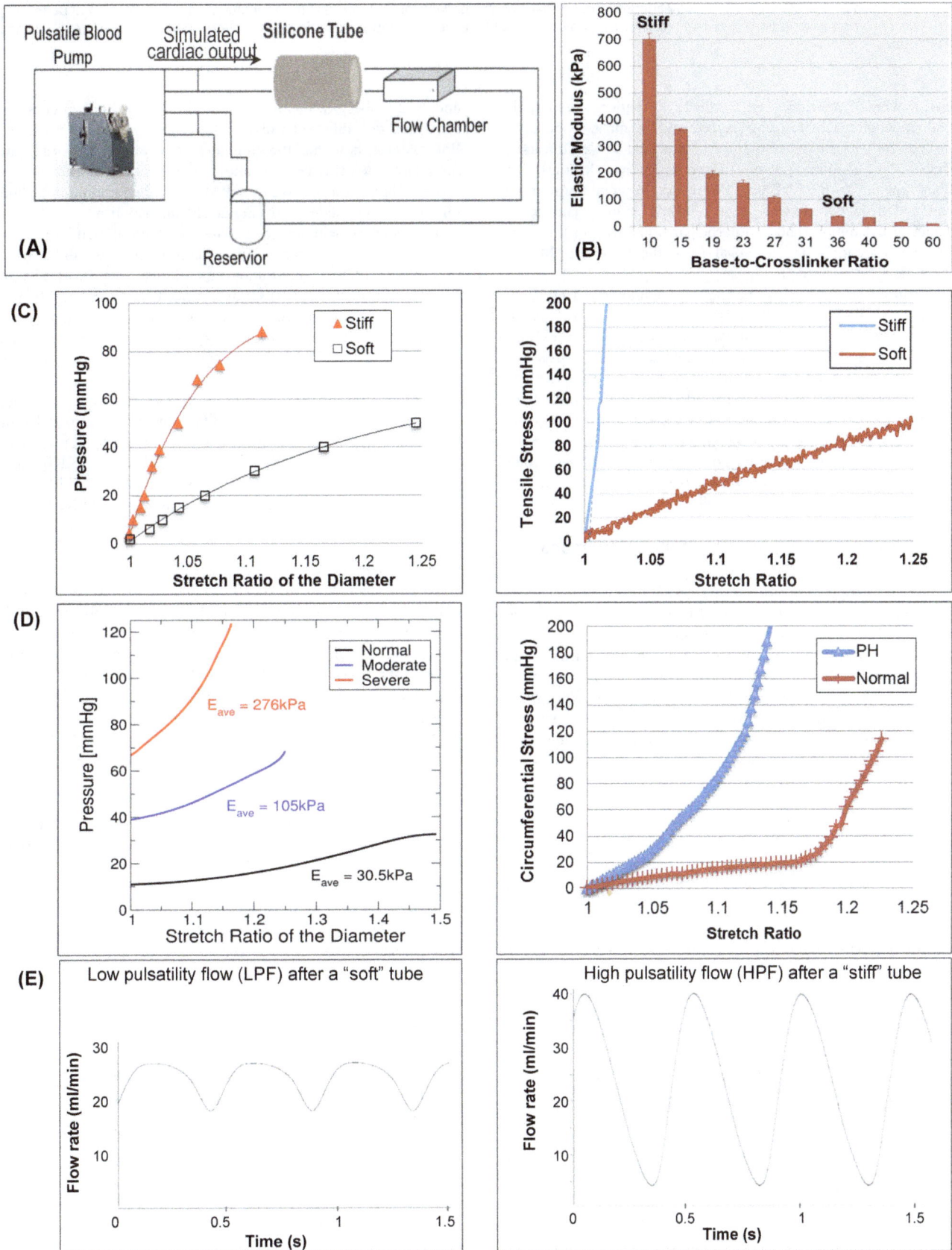

Figure 1. Experimental setup for flow studies. (A) Illustration of the flow circulation system. (B) Silicone tubes with various elastic moduli were prepared with varying the base-to-crosslinker ratio. (C) Pressure-diameter relationship curves of "soft" and "stiff" tubes showing their difference in compliance (left) and representative tensile stress-strain curves of "soft and "stiff" silicone materials (right). (D) Representative biomechanical

characterization curves of human pulmonary arteries from normal (control) patients or from those with moderate or severe pulmonary hypertension (PH) using *in vivo* measures (left) or *ex vivo* tensile stress-strain tests (right). (E) Representative pulsatile flow waveforms taken at the exit of "soft" and "stiff" tubes.

assent when applicable, we studied 36 patients undergoing evaluation of reactivity using oxygen and/or nitric oxide in the cardiac catheterization laboratory at the Children's Hospital in Denver, CO. Pediatric patients ranged in age from 1 month to 19 years (mean = 6.5 ± 5.2 yrs, 19 males). Written consent was obtained from the next of kin, caretakers, or guardians on the behalf of the minors/children participants involved in this study. All clinical studies had approval from the Colorado Multiple Institutional Review Board.

Pressure was obtained within the right pulmonary artery (RPA) using 5- or 6-fr Swan-Ganz catheters (Transpac IV, Abbott Critical Care Systems, Abbott Park, IL), while CMM-TDI was obtained of the RPA wall from the suprasternal short-axis view, which provides a long-axis representation of the RPA with the walls perpendicular to the ultrasound beam angle. Immediately prior to acquisition, the ultrasound beam was swept through the long axis of the RPAs to locate maximal diameter; acquisition then occurred along this beamline. For each patient, measurements were typically obtained at room air, considered the baseline, and toward the end of each clinical challenge.

Tensile testing of silicone elastomers and pulmonary arteries

Tensile testing was performed using an MTS Insight2 electromechanical testing system (MTS Systems Corp., Eden Prairie, MN, USA). For testing of silicone elastomers, all materials were cut to 5 mm wide by 25 mm long. Uniaxial tensile testing with a strain rate of 5 mm per min was performed on samples. All elastomers showed linear behavior, and a linear fit of the stress–strain curve was used to determine the modulus. For testing of main pulmonary arteries from human, stress-strain data was acquired with an MTS Insight2 system with a 5 N load cell. Tissue strip widths were measured with digital calipers. The circumferential strips were tested in an auxiliary environmental chamber with the same buffer solution as storage and pressure diameter testing. Tissues were prestrained by applying nine extension-relaxation cycles, and data was collected on the tenth cycle. Arteries cut in the circumferential direction were strained at a rate of 10% strain per second.

Experimental setup and protocol for flow studies on cells

The flow system used for examining PAECs under mimetic pulse flow conditions is demonstrated in Figure 1A. The circulating medium contained 7% Dextran (MP-products Inc, Solon, OH) and 1% penicillin/streptomycin, as its viscosity was close to blood viscosity. A pulsatile blood pump (Harvard Apparatus Inc; Holliston, MA) was used to circulate the medium, going through a silicone tube, a flow chamber with cell culture, a medium reservoir, and then back to the pump. Herein, the pump simulates the heart function generating cardiac output, while the silicone tube simulates the flow buffering or cushion function of proximal large arteries, and the flow chamber holds the endothelium to simulate the distal pulmonary vascular bed. Each component was connected by stiff polystyrene tubing. For flow measurements, a flow meter (Alicat Inc, Tucson, AZ) was placed before the flow chamber. Silicone tubes expanded during the systolic stage and contracted during the diastolic stage in response to the simulated cardiac output, behaving like large elastic arteries (Movie S1 and Movie S2). Tubes different in distensibility, "soft"

and "stiff" tubes, were in use (Figure 1B). Through these tubes, we generated two different pulsatile flows for the cell experiments. Both pulsatile flows had the same mean flow rate with a mean flow shear stress of 14 dynes/cm^2 and run at the same frequency.

To examine the response of PAECs to flow conditions, plain microscope glass slides were chemically functionalized with 20% of aqueous sulfuric acid and then coated with 6% of 3-aminopropyl-triethoxysilane in acetone. After silanization, glass slides were treated with 1.5% of glutaraldehyde and then coated with 25 μg/ml fibronectin. Bovine PAECs at a concentration of 6.0×10^5 per ml were seeded on the fibronectin-coated slides that were transferred to the flow chamber apparatus after cells reached confluence. Then, PAECs were exposed to either high or low pulsatility flow for 24 h with 4 h preconditioning under steady flow. PAECs grown in the absence of flow (the static condition) were used as a control. After PAECs were exposed to different flows, they were collected and analyzed for gene expression of ICAM-1, VCAM-1, MCP-1, E-selectin, IKKα and IKKβ using real-time PCR and for protein expression of MCP-1, TLR2 and TLR4 using western blotting. Nuclear translocation of NF-κB was analyzed by immunofluorescence.

Pharmacological treatments on cells

To determine the role of TLR2 and/or NF-κB in the flow-induced inflammatory response, BPAECs were incubated for 2 h with TLR2/4 inhibitor OxPAPC (Invivogen, San Diego, CA, 30 μg/ml), TLR4 inhibitor CLI-095 (Invivogen, 1 μg/ml) and NF-κB inhibitor BAY11-7082 (Enzo Life Sciences Inc, Farming-dale, NY, 5 μmol/l), respectively. After pretreatment with drugs, cells were exposed to the pulsatile flow conditions, using the medium containing OxPAPC (30 μg/ml), CLI-095 (1 μg/ml) and BAY11-7082 (5 μmol/l), respectively.

Gene knockdown with siRNA

Short interfering (si) RNA targeting TLR-2 (5'-rGrArArUrUr-ArGrArCrArCrCrUrArGrGrUr ArArUrGrUrGGA-3' and 5'-rUr-CrCrArCrArUrUrArCrCrUrArGrGrUrGrUrCrUrArArUrUrCr-UrG-3') and TLR-4 (5'-rGrGrArGrCrArArArGrArArCrUrArCrAr-GrArArUrUrUrGrCCA-3' and 5'-rUrUrCrCrUrCrGrUrUrCrUr-UrGrArUrGrUrCrUrArArArCrGrGrU-3') were obtained from IDT (Integrated DNA Technologies, Coralville, IA). Scrambled siRNA (5'- rCrCrArGrUrCrGrCrArArArACrGrCrGrAr CrU -3' and 5'- rArArCrArGrUrCrGrCrGrUrUrUrGrCrGrArC -3') was used as a control. Cells were seeded for transfection at a density of 6.0×10^5 per ml on a fibronectin-coated slide and cultured for 16 h. Cells were transfected with siTLR2 at a concentration of 50 nmol/L, using DharmaFECT siRNA transfection reagents (Dharmacon Inc., Lafayette, CO) according to the manufacturer's instruction. Culture medium was changed after 8 h to remove the transfection reagent. Transfected cells (after 48 h) were used in flow experiments.

Real-time qPCR

Total cellular mRNA from each sample was extracted using RNeasy Mini Kit (Qiagen; Hilden, Germany) according to the manufacturer's instructions. Complementary DNA was synthesized from 1 μg of total cellular mRNA using iScript cDNA Synthesis Kit (Bio-Rad, Hercules, CA). Real-time quantitative PCR primers are designed using Primer 3 Software to target bovine species for genes related to pro-inflammatory adhesion molecules including ICAM-1, VCAM-1 and E-selectin, chemokines such as MCP-1, and signaling molecules such as TLR2, TLR4, IKKα and IKKβ. The sequences of these genes are listed in Table 1. The SYBR Green I assay and the iCycler iQ real-time PCR detection system (Bio-Rad MyiQ; Hercules, CA) were used for quantitatively detecting real-time PCR products from 12 ng of reverse-transcribed cDNA. PCR thermal profile consisted of 94°C for 3 min, followed by 42 cycles of 94°C for 45 s, 50°C for 45 s and 77°C for 1 min. Genes were normalized to the housekeeping gene hypoxanthine-xanthine phosphoribosyl transferase (HPRT) and the fold change relative to static condition was determined using the ΔΔCT method.

Western blotting

Western blot analyses were performed as per the manufacturer's suggestions (Invitrogen, Carlsbad, CA). Antibodies used here include: rabbit polyclonal antibody against bovine MCP-1 (1:500 dilution; Kingfisher Biotech, St. Paul, MN), rabbit polyclonal antibody against TLR2 (1:100 dilution; Bioss Inc, Woburn MA), mouse monoclonal antibody against TLR4 (1:100 dilution; Acris Antibodies Inc, San Diego, CA) and mouse monoclonal antibody against GAPDH (1:20,000 dilution; Sigma Inc, Saint Louis, MO). The molecular sizes for MCP-1, TLR2, TLR4 and GAPDH are 8.8 kDa, 84 kDa, 96 kDa and 36 kDa, respectively.

Immunofluorescent staining

Cells were fixed in PBS-buffered 4% paraformaldehyde at room temperature, and then blocked with 3% BSA in PBS for 30 min. Subsequently, they were incubated with a primary antibody overnight at 4°C. NF-κB p105/p50 (specificity to p65, 1:500 dilution; Novus, Littleton, CO) were used. After washing with PBS, cells were incubated with a secondary antibody. Nuclei were counterstained with DAPI. Microscopic imaging was performed with a Zeiss fluorescent microscope and/or a Leica DMRXA microscope (Solms, Germany). Tissue cryosections were similarly stained with human TLR2 (1:50 dilution; Imgenex).

Data and statistical analysis

All data are expressed as mean ± SEM, and the number of sample studied (n) is ≥3. Using the power analysis with Graphpad StateMate, the power values of all data were found to be greater than 80%. One-Way ANOVA was used to determine effects of flow pulsatility on gene expression. If significant difference exists, Student's t-test for one-to-one comparison and Tukey for post-hoc analysis were used to compare means of each individual group. A P value <0.05 was considered significantly different.

Results

Development of the mimetic flow circulatory system

To determine the effects of upstream compliance and flow pulsatility on proinflammatory responses and underlying molecular signaling in downstream PAECs, we stimulated PAECs with pulsatile flows downstream to "soft" or "stiff" tubes which, by virtue of differences in tube deformation, dampened the pulsatile flow from the pump to various degrees (Figure 1). Silicone elastomers with various elastic moduli were constructed and then utilized to form tubes, and placed upstream to the flow chambers where PAECs were cultured (Figure 1A). As shown in Figure 1B, the elastic modulus of silicone tubes decreased with the increase of the base-to-crosslinker ratio. Two tube conditions were chosen as representatives to respectively simulate buffering function of normotensive and hypertensive proximal pulmonary arteries, as it was previously shown that the elastic modulus of large pulmonary arteries in normotensive subjects (calf or human) was in the range of 20–50 kPa, whereas that in hypertensive subjects could increase anywhere from 2–10 fold [17–21]. To illustrate the different cushion functions and mechanical properties of "stiff" and "soft" tubes, Figure 1C (left) shows tube distensibility with pressure-diameter relationship curves obtained with a series of static flow pressures and Figure 1C (right) illustrates their elasticity with representative stress-strain curves. Using ultrasonic imaging and tensile testing on artery strips obtained in the circumferential direction, we also showed representative pressure-diameter relationship and tensile stress-strain curves for human pulmonary arteries from different patient groups (Figure 1D). Though mechanical behaviors of pulmonary arteries are more complicated, the results showed that the tubes could serve as good mechanical equivalents to upstream arteries. Earlier studies on the relationship between arterial compliance and arterial elastic modulus showed that the thickness of the arterial wall plays an important role in determining the arterial compliance in addition to elastic modulus. Though hypertensive arteries exhibited both tissue thickening and progressive matrix remodeling such as increased collagen content which increases arterial elastic modulus, we simplified the tube preparation by making tube thickness constant while using the tube distensibility and flow buffering function as the mimetic criteria. Figure 1E demonstrates cushion function of the tubes by showing varied pulsatile flows at the exit of the tubes which modulate the input flow waveform of simulated

Table 1. Bovine primer sequences for real-time RT-PCR.

	FWD	REV
MCP-1:	CGCCTGCTGCTATACATTCA	ACACTTGCTGCTGGTGACTC
VCAM-1:	GAGCTTGGACGTGACCTTCT	TGGGTGGAGAATCATCATCA
ICAM-1:	GACTTCTTCAGCTCCCCAAG	CCCACATGCTATTTGTCCTG
E-Selectin:	CTCCCCGTCCAAGAACTACA	CGCCTCTACCTGTCCTTGAG
TLR 2:	TTCTGAATGCCACAGGGCGG	TGCAGCCACGCCCACATCAT
TLR 4:	ATGCCAGGATGATGGCGCGT	ACCTGTACGCAAGGGTCCCA
IKKa:	CCGGAATTCGAGCGGCCCCCGGGGCTG	AAACTCGAGTTATTCTGTTAACCAACTCCAATC
IKKβ:	CCGGAATTCAGCTGGTCACCTTCCCTGCC	AAAGTCGACTTACGAGGCCCGCTCCAGGCT
HPRT:	CTGGCTCGAGATGTGATGAA	CAACAGGTCGGCAAAGAACT

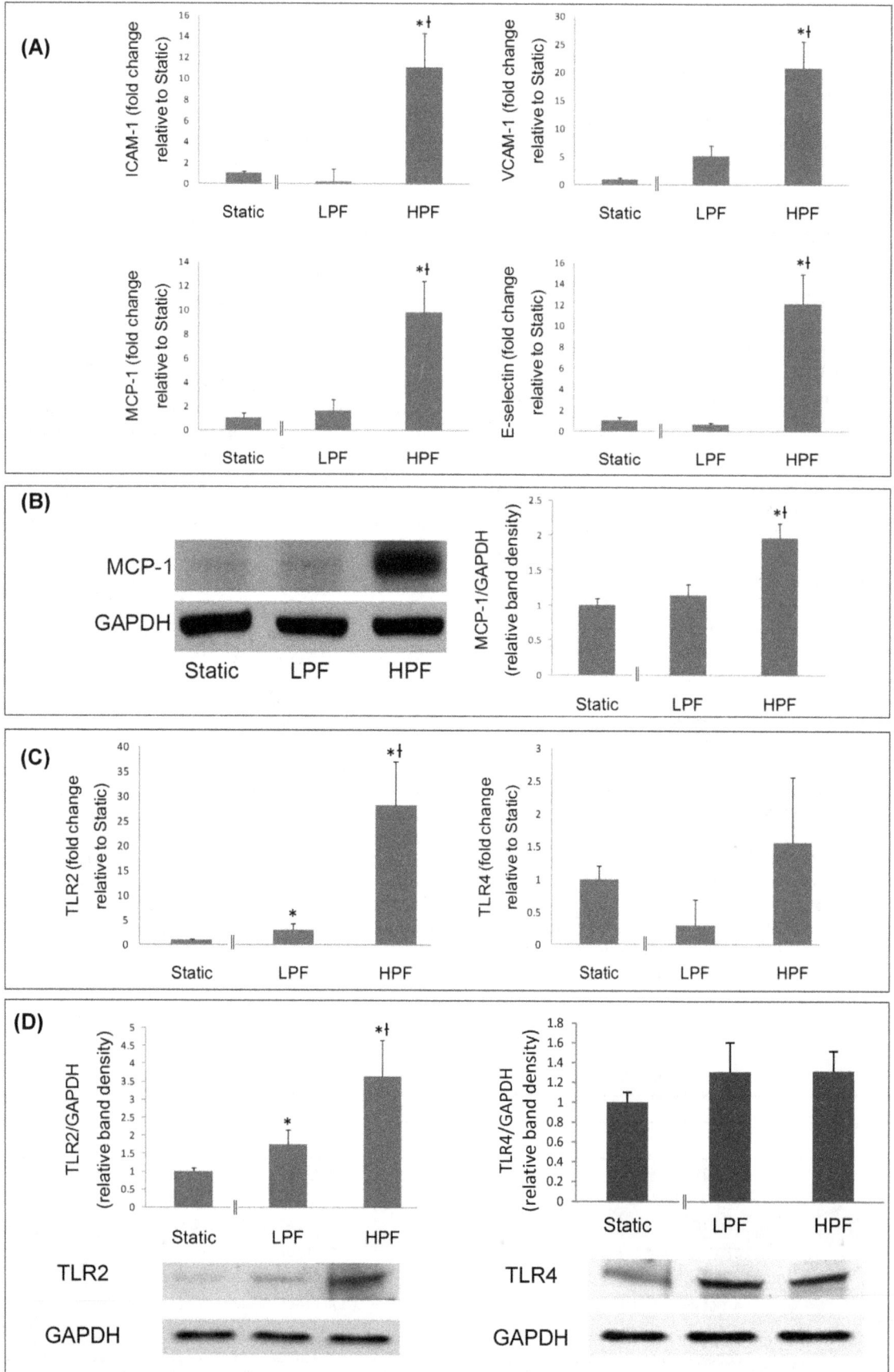

Figure 2. Proximal stiffening induces proinflammatory response and upregulates TLR2 expression in downstream bovine PAECs.
(A-B) High pulsatility flow (HPF), due to the use of a "stiff" tube upstream to cell culture, upregulated proinflammatory molecule mRNA (ICAM-1, VCAM-1, MCP-1 and E-selectin) and protein (MCP-1) in healthy PAECs, compared to low pulsatility flow (LPF) or to static conditions. (C-D) The mRNA and protein expression of TLR2 but not TLR4 in PAECs was highly upregulated by HPF. *: p<0.05 versus Static, †: p<0.05 versus LPF.

cardiac output. Both pulsatile flows had the same mean flow rate with a mean flow shear stress of 14 dynes/cm^2 and run at the same frequency. Figure 1E shows the flow pulsatility indices after the "stiff" and "soft" silicone tubes are 1.5 and 0.5, respectively. The pulsatility levels *in vivo* fall within a close range of pulsatility levels used here. Previous studies showed that the mean flow pulsatility in the large PAs ranged from 4.4 to 5.1 *in vivo*, while the flow pulsatility in the pulmonary capillaries decreased to ~1 [22,23]. When there is no elastic deformation on the wall, a pulsatility value greater than 1 could exert detrimental effects on the endothelium.[24]

Proximal stiffening increases flow pulsatility and augments inflammatory responses in downstream PAECs

As shown in Figure 2A, endothelial cells exposed to HPF (with a pulsatility index of 1.5 for 24 h), induced by increased stiffness of the proximal silicone tube, exhibited markedly higher levels of ICAM-1, VCAM-1, E-selectin and MCP-1 expression than cells exposed to low pulsatility flow (LPF). Changes in gene expression were confirmed at the protein level by western blot analyses for MCP-1 (Figure 2B). Limitations on the availability of bovine-specific antibodies prevented evaluation of protein expression of other gene products ICAM-1, VCAM-1 and E-selectin. No significant changes in the expression of these genes were found between cells exposed to LPF (with a pulsatility index of 0.5) generated by "soft" tube, when compared to those maintained under the static condition (Figure 2A).

HPF upregulates TLR2 expression but not TLR4 expression in PAEC

To explore whether HPF alters TLR expression, PAECs exposed to LPF or HPF were analyzed for TLR2/4 expression using real-time PCR and western blot analysis, after 24 h of flow stimulation. Figures 2C-D show that both gene and protein expression of TLR2 was significantly upregulated in the cells exposed to HPF, compared to those exposed to static or LPF conditions. No statistically significant changes in TLR4 protein levels were observed in cells stimulated by different flow conditions. Hereafter, LPF condition was used as control for HPF in order to illuminate the differences in flow conditions related to upstream artery stiffness in the normal vs hypertensive subjects.

Inhibition or knockdown of TLR2 results in suppression of HPF-induced endothelial inflammation

To determine whether TLR2- or TLR4- mediated signaling contributed to the inflammatory responses induced by HPF, the TLR4 inhibitor CLI-095 and the TLR2/TLR4 inhibitor OxPAPC (a TLR2 specific pharmacological inhibitor is not available) were used. As shown in Figures 3A-B, PAECs treated with OxPAPC (inhibiting both TLR2 and TLR4) but not CLI-095 dramatically reduced proinflammatory adhesion molecule (ICAM-1, VCAM-1, E-selectin) and cytokine (MCP-1) gene expression in response to HPF. To further validate the role of TLR2 signaling in mediating the effects of HPF, we performed studies using ECs pretreated with TLR2 siRNA. Knockdown of TLR2 expression was confirmed with real-time PCR by showing decreased TLR2

expression in the cells treated with TLR2 siRNA compared to those treated with scrambled siRNA (data not shown). siRNA knockdown of TLR2 resulted in significant downregulation of inflammatory gene expression in PAECs exposed to HPF (Figures 3C-D). Similarly, to validate the role of TLR4 signaling in mediating the effects of HPF, we performed studies using ECs pretreated with TLR4 siRNA. Knockdown of TLR4 expression was confirmed with real-time PCR by showing decreased TLR4 expression in the cells treated with TLR4 siRNA, compared to those treated with scrambled siRNA (data not shown). As shown in Figures 3C-D, we found that siRNA knockdown of TLR4 reduced the mRNA levels of some pro-inflammatory molecules (ICAM-1 and E-selectin) under HPF, but not VCAM-1 or MCP-1. This is an interesting finding, because the different results from different TLR4 inhibition approaches, pharmacological inhibitor (CLI-095) which blocks the signaling mediated by the intracellular domain of TLR4 and a more effective inhibitor with siRNA gene silencing, may suggest possible TLR4 mechanisms for future studies. Because TLR4 has more complicated role and relatively minor effects on HPF-mediated responses compared to TLR2, we have focused on illuminating TLR2-mediated signaling underlying endothelial mechanotransduction of flow pulsatility.

Activation of NF-κB in PAECs is induced by HPF and attenuated by TLR2 inhibition or siRNA knockdown

To examine signaling downstream of TLR2 activation caused by HPF, we studied nuclear translocation or activation of NF-κB. As shown in Figure 4A, inhibition of TLR2 with OxPAPC or siTLR2 treatment decreased intranuclear translocation of NF-κB in the cells stimulated with HPF. Also, as the IkappaB kinase complex (IKK) contains two kinase subunits, IKKalpha (IKKα) and IKKbeta (IKKβ), necessary for IkappaB phosphorylation and NF-κB activation, we also examined flow and drug effects on PAEC expression of IKKα and IKKβ. As shown in Figure 4B, HPF enhanced IKKα and IKKβ gene expression and knockdown of TLR2 attenuated this effect. To further examine the role of NF-κB in the inflammatory response of cells to HPF stimulation, the NF-κB inhibitor BAY11-7082 was used. BAY 11–7082 treatment of PAECs led to a reduction in MCP-1 protein expression in response to HPF (Figure 4C).

Circulating media from cells exposed to HPF upregulate the inflammatory responses in normal PAECs through the TLR2/NF-κB pathway

To determine whether TLR2-mediated PAEC inflammation in response to HPF is mediated, at least in part, through endothelial release of damage-associated molecules, we investigated whether there were endogenous signals released from ECs exposed to HPF, which could activate TLR2 triggering an inflammatory response in the absence of flow. We collected the conditioned circulating media from cell cultures under the HPF and LPF conditions (labeled as HPF-FM and LPF-FM, respectively), and then exposed normal bovine PAECs to the conditioned media for 24 h under static conditions. As shown in Figure 5A, cells exposed to HPF-FM produced markedly higher mRNA levels of ICAM-1, VCAM-1, E-selectin and MCP-1 than cells exposed to LPF-FM. Inhibition of TLR2 with OxPAPC or siTLR2 treatment decreased endothelial

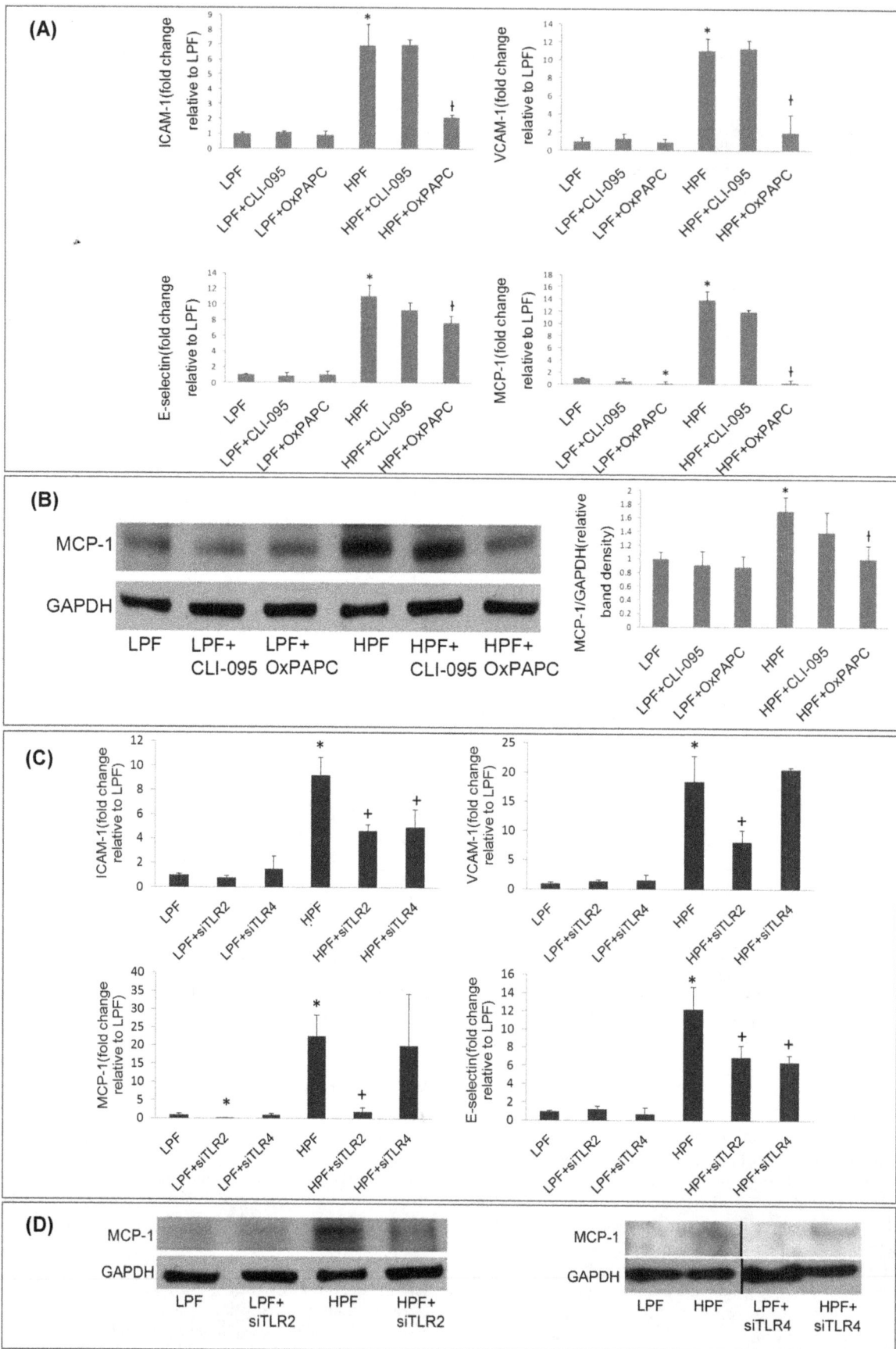

Figure 3. Pharmacological or siRNA inhibition of TLR2 results in suppression of PAEC proinflammatory responses caused by stiffening-induced HPF. (A, C) At the mRNA level, TLR2/4 inhibitor OxPAPC or TLR2 siRNA but not TLR4 inhibitor CLI-095, decreased PAEC expression of ICAM-1, VCAM-1, MCP-1 and E-selectin mRNAs under HPF; TLR4 siRNA decreased ICAM-1 and E-selectin but not VCAM-1 and MCP-1 mRNAs. "*": $p<0.05$ versus LPF, "†": $p<0.05$ versus HPF. (B, D) At the protein level, the MCP-1 expression in PAECs exposed to HPF was inhibited by OxPAPC or TLR2 siRNA treatment but not CLI-095 or TLR4 siRNA. The black line in the blot images (D, right) shows separated lanes obtained on the same gel.

expression of ICAM-1, VCAM-1, E-selectin and MCP-1 mRNAs in response to HPF-FM conditioned media. OxPAPC and siTLR2 also decreased HPF-FM induced increases in MCP-1 protein in ECs (Figure 5B). As shown in Figure 5C, inhibition of TLR2 with OxPAPC or siTLR2 treatment also decreased intranuclear translocation of NF-κB in the cells stimulated with HPF-FM.

TLR2 and TLR4 are upregulated in hypertensive pulmonary arterial endothelium

To verify the results obtained in our ex-vivo model system and to confirm that the expression of TLRs and MCP-1 in pulmonary arterial endothelial changes with hypoxia-induced pulmonary hypertension characterized by proximal vascular stiffening [17], we analyzed protein levels in fresh cell lysates of PAECs derived from normal and hypertensive calves using western blotting. Figures 6A and 6B show that distal PAECs from pulmonary hypertensive calves (PH-ECs) exhibited higher levels of MCP-1, TLR2 and TLR4 than control ECs. We also observed that TLR2 expression was upregulated in vivo in the endothelium of human patients with IPAH (Figure 6C); as we could not locate bovine TLR antibodies that specifically worked for immunofluorescence.

Discussion

Using a new in vitro system, a model illustrating the proximal-distal vascular coupling, we have examined the effects of upstream stiffening on biological changes in downstream endothelium. Herein, silicone tubes with varied moduli and compliances were used to mimic the flow buffering function of proximal pulmonary arteries and resultant hemodynamic effects on changes in downstream arterial endothelium. Using the flow model as well as the hypoxia-induced pulmonary hypertension neonatal calf model characterized by proximal arterial stiffening [17], we have shown that stiffening-induced HPF caused pro-inflammatory responses and upregulated expression of TLRs (TLR2 and TLR4) in "downstream" ECs. We further demonstrated a causal relationship between HPF, TLR2/NF-kB expression and proinflammatory responses in PAECs. The results show that reduced upstream artery compliance induced pro-inflammatory signaling through TLR2. It was also found that TLR2 was upregulated in the freshly separated hypertensive PAECs. Using pharmacologic and siRNA approaches, a role for TLR2 in mediating proinflammatory responses in PAECs in response to HPF was confirmed. To identify the nuclear transcription factor mediating TLR2 flow sensing and pro-inflammatory gene expression, we evaluated the activation of NF-κB in response to low or high flow pulsatility in the presence or absence of a TLR2 inhibitor or gene knockdown and found that TLR2/NF-κB pathway mediated PAEC pro-inflammatory responses. In addition, the finding that conditioned flow media from HPF-stimulated PAEC enhanced TLR2 expression in the normal endothelium suggest that cells under HPF could generate autocrine/paracrine signaling through release of damage-associated molecular patterns (DAMPs) and thus perpetuate endothelial dysfunction through TLR2. Collectively, our findings support the idea that large vascular stiffening could initiate and/or perpetuate inflammatory responses in "downstream" vessels through the TLR2/NF-κB pathway.

Increasing evidence shows that artery stiffening or reduced arterial compliance is a prominent feature of systemic hypertension, pulmonary hypertension and other vascular-related diseases. Only recently have researchers started to relate the coupling of arterial stiffening and consequent flow changes to vascular cell dysfunction [3,5]. However, the mechanisms underlying such coupling remain elusive. Our study illustrates a new potential mechanism in that defective buffering function of a stiffened vessel causes downstream endothelial inflammation by activating TLR2/NF-?B signaling. Using bioengineering principles and polymer technology, we have developed a new flow circulatory system, which reproduces physiological functions of both normal and stiff large arteries in the pulmonary (and perhaps systemic), circulation, provides a physiological link between proximal artery stiffening and hemodynamic environments for distal vascular cells. The mimetic circulatory model, in parallel with animal models, allows investigation of the effects of artery stiffening and flow pulsatility on distal PA remodeling. In pulmonary hypertension, though pulmonary arterial stiffening is increasingly believed to significantly increase right ventricular afterload [6], few have explored its influence on the progression of pulmonary vascular disease which is characterized by progressive endothelial dysfunction and remodeling of downstream small arteries [25]. We previously showed the proinflammatory effects of flow pulsatility on PAECs using a compliance-adjustment chamber [12]. The present study provides more direct in vitro and in vivo evidence regarding stiffening-induced proinflammatory responses in PAECs, by designing mechanical equivalents of pulmonary arteries to modulate pulse flow waves from a simulated cardiac output, in addition to mechanical and histological characterizations of native human pulmonary arteries. The mechanical properties of blood vessels are designed such that the wall compliance and flow pulsatility are well coupled to maintain vascular homeostasis. Previous studies showed that high distensibility of proximal arteries protects ECs under HPF, but the same flow stimulus has an adverse effect in less compliant vessels such as distal arteries [26].

Consistent with recent studies highlighting on the novel roles of TLR2/4 signaling in cardiovascular diseases such as atherosclerosis and hypertension via endogenous signals from damaged or stressed cells [16,27–30], known as DAMPs, the present study is the first to show that TLR2 was highly upregulated in the small PA endothelium of both calf and human subjects with pulmonary hypertension and stiffened proximal PAs. The mechanistic studies here demonstrate that the underlying mechanism involved in stiffening-induced HPF effects on PAECs is at least partly through flow-induced cell damage that leads to release of TLR ligands. It is possible that these DAMPs could participate in the right heart dysfunction observed in pulmonary hypertension. This proximal-distal coupling mechanism is consistent with the observations of Voelkel et al. that elevated pulmonary vascular pressure alone, without perturbed lung vasculature or involved mediators, do not cause right ventricular failure [31]. These molecules might also contribute to dysfunction of other organs such as kidney and liver, which is also one of characteristics of late stage pulmonary

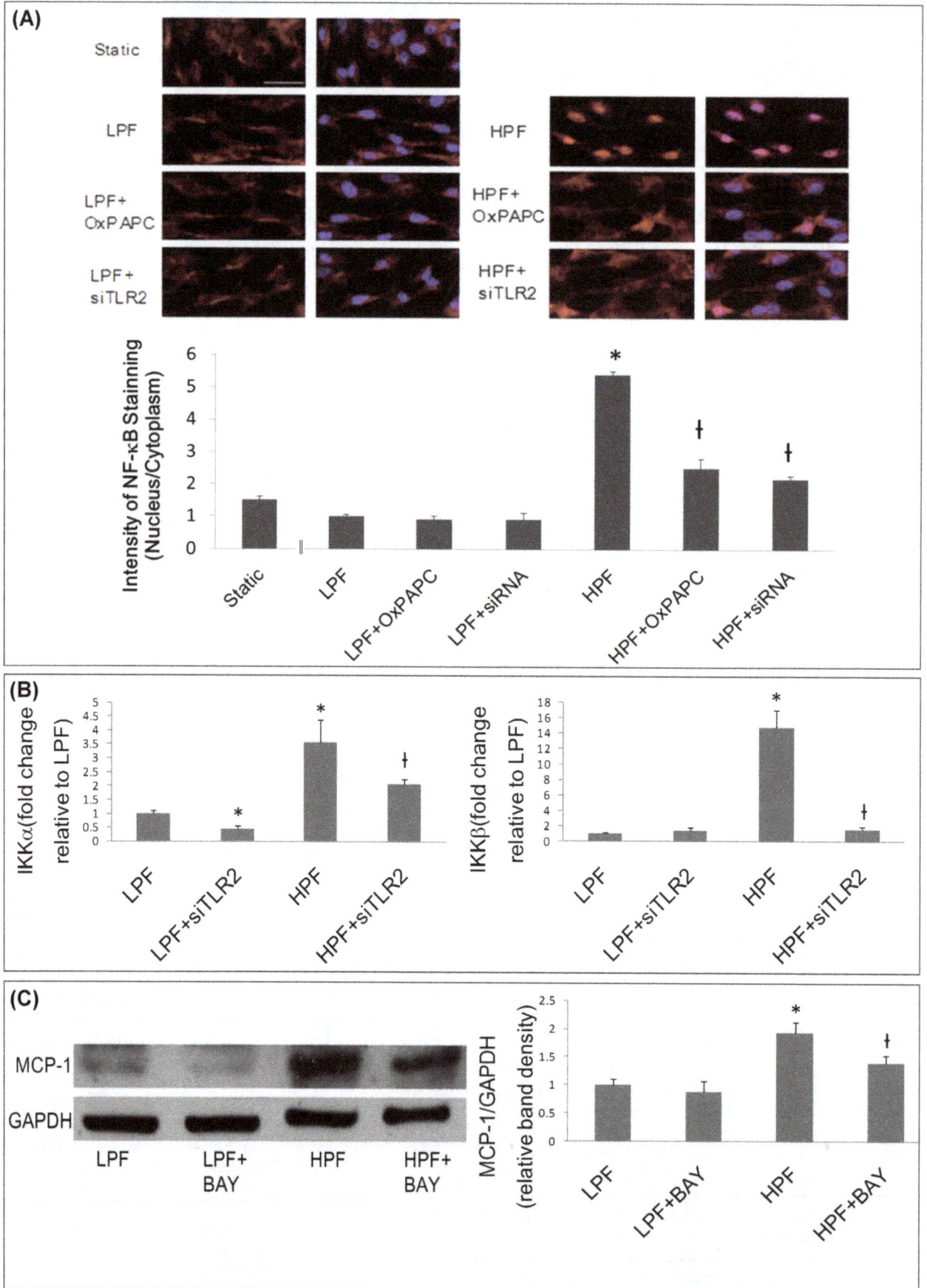

Figure 4. Activation of TLR2/NF-κB pathway mediated pro-inflammatory responses of PAECs exposed to stiffening-induced HPF. Pulse flow modulates TLR2-induced NF-κB activation in BPAECs. (A) Representative fluorescent images and quantitative measures of NF-kBp65 staining (red) in PAECs show HPF stimulation of PAECs led to increased intranuclear translocation or activation of NF-κB, which was reduced by TLR2/4 inhibitor OxPAPC and TLR2 siRNA. Blue stains show the nuclei. The scale bar shows 50 μm. (B) HPF stimulation of PAECs increased the mRNA levels of IKKα and IKKβ, both of which were attenuated in siRNA-transfected cells with knockdown of TLR2. (C) NF-κB inhibitor (BAY 11–7082) decreased the MCP-1 expression by PAECs exposed to HPF. *: p<0.05 versus LPF, †: p<0.05 versus HPF.

hypertension. We further established the role of TLR2 in HPF induced endothelial inflammation. Inhibition of TLR2 using pharmacologic (OxPAPC) and molecular (siRNA – siTLR2) approaches reduced NF-kB activation and endothelial inflammation in response to HPF. Though we did not identify specific DAMP ligands induced by HPF, our results using conditioned circulating media to culture normal PAECs demonstrated that molecules released by PAECs stressed under HPF activated PAEC inflammation through TLR2/NF-κB, which could be a mechanism for the endothelium to initiate autocrine signaling. The possible content of the endogenous ligands secreted by PAECs under flow might include heat shock proteins (or HSPs), because HSPs were known as endogenous ligands for TLR2 [32,33] and could be upregulated by pulsatile flow. Damage or stress-induced endogenous TLR2 ligands likely provide continuous support to PAEC dysfunction via autocrine signaling through endogenous TLR2 ligands. In addition to mechanical stimulation with flow, we also used TLR ligands of TLR-2 (peptidoglycan, 10 μg/mL) and TLR-4 (lipopolysaccharide, 200 ng/mL), which similarly upregulated pro-inflammatory stimulation of TLR-2 and TLR-4 pathways (data not shown). Taken together, our findings here, together with new insights into the TLR regulation of inflammation or tissue-damaging responses, provide strong evidence to support evaluation of TLRs as potential targets for the develop-

ment of new therapies in chronic vascular inflammatory disease where large vessel stiffening is observed. TLR2 and TLR4 are the only TLRs ubiquitously expressed in normal human arteries [34]. Because TLR2 in the endothelium can be upregulated by disturbed flow in atherogenic regions [35] [14], by HPF in distal pulmonary arteries as shown in this study, and by saturated fatty acids [36], targeting TLR2 may be an exciting prospect for the treatment of certain cardiovascular diseases [37,38], especially those characterized by large vessel stiffening.

Compared to TLR2, the role of TLR4 in HPF-mediated proinflammatory responses appears more complicated. Knockdown of TLR4 with specific siRNA, but not TLR4 pharmacological inhibitor CLI-095, decreased part of HPF-induced proinflammatory gene expression. The discrepancy in PAEC responses of different TLR4 inhibitors might be caused by different inhibition mechanisms. CLI-095, also known as TAK-242, is a cyclohexene derivative that suppresses TLR4 signaling mediated by the intracellular domain of TLR4, whereas siRNA gene silencing effectively down-regulates overall TLR4 protein expression, which thus reduces TLR4 signaling through both intracellular and extracellular domains. TLR4 signaling might contribute to the flow-induced inflammation predominantly via extracellular domain. As ECs normally express TLR4 and a very low level of TLR2 [14], absence of TLR4 might also influence EC physiology. Additionally, the discrepancy between TLR4 expression under HPF in the experimental set-up and human situation further suggested the complicated roles of TLR4 in flow-mediated mechanotransduction. TLR4-mediated mechanotransduction of HPF requires further exploration. Recent studies suggested a close relationship between TLR4 and pulmonary hypertension [39].

The present study highlights an important role of TLR2 in regulation of HPF-induced inflammatory response in PAECs. It also shows upregulated expression of TLR4 in hypertensive PAECs; TLR4 reduction inhibited some proinflammatory genes. This is consistent with studies that found greater TLR expression in clinical phenotypes of human pulmonary hypertension [40], and is also consistent with recent literatures showing relevance of TLR to cardiovascular diseases. But it remains unclear from this study why the level of TLR4 is higher in hypertensive PAECs and how it contributes to pathogenesis. In addition, the exact mechanisms underlying DAMP-mediated endothelial inflammation through TLR/NF-κB pathway requires further investigation.

Conclusions

To our knowledge, this is the first report to evaluate the effects of flow pulsatility on TLR signaling in the endothelium and the first to unravel molecular events underlying endothelial mechanotransduction of flow pulsatility. The TLR2/NF-κB pathway in PAECs likely mediates downstream inflammatory responses induced by reduced compliance of upstream vessels which are less capable of dampening HPF, and thus TLR2 might be a potential target for endothelial inflammation of pulmonary hypertension.

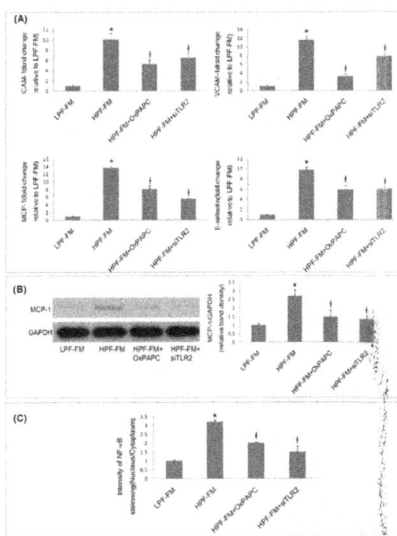

Figure 5. The circulating media from the cells exposed to HPF upregulate the inflammatory responses in normal PAECs through the TLR2/NF-κB pathway. The conditioned circulating media collected from cell cultures under the HPF and LPF conditions, respectively labeled as LPF-FM and HPF-FM, were used to culture normal PAECs for 24 h. (A) The mRNA expressions of ICAM-1, VCAM-1, MCP-1 and E-selectin were upregulated by HPF-FM condition, which were then reduced by OxPAPC and siTLR2. (B) Similar changes were shown in the MCP-1 protein expression. (C) NF-κB intranuclear translocation increased in PAECs stimulated with HPF-FM, which was reduced by OxPAPC and siTLR2. *: p<0.05 versus LPF-FM, †: p<0.05 versus HPF-FM.

(A)

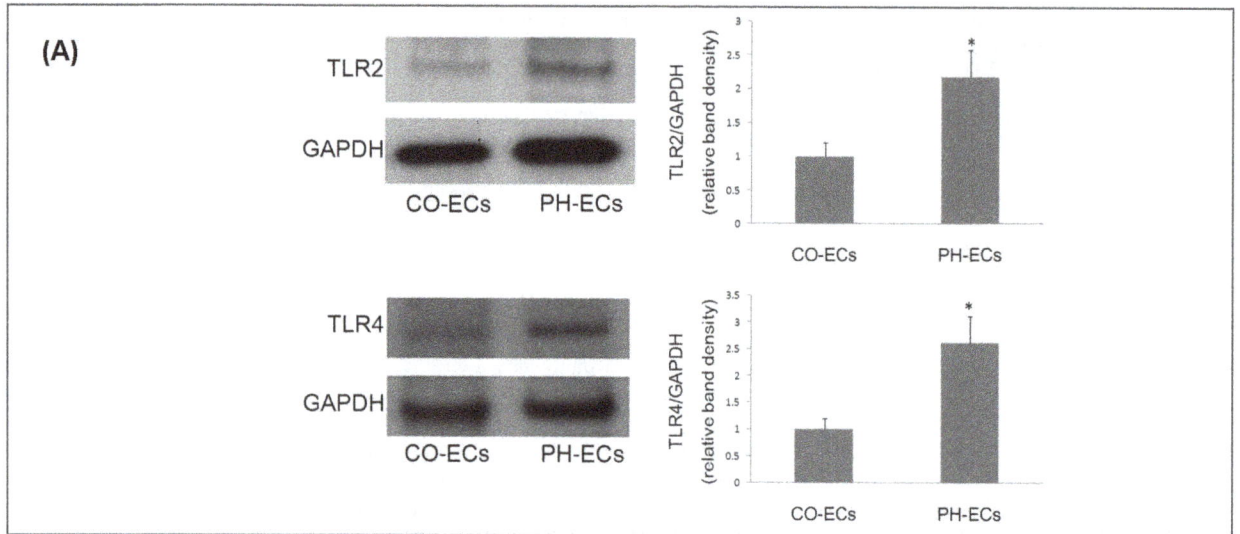

(B)

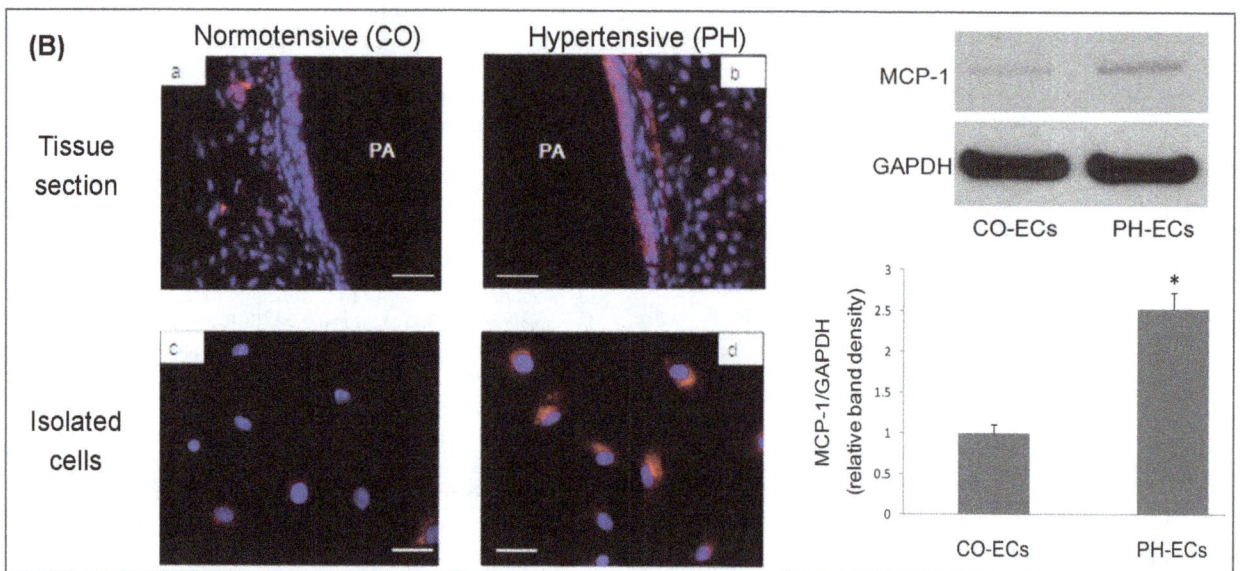

(C)

TLR2 / DAPI / elastic lamellae

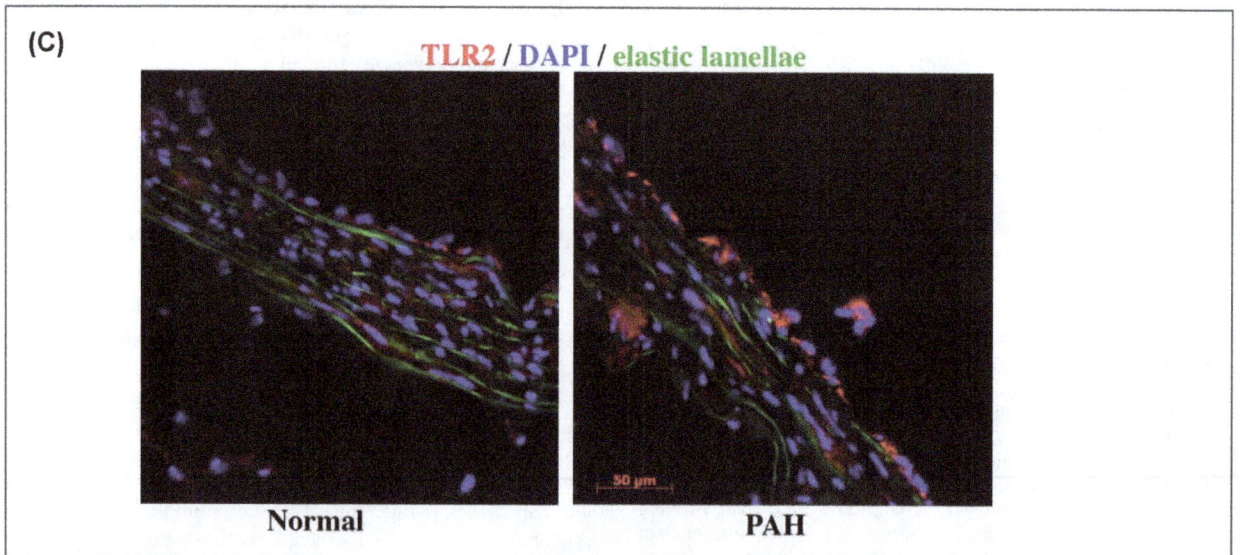

Normal   PAH

Figure 6. Enhanced TLR and MCP-1 expression in the distal pulmonary artery endothelium *in vivo*. (A) PAECs from calves with hypoxia-induced pulmonary hypertension (PH) show elevated expression of TLR2 and TLR4, compared to control (CO). *:p<0.05. (B) Both immunostaining and western blotting results show elevated MCP-1 expression by PH-ECs compared to CO-ECs from calves. "PA" indicates the lumen of a pulmonary artery. *:p<0.05. (C) Enhanced TLR2 expression in the pulmonary arterial endothelium of human with pulmonary arterial hypertension (PAH). Cryosections of human intra-lobar pulmonary arteries were immunostained with TLR2 (red fluorescence) and counterstained with DAPI (cell nuclei, blue). Elastic lamellae showed green auto-fluorescence.

Supporting Information

Movie S1   The video illustrating the deformation of a "soft" tube under the normal physiological pulsatile flow condition.

Movie S2   The video illustrating the deformation of a "stiff" tube under the normal physiological pulsatile flow condition.

Acknowledgments

The authors would like to thank Dr. Maria Frid for her help with tissue samples, Dr. Xianzhong Meng for his advice on TLR signaling and for providing human TLR antibodies and Qingchun Zeng for his help with experiments. Lung tissues from idiopathic PAH patients and control subjects were kindly provided by Dr. Barbara Meyrick and obtained from the Pulmonary Hypertension Breakthrough Initiative (PHBI), which is funded by the Cardiovascular Medical Research Education Fund (CMREF). The tissues were procured at the Transplant Procurement Centers at Stanford University, University of California, San Diego, Vanderbilt University and Allegheny General Hospital.

Author Contributions

Conceived and designed the experiments: YT DW HZ KS JH WT. Performed the experiments: YT HZ PT. Analyzed the data: KH WT. Contributed reagents/materials/analysis tools: WT. Wrote the paper: YT WT KS.

References

1. Adji A, O'Rourke MF, Namasivayam M (2011) Arterial stiffness, its assessment, prognostic value, and implications for treatment. Am J Hypertens 24: 5–17.
2. Hashimoto J, Ito S (2011) Central pulse pressure and aortic stiffness determine renal hemodynamics: pathophysiological implication for microalbuminuria in hypertension. Hypertension 58: 839–846.
3. Mitchell GF, van Buchem MA, Sigurdsson S, Gotal JD, Jonsdottir MK, et al. (2011) Arterial stiffness, pressure and flow pulsatility and brain structure and function: the Age, Gene/Environment Susceptibility—Reykjavik study. Brain 134: 3398–3407.
4. Lammers S, Scott DE, Hunter K, Tan W, Shandas R, et al. (2012) Mechanics and function of the pulmonary vasculature: Implications for pulmonary vascular disease and right ventricular function. Compr Physiol 1: 1–25.
5. Zachariah JP, Xanthakis V, Larson MG, Vita JA, Sullivan LM, et al. (2012) Circulating vascular growth factors and central hemodynamic load in the community. Hypertension 59: 773–779.
6. Wang Z, Chesler NC (2011) Pulmonary vascular wall stiffness: An important contributor to the increased right ventricular afterload with pulmonary hypertension. Pulm Circ 1: 212–223.
7. Burton A, editor (1966) Physiology and biophysics of the circulation. Chicago: Year Book.
8. Chiu RCJ (1995) Biophysics of pulsatile perfusion. J Thorac Cardiovas Surg 109: 810.
9. Chiu JJ, Chien S (2011) Effects of disturbed flow on vascular endothelium: pathophysiological basis and clinical perspectives. Physiological reviews 91: 327–387.
10. Davies PF (2009) Hemodynamic shear stress and the endothelium in cardiovascular pathophysiology. Nature clinical practice Cardiovascular medicine 6: 16–26.
11. Hahn C, Schwartz MA (2009) Mechanotransduction in vascular physiology and atherogenesis. Nature reviews Molecular cell biology 10: 53–62.
12. Li M, Scott DE, Shandas R, Stenmark KR, Tan W (2009) High pulsatility flow induces adhesion molecule and cytokine mRNA expression in distal pulmonary artery endothelial cells. Ann Biomed Eng 37: 1082–1092.
13. Curtiss LK, Tobias PS (2009) Emerging role of Toll-like receptors in atherosclerosis. J Lipid Res 50 Suppl: S340–345.
14. Dunzendorfer S, Lee HK, Tobias PS (2004) Flow-dependent regulation of endothelial Toll-like receptor 2 expression through inhibition of SP1 activity. Circ Res 95: 684–691.
15. Li X, Jiang S, Tapping RI (2010) Toll-like receptor signaling in cell proliferation and survival. Cytokine 49: 1–9.
16. Erridge C (2009) The roles of Toll-like receptors in atherosclerosis. J Innate Immun 1: 340–349.
17. Tian L, Lammers SR, Kao PH, Reusser M, Stenmark KR, et al. (2011) Linked opening angle and histological and mechanical aspects of the proximal pulmonary arteries of healthy and pulmonary hypertensive rats and calves. Am J Physiol Heart Circ Physiol 301: H1810–1818.
18. Lau EM, Iyer N, Ilsar R, Bailey BP, Adams MR, et al. (2012) Abnormal pulmonary artery stiffness in pulmonary arterial hypertension: in vivo study with intravascular ultrasound. PLoS One 7: e33331.
19. Sanz J, Kariisa M, Dellegrottaglie S, Prat-Gonzalez S, Garcia MJ, et al. (2009) Evaluation of pulmonary artery stiffness in pulmonary hypertension with cardiac magnetic resonance. JACC Cardiovasc Imaging 2: 286–295.
20. Hunter KS, Albietz JA, Lee PF, Lanning CJ, Lammers SR, et al. (2010) In vivo measurement of proximal pulmonary artery elastic modulus in the neonatal calf model of pulmonary hypertension: development and ex vivo validation. J Appl Physiol 108: 968–975.
21. Grignola JC, Domingo E, Aguilar R, Vazquez M, Lopez-Messeguer M, et al. (2011) Acute absolute vasodilatation is associated with a lower vascular wall stiffness in pulmonary arterial hypertension. Int J Cardiol.
22. Paz R, Mohiaddin RH, Longmore DB (1993) Magnetic resonance assessment of the pulmonary arterial trunk anatomy, flow, pulsatility and distensibility. Eur Heart J 14: 1524–1530.
23. Reuben SR (1971) Compliance of the human pulmonary arterial system in disease. Circ Res 29: 40–50.
24. Li M, Scott DE, Shandas R, Stenmark KR, Tan W (2009) High pulsatility flow induces adhesion molecule and cytokine mRNA expression in distal pulmonary artery endothelial cells. Ann Biomed Eng 37: 1082–1092.
25. Stenmark KR, McMurtry IF (2005) Vascular remodeling versus vasoconstriction in chronic hypoxic pulmonary hypertension: a time for reappraisal? Circ Res 97: 95–98.
26. Peng X, Haldar S, Deshpande S, Irani K, Kass DA (2003) Wall stiffness suppresses Akt/eNOS and cytoprotection in pulse-perfused endothelium. Hypertension 41: 378–381.
27. McCarthy CG, Goulopoulou S, Wenceslau CF, Spitler K, Matsumoto T, et al. (2014) Toll-like receptors and damage-associated molecular patterns: novel links between inflammation and hypertension. American journal of physiology Heart and circulatory physiology 306: H184–196.
28. Mian MO, Paradis P, Schiffrin EL (2014) Innate immunity in hypertension. Current hypertension reports 16: 413.
29. Singh MV, Chapleau MW, Harwani SC, Abboud FM (2014) The immune system and hypertension. Immunologic research.
30. Spirig R, Tsui J, Shaw S (2012) The Emerging Role of TLR and Innate Immunity in Cardiovascular Disease. Cardiology research and practice 2012: 181394.
31. Bogaard HJ, Natarajan R, Henderson SC, Long CS, Kraskauskas D, et al. (2009) Chronic pulmonary artery pressure elevation is insufficient to explain right heart failure. Circulation 120: 1951–1960.
32. Erridge C (2010) Endogenous ligands of TLR2 and TLR4: agonists or assistants? Journal of leukocyte biology 87: 989–999.
33. Hochleitner BW, Hochleitner EO, Obrist P, Eberl T, Amberger A, et al. (2000) Fluid shear stress induces heat shock protein 60 expression in endothelial cells in vitro and in vivo. Arteriosclerosis, thrombosis, and vascular biology 20: 617–623.
34. Pryshchep O, Ma-Krupa W, Younge BR, Goronzy JJ, Weyand CM (2008) Vessel-specific Toll-like receptor profiles in human medium and large arteries. Circulation 118: 1276–1284.
35. Mullick AE, Soldau K, Kiosses WB, Bell TA 3rd, Tobias PS, et al. (2008) Increased endothelial expression of Toll-like receptor 2 at sites of disturbed blood flow exacerbates early atherogenic events. J Exp Med 205: 373–383.
36. Jang HJ, Kim HS, Hwang DH, Quon MJ, Kim JA (2013) Toll-like receptor 2 mediates high-fat diet-induced impairment of vasodilator actions of insulin.

American journal of physiology Endocrinology and metabolism 304: E1077–1088.

37. Bertocchi C, Traunwieser M, Dorler J, Hasslacher J, Joannidis M, et al. (2011) Atorvastatin inhibits functional expression of proatherogenic TLR2 in arterial endothelial cells. Cellular physiology and biochemistry : international journal of experimental cellular physiology, biochemistry, and pharmacology 28: 625–630.

38. Higashikuni Y, Tanaka K, Kato M, Nureki O, Hirata Y, et al. (2013) Toll-like receptor-2 mediates adaptive cardiac hypertrophy in response to pressure overload through interleukin-1beta upregulation via nuclear factor kappaB activation. Journal of the American Heart Association 2: e000267.

39. Bauer EM, Chanthaphavong RS, Sodhi CP, Hackam DJ, Billiar TR, et al. (2014) Genetic deletion of toll-like receptor 4 on platelets attenuates experimental pulmonary hypertension. Circulation research 114: 1596–1600.

40. Broen JC, Bossini-Castillo L, van Bon L, Vonk MC, Knaapen H, et al. (2011) A rare polymorphism in the gene for Toll-like receptor 2 is associated with systemic sclerosis phenotype and increases the production of inflammatory mediators. Arthritis Rheum 64: 264–271.

14

Increased CD39 Nucleotidase Activity on Microparticles from Patients with Idiopathic Pulmonary Arterial Hypertension

Scott H. Visovatti[1]*, **Matthew C. Hyman**[2], **Diane Bouis**[1], **Richard Neubig**[3], **Vallerie V. McLaughlin**[1], **David J. Pinsky**[1]

1 Division of Cardiology, Department of Medicine, University of Michigan, Ann Arbor, Michigan, United States of America, 2 Department of Medicine, University of Pennsylvania, Philadelphia, Pennsylvania, United States of America, 3 Department of Pharmacology, University of Michigan, Ann Arbor, Michigan, United States of America

Abstract

Background: Idiopathic pulmonary arterial hypertension (IPAH) is a devastating disease characterized by increased pulmonary vascular resistance, smooth muscle and endothelial cell proliferation, perivascular inflammatory infiltrates, and *in situ* thrombosis. Circulating intravascular ATP, ADP, AMP and adenosine activate purinergic cell signaling pathways and appear to induce many of the same pathologic processes that underlie IPAH. Extracellular dephosphorylation of ATP to ADP and AMP occurs primarily *via* CD39 (ENTPD1), an ectonucleotidase found on the surface of leukocytes, platelets, and endothelial cells [1]. Microparticles are micron-sized phospholipid vesicles formed from the membranes of platelets and endothelial cells. *Objectives:* Studies here examine whether CD39 is an important microparticle surface nucleotidase, and whether patients with IPAH have altered microparticle-bound CD39 activity that may contribute to the pathophysiology of the disease.

Methodology/ Principal Findings: Kinetic parameters, inhibitor blocking experiments, and immunogold labeling with electron microscopy support the role of CD39 as a major nucleotidase on the surface of microparticles. Comparison of microparticle surface CD39 expression and nucleotidase activity in 10 patients with advanced IPAH and 10 healthy controls using flow cytometry and thin layer chromatograph demonstrate the following: 1) circulating platelet ($CD39^+CD31^+CD42b^+$) and endothelial ($CD39^+CD31^+CD42b^-$) microparticle subpopulations in patients with IPAH show increased CD39 expression; 2) microparticle ATPase and ADPase activity in patients with IPAH is increased.

Conclusions/ Significance: We demonstrate for the first time increased CD39 expression and function on circulating microparticles in patients with IPAH. Further research is needed to elucidate whether these findings identify an important trigger for the development of the disease, or reflect a physiologic response to IPAH.

Editor: Holger K. Eltzschig, University of Colorado Denver, United States of America

Funding: This work was supported by the Pulmonary Hypertension Breakthrough Initiative (DJP), and NIH grants P01HL089407-04 (DJP), R01HL086676-05 (DJP), R01HL085149-04 (DJP), T32HL007853-14 (SHV. and DJP), and the Taubman Medical Research Institute of the University of Michigan. Funding for the PHBI is provided by the Cardiovascular Medical Research and Education Fund (CMREF). The funders had no role in study design, data collection and analysis, decision to publish, or preparation of the manuscript.

Competing Interests: The authors have declared that no competing interests exist.

* E-mail: shv@med.umich.edu

Introduction

Idiopathic pulmonary artery hypertension (IPAH) is a devastating disease of unclear etiology that ultimately results in right-sided heart failure, low cardiac output and death. Though the exact etiology of IPAH remains unclear, the disease is characterized by increased pulmonary vascular resistance, smooth muscle and endothelial cell proliferation, perivascular inflammatory infiltrates, and *in situ* thrombosis. The contributions of prostanoids, endothelin-1, nitric oxide, BMPR-II signaling, endothelial dysfunction, and inflammation to the pathobiology of IPAH have been studied extensively, and such investigations form the basis of current treatment options [2]. Despite such advances, median survival in the modern treatment era is 3.6 years [3], increased from a mean survival of 2.8 years in untreated patients [4]. Thus,

continued investigation into the mechanisms leading to the development of IPAH is of paramount importance.

In addition to their roles as intracellular energy transporters, the purine nucleotides ATP, ADP, and AMP are important extracellular signaling molecules [5]. Such purinergic signaling is vital to the regulation of processes including vessel tone [6], apoptosis [7], smooth muscle and endothelial cell proliferation [8], platelet aggregation [9], and inflammation [10]; many of the same processes that are dysregulated in IPAH. Thus, it is possible that a perturbation in purinergic signaling due to a disruption in the normal intravascular nucleotide balance may play a role in the pathophysiology of IPAH.

Regulation of nucleotides within the extracellular, intravascular milieu is regulated in large part through the enzymatic activity of the transmembrane ectonucleotidase CD39 (ENTPD1) [11,12].

Studies have shown that CD39-mediated dephosphorylation of ATP and ADP into AMP plays a central role in vital homeostatic processes including thromboregulation [13], inflammation, stroke and the immune response [14], and apoptosis [15]. CD39 localizes to the surface of endothelial cells, circulating platelets, and some leukocytes [1]. Recently, CD39 activity has also been reported on circulating microparticles [16]. Microparticles are micron-sized phospholipid vesicles shed from cell membranes in response to activation or apoptosis [17]. The majority of circulating microparticles are thought to derive from platelets, with endothelial cell-, erythrocyte-, and leukocyte-derived microparticles contributing smaller percentages to the total circulating pool [18]. Each microparticle carries on it surface proteins specific to the membranes of the parent cell. The composition and structure of microparticles make them a unique circulating repository of potentially bioactive molecules, and studies have supported the participation of microparticles in diverse biological functions including thrombosis [19], hematopoiesis [20], and inflammation [21].

We hypothesize that circulating platelet and endothelial microparticles in patients with IPAH exhibit altered surface CD39 expression and function. If this hypothesis is validated, it would implicate altered purinergic signaling in the pathogenesis of IPAH, or activation of associated compensatory mechanisms.

Methods

Reagents used

HEPES buffer, TWEEN-20, isobutanol, isoamyl alcohol, 2-ethoxyethanol, ammonia, β-glycerophosphate, ammonium molybdate, levamizole, ouabain, oligomycin, and formic acid were obtained from Sigma-Aldrich (St. Louis, MO). M-270 epoxy Dynabeads, phosphate buffered saline, and RPMI containing 2.05 mM L-glutamine were purchased from Invitrogen (Carlsbad, CA). Six nanometer gold particles and gluteraldehyde phosphate buffer were purchased from Electron Microscopy Sciences (Hatfield, PA). Antibodies were purchased from the following vendors: mouse anti-human CD42b, FITC-conjugated mouse anti-human CD42b, APC-conjugated mouse anti-human CD31 and appropriate isotype controls (eBioscience, San Diego, CA); PE-conjugated mouse anti-human CD39 antibody and isotype control (Ancell, Bayport, MN); anti-CD39 clone A1, anti-ENTPD2 clone EPR3885, polyclonal anti-ENTPD3 and polyclonal anti-ENTPD8 (Abcam, Cambridge, MA). The inhibitors suramin, ARL 67156, and POM-1 were purchased from R&D

Table 2. Clinical, Functional and Hemodynamic Characteristics of IPAH Patients (N = 10).

World Health Organization Class		
	Class IV	100%
IPAH-specific Therapy		
	Parenteral Prostacyclin Therapy	100%
	Phosphodiesterase-5 Inhibitor	43%
	Endothelin-1 receptor Blocker	57%
Anticoagulation Therapy		
	Aspirin	16%
	Warfarin	59%
Functional		
	6-minute walking distance	170±33 meters
Hemodynamic		
	Mean Right Atrial Pressure	13.0±2.9 mm Hg
	Mean Pulmonary Arterial Pressure	54.8±5.7 mm Hg
	Mean Pulmonary Capillary Wedge Pressure	12.1±1.0 mm Hg
	Cardiac Output*	4.4±0.9L/min
	Cardiac Index*	1.84±0.4 L/min/m²
	Pulmonary Vascular Resistance	11.8±1.7 Wood Units

*Thermodilution method used. All values are expressed as mean ± standard error of the mean.

Systems (Minneapolis, MN). HistoGel was obtained from Thermo Scientific (Asheville, NC). For flow cytometry experiments CaliBRITE beads, FluoSphere fluorescent beads, Annexin V Binding Buffer, APC-conjugated annexin V, and TruCOUNT tubes were purchased from BD Biosciences (San Jose, CA). 14C-radiolabeled radiochemicals were purchased from the following vendors: ATP and ADP (MP Biomedicals, Solon, OH); ADP and adenosine (Perkin Elmer, Waltham, MA).

Patients and control subjects

The study protocol was approved by the Institutional Review Boards (IRBs) of the University of Michigan, Baylor University, Stanford University and the Cleveland Clinic. All subjects provided written informed consent. Patients who had been diagnosed with IPAH, and who were active on lung or heart-lung transplant lists, were approached for participation in the project. Inclusion criteria for patient participants were as follows: 1) a diagnosis of IPAH; 2) mean pulmonary artery pressure (mPAP) >25 mm Hg; 3) pulmonary capillary wedge pressure or left ventricular end diastolic pressure ≤15 mmHg; 4) pulmonary vascular resistance >3.0 Wood units; 5) total lung capacity >60% predicted; 6) Doppler echocardiogram demonstrating no significant mitral valve, aortic valve, or left heart disease; 7) pulmonary function testing demonstrated the absence of significant obstructive lung disease. Ten patients with idiopathic pulmonary arterial hypertension were recruited. The comparison control group

Table 1. Sample Characteristics.

		Controls (N = 10)	IPAH (N = 10)
Age (in years, Mean, Range)		41 (28 – 55)	47 (15 – 63)
Gender (N)			
	Males	0	0
	Females	10	10
Current Tobacco Use (N)			
	Yes	0	0
	No	10	10
Platelet Count (Mean, SEM)		197±31×10⁹	183×10⁹±34×10⁹

Table 3. Influence of inhibitors on relative ATPase and ADPase activity.

Inhibitor	Concentration	ATPase		ADPase	
		Control	IPAH	Control	IPAH
No inhibitor	-	100±3.2	100±1.2	100±2.4	100±6.8
β-glycerophosphate	10 mM	136±5.6	124±3.5	110±3.2	114±5.4
Ammonium molybdate	1 mM	101±4.7	92±6.2	98±6.7	94±4.9
Levamizole	1 mM	82±2.9	89±4.7	90±7.1	88±3.2
Ouabain	1 mM	117±5.1	104±2.7	102±4.8	92±8.8
Oligomycin	10 μg mL⁻¹	142±6.1	104±4.4	132±8.4	107±7.7
Suramin	0.5 mM	20±.0.1*	12±0.1*	15±0.5*	9±1*
ARL 67156	100 μM	22±0.1*	9±02*	14±0.3*	4±0.2*
POM-1	100 μM	7±0.1*	6±0.1*	1±0.1*	7±0.2

Relative nucleotidase activities expressed as percentage of available substrate dephosphorylated, and is normalized to reactions without inhibitors. The experiment was performed in triplicate using isolated microparticles from three healthy controls and three IPAH patients. *Significant difference from the sample without inhibitor ($P<0.05$).

consisted of ten gender- and race-matched controls recruited from the University of Michigan, Ann Arbor, Michigan.

Clinical and hemodynamic data

Age, race, gender, diagnosis, right heart catheterization pressures, 6-minute hall walk (6MHW) distances, World Health Organization functional capacity classification, platelet counts, and current medication for patients with IPAH were obtained through the PHBI network (Tables 1 and 2).

Whole blood collection

Antecubital venipuncture using a 21-gauge butterfly needle was used to collect 4.5 mL of whole blood in venous blood collection tubes with 0.5 mL of citrate solution (Becton Dickinson, Franklin Lakes, NJ). In the case of IPAH patients, collection of whole blood occurred at remote sites immediately prior to transplant. The collection tubes were placed in an insulated container containing wet ice, and transferred to our laboratory via overnight courier. To create similar conditions for control samples obtained locally, tubes containing whole blood samples from control patients were placed in insulated containers with wet ice for 16 hours, the average transportation time for IPAH samples.

Preparation of plasma

Platelet-poor plasma (PPP) was obtained by double centrifugation at room temperature (1,500× g for 25 minutes followed by 15,000× g for 45 minutes). The supernatant containing platelet-poor plasma was transferred to tubes, snap frozen using liquid nitrogen, and stored at −80 degrees Celsius.

Isolation of plasma microparticles

Frozen samples were thawed at 37 degrees Celsius. Platelet-poor plasma was added to 11×60 mm tubes (Seton Scientific, Los Gatos, California), and ultracentrifuged (ThermoFisher Scientific, Asheville, North Carolina) at 100,000× g for 75 minutes. For each tube, all but 100 μl of the supernatant was removed, and the remaining 100 μl was resuspended in a calcium-free HEPES buffer (10 mM/L HEPES, 5 mM/L KCl, 1 mM/L MgCl₂, 136 mM/L NaCl) at a pH of 7.4 and used for the experiments described.

Transmission electron microscopy (TEM)

Dynabeads were used to capture platelet microparticles from platelet poor plasma (PPP). The magnetic properties of the Dynabeads ensured a high yield of platelet microparticles despite multiple washing steps. M-270 epoxy Dynabeads were coated with mouse anti-human CD42b antibody to detect the glycoprotein Ib platelet surface antigen. PPP from a human control and coated Dynabeads were added to each of three Eppendorf tubes and mixed. Beads without capture antibody, as well as beads coated with IgG isotype control to correct for Fc binding, were also incubated with PPP as controls. A DynaMag-2 magnet (Invitrogen, Carlsbad, CA) was used to separate the Dynabeads coated with CD42b linked to microparticles from the PPP. The sample was resuspended in phosphate buffered saline (PBS) containing 0.01% TWEEN-20 and biotinylated mouse anti-human CD39 antibody was added. The sample was mixed and the Dynabeads removed using the magnet. The Dynabeads were resuspended in PBS, and Aurion streptavidin-linked 6 nanometer gold particles were added. The sample was mixed on a roller, and the Dynabeads were then separated from the supernatant using the magnet. The sample was resuspended in 0.25% gluteraldehyde phosphate buffer. Each sample was added to an Eppendorf tube containing HistoGel in such a way as to isolate the bulk of the Dynabeads at the tip of the tube. The hardened HistoGel sample was removed and stored in the gluteraldehyde phosphate buffer. Dynabead samples and controls were visualized using a Philips CM-100 electron microscope (FEI, Hillsboro, OR) at magnifications of 10,500 to 180,000X. Processing of samples and TEM imaging was performed by the University of Michigan Microscopy and Image Analysis Laboratory.

Flow cytometry

A flow cytometer (FACSCalibur, BD Biosciences, San Jose, CA) was used to count the number of microparticle events per milliliter of PPP, and to measure the expression of CD39 on platelet- and endothelial cell-derived microparticles. CaliBRITE beads and FACSComp software (BD, San Jose, CA) were used to check flow cytometer sensitivity and set the voltages and compensation prior to sample evaluation. All samples from patients and controls were processed during the same session using the following protocol. In order to identify the region containing microparticles, FluoSphere fluorescent beads with diameters of 0.5 and 1.5 microns were run using a forward versus side scatter dot plot, and the region between the two bead populations was gated as the population of interest. For total microparticle counts, microparticles isolated from 250 μL of PPP were resuspended in 500 μL of Annexin V Binding Buffer containing calcium. APC-conjugated annexin V was added to the sample and incubated for 30 minutes. The sample was transferred to a TruCOUNT tube containing a lyophilized pellet composed of a known number of fluorescent beads. The previously determined microparticle size gate and a gate around the TruCOUNT beads were used to determine the concentration of annexin-V⁺ microparticles per microliter of PPP using the following equation:

(number of events in microparticle region/number of events in count bead region) × *(number of beads per test/test volume)* × *a dilution factor of 2 = absolute microparticle count.*

Surface CD39 expression on endothelial and platelet microparticles was identified using triple flurophore-conjugated antibody labeling utilizing FITC-conjugated mouse anti-human

A

B

C

D

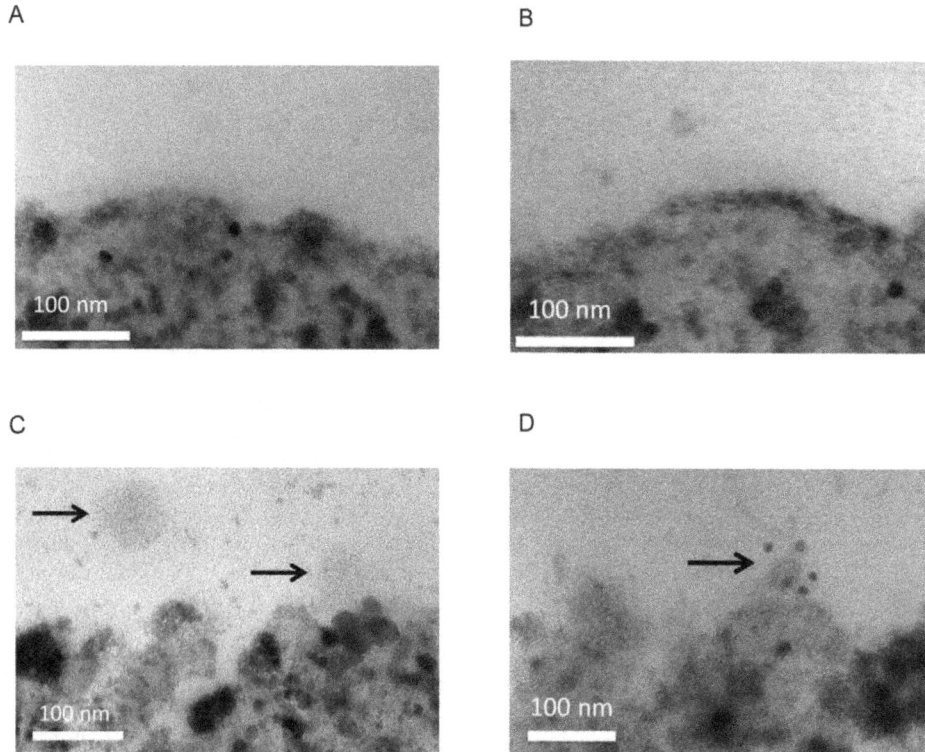

Figure 1. Transmission electron micrographs (TEM) of platelet microparticles (CD31⁺CD42b⁺) with immunogold labeling of surface CD39. (A) shows the surface of Dynabeads without CD42b capture antibody after exposure to PPP and (B) shows the surface of Dynabeads coated with IgG isotype control after PPP exposure. No microparticles adhered to the surfaces of these Dynabeads. Subsequent lack of immunogold staining for CD39 was also noted. Platelet microparticles were captured by Dynabeads coated with CD42b antibody (arrows on C, D). The sample imaged in C was not incubated with mouse anti-CD39 antibody conjugated to biotin prior to the addition of streptavidin-linked immunogold. (D) shows positive SA-immunogold labeling of a microparticle which was previously incubated with biotinylated anti-CD39. (all at 180,000× magnification).

CD42b, APC-conjugated mouse anti-human CD31, and PE-conjugated mouse anti-human CD39 antibody added to calcium-free HEPES buffer containing microparticles isolated by ultracentrifugation from 250 μL of PPP. After 30 minutes, 400 μL of HEPES buffer without calcium was added to the sample, and flow cytometry performed. A forward versus side scatter dot plot was used to gate microparticles based on size, as described previously. Triple staining was used to identify CD39 on platelet microparticles (CD39⁺CD31⁺CD42b⁺) and endothelial microparticles

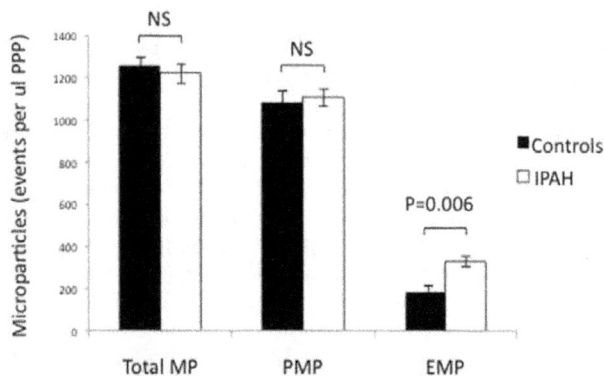

Figure 2. Quantification of circulating microparticles in healthy controls compared to IPAH patients. No difference was found in total microparticle (annexin V⁺) or platelet microparticle (CD31⁺CD42b⁺) levels. Patients with IPAH had a statistically significant increase in circulating endothelial microparticle (CD31⁺CD42b⁻) levels compared to controls. Results expressed as flow cytometric events per ul of platelet poor plasma (PPP) and presented as mean ± SEM. NA = not significant, MP = microparticles, PMP = platelet microparticles, EMP = endothelial microparticles.

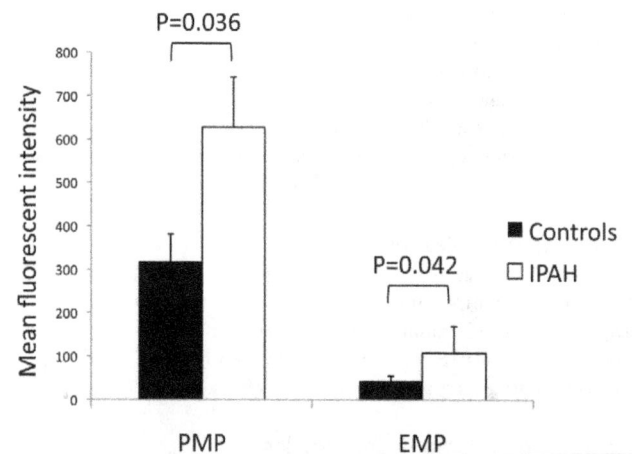

Figure 3. CD39 expression on platelet and endothelial microparticles. Flow cytometry revealed significantly increased surface CD39 expression on platelet (CD31+CD42b⁺) and endothelial (CD31⁺CD42b⁻) microparticles. PMP = platelet microparticles, EMP = endothelial microparticles.

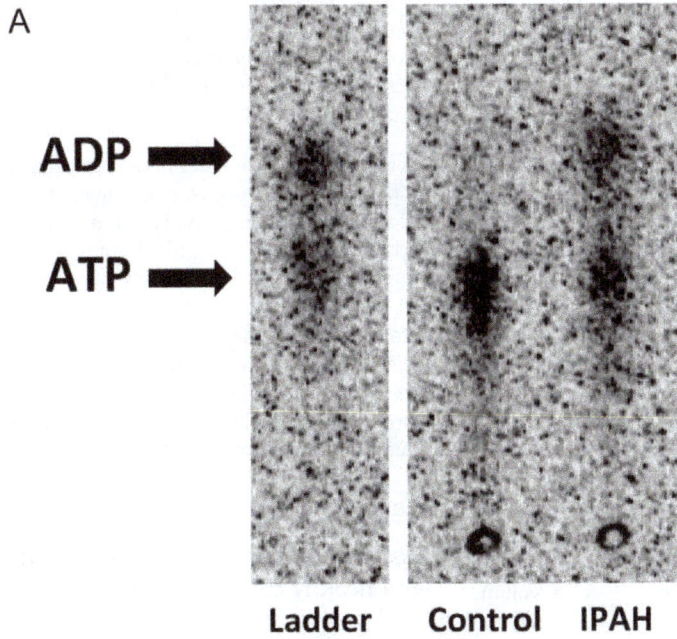

A

ADP ➡

ATP ➡

Ladder   Control   IPAH

B

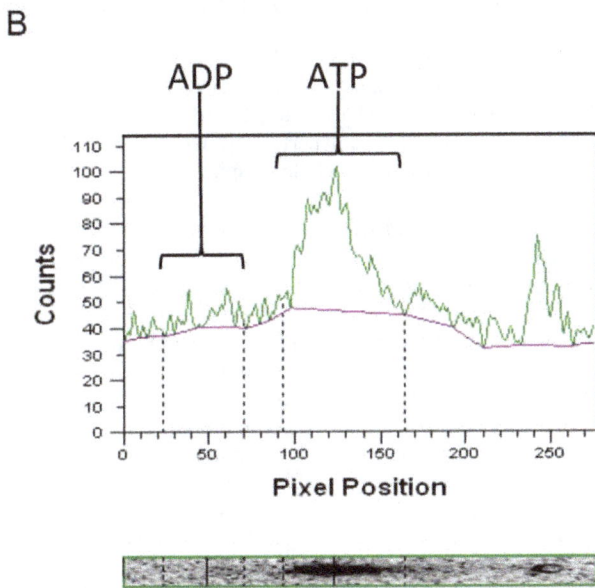

C

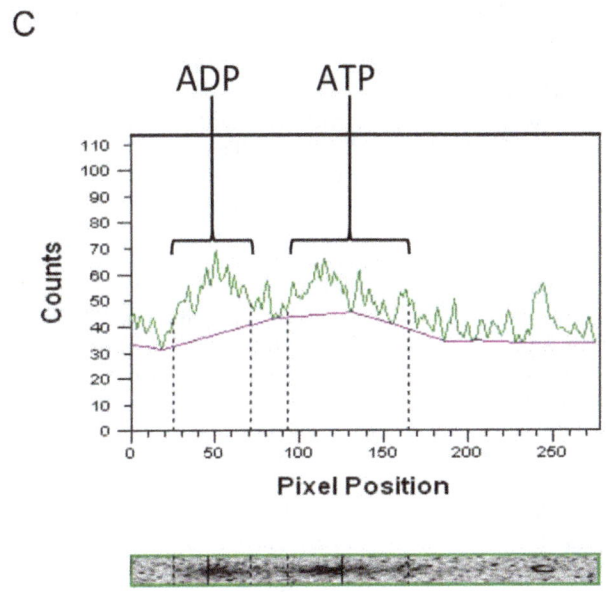

D

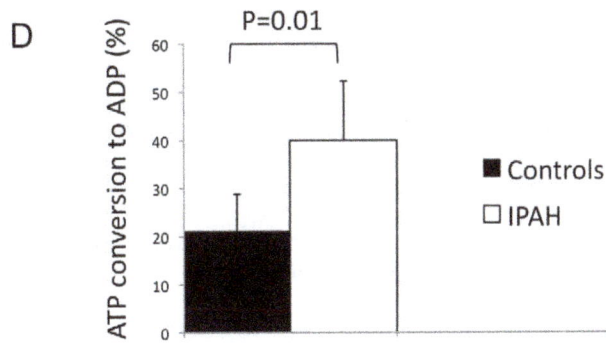

Figure 4. Measurement of CD39 ATPase activity on microparticles from healthy controls compared with IPAH patients. Representative thin layer chromatography (A) shows increased dephosphorylation of 14C-labeled ATP to ADP in samples incubated with microparticles isolated from a patient with IPAH compared to a healthy control. Quantification of radiolabeled ATP and ADP in TLC samples from Controls (B) and IPAH patients (C) revealed a significant increase in the percentage of ATP dephosphorylated to ADP, as shown in (D).

(CD39$^+$CD31$^+$CD42b$^-$). The mean fluorescent intensity (MFI) of CD39 was measured on both platelet and endothelial microparticles.

Thin layer chromatography

Thin layer chromatography (TLC) was used for enzyme kinetics and inhibitor assays. A previously described liquid phase consisting of isobutanol/isoamyl alcohol/2-ethoxyethanol/ammonia/H$_2$O in a 9:6:18:9:15 ratio [22] was added to a 20cm × 20cm rectangular thin layer chromatography tank (Fisher Scientific, Waltham, MA) and allowed to equalize. For each patient and control sample, microparticles were isolated from 250 µL of PPP using ultracentrifugation (100,000× g at 4 degrees Celsius for 70 minutes), and the concentrated microparticles were resuspended in HEPES buffer. Based on the microparticle count performed for each patient sample (described above), a volume containing 250,000 microparticles was placed in a 1.5 milliliter tube, and the total volume was brought to 25 µL by the addition of PBS, if needed. A substrate mix was created by mixing RPMI containing 2.05 mM L-glutamine with 40–60 mCi/mmol 14C-radiolabeled ATP or ADP. 25 µL of substrate mix was combined with each 25 µL microparticle sample. All tubes were incubated in a water bath at 37 degrees Celsius. Based on time course experiments that identified the linear phase of ATPase and ADPase reactions, 35 minutes was selected as the optimal water bath incubation time for the kinetics and inhibitor assays. A radiolabeled substrate concentration range of 0 to 500 mM was used to determine Km and Vmax for ATPase and ADPase activity. For inhibition assays, 5 µL of each inhibitor (Table 3) was added to the microparticle samples 60 minutes prior to the addition of the radiolabeled substrate. Inhibitors were used at the concentrations shown in Table 3, consistent with other published studies [23,24]. Each antibody blocking experiment was performed by pre-treating 250,000 isolated microparticles in 5 µL of reaction mixture with 5 µL of one of the following antibodies: anti-CD39 (clone A1, 0.025 mg/mL), anti-ENTPD2 (clone EPR3885, 0.25 mg/mL), anti-ENTPD3 (polyclonal, 0.23 mg/mL), anti-ENTPD8 (polyclonal, 0.25 mg/mL). The remainder of the assay was performed as described above. All steps were performed on ice prior to incubation in the water bath. Kinetic and inhibition assays were performed in triplicate using microparticles isolated from 3 healthy controls and 3 IPAH patients.

Following incubation, 8N formic acid was added to each tube to terminate enzymatic activity. One microliter of each sample, as well as a ladder containing 14C-radiolabeled ATP, ADP, AMP and (in some cases) adenosine were applied to a silica-based TLC plate (Sigma, St Louis, MO) and allowed to dry. The TLC plate was placed in the TLC tank containing the liquid phase, and removed 5 hours later. After drying, the TLC plate was covered in plastic wrap and placed on a storage phosphor screen for two hours. The phosphor screen was then scanned using a phosphor-imager (Typhoon, GE Life Sciences, Piscataway, NJ). Quantification of the intensity of TLC spots was performed using ImageQuant software (GE Healthcare, Piscataway, NJ). In order to determine the effects of needle size on nucleotidase activity phlebotomy utilizing antecubital vein access was performed on 3 healthy volunteers using three needle sizes (21G, 23G, 25G). Radiolabeled C-14 ADP was added to one set of reaction mixtures

to assess needle size effect on ADPase activity and C-14 ATP was added to another set of reaction mixtures to assess needle size effect on ATPase activity. Km and Vmax were determined using Prism 5.0 software (GraphPad Software, La Jolla, CA) to create a curve based upon the Michaelis-Menten equation.

Statistical analysis

All data were analyzed using SPSS Statistics (IBM, Somers, NY). Student's t-test was used to compare the mean ± standard error of the mean for variables between groups. Differences were considered significant at $p < 0.05$.

Results

Demographic and Medical Characteristics of IPAH patient and healthy controls

There were no significant differences in age ($M = 41$ years for controls, $M = 47$ years for IPAH, $p = 0.7$), race, or gender, and no subject was actively using tobacco (Table 1). There was no significant difference in platelet count between the two groups ($M = 197$ for controls, $M = 183$ for IPAH, $p = 0.72$). The medical, functional and hemodynamic characteristics of individuals with IPAH are described in Tables 1 and 2 and are consistent with advanced pulmonary arterial hypertension. Healthy controls were not taking any medications, including aspirin.

Transmission electron microscopy of microparticles

Circulating platelet microparticles were covalently linked to superparamagnetic Dynabeads. Figure 1A is a 180,000× magnification of a stock Dynabead without capture antibody coating, and Figure 1B is a 180,000× magnification of a Dynabead coated with IgG isotype control. Note the lack of microparticles bound to the surfaces, indicating that non-specific binding of platelet microparticles does not occur. These samples were also incubated with immunogold particles linked to streptavidin (SA). The lack of gold particles shows that nonspecific binding of SA to the bead surface does not occur. Figure 1C is a 180,000x magnification of a Dynabead coated with mouse anti-human CD42b antibody against platelet GP1b platelet surface antigen and then incubated with microparticles. The arrows identify a microparticle in the vicinity of the Dynabead (left) as well as a platelet microparticle captured on the surface (right). The sample was also exposed to SA-linked immunogold particles without having first been incubated with biotinylated mouse anti-human CD39. Note the lack of immunogold labeling of the microparticles in this figure, indicating that nonspecific binding of SA to microparticles does not occur. Figure 1D illustrates the result of pretreating platelet microparticles bound to Dynabeads with biotinylated mouse anti-human CD39 prior to the addition of SA-linked immunogold particles. The arrow identifies a bound microparticle with 6nm gold particles linked to surface CD39 through streptavidin-biotin interaction.

Quantification of circulating microparticles by flow cytometry

Measurements of circulating total microparticles, as well as platelet and endothelial microparticle subtypes, are shown in Figure 2. The results are given in units of flow cytometric "events

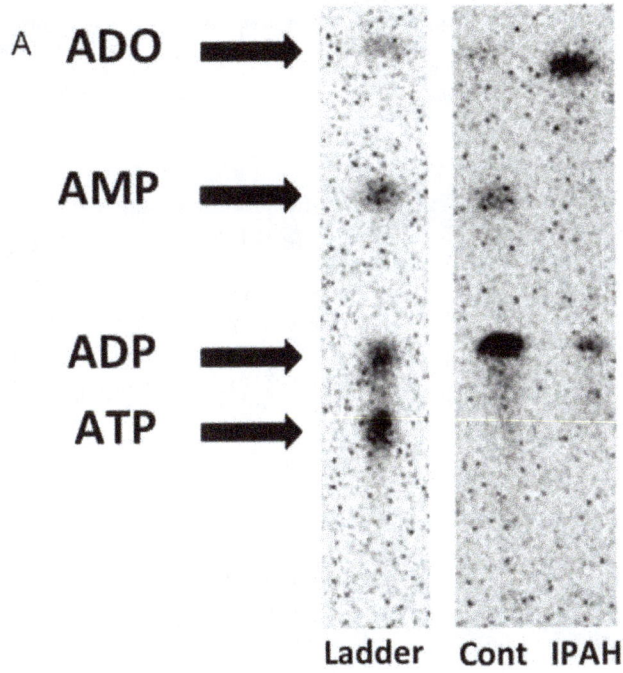

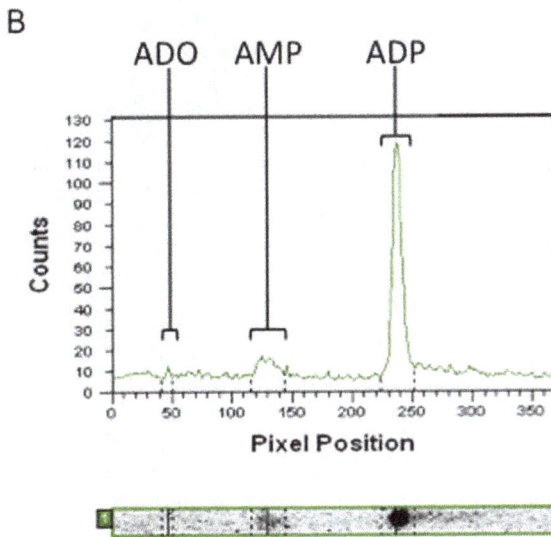

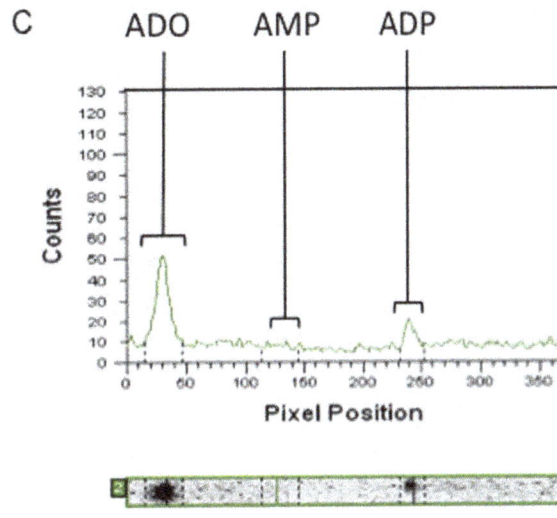

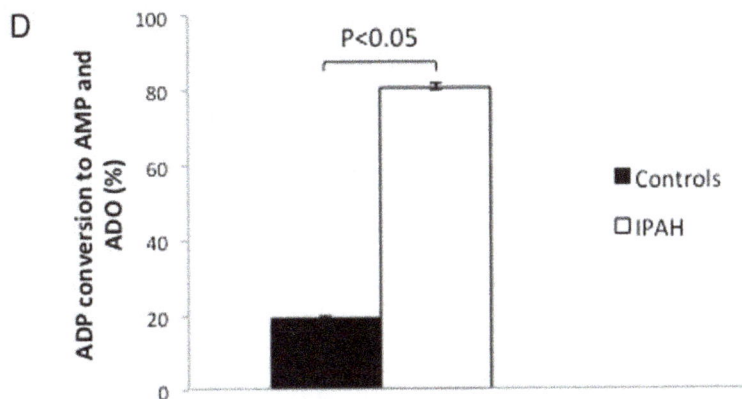

Figure 5. Measurement of CD39 ADPase activity on microparticles from healthy controls compared with IPAH patients.
Representative thin layer chromatography (A) shows increased dephosphorylation of 14C-labeled ADP to AMP and adenosine (ADO) in samples incubated with microparticles isolated from a patient with IPAH compared to a healthy control. Quantification of radiolabeled ADP, AMP and ADO in TLC samples from Controls (B) and IPAH patients (C) revealed a significant increase in the percentage of ADP dephosphorylated to AMP and adensoine, as shown in (D).

per microliter of PPP." In the case of the first pairing of bars on the left side of Figure 2, total microparticles were identified using annexin-V conjugated to the allophycocyanin fluorophore. Note that there is no statistically significant difference in the number of total microparticles circulating in patients with IPAH versus controls (1224±205 events/μl PPP vs. 1257±89 events/μl PPP). The number of circulating platelet microparticles ($CD31^+CD42b^+$) in IPAH patients and controls was also similar (1109±174 events/μl PPP vs. 1085±73 events/μl PPP). A statistically significant increase in circulating endothelial microparticles ($CD31^+CD42b^-$) was identified in patients with IPAH compared to healthy controls (330±32 events/μl PPP vs. 185±27 events/μl PPP), as shown by the pairing of bars to the right in Figure 2.

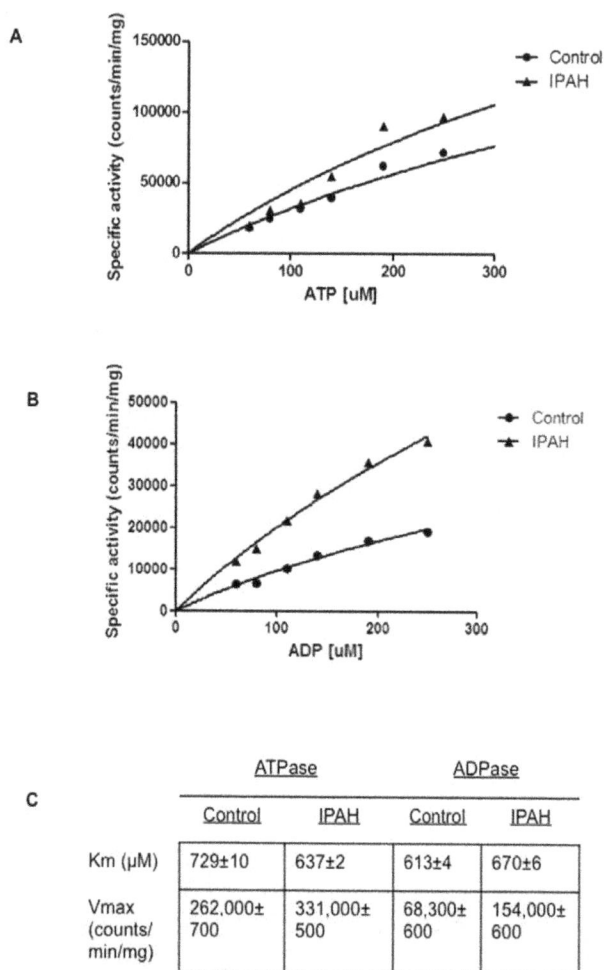

Flow cytometric comparison of microparticle surface CD39 expression

Figure 3 shows the mean fluorescent intensity of CD39 on circulating platelet microparticles ($CD39^+CD31^+CD42b^-$) and endothelial microparticles ($CD39^+CD31^+CD42b^+$), as determined by flow cytometry. As shown in the pairing of bars on the left, platelet microparticles from patients with IPAH have a statistically significant two-fold increase in CD39 expression compared to controls. The bars on the right of Figure 3 reflect the significant 2.5-fold increase in CD39 expression found on circulating endothelial microparticles from patients with IPAH compared to healthy controls.

Measurement of microparticle nucleotidase kinetics and inhibition by thin layer chromatography

Thin layer chromatography was used to separate carbon-14-labeled nucleotides after varying degrees of dephosphorylation by microparticle nucleotidase activity. Subsequent scanning of the TLC plates with a phosphorimager allowed for the quantification of ATP, ADP, AMP, and adenosine in each sample. As shown in Figure S1, differences in needle gauge did not produce a significant difference in the percentage of radiolabeled ATP or ADP dephosphorylayted. Figure 4 shows a representative plate assessing the ATPase activity of microparticles from one healthy control and one IPAH patient. No AMP or ADO signals were detected. Each of the processed plates containing samples from the remaining healthy controls and IPAH patients had similar results. The narrow left panel shows the ladder containing known radiolabeled nucleotides to facilitate identification of each nucleotide in the patient samples. The ladder mixture contains 14C-labeled nucleotides and adenosine, and is added to the plate at the same time as the patient samples. In Figure 4A, ADP has migrated more rapidly than ATP, and is thus closer to the top of the plate. The wider dual-lane panel on the right of Figure 4A shows the migration of samples from healthy controls and patients with IPAH. The left lane contains the nucleotide mixture that had been incubated with 250,000 microparticles from a healthy control. The lane containing the reaction mixture incubated with microparticles from a patient with IPAH shows spots with similar intensity in both the ATP and ADP regions. Thus, more ATP was dephosphorylated to ADP in the IPAH sample compared to the control sample, indicating increased ATPase activity. Figure 4B illustrates a quantitative scan of the data shown in 4A. The line running continuously underneath the contours of the histogram represents the background signal of the TLC plates, and is subtracted from the final volumes calculated for each nucleotide spot. The narrow, horizontal rectangle beneath the histogram is a smaller version of the TLC lane from Figure 4A, and aids in identifying the region of the spot to be quantified. Figure 4C shows the quantification of the ADP and ATP peaks for the IPAH lane shown in Figure 4A. Figure 4D shows the mean percentage of ATP dephosphorylated to ADP over the course of 35 minutes by microparticles for the ten healthy controls and ten IPAH patients studied. There is a statistically significant (50%) increase in microparticle ATPase activity in IPAH patients compared to controls (43.8±11.0% vs. 29.9±7.6%, p=0.01). Figure 5 compares ADPase activity of a healthy control versus that of an IPAH

	ATPase		ADPase	
	Control	IPAH	Control	IPAH
Km (μM)	729±10	637±2	613±4	670±6
Vmax (counts/ min/mg)	262,000± 700	331,000± 500	68,300± 600	154,000± 600

Figure 6. A comparison of ATPase (A) and ADPase (B) activities of microparticles from healthy controls and IPAH patients. Km and Vmax values are shown (C). Non-linear regression was used to fit experimental data to the curves using the Mihaelis-Menten equation. Data are means ± SEM from triplicate experiments using microparticles isolated from three healthy controls and three IPAH patients.

A

B

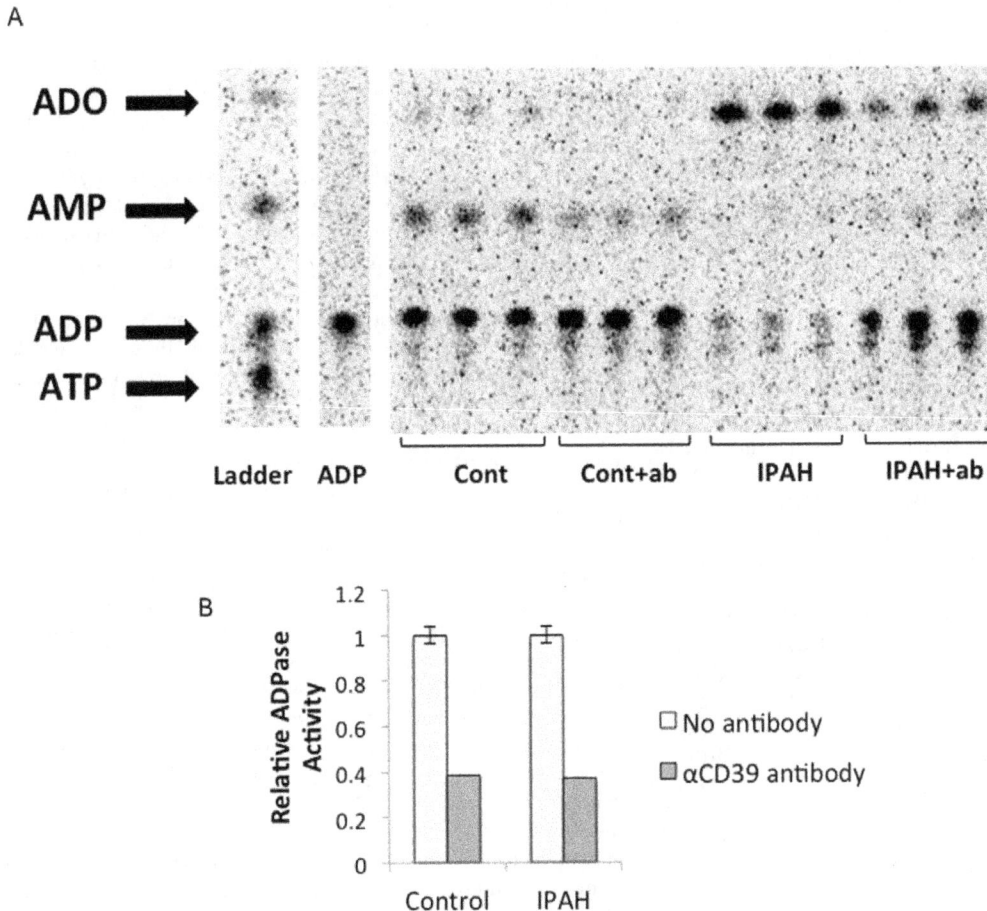

Figure 7. Microparticle ADPase inhibition using anti-CD39 monoclonal antibody. (**A**) TLC performed following anti-CD39 pre-treatment of microparticles from healthy controls and IPAH patients (**Cont+ab** and **IPAH+ab**) shows a decrease in the dephosphorylation of 14C ADP to AMP and adenosine (ADO) in both groups compared to samples without antibody pre-treatment (**Cont** and **IPAH**). The ADP lane contains 14C ADP subjected to the same experimental conditions but without microparticles. Quantification of the percent of available 14C ADP converted to AMP and ADO (**B**) reveals a relative decrease in nucleotidase activity of 62% in controls and 63% in IPAH patients (normalized to samples not pre-treated with antibody).

patient following the addition of 14C ADP to a reaction mixture containing 250,000 microparticles. As shown, microparticles from IPAH patients dephosphorylated 400% more 14C ADP to AMP and adenosine than the control ($80.8 \pm 0.8\%$ vs. $19.0 \pm 0.83\%$, $p < 0.05$).

The results of ATPase and ADPase kinetic assays are shown in Figure 6. At the chosen incubation time of 35 minutes about 28% of ATP and 25% of ADP are dephosphorylated, indicating that near-initial rate conditions are satisfied. Figures 6A and 6B show the data fit to Michaelis-Menten curves. The apparent K_m for the dephosphorylation of ATP by microparticles from controls and IPAH patients was of essentially the same magnitude (729 ± 10 µM and 637 ± 2 µM, respectively). Similarly, the apparent K_m for the dephosphorylation of ADP by microparticles from controls and IPAH patients was 613 ± 4 µM and 670 ± 6 µM, respectively. The V_{max} for the dephosphorylation of ATP by microparticles from IPAH patients was significantly greater than the Vmax for controls ($331,000 \pm 500$ versus $262,000 \pm 700$ counts per minute per mg of microprticles, respectively). Similarly, the V_{max} for the dephosphorylation of ADP by microparticles from IPAH patients and controls was quite different ($154,000 \pm 600$ versus $68,300 \pm 600$ counts per minute per mg of microprticles, respectively). A comparison of the kinetics data in Figure 6C shows that the difference in ATP and ADP nucleotidase activity in controls versus patients with IPAH result in a substantial increase in V_{max} with minimal change in K_m.

To determine whether the predominant microparticle nucleotidase is consistent with an ectonucleoside triphosphate diphosphohydrolase (ENTPD), specifically CD39 (ENTPD-1), inhibitor studies were performed. Ouabain [25] was used to inhibit Na^+/K^+ ATPase activity, and the mitochondrial ATPase was inhibited with sodium azide and oligomycin [26]. The acid phosphatase inhibitor ammonium molybdate (also an inhibitor of 5′-nuceotidases), the Ser/Thr phosphatase inhibitor beta-glycerophosphate, and the alkaline phosphatase inhibitor levamizole were also tested. As shown in Table 3, there was no effect of any of these inhibitors on either ATPase or ADPase activity. However, the addition of the non-penetrating ectonucleotidase inhibitor suramin [27], the selective ecto-ATPase inhibitor ARL 67156 [28] or POM-1, a selective inhibitor of ENTPD-1, -2, and -3 [29], significantly decreased ATPase and ADPase activity on both control and IPAH microparticles.

To further identify CD39 as the predominant microparticle ectonucleotidase, antibody blocking experiments were performed using antibodies against ENTPD-1 (CD39), ENTPD-2, ENTPD-3, and ENTPD-8. The chromatogram in Figure 7A shows ADPase activity after 60 minutes of pre-treatment of microparticles with the anti-CD39 antibody. Microparticles from both healthy controls (**Cont**) and IPAH patients (**IPAH**) dephosphorylated less 14C ADP to AMP and adenosine (**ADO**) after pre-treatment with the anti-CD39 antibody. The relative ADPase activity of microparticles isolated from control and IPAH patients decreased by 62% and 63%, respectively, after pre-treatment with αCD39 antibody (Figure 7B). In order to rule out a significant role for related ENTPDases, experiments were performed using pre-treatment with antibodies against ENTPD-2, -3, and -8. These antibodies produced no change in ADPase or ATPase activity (data not shown).

Discussion

The current study characterizes, for the first time, the nucleotidase activity of microparticles isolated from healthy controls and patients with IPAH. In addition, we demonstrate that microparticles isolated from IPAH patients have increased ATPase and ADPase activity, as well as increased surface CD39 expression. Our finding of similar ATPase and ADPase apparent Km values for control and IPAH microparticles suggests that it is the same enzyme present on the surface of microparticles of both groups. Additionally, the ratio of ATPase to ADPase Vmax values of 3.9 (control) and 2.1 (IPAH) is similar to the 2.5-fold difference found by Zebisch et al in their characterization of CD39 refolded from bacterial inclusion bodies [30]. This is consistent with CD39 being the primary ATP and ADP nucleotidase on the microparticles. The role of an ENTPDase is more directly supported by inhibitor blocking studies. Antibody blocking experiments further identify CD39 as a significant microparticle ENTPDase. TEM showing positive immunogold labeling of CD39 on the surface of circulating platelet microparticles also supports the presence of CD39 on the surface of microparticles. We chose to capture the platelet-derived subtype of microparticle for TEM because it comprises the majority of circulating microparticles [18].

The finding of a significant increase in microparticle CD39 may have clinical implications. Earlier work by Banz et al [16] and Bakouboula et al [31] support the hypothesis that microparticle compositions have systemic effects, and that alterations in microparticle phenotype may be related to pathological states. In the case of IPAH, an increase in circulating microparticle CD39 activity may result in a shift in the intravascular nucleotide/nucleoside milieu away from an ATP- and ADP-laden environment. ATP has been shown to have a potent endothelium-dependent vasodilatory effect on human pulmonary arteries *via* its ability to stimulate nitric oxide [32] and prostacyclin [33] release from vascular endothelium. Treatment with infusions of ATP-MgCl$_2$ has been shown to be a safe and effective treatment for pulmonary hypertension associated with congenital heart defects in children [6]. Decreased levels of both prostacyclin and nitric oxide have been found in patients with IPAH, and exogenous administration of them are validated therapies for patients with the disease.[2] Thus, a decrease in intravascular ATP concentration through increased microparticle ATPase activity may contribute to the increased pulmonary vascular resistance measured in patients with IPAH.

The increased microparticle surface CD39 described in our study may instead reflect a compensatory mechanism activated by the body in an attempt to mitigate the pro-inflammatory, pro-thrombotic, hyper-proliferative processes associated with IPAH. An increase in ATP and ADPase activity shifts the intravascular nucleotide composition towards increased AMP. AMP is the substrate for ecto-5′ nucleotidase (CD73), a membrane bound glycoprotein that dephosphorylates AMP into adenosine [34]. Adenosine is a known vasodilator [35] that also modulates platelet

aggregation [36], inflammation [37], and cell proliferation [38]. Platelet-derived ADP is a potent stimulator of platelet aggregation [9] and thrombus formation [39], and acts in a synergistic fashion with peptide growth factors to induce SMC proliferation [40]. Thus, CD39- and CD73-mediated conversion of ATP and ADP into AMP and ultimately adenosine may at once deprive the intravascular milieu of pro-thrombotic, pro-inflammatory nucleotides and increase the availability of a vasodilatory, anti-inflammatory, anti-thrombotic, and anti-proliferative nucleoside.

Our studies show an increase in the number of circulating endothelial microparticles, but no difference in total or platelet microparticles in patients with IPAH compared to healthy controls. These findings are consistent with those of Amabile et al, who identified circulating endothelial microparticles as CD31$^+$CD41$^-$ (glycoprotein IIB negative) by flow cytometry [41]. Our measured total, endothelial, and platelet microparticle concentrations are lower than those in this earlier study, and may be secondary to differences in flow cytometric technique or a lesser degree of systemic activation.

Our study has several limitations. Our sample size of ten patients with IPAH reflects the rarity of this disease. The creation of the PHBI network has enabled researchers to share invaluable tissue from patients, and continued collaboration through the network will allow us to increase the sample size of future experiments. Our IPAH samples were shipped to our laboratory, arriving one day after phlebotomy. While this did not affect microparticle concentration or nucleotidase activity, intravascular nucleotides are known to degrade rapidly. Thus, the actual concentrations of nucleotides in the blood samples were not measured in these studies. Future investigations will measure intravascular nucleotide concentrations in IPAH patients recruited from our institution, allowing for rapid measurement soon after phlebotomy.

In conclusion, our investigation utilizes kinetic, inhibition, and TEM studies to identify CD39 as an important nucleotidase on circulating microparticles. We also demonstrate increased CD39 expression on the surface of circulating platelet (CD31$^+$CD42b$^+$) and endothelial (CD31$^+$CD42b$^-$) microparticle subpopulations in patients with IPAH. We have shown increased microparticle ATPase and ADPase activity in patients with this disease, indicating that the increased surface CD39 is functional. Further studies are needed to determine whether the increase in functional microparticle-bound CD39 contributes to the pathogenesis of IPAH, or whether it represents a compensatory mechanism aimed at mitigating the devastating effects of this rapidly fatal disease.

Supporting Information

Figure S1 Needle gauge used for phlebotomy does not alter CD39 activity on microparticles. Phlebotomy utilizing antecubital vein access was performed on 3 healthy volunteers using three needle sizes (21G, 23G, 25G). Radiolabeled 14C ADP was added to one set of reaction mixtures to assess needle size effect on CD39 **ADPase** activity and 14C ATP was added to another set of reaction mixtures to assess needle size effect on CD39 **ATPase** activity (**A**). Differences in needle gauge did not produce a significant difference in the percentage of radiolabeled ADP (**B**) or ATP (**C**) dephosphorylayted. Isolation of microparticles, TLC, and quantification of enzyme activity were performed as described in the Methods section of primary manuscript.

Increased CD39 Nucleotidase Activity on Microparticles from Patients with Idiopathic Pulmonary Arterial...

149

Acknowledgments

We wish to thank Dotty Sorenson; Kevin Bobbitt, PhD; Linda Thompson, PhD; and Angela Hawley for methodologic advice. Patient samples were provided by Baylor University, Stanford University and the Cleveland Clinic under the Pulmonary Hypertension Breakthrough Initiative (PHBI).

References

1. Koziak K, Sevigny J, Robson SC, Siegel JB, Kaczmarek E (1999) Analysis of CD39/ATP diphosphohydrolase (ATPDase) expression in endothelial cells, platelets and leukocytes. Thromb Haemost 82: 1538–1544.

2. McLaughlin VV, Archer SL, Badesch DB, Barst RJ, Farber HW, et al. (2009) ACCF/AHA 2009 expert consensus document on pulmonary hypertension a report of the American College of Cardiology Foundation Task Force on Expert Consensus Documents and the American Heart Association developed in collaboration with the American College of Chest Physicians; American Thoracic Society, Inc.; and the Pulmonary Hypertension Association. J Am Coll Cardiol 53: 1573–1619.

3. Thenappan T, Shah SJ, Rich S, Gomberg-Maitland M (2007) A USA-based registry for pulmonary arterial hypertension: 1982–2006. Eur Respir J 30: 1103–1110.

4. D'Alonzo GE, Barst RJ, Ayres SM, Bergofsky EH, Brundage BH, et al. (1991) Survival in patients with primary pulmonary hypertension. Results from a national prospective registry. Ann Intern Med 115: 343–349.

5. Burnstock G (1972) Purinergic nerves. Pharmacol Rev 24: 509–581.

6. Brook MM, Fineman JR, Bolinger AM, Wong AF, Heymann MA, et al. (1994) Use of ATP-MgCl2 in the evaluation and treatment of children with pulmonary hypertension secondary to congenital heart defects. Circulation 90: 1287–1293.

7. Dawicki DD, Chatterjee D, Wyche J, Rounds S (1997) Extracellular ATP and adenosine cause apoptosis of pulmonary artery endothelial cells. Am J Physiol 273: L485–494.

8. McAuslan BR, Reilly WG, Hannan GN, Gole GA (1983) Angiogenic factors and their assay: activity of formyl methionyl leucyl phenylalanine, adenosine diphosphate, heparin, copper, and bovine endothelium stimulating factor. Microvasc Res 26: 323–338.

9. Dorsam RT, Kunapuli SP (2004) Central role of the P2Y12 receptor in platelet activation. J Clin Invest 113: 340–345.

10. Chen Y, Corriden R, Inoue Y, Yip L, Hashiguchi N, et al. (2006) ATP release guides neutrophil chemotaxis via P2Y2 and A3 receptors. Science 314: 1792–1795.

11. Kaczmarek E, Koziak K, Sevigny J, Siegel JB, Anrather J, et al. (1996) Identification and characterization of CD39/vascular ATP diphosphohydrolase. J Biol Chem 271: 33116–33122.

12. Marcus AJ, Broekman MJ, Drosopoulos JH, Islam N, Alyonycheva TN, et al. (1997) The endothelial cell ecto-ADPase responsible for inhibition of platelet function is CD39. J Clin Invest 99: 1351–1360.

13. Pinsky DJ, Broekman MJ, Peschon JJ, Stocking KL, Fujita T, et al. (2002) Elucidation of the thromboregulatory role of CD39/ectoapyrase in the ischemic brain. J Clin Invest 109: 1031–1040.

14. Berchtold S, Ogilvie AL, Bogdan C, Muhl-Zurbes P, Ogilvie A, et al. (1999) Human monocyte derived dendritic cells express functional P2X and P2Y receptors as well as ecto-nucleotidases. FEBS Lett 458: 424–428.

15. Goepfert C, Imai M, Brouard S, Csizmadia E, Kaczmarek E, et al. (2000) CD39 modulates endothelial cell activation and apoptosis. Mol Med 6: 591–603.

16. Banz Y, Beldi G, Wu Y, Atkinson B, Usheva A, et al. (2008) CD39 is incorporated into plasma microparticles where it maintains functional properties and impacts endothelial activation. Br J Haematol 142: 627–637.

17. Freyssinet JM (2003) Cellular microparticles: what are they bad or good for? J Thromb Haemost 1: 1655–1662.

18. Horstman LL, Ahn YS (1999) Platelet microparticles: a wide-angle perspective. Crit Rev Oncol Hematol 30: 111–142.

19. Combes V, Simon AC, Grau GE, Arnoux D, Camoin L, et al. (1999) In vitro generation of endothelial microparticles and possible prothrombotic activity in patients with lupus anticoagulant. J Clin Invest 104: 93–102.

20. Baj-Krzyworzeka M, Majka M, Pratico D, Ratajczak J, Vilaire G, et al. (2002) Platelet-derived microparticles stimulate proliferation, survival, adhesion, and chemotaxis of hematopoietic cells. Exp Hematol 30: 450–459.

21. Distler JH, Pisetsky DS, Huber LC, Kalden JR, Gay S, et al. (2005) Microparticles as regulators of inflammation: novel players of cellular crosstalk in the rheumatic diseases. Arthritis Rheum 52: 3337–3348.

22. Yegutkin GG, Samburski SS, Jalkanen S (2003) Soluble purine-converting enzymes circulate in human blood and regulate extracellular ATP level via counteracting pyrophosphatase and phosphotransfer reactions. FASEB J 17: 1328–1330.

23. Kiffer-Moreira T, Fernandes Sampaio ME, Alviano DS, Axelband F, Cesar GV, et al. (2010) Biochemical characterization of an ecto-ATP diphosphohydrolase activity in Candida parapsilosis and its possible role in adenosine acquisition and pathogenesis. FEMS yeast research 10: 735–746.

24. Wall MJ, Wigmore G, Lopatar J, Frenguelli BG, Dale N (2008) The novel NTPDase inhibitor sodium polyoxotungstate (POM-1) inhibits ATP breakdown but also blocks central synaptic transmission, an action independent of NTPDase inhibition. Neuropharmacology 55: 1251–1258.

25. Blaustein MP, Juhaszova M, Golovina VA (1998) The cellular mechanism of action of cardiotonic steroids: a new hypothesis. Clinical and experimental hypertension 20: 691–703.

26. Meyer-Fernandes JR, Dutra PM, Rodrigues CO, Saad-Nehme J, Lopes AH (1997) Mg-dependent ecto-ATPase activity in Leishmania tropica. Archives of biochemistry and biophysics 341: 40–46.

27. Voogd TE, Vansterkenburg EL, Wilting J, Janssen LH (1993) Recent research on the biological activity of suramin. Pharmacological reviews 45: 177–203.

28. Crack BE, Pollard CE, Beukers MW, Roberts SM, Hunt SF, et al. (1995) Pharmacological and biochemical analysis of FPL 67156, a novel, selective inhibitor of ecto-ATPase. British journal of pharmacology 114: 475–481.

29. Muller CE, Iqbal J, Baqi Y, Zimmermann H, Rollich A, et al. (2006) Polyoxometalates–a new class of potent ecto-nucleoside triphosphate diphosphohydrolase (NTPDase) inhibitors. Bioorganic & medicinal chemistry letters 16: 5943–5947.

30. Zebisch M, Strater N (2007) Characterization of Rat NTPDase1, -2, and -3 ectodomains refolded from bacterial inclusion bodies. Biochemistry 46: 11945–11956.

31. Bakouboula B, Morel O, Faure A, Zobairi F, Jesel L, et al. (2008) Procoagulant membrane microparticles correlate with the severity of pulmonary arterial hypertension. Am J Respir Crit Care Med 177: 536–543.

32. Bogle RG, Coade SB, Moncada S, Pearson JD, Mann GE (1991) Bradykinin and ATP stimulate L-arginine uptake and nitric oxide release in vascular endothelial cells. Biochem Biophys Res Commun 180: 926–932.

33. Boeynaems JM, Galand N (1983) Stimulation of vascular prostacyclin synthesis by extracellular ADP and ATP. Biochem Biophys Res Commun 112: 290–296.

34. Zimmermann H (1992) 5′-Nucleotidase: molecular structure and functional aspects. Biochem J 285 (Pt 2): 345–365.

35. Edmunds NJ, Marshall JM (2003) The roles of nitric oxide in dilating proximal and terminal arterioles of skeletal muscle during systemic hypoxia. J Vasc Res 40: 68–76.

36. Bullough DA, Zhang C, Montag A, Mullane KM, Young MA (1994) Adenosine-mediated inhibition of platelet aggregation by acadesine. A novel antithrombotic mechanism in vitro and in vivo. The Journal of clinical investigation 94: 1524–1532.

37. Cronstein BN, Kramer SB, Weissmann G, Hirschhorn R (1983) Adenosine: a physiological modulator of superoxide anion generation by human neutrophils. J Exp Med 158: 1160–1177.

38. Dubey RK, Gillespie DG, Mi Z, Jackson EK (1998) Adenosine inhibits growth of human aortic smooth muscle cells via A2B receptors. Hypertension 31: 516–521.

39. Marcus AJ, Broekman MJ, Drosopoulos JH, Islam N, Pinsky DJ, et al. (2003) Heterologous cell-cell interactions: thromboregulation, cerebroprotection and cardioprotection by CD39 (NTPDase-1). J Thromb Haemost 1: 2497–2509.

40. Crowley ST, Dempsey EC, Horwitz KB, Horwitz LD (1994) Platelet-induced vascular smooth muscle cell proliferation is modulated by the growth amplification factors serotonin and adenosine diphosphate. Circulation 90: 1908–1918.

41. Amabile N, Heiss C, Real WM, Minasi P, McGlothlin D, et al. (2008) Circulating endothelial microparticle levels predict hemodynamic severity of pulmonary hypertension. Am J Respir Crit Care Med 177: 1268–1275.

Author Contributions

Conceived and designed the experiments: SHV MCH DB RRN VVM DJP. Performed the experiments: SHV MCH. Analyzed the data: SHV MCH DB RRN VVM DJP. Wrote the paper: SHV DJP.

15

Pressure Load: The Main Factor for Altered Gene Expression in Right Ventricular Hypertrophy in Chronic Hypoxic Rats

Jonas D. Baandrup[1,⑨], **Lars H. Markvardsen**[1,⑨], **Christian D. Peters**[2], **Uffe K. Schou**[2], **Jens L. Jensen**[3], **Nils E. Magnusson**[1], **Torben F. Ørntoft**[4], **Mogens Kruhøffer**[4], **Ulf Simonsen**[1]*

1 Department of Pharmacology, Aarhus University, Aarhus, Denmark, **2** The Water and Salt Research Center, Department of Anatomy, Aarhus University, Aarhus, Denmark, **3** Department of Theoretical Statistics, Institute of Mathematics, Aarhus University, Aarhus, Denmark, **4** Molecular Diagnostic Laboratory, Department of Clinical Biochemistry, Aarhus University Hospital, Aarhus, Denmark

Abstract

Background: The present study investigated whether changes in gene expression in the right ventricle following pulmonary hypertension can be attributed to hypoxia or pressure loading.

Methodology/Principal Findings: To distinguish hypoxia from pressure-induced alterations, a group of rats underwent banding of the pulmonary trunk (PTB), sham operation, or the rats were exposed to normoxia or chronic, hypobaric hypoxia. Pressure measurements were performed and the right ventricle was analyzed by Affymetrix GeneChip, and selected genes were confirmed by quantitative PCR and immunoblotting. Right ventricular systolic blood pressure and right ventricle to body weight ratio were elevated in the PTB and the hypoxic rats. Expression of the same 172 genes was altered in the chronic hypoxic and PTB rats. Thus, gene expression of enzymes participating in fatty acid oxidation and the glycerol channel were downregulated. mRNA expression of aquaporin 7 was downregulated, but this was not the case for the protein expression. In contrast, monoamine oxidase A and tissue transglutaminase were upregulated both at gene and protein levels. 11 genes (e.g. insulin-like growth factor binding protein) were upregulated in the PTB experiment and downregulated in the hypoxic experiment, and 3 genes (e.g. c-kit tyrosine kinase) were downregulated in the PTB and upregulated in the hypoxic experiment.

Conclusion/Significance: Pressure load of the right ventricle induces a marked shift in the gene expression, which in case of the metabolic genes appears compensated at the protein level, while both expression of genes and proteins of importance for myocardial function and remodelling are altered by the increased pressure load of the right ventricle. These findings imply that treatment of pulmonary hypertension should also aim at reducing right ventricular pressure.

Editor: Carlo Gaetano, Istituto Dermopatico dell'Immacolata, Italy

Funding: Jonas Baandrup was supported by the Danish Heart Foundation, and Ulf Simonsen was supported by the Danish Lung Foundation and the Danish Research Council. The funders had no role in study design, data collection and analysis, decision to publish, or preparation of the manuscript.

Competing Interests: The authors have declared that no competing interests exist.

* E-mail: us@farm.au.dk

⑨ These authors contributed equally to this work.

Introduction

Pulmonary arterial hypertension is a heterogeneous group of disorders characterized by increased pulmonary artery pressure and resistance as a result of pulmonary vascular remodeling, active vasoconstriction, and in-situ thrombosis. The increased pressure load results in right ventricular hypertrophy representing an initial stage which can progress to failure and death [1]. The current treatments with prostaglandin (PGI_2) analogues (e.g. epoprostenol), endothelin receptor antagonists (e.g. bosentan), and phosphodiesterase 5 inhibitors (e.g. sildenafil) have markedly improved the prognosis of the disease [2]. Direct inotropic effects of epoprostenol on the right ventricle was described [3,4] and that bosentan reduces cardiac fibrosis and hypertrophy [5]. However, these treatments are mainly vasodilatory and antiproliferative, and hence targeting the vasculature rather than the right ventricle in pulmonary hypertension.

Parameters of right ventricular function such as cardiac index and mean right atrial pressure are the most important determinants of survival in pulmonary arterial hypertension [1]. Multiple signal transduction pathways are known to be involved in the remodeling of the heart [6]. Although it is a matter of debate which mechanisms are important for transition to failure and hypertrophy, failure of the left ventricle are characterized to varying degrees by changes in extracellular matrix composition, energy metabolism, contraction, adrenergic signaling, and calcium handling [7]. In the right ventricle from chronic hypoxic rats gene expression studies have suggested a switch of metabolic genes suggesting that the hypertrophic right ventricle changes from fatty acid to glucose oxidation [8], and a recent microarray study of the right ventricle from rats with monocrotaline-induced pulmonary hypertension suggested that pro-apoptotic pathways and intracellular calcium handling enzymes play a role for development of failure [9–11] while growth genes such as mitogen activated protein kinase (MAPK) are pivotal in compensated hypertrophy [9]. However, in contrast to the thick-walled left ventricle, the right ventricle has a concave thin wall opposite to the convex interventricular septum, and the anatomic response to pressure overload of the right ventricle is different from the left ventricle [1], hence suggesting that other signaling pathways may play a role for development of right ventricular hypertrophy in response to pressure load.

Global gene analysis has been employed to map the expression profile of cardiac hypertrophy in man [12] and in the lungs and peripheral blood cells from patients with severe pulmonary arterial hypertension [13,14] as well as in lungs of mice with hypoxic pulmonary hypertension [15]. These types of global gene analyses are believed to be of significant value both for understanding and predicting disease processes also in pulmonary hypertension [16].

The present study investigated the changes in global gene expression by gene chip analysis during the development of right ventricular hypertrophy induced by chronic hypoxic pulmonary hypertension in rats. Most of the regulated genes in the hypoxic model were expected to be associated to the adaptive response to sustain right ventricular output, but some may be exclusively associated to hypoxia. Therefore, gene expression changes were also analyzed in rats undergoing pulmonary trunk banding (PTB), another animal model for pressure loading of the right ventricle. The alterations in expression of a subset of genes were confirmed by quantitative realtime polymerase chain reaction (qPCR), immunoblotting, and immunohistochemistry.

Methods

Ethics Statement

All animal procedures followed the revised NIH publication no. 86–23, entitled: "Principle of laboratory animal care", and were performed according to the Danish legislation with permission (no. 2006/561–1160) from the Animal Surveillance Committee, The Danish Ministry of Justice.

Animal models of right ventricular hypertrophy

48 male Wistar rats (10 weeks, weight approximately 290 grams) were divided into two groups of 24 animals. Each group was divided into subgroups of six animals. Four subgroups were maintained at hypobaric, hypoxic pressure. Four subgroups were maintained at normobaric, normoxic pressure and served as controls (Table 1). The hypoxic group was placed in a hypobaric chamber, where the ambient pressure was continuously held at 500 mbar which was equivalent to rats breathing 10% oxygen at standard pressure. The temperature in the chamber was maintained at 21–22°C and the chamber was ventilated with air at approximately 45 l min^{-1} through an inlet valve with the aid of a vacuum pump. The four subgroups were maintained in these hypoxic, hypobaric conditions for 1, 2, 3 or 4 weeks and studied immediately after removal from the chamber. The hypoxic chamber was opened once a week for approximately 30–40 minutes for cleaning and supplying purposes. Age-matched controls were maintained in similar but normoxic, normobaric chambers. All animals were provided with chow and water ad libitum.

For the PTB experiment, 46 male Wistar rats were divided into two groups. One group underwent PTB operation, and the other group underwent sham operation. Sham operated animals underwent the same procedure as PTB rats except for banding of the pulmonary trunk. Animals were subdivided into 4 groups and examined 2, 3, 5 and 6 weeks after the operation. 4 Sham and 4 PTB animals were randomly selected for gene chip analysis (Table 1). The animal model for pressure loading of the right ventricle using PTB has been described in detail in a previous publication [17].

In the experiment with chronic hypoxic rats, body weight (BW) and systemic systolic blood pressure (SSBP) of the animals were measured on the day of sacrifice. SSBP was measured using the tail cuff method with a plethysmograph (Digital Pressure Meter LE 5000 with tail cuff). Before measurements, rats were preheated for 20 minutes at 35°C in their cages. Rats were then placed in a heated Plexiglas tube (35°C). In each rat, three subsequent measurements within a difference of 5 mmHg were made, and the mean values were used. For measurement of right ventricular systolic pressure (RVSBP), rats were fully anaesthetized with an intraperitoneal injection of Midazolam 0.825 ml/kg, Fentanyl 0.825 ml/kg and sterilized water 0.825 ml/kg. For maintenance, intraperitoneal injection of 100 µL Fentanyl was given every 30 minutes. The external jugular vein was isolated by blunt dissection and ligated (using Seralon® 3/0 – Serag Wiessner). A small hole was cut in the vein and through this a catheter (30 cm. Tygon micropore, OD: 0.76 mm, ID: 0.25 mm, Norton performance plastics, OH, USA) slightly bended in one end, was inserted and led into the right ventricle through the right atrium (marks on the catheter at four to five cm indicates this location). The pressure profile was simultaneously registered via a pressure transducer (MLT0699 Disposable BP Transducer, ADInstruments, CO, USA), an amplifier (ML118G Quad Bridge Amp, ADInstruments) and through a signal box (PowerLab 4/20, ADInstruments) registered on a computer (software: Chart v5.0, ADInstruments). Once the catheter was in place, the pressure was left to stabilize over a period of approximately 5 to 10 minutes. The rats were

Table 1. Experimental design.

Animal groups	Week 1	Week 2	Week 3	Week 4	Total	GeneChip
Intervention (hypoxia)	6	6	6	6	24	16*
Control (normoxia)	6	6	6	6	24	12*
	Week 2	Week 3	Week 5	Week 6	Total	GeneChip
Intervention (PTB)	5	6	6	6	23	4*
Control (Sham)	5	6	6	6	23	4*

*Three animals from each control and four animals from each hypoxic subgroup were used for GeneChip analysis. Four animals from each group either pulmonary trunk banded (PTB) or sham at week 5 were used for GeneChip analysis.

sacrificed by decapitation. The hematocrit was measured post mortem by centrifuging the blood (Micro-Hematocrit Centrifuge, model MB, 11,700 RPM, 13,700 × g, International Equipment Company, MA, USA) for 10 minutes.

In the PTB experiment, invasive pressure measurements were performed as previously described [17].

Assessment of right ventricular hypertrophy

Immediately after the rat was decapitated, the heart was removed and placed in diethylpyrocarbonate (DEPC) treated water. For gene expression analysis a piece of four times four mm of the free wall of the right ventricle was cut out, and placed in RNA*later* (Ambion Inc., TX, U.S.A.). The atria of the heart were removed and the right ventricle separated from the left ventricle and septum. Right ventricle (including the piece cut out for gene expression analysis) and left ventricle was weighed separately. Right ventricular weight to body weight ratio (RV/BW) and the entire heart weight to body weight (HW/BW) were calculated.

Morphometric measurements

Tissue from the right ventricle was stained with reticulin that is useful to outline the architecture. The myocardial cell was considered to represent a near cylinder with a nucleus placed in the centre of the cell. Measurements were restricted to the nuclear areas. The smallest diameter was chosen as the one representing the actual diameter. The measurements were done on as many cells as possible in a field of vision. Only cells represented by a nucleus were measured. The fields of vision were randomly picked.

Gene chip analysis

The gene expression profiles was obtained by the use of Affymetrix GeneChips (GeneChip® Rat Genome 230 2.0 Array, Affymetrix Inc., CA, U.S.A.). Protocols for the analysis of Affymetrix GeneChips and the evaluation of the sensitivity and quantitative aspects of the method have been previously described [18]. The raw data files are available in European Molecular Biology Laboratory, European Bioinformatic Institute, Microarray Informatics, (http://www.ebi.ac.uk/miamexpress). 293 genes were chosen for analysis in the hypoxic and PTB experiment (see details in the statistical analysis section).

qPCR analysis

In the present project we used an Applied Biosystems 7000 Real-Time PCR System (Applied Biosystems, CA, U.S.A.) and probes composed of LNA^{TM} molecules (Exiqon, Denmark). LNA (Locked Nucleic Acid) is a bicyclic nucleic acid where a ribonucleoside is linked between the 2′-oxygen and the 4′-carbon atoms with a methylene unit (CH_2). As with the DNA probes each of the 90 LNA probes in the ProbeLibrary^{TM} kit is labeled with fluorescein (*reporter*) and a non-fluorescent *quencher*.

Primers (forward and reverse) and probes used were: adrenergic receptor, alpha 1B (α_{1B}-AR): 5′-cgtatccttgggtgccagt-3′, 5′-cacg-gccggtaggtgtaa-3′, probe #22; aquaporin 7: 5′-tccccggttcttc-actttc-3′, 5′-acccaccaccagttgttcc-3′, probe #15; triadin 1: 5′-gtg-gactacaaaaacttttcagca-3′, 5′-cagcatcgttcactagtttagagg-3′, probe #20; CD151 antigen: 5′-acggaacctgttacgcttgt-3′, 5′-cagca-at-gatctccagaagga-3′, probe #5; tissue transglutaminase (tTG): 5′-agctggagagcaacaagagc-3′, 5′-gcctggtcatccaggactc-3′, probe #9; transforming growth factor, beta 1 (TGF-β1): 5′-cctgcc-cctac-atttgga-3′, 5′-tggttgtagagggcaaggac-3′, probe #73; Ubiquitin C: 5′-caggacaaggagggcatc-3′, 5′-gccatcttccagctgctt-3′, probe #90; myosin regulatory light chain: 5′-cttcgcttgcttcgatgag-3′,5′-gtgag-cagctccctcaggt-3′ , probe #31; clathrin, light polypeptide (Lcb):

5′-tggagagaggagc-agaagaaa-3′, 5′-cactcctgttcggtcacctt-3′, probe #89; Similar to C11orf17 protein: 5′-ctcagactc-ggggcacag-3′, 5′-atgcttcctggaccaacaga-3′, probe #40.

Immunoblotting

Frozen samples of the right ventricle from chronic hypoxic and normoxic rats were homogenized, extracted in 300 μl lysis buffer (20 mM Tris-HCl, 5 mM EGTA, 150 mM NaCl, 20 mM glycerolphosphate, 10 mM NaF, 1% Triton X-100, 0.1% tween-20, 0.02 mM ortho-vanadate, 40 nM PMSF, PIM) and centrifuged at 3000 rpm at 4°C for 15 minutes. The supernatant was removed and protein concentration was measured by double determination of the samples against a standard curve with known concentration of albumin using Bio-Rad Protein Assay (Bio-Rad Laboratories, CA, USA). Protein lysate was mixed with sample buffer (350 mM Tris-HCl, 10% dithiothreitolsodium-laurylsulfate, 30% glycerol, 0.123% bromphenol blue). Samples, containing equal amounts of protein, and Protein Stain marker (Bio-Rad Laboratories) were loaded to the gel (Criterion XT Bis-Tris gel 4–12%, Bio-Rad Laboratories) and separation was carried out in the Criterion Electrophoresis System (Bio-Rad Laboratories) using XT-MOPS as a running buffer. The proteins were transferred from the gel to a polyvinylidine difluoride membrane for 1 hour at 100 V. The membrane was blocked in 5% milk for 2 hours at 20°C and afterwards incubated with primary antibody diluted in 5% milk over night at 4°C. The membrane was washed four times in TBS-T (stock: 10 mM tris/base, 2M NaCl, 1 mM EDTA 0.1% tween-20–200 ml stock, 1800 ml MQ-water, pH adjusted to 7.5) and then incubated in secondary antibody for 2 hours at 20°C. Then again washed four times in TBS-T and finally the blots were detected by enhanced chemiluminiscence system (ECL Plus Western Blotting Detection System, GE Healthcare UK Ltd., UK). Differences in protein abundance were determined by densitometry (Image Quant TL; Amersham Biosciences, UK). The known amount of loaded protein was used as loading control.

Table 2. Parameters describing the pulmonary and systemic impact of hypoxia.

	Week 1	Week 2	Week 3	Week 4
Hematocrit (%)				
Normoxia	38.7±0.9	39.0±2.6	39.0±1.5	39.0±1.4
Hypoxia	50.2±1.3*	54.3±1.7*	51.5±1.9*	51.8±1.5*
SSBP (mmHg)				
Normoxia	131.3±2.2	127.8±2.4	124.7±4.9	124.7±2.3
Hypoxia	128.7±2.8	124.3±2.8	129.5±2.5	122.2±3.6
Body weight (gram)				
Normoxia	331±12	342±11	334±12	364±10
Hypoxia	298±11	300±11	342±10	310±19*
HW/BW (%)				
Normoxia	0.27±0.005	0.26±0.009	0.25±0.009	0.24±0.007
Hypoxia	0.29±0.004	0.31±0.008*	0.33±0.014*	0.32±0.010*

SSBP: Systemic systolic blood pressure; HW/BW: Heart weight to body weight ratio.
n=6 in both groups at all time points. Values are means ± SE. *P<0.05 vs. normoxia at same time point.

Antibodies

Primary antibodies used were: anti-acetyl-Coenzyme A acyltransferase 2 (ACAA2) (cat.nr. 11111-1-AP, Ptg.Lab, IL, USA), anti-hydroxyacyl-Coenzyme A dehydrogenase/3-ketoacyl-Coenzyme A thiolase/enoyl-Coenzyme A hydratase (trifunctional protein), alpha subunit (HADHA) (cat.nr. 10758-1-AP, Ptg.Lab, IL, USA), anti-aquaporin 7 (cat.nr. AB3076, Chemicon International, MA, USA), anti-monoamine oxidase A (MAOA) (cat.nr. 10359-1-AP, Ptg.Lab, IL, USA), anti-tissue transglutaminase (tTG) (TGase II Ab-2 (TG-100), Thermo Scientific, CA, USA), anti-endothelin receptor B (ET$_B$) (cat.nr. ab1921, Abcam, UK).

Secondary antibodies used were: horse radish peroxidase (HRP) conjugated goat anti-rabbit IgG (Santa-Cruz biotechnology, CA, USA), HRP conjugated goat anti-mouse IgG (Zymed, CA, USA), HRP conjugated rabbit anti-chicken (ab6753, Abcam).

Immunohistochemistry

Pieces from the right ventricle from normoxic and hypoxic rats were stored in formalin 4% until they were embedded into paraffin. Slices of approximately 3 μm were made from each piece. Removing paraffin from the slices was done by washing in different solutions each for 5 minutes following the schedule: 2 x xylene (Xylene – mixture of isomers (AppliChem, Germany)), 2×99% ethanol, 96% ethanol, 50% ethanol and water. The slices were incubated in 3% H_2O_2 for 10 minutes and afterwards washed 2×5 minutes in Coon's buffer (Na$_2$H$_2$PO$_4$ (2H$_2$O), NaH$_2$PO$_4$ (H$_2$O), NaCl – ad. 10,000 ml H$_2$O). Slices were then pretreated with either citrat buffer (10 mM (Tri-sodiumcitrate dihydrat 5 mM, dinatriumhydrogencitrat 5 mM, pH adjusted to 6.0)) or TEG buffer (Tris 10 mM, EGTA 0.5 mM, pH adjusted to 9.0) for 2×5 minutes in microwave at 650 W and afterwards washed in Coon's buffer. 10% bovine serum in solution of 1% bovine serum albumin dissolved in Coon's Buffer (BSA1%) was added to avoid unspecific binding of the antibodies. The serum was removed and the primary antibody, the same as used for immunoblotting, diluted in BSA1% was added and incubating over night at 4°C in a moisture chamber.

The slices were washed in Coon's buffer and then incubating with secondary antibody (Bionylated Link - Universal LSAB^{TM}2 Kit/HRP, Rabbit/Mouse, Dako, CA, USA) for 20 minutes at 20°C in a moisture chamber. Again washing with Coon's buffer and incubation with streptavidin (Streptavidin, Dako) for 20 minutes at 20°C in a moisture chamber. After washing with Coon's buffer DAB (DAB Chromogen (tablets dissolved in Coon's buffer), Dako) was added and incubating for 5 minutes. Slices were incubated with Mayer's hematoxylin for 1 minute, washed in H$_2$O and incubating for 5 minutes in each solution: 50% ethanol, 96% ethanol and 99% ethanol. Negative controls were made exactly identical but without incubation with primary antibody.

Statistical analysis

The data obtained in the hypoxic experiment was firstly filtered to include probe sets with at least one present call in all 28 chips and secondly logarithmic transformed. A t-test for difference between the hypoxic and the normoxic groups, that adds the effects from the four time points (allowing for different general levels at the four time points) was calculated. The corresponding P-value from the appropiate t-distribution was calculated for each gene.

The calculated P-values were used to rank the genes within each test. To estimate how many of the called genes that were falsely positively called, we estimated a false discovery rate (FDR), avoiding the assumptions of the data being independent and

normally distributed. The FDR was calculated by comparing the original data to a reference distribution based on permutated data. Permutation consists in permutating group labels while keeping the size of the two groups. In this experiment we generated alternative arrangements by exchanging two individuals between the control and the intervention group for each of the four time points. For the whole experiment, there were a total of 104.976 different permutations. 500 randomly picked permutations were chosen, and for each of the 500 permutated experiments a t$_{sum}$ perm. test was calculated, and the corresponding P-values were found. FDR was found by calculating the ratio between the median number of genes based on the permutated datasets with P<0.0001 and the number of genes based on the original dataset with P<0.0001.

In the PTB experiment, the genes that were found to be significantly differentially expressed in the hypoxic experiment,

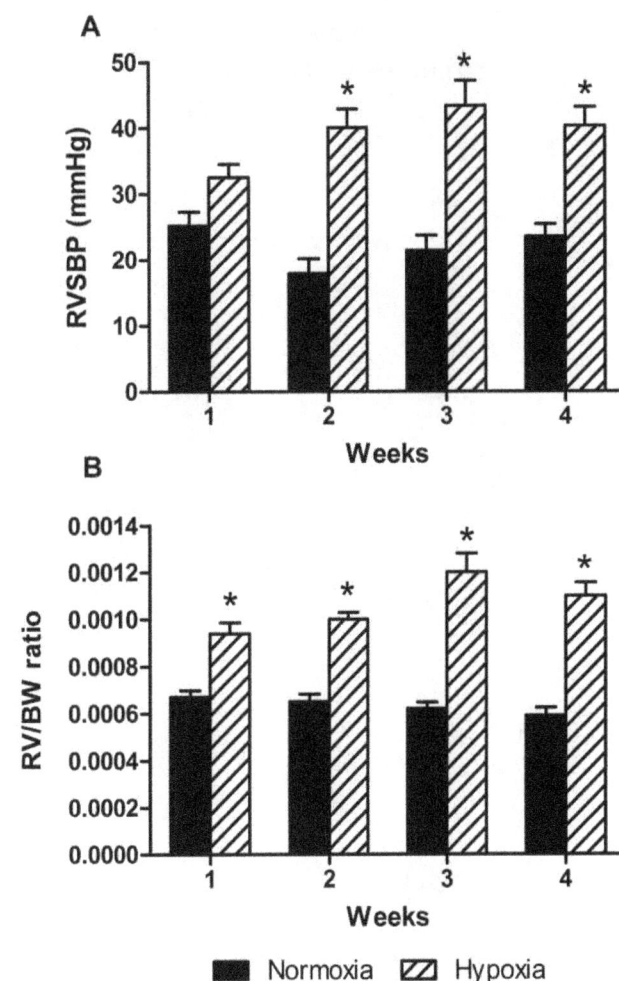

Figure 1. Right ventricular systolic blood pressure (RVSBP) and right ventricular hypertrophy in hypoxic experiment. A: changes in RVSBP in the normoxic and hypoxic groups at the four time points. RVSBP was constant in the normoxic group and significantly increased in the hypoxic groups after 2 weeks. B: temporal change in right ventricular hypertrophy in the hypoxic experiment assessed by right ventricular weight relative to body weight ratio (RV/BW) shows significant increase due to hypoxia. n = 6 in both groups at all time points. Values are means ± SE. *P<0.05 vs. normoxia at same time point.

were selected in the gene expression dataset belonging to the PTB experiment, and differences between the two groups were analysed using Student's t test.

Results from immunoblotting, qPCR, morphometric and hemodynamic measurements from both the PTB and hypoxic experiment were analyzed separately by using two-way analysis of variance (ANOVA) comparing hypoxia or PTB to time. In case of significance a Bonferroni post hoc test was made. Statistical calculations were made by using GraphPad Prism version 4.03 (GraphPad Software Inc, San Diego, CA, USA).

All over, P-values of less than 0.05 were considered significant.

Results

Functional Data

Hematocrit, SSBP, BW and HW/BW are listed in Table 2. The hematocrit was 39% in the normoxic group. Hypoxia increased the hematocrit to 50–54%. SSBP was unaltered by hypoxia. The normoxic animals gained weight during the four weeks, while the hypoxic rats had a significant lower body weight after four weeks of experiment. HW/BW in the hypoxic group showed a significant increase at week two, three and four.

RVSBP was constant in the normoxic group (18–25 mmHg) but raised by hypoxia from 32 mmHg at week one to 40–

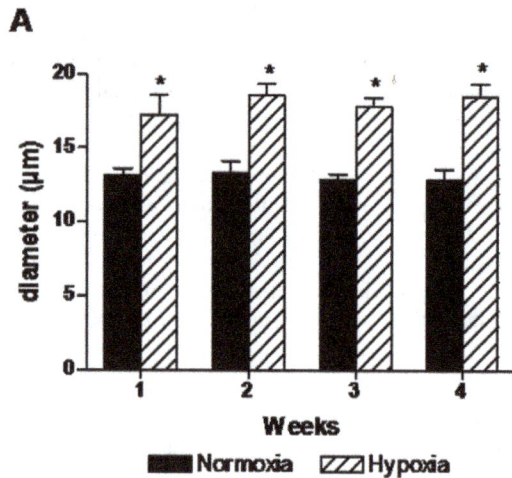

Figure 2. Morphometric measurements of the right ventricle. A: cardiomyocyte diameter was significantly increased by hypoxia compared to normoxic controls. B: examples of staining with reticulin in right ventricle samples from normoxic and hypoxic rats. n = 5–6 in both groups at all time points. Values are means ± SE. *P<0.05 vs. normoxia at same time point.

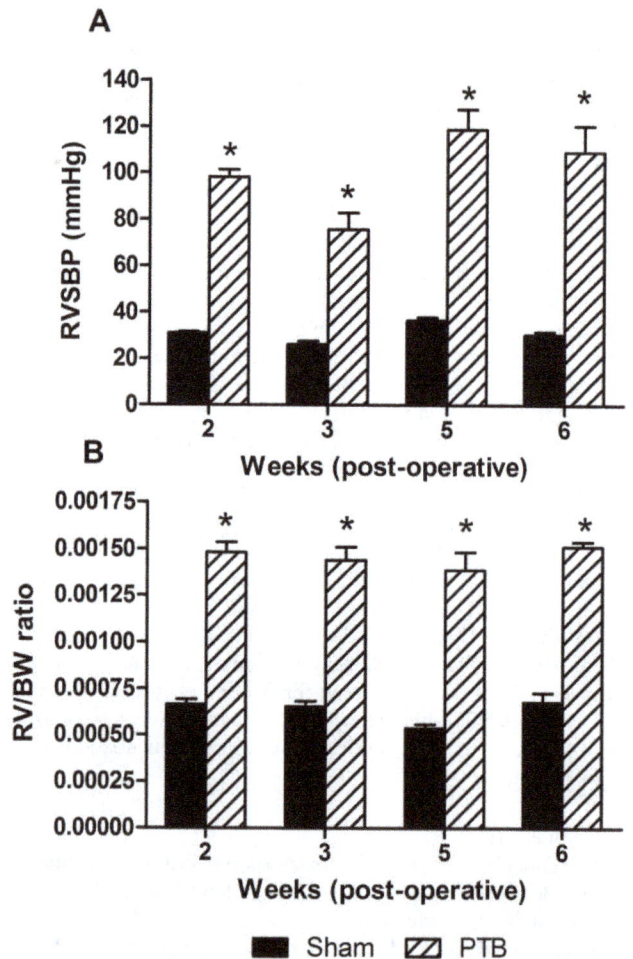

Figure 3. RVSBP and RV/BW in the pulmonary trunk banding (PTB) experiment. A: RVSBP was significantly increased due to PTB compared to sham operated animals. B: temporal change in right ventricular hypertrophy in the PTB experiment assessed by RV/BW and compared to the sham group shows a significant increasing effect of PTB. n = 4–7 in both groups at all time points. Values are means ± SE. *P<0.05 vs. sham at same time point.

Table 3. Changes in gene expression by gene chip analysis – hypoxia compared to normoxia.

Public ID	Encoded protein	Fold changes[a]
NM_012612	natriuretic peptide precursor type A	+50.13
NM_019296	cell division cycle 2 homolog A (S. pombe)	+6.21
NM_031131	transforming growth factor, beta 2	+5.60
NM_012843	Epithelial membrane protein 1	+5.25
AI145313	thymus cell antigen 1, theta	+4.64
AB026903	decay-accelerating factor	+2.31
D00688	monoamine oxidase A	+3.44
BI298356	four and a half LIM domains 1	+3.07
M14400	creatine kinase, brain	+2.95
AF413212	guanine nucleotide binding protein, alpha o	+2.91
NM_019212	actin alpha 1	+2.85
NM_012886	tissue inhibitor of metalloproteinase 3	+2.72
NM_031545	natriuretic peptide precursor type B	+2.68
L09752	cyclin D2	+2.52
AA851939	FXYD domain-containing ion transport regulator 6	+2.50
U54791	Chemokine receptor (LCR1)	+2.47
AA945643	Chitinase 3-like 1 (cartilage glycoprotein-39)	+2.38
AF095585	enigma (LIM domain protein)	+2.38
Z78279	collagen, type 1, alpha 1	+2.37
AI227742	Bcl-2-related ovarian killer protein	+2.29
NM_019237	procollagen C-proteinase enhancer protein	+2.25
BM389019	fibrillin-1	+2.23
X57764	endothelin receptor B	+2.23
AW143798	cyclin D1	+2.21
AF072892	chondroitin sulphate proteoglycan 2 (versican)	+2.16
NM_019341	Regulator of G-protein signaling 5	+2.16
NM_134452	collagen, type V, alpha 1	+2.11
AB026665	peptide/histidine transporter PHT2	+2.11
NM_019386	tissue transglutaminase	+2.08
AW253722	RAB13	+2.01
AI009597	FXYD domain-containing ion transport regulator 3	−8.67
NM_031543	cytochrome P450, subfamily 2E, polypeptide 1	−5.60
AF385402	Potassium channel, subfamily K, member 2	−4.15
AI535411	myosin heavy chain, polypeptide 7	−3.63
AJ243304	triadin 1	−3.04
NM_019157	Aquaporin 7	−2.82
BE103537	tropomyosin 1, alpha	−2.81
U31554	limbic system-associated membrane protein	−2.76
AI137995	sodium channel, voltage-gated, type IV, beta	−2.50
NM_012505	ATPase, Na+K+ transporting, alpha 2	−2.37
NM_080399	Smhs1 protein	−2.18
NM_057197	2,4-dienoyl CoA reductase 1, mitochondrial	−2.14
NM_030865	Myocilin	−2.14
AF322216	immunoglobulin superfamily, member 1	−2.14
NM_017079	CD1d1 antigen	−2.13
NM_012793	guanidinoacetate methyltransferase	−2.08
AA899304	acetyl-coenzyme A acetyltransferase 1	−2.05
AW528891	potassium voltage gated channel, Shal-related family, m...	−2.03
NM_016991	adrenergic receptor, alpha 1B	−2.03

[a]Values are the average of a four-way analysis as described in Methods. Only genes with fold changes larger than 2 are included in this table.

43 mmHg at week two, three and four (Figure 1A). RV/BW was almost unaltered in the normoxic group, while in the hypoxic group RV/BW was increasing during the four weeks (Figure 1B). There was a strong positive correlation between RVSBP and RV/BW in the hypoxic experiment (n = 48, $R^2 = 0.66$, P<0.0001).

The diameter of the cardiomyocytes increased significantly (31 to 64%) in the hypoxic group but within each group there was no significant difference between the four different time points (Figure 2A). Staining with reticulin did not reveal any other differences between hypoxic and normoxic rats (Figure 2B).

In the PTB experiment, RVSBP was approximately constant in the sham group (26 to 38 mmHg). RVSBP was significantly raised in the PTB group at all time points (76 to 118 mmHg) (Figure 3A). Temporal change in right ventricular hypertrophy was assessed by RV/BW ratio. The degree of right ventricular hypertrophy in the PTB group was increased significantly at all time points compared to the sham group (Figure 3B). There was a strong correlation between RVSBP and RV/BW (n = 46, $R^2 = 0.76$, P<0.0001).

Gene expression data

Table 3 contains results for 49 genes from gene chip analysis for genes up- or down-regulated with a fold change greater than two.

The validation of the gene expression profiles was done by qPCR. We chose four upregulated (CD 151 antigen, tTG, TGF-β1 and Similar to C11orf17 protein), three downregulated (α_{1B}-AR, aquaporin 7, and triadin 1) and two genes without change (myosin regulatory light chain and clathrin – light polypeptide). Ubiquitin C was used for normalization. The qPCR results were in accordance with the gene chip data (Figure 4A,B), exemplified by aquaporin 7 and tTG. The correlation between the gene chip and qPCR results was tested by comparing 3 up-regulated, 4 down-regulated and 2 genes with no change in expression according to the gene chip tsum analysis. There is a strong positive correlation between gene chip detection (normalized to 0) values and the qPCR detection values (normalized to 0) and in the hypoxic experiment (n = 72, $R^2 = 0.70$) (Figure 5).

The signal log ratio estimates the magnitude and direction of change of a transcript when two arrays are compared (experiment versus control). Signal log ratios from the hypoxic and the PTB experiments were plotted for 288 genes (5 genes were excluded of the original 293 genes tested because they showed absent calls in the PTB experiment). 266 were regulated in the same direction or were unchanged in the two experiments (Wilcoxon signed rank test: $P<2.2\times10^{-16}$). Of these genes, 172 were non-expressed sequence tags (non-EST) involved in apoptosis, inflammation, heart function, and growth and the remaining 94 were EST. Of the 22 genes regulated differently, 11 were up-regulated and 5 unaltered in the PTB experiment but down-regulated in the hypoxic experiment, 3 were down-regulated in PTB and up-regulated in hypoxia and 3 were EST (Table 4). There is a strong positive correlation between the log ratios of gene expression in the hypoxic and the PTB experiment ($R^2 = 0.69$, P<0.05, n = 288) (Figure 6). Limiting the analysis to genes where the fold change is larger than 2 yielded an even stronger correlation ($R^2 = 0.84$, P<0.05, n = 125) of gene expression in the hypoxic and PTB experiment.

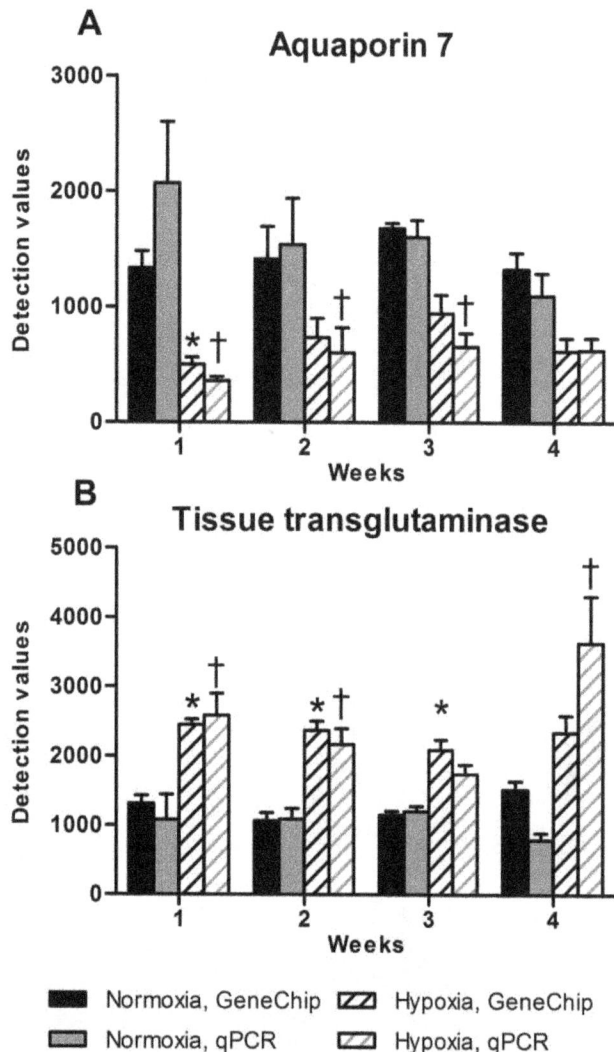

Figure 4. qPCR analysis of aquaporin7 and tissue transgluta-minase. A: gene expression of the aquaporin 7 mRNA by use of gene chip and qPCR shows a decrease in gene expression according to hypoxia. B: gene expression of tissue transglutaminase mRNA by use of gene chip and qPCR shows the opposite impact of hypoxia by increasing gene expression. n = 6 in both groups at all time points.

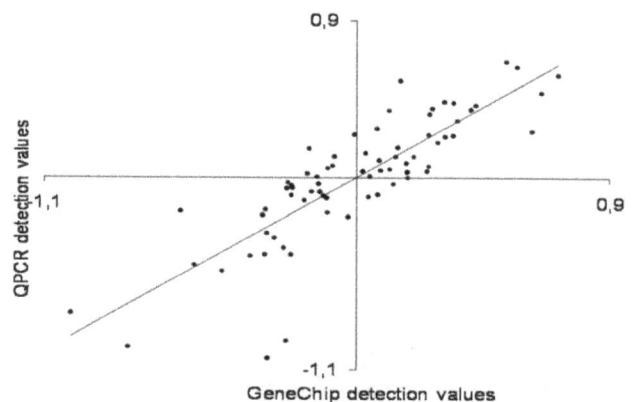

Figure 5. Correlation of the gene chip and qPCR gene expression results. The correlation is tested by comparing three upregulated, four downregulated and two not regulated genes (according to the gene chip, tsum analysis). There was found significant correlation between qPCR and gene chip analysis. Values are means ± SE. *P<0.05 vs. normoxia, gene chip at same time point, †P<0.05 vs. normoxia, qPCR at same time point.

Table 4. Differentially regulated genes in the right ventricle of pulmonary trunk banded (PTB) rats versus chronic hypoxic rats.

Public ID	Encoded protein	Fold change	
		PTB	Hypoxia
NM_024400	A disintegrin and metalloproteinase with thrombospondin motifs 1 (ADAMTS-1)	0.60	−0.61
BG671506	avian sarcoma virus CT10 (v-crk) oncogene homolog	0.38	−0.41
AI454911	endothelial monocyte activating polypeptide 2	0.15	−0.28
BF282186	eukaryotic initiation factor 5 (eIF-5)	0.35	−0.35
AI713966	insulin-like growth factor binding protein 3	0.41	−0.84
NM_012588	insulin-like growth factor binding protein 3	0.33	−0.78
NM_053713	Kruppel-like factor 4 (gut)	0.48	−0.68
AA818911	mob protein	0.21	−0.39
AI409862	protein phosphatase 1, catalytic subunit, beta isoform	0.22	−0.37
NM_033096	protein phosphatase 1B, magnesium dependent, beta isoform	0.12	−0.36
AY043246	regulator of G-protein signaling protein 2	0.44	−0.99
AI454052	c-kit receptor tyrosine kinase	−0.24	0.91
AW914928	DEAD (aspartate-glutamate-alanine-aspartate) box polypeptide 25	−0.36	0.51
BI275583	lectin, galactoside-binding, soluble, 2 (galectin 2)	−0.17	0.15

In addition 4 genes (LYRIC, glioma tumor suppressor candidate region gene 2, splicing factor (arginine/serine-rich 5), transducer of ERBB2 1, and TRAP-complex gamma subunit) were unaltered in PTB, but down-regulated in hypoxia, but with fold changes less than 0.5.

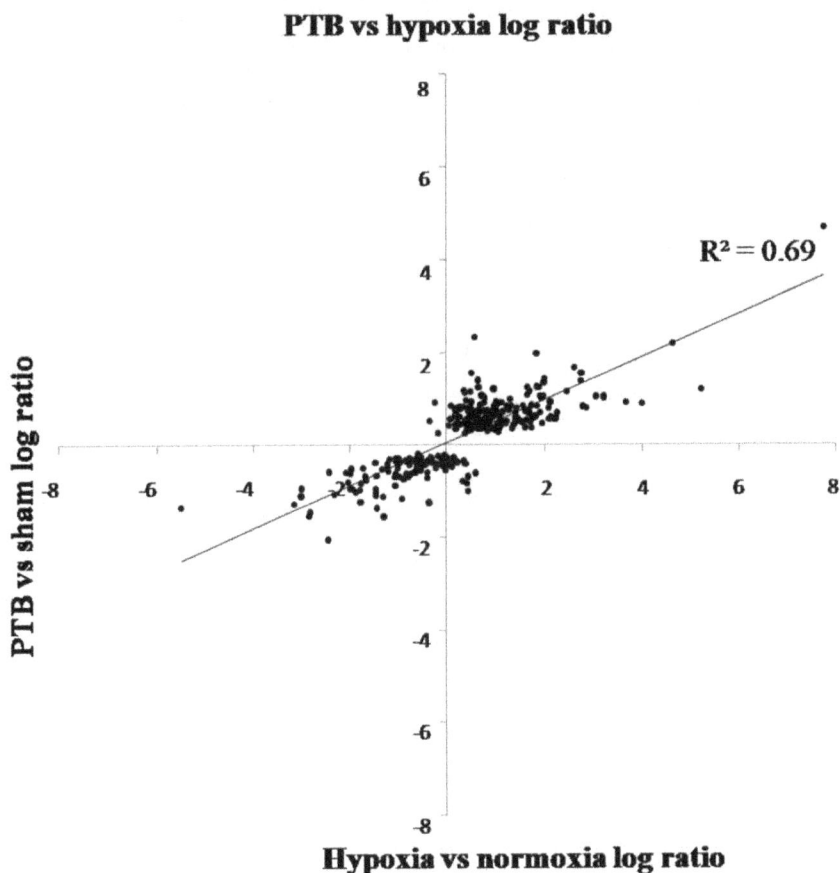

PTB vs hypoxia log ratio

$R^2 = 0.69$

PTB vs sham log ratio

Hypoxia vs normoxia log ratio

Figure 6. Log ratio of gene chip data obtained in the right ventricle of chronic hypoxic compared to normoxic rats versus pulmonary trunk banded (PTB) compared to sham-operated rats. There was found a positive correlation between regulation of the genes in the two experiments with a significant correlation coefficient $R^2 = 0.69$ (P<0.05, n = 288).

Immunoblotting

Figure 7 shows the representative immunoblots. Six proteins were chosen for immunoblotting based on the gene chip that showed three genes were downregulated (ACAA2, HADHA and aquaporin 7) and three were upregulated (tTG, MAOA and ET$_B$). By use of antibodies against these proteins we showed that some of the changes found on gene levels are also reflected at protein level. ACAA2, HADHA and aquaporin 7 were not significantly downregulated, but the tendency is clear (Figure 8A–C). MAOA and tTG were significantly upregulated in hypoxic rats after 2, 3 or 4 weeks when compared to normoxic controls (Figure 8D–E). Finally, ET$_B$ was only significantly upregulated after 3 weeks of hypoxia (Figure 8F).

Immunohistochemistry

By incubating slides from the right ventricle from hypoxic and normoxic rats with antibodies used for immunoblotting we were able to evaluate the localization of the proteins. Controls were made without primary antibody incubation (Figure 9A). For the proteins participating in beta-oxidation, ACAA2 and HADHA, the localization is intracellular in the cardiomyocyte (Figure 9B–C). Aquaporin 7 was also located in the cardiomyocyte at the cellular membrane (Figure 9D). MAOA was also upregulated on the immunostainings when compared to normoxic controls and the location is intracellular (Figure 9E). Finally, tTG was also located to the cardiomyocyte mainly in the cytosol (Figure 9F).

Discussion

The main findings of the present study are addressing gene expression common for the pressure loading of the right ventricle in both chronic hypoxic rats and rats with banding of the pulmonary trunk. The present study revealed alterations in expression of 172 genes involved in apoptosis, inflammation, heart function, and growth. A small subset of differentiated genes in the hypoxia and PTB groups suggests pressure load as the main contributer to development of right ventricular hypertrophy. GeneChip analysis of the right ventricle was confirmed by qPCR for a subgroup of genes and was further substantiated by measuring protein expression showing a marked upregulation of tTG due to right ventricular hypertrophy.

Role of hypoxia versus pressure load in right ventricular hypertrophy in pulmonary hypertension

The hypobaric hypoxia model has been used in several studies for induction of pulmonary hypertension in rats and has shown increase of RVSBP and right ventricular weight [19]. Another approach to induce high RVSBP and to increase right ventricular weight is by PTB [17,20]. By comparing these two animal models, it is possible to distinguish the isolated effect of respectively pressure load and hypoxia. There was a significant correlation of genes changed in the right ventricle of chronic hypoxic rats with the changes observed in the PTB experiment and this correlation was even stronger when only genes regulated more than two-fold were considered. These findings suggest that pressure load is the main factor altering gene expression in the right ventricle in rats with pulmonary hypertension induced by hypoxia.

Comparing chronic hypoxia and PTB identified a small subgroup of genes changing in opposite directions suggesting that hypoxia alone has an impact on the gene expression in the right ventricle. Thus, c-kit receptor tyrosine kinase and DEAD (asparatate-glutamate-alanine-asparatate) box polypeptide 25 were upregulated in hypoxia and downregulated in the PTB experiments, while insulin-like growth factor binding protein 3 and

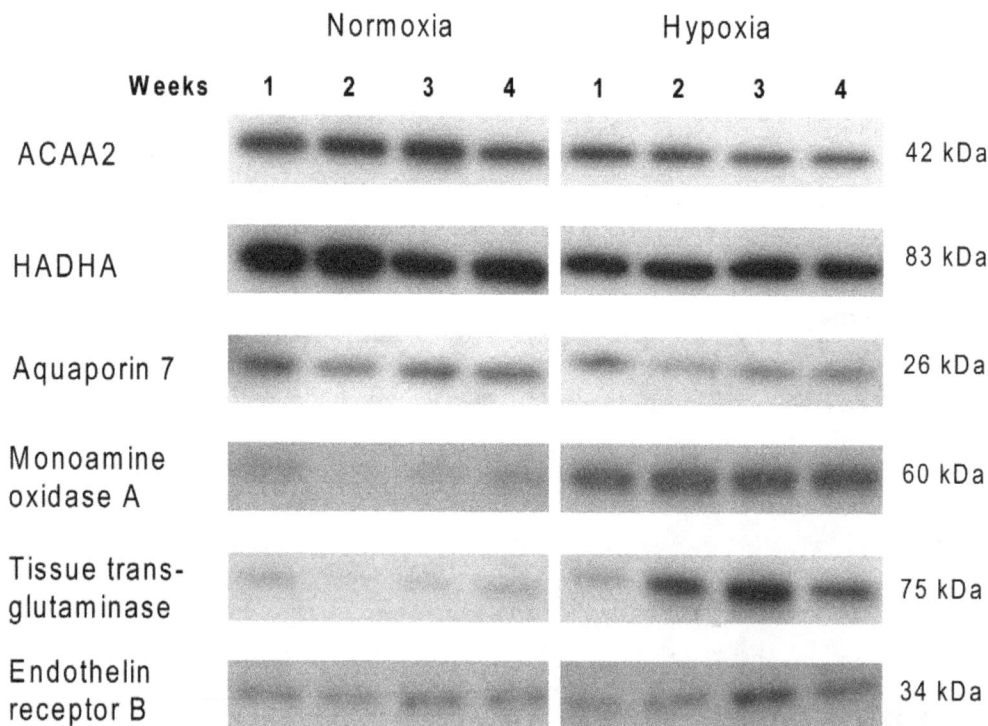

Figure 7. Representative immunoblots for proteins measured in the right ventricle from normoxic and hypoxic rats. ACAA2: acetyl-Coenzyme A acyltransferase 2, HADHA: hydroxyacyl-Coenzyme A dehydrogenase/3-ketoacyl-Coenzyme A thiolase/enoyl-Coenzyme A hydratase (trifunctional protein), alpha subunit.

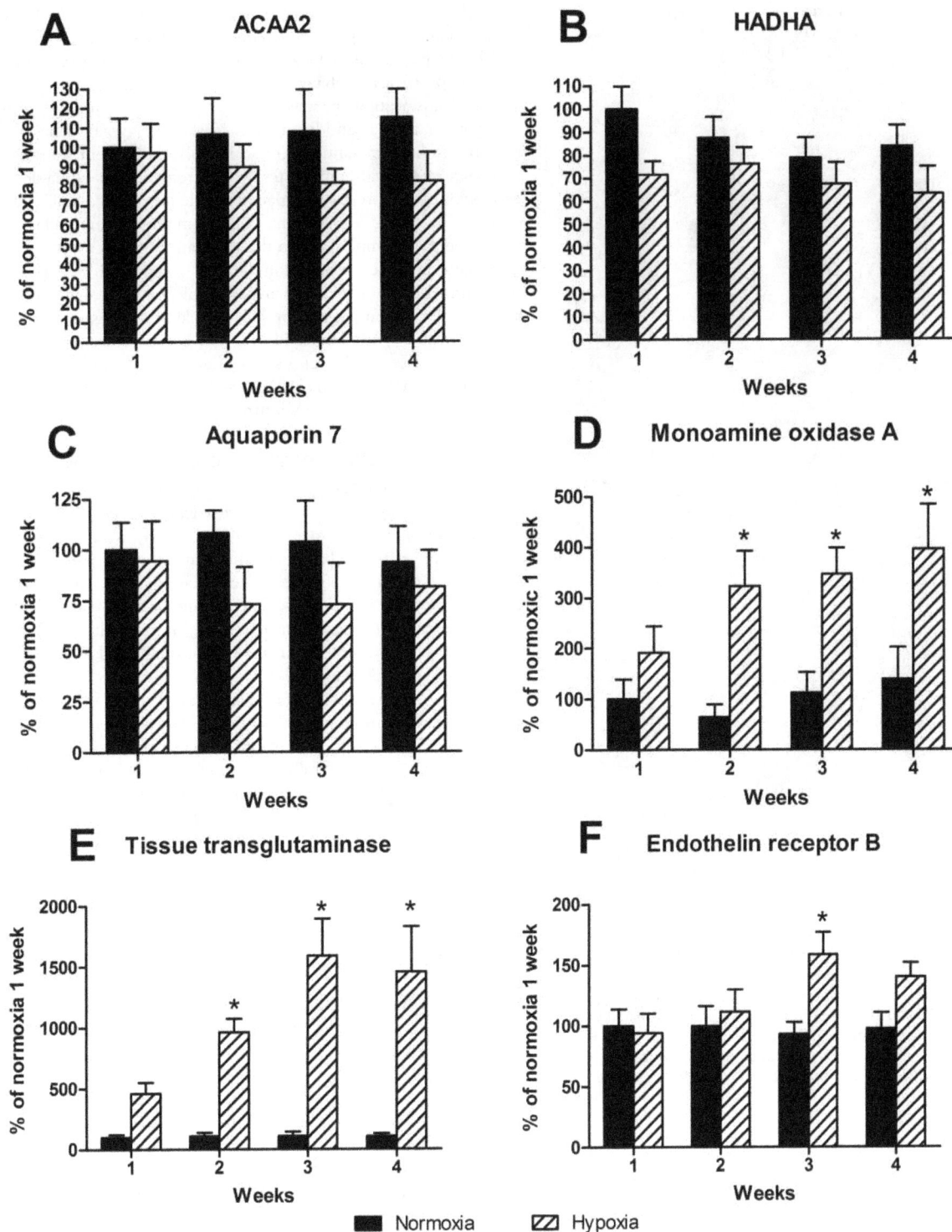

Figure 8. Immunoblottings of right ventricle samples from normoxic and hypoxic rats. Proteins participating in metabolism A: ACAA2, B: HADHA and C: aquaporin 7 show tendency to downregulation by hypoxia. D: monoamine oxidase A, E: tissue transglutaminase and F: endothelin receptor B were all upregulated by hypoxia. ACAA2: acetyl-Coenzyme A acyltransferase 2, HADHA: hydroxyacyl-Coenzyme A dehydrogenase/3-ketoacyl-Coenzyme A thiolase/enoyl-Coenzyme A hydratase (trifunctional protein), alpha subunit. Values are means ± SE and are calculated as percent of normoxia 1 week. n = 6 in both groups at all time points. *P<0.05 vs. normoxia at same time point.

regulator of G-protein signaling protein 2 were upregulated. Both c-kit receptor tyrosine kinase and insulin-like growth factor binding protein 3 have previously been described to be involved in hypoxia-induced angiogenesis [21,22], and insulin growth factor 1 stimulation in mouse fibroblasts resulted in upregulation of DEAD [23]. Therefore, hypoxia seems to directly affect gene expression in the right ventricle. However, in all cases the fold changes in gene expression comparing the PTB and hypoxic

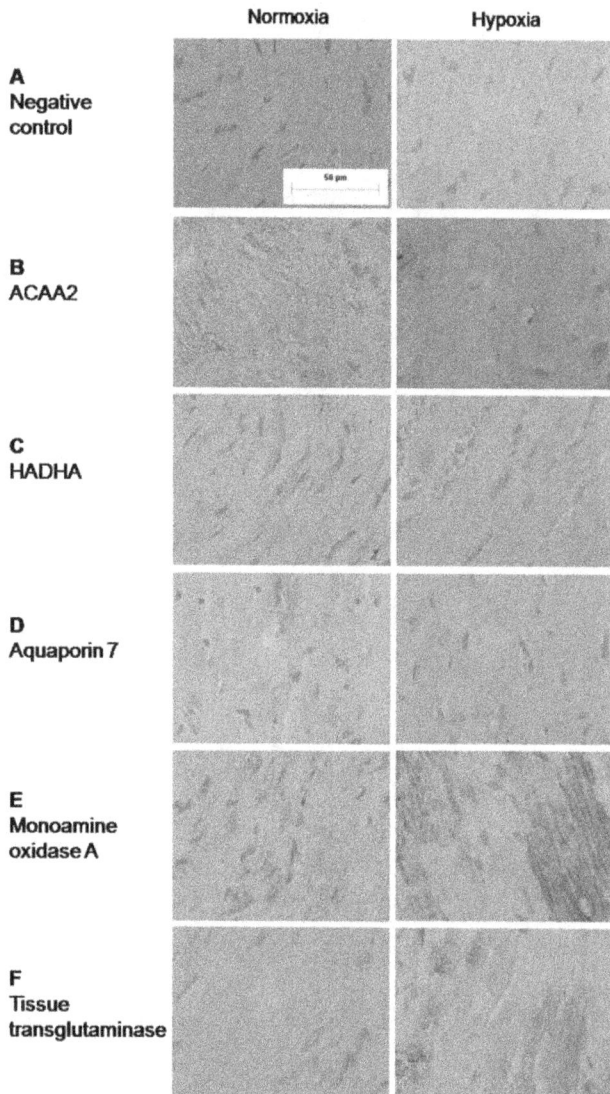

Figure 9. Immunostainings of slides from the right ventricle from rats exposed to normoxia or hypoxia for 2 weeks. A: Negative controls without incubation with the primary antibody. The bar on control picture shows the size reference (50 μm) for all pictures. B: ACAA2 C: HADHA, D: aquaporin 7, E: monoamine oxidase A, F: tissue transglutaminase. All proteins were found to be located to the cardiomyocyte and only aquaporin 7 was thought to be located to the cellular membrane whereas the other proteins is located to the cytosol.

experiments with regard to differentially expressed genes are small (Table 4), and it cannot be excluded that differences in pressure load comparing chronic hypoxic rats and PTB rats may also contribute to the differential gene regulation.

Previous studies have also provided evidence suggesting that mechanical load of the right ventricle from rats with pulmonary hypertension influences gene expression [11]. Thus, atrial natriuretic peptide expression, probably induced by stretch of the myocardium, was upregulated in the right ventricle from rats with pulmonary hypertension induced by either moncrotaline or hypoxia [8,9], and in agreement with these findings, both natriuretic peptide precursor type A and B were markedly increased in the present study. Genes involved in cell proliferation, the cyclin family of genes and BCl2, were upregulated in the right

ventricle of rats with pulmonary hypertension induced by monocrotaline [9,10], and the same was the case for cyclin D1 and D2 as well as BCl2 in the present study. In addition, several signaling processes involving fetal gene re-expression, activation of protein translocation, increase in mass, and enlargement of cell size/volume have been identified as markers of hypertrophy as a response to hemodynamic overload [24]. In the present study the diameter of the cardiomyocytes was increased, and alpha-actin expression was upregulated together with four and a half LIM domains 1 (FHL), and enigma (LIM domain protein). FHL is contained in a complex within the cardiomyocyte sacromere and mice lacking FHL displayed a blunted hypertrophic response suggesting FHL1 to mediates hypertrophic biomechanical stress responses in the myocardium [25], while the Enigma protein family are Z-line proteins at the border between two sarcomers [26]. Thus, upregulation of a series of genes in the present study also suggest that mechanical load regulate gene expression and results in right ventricular hypertrophy.

Role of specific signal pathways changed in right ventricular hypertrophy

During development of right ventricular hypertrophy the myocardium changes metabolism to avoid ischemia [27]. Normally the major substrate for heart metabolism is free fatty acids that account for 60–80%. The remaining part comes from metabolism of carbohydrates, but during development of left ventricular hypertrophy and heart failure the ratio alters towards increased carbohydrates as cardiac fuel substrate and augmented mitochondrial respiratory capacity which is considered to play a central role in hypoxia-mediated cardioprotection [27]. A study of gene expression from chronic hypoxic rats showed increased expression of genes associated to glucose metabolism and they also found changes in the left ventricle, which indicates that not only myocardial hypertrophy causes changes, but also chronic hypoxia contributes to altered gene expression [8]. Indeed, in the present study genes encoding for enzymes participating in beta-oxidation of fatty acids (ACAA2 and HADHA) were downregulated in right ventricles from hypoxic rats. The tendency was reflected at protein level, although not significantly and supports that pressure load by itself is able to cause a shift in genes related to myocardial metabolism from free fatty acids to carbohydrates.

Aquaporin 7 is a water and glycerol channel that has been found especially in adipocytes and skeletal muscle cells in the human body. The overall function of aquaporins is to maintain cellular water homeostasis [28,29]. Studies of aquaporin 7 showed that it is expressed in cardiac tissue from mice, rats and humans [30]. Our results confirmed these findings both by gene chip, qPCR and immunoblotting. Moreover, we found that hypoxia decreases gene expression for aquaporin 7, although this was not confirmed at protein level. Skowronski et al. found that aquaporin 7 is only localized in small vessels in cardiac tissue, and these observations agree with our findings [31]. A downregulation of aquaporin 7 in hypoxic rats may reflect reduced glycerol transport as a consequence of a shift of the metabolism from fatty acids to carbohydrates.

Hypertrophy of the ventricle also leads to remodeling of the ventricular wall and altered expression of structural proteins in the myocardium and in the surrounding tissue. Studies of tTG in left the ventricle show association between the expression of tTG and development of ventricular hypertrophy [32,33]. The mechanism is primarily through its action as TGase leading to structural changes of actin and myosin, but also more or less through the GTPase activity. tTG is coupled to the α_{1B}-AR as Gα-protein [34]. Overexpression of α_{1B}-AR is known to induce cardiac hypertrophy [35] and studies of the expression of the α_{1B}-AR have shown that it is downregulated on mRNA level in vascular smooth muscle cells from chronic hypoxic animals [36], and that knockout of the receptor did not alter development of right ventricular hypertrophy and the increase in RVSBP [37]. The conclusion of these studies is that α_{1B}-AR is associated to vascular smooth muscle cell proliferation. Our findings show that the α_{1B}-AR is downregulated in the right ventricle at mRNA level, while the potential coupling protein tTG is markedly upregulated and associated to right ventricular hypertrophy in rats with pulmonary hypertension. The exact role of α_{1B}-AR is still unknown but it seems to play an adaptional role to avoid development of cardiac hypertrophy according to pulmonary hypertension.

Transforming growth factor beta 1 (TGF-β1) is thought to be associated with proliferation of cells during development of hypertrophy and cell division. Studies of rats with pulmonary hypertension and right ventricular hypertrophy induced by monocrotaline showed by qPCR analysis increased levels of TGF-β1 in the right ventricle but not in the left ventricle indicating association to right ventricular hypertrophy [38]. Also immunoblottings of pulmonary arteries from chronic hypoxic rats showed association between TGF-β1 and increased proliferation of vascular smooth muscle cells [39]. These findings indicate that TGF-β1 is associated both to right ventricular hypertrophy and vascular smooth muscle cell proliferation. Our studies support that TGF-β1 appears to play a role in development of right ventricular hypertrophy.

MAOA is an enzyme located to the mitochondria of the cardiomyocytes and metabolizes epinephrine, norepinephrine, and serotonin (5-HT). Studies have shown that 5-HT is associated to ventricular hypertrophy by binding to its receptor 5-HT$_{2B}$, and that it induces oxidative stress and apoptosis [40]. It has been found that blocking of the 5-HT$_{2B}$ receptor only partly inhibited the effect of 5-HT, and that inhibition of MAOA prevented the hypertrophic effect of 5-HT [41]. Overexpression of the 5-HT$_{2B}$ receptor leads to left ventricular hypertrophy. The localization of MAOA has been found to be intracellular [42,43]. Our findings indicate an association between right ventricular hypertrophy and the expression of MAOA. Moreover, we evaluated the localization of MAOA and found that it is located to the cardiomyocytes and probably to the mitochondria, which are highly expressed in

cardiomyocytes and is the place where catecholamines and 5-HT are metabolized. Reactive oxygen species (ROS), a product from oxidation of 5-HT catalyzed by MAOA, is related to right ventricular hypertrophy and ROS has been found to be located to the mitochondria [44]. This indicates that metabolization of 5-HT and thereby MAOA is located here.

The effects of endothelin are mediated by two distinct receptors termed ET$_A$ and ET$_B$, where 90% of endothelin receptors belong to the ET$_A$ subtype in cardiomyocytes, and their stimulation has a positive inotropic effect [45]. Cardiac ET$_B$ receptors may contribute to clearance of circulating endothelin and together with the ET$_A$ to cardiac fibrosis and cardiomyocyte hypertrophy [45,46]. In the present study only the ET$_B$ receptor expression was elevated in the right ventricle as well as expression of several collagens e.g. collagen type 1 alpha 1 and collagen type V alpha 1 (Table 3). The dual ET$_A$/ET$_B$ receptor antagonist, bosentan reduces right ventricular hypertrophy in pulmonary hypertension in chronic hypoxic rats [47], but at present it is unclear whether the block of endothelin clearance and pulmonary vascular dilation by ET$_B$ receptors outweigh the beneficial effects of blocking both the ET$_A$ and ET$_B$ receptors in pulmonary hypertension due to hypoxia.

In conclusion, we have found that several genes are altered during development of right ventricular hypertrophy induced by pulmonary hypertension in chronic hypoxic rats. In case of the metabolic genes the effect of high pressure on the right ventricle appears compensated at the protein level, while both expression of genes and proteins of importance for myocardial function and remodelling are altered by the increased pressure load of the right ventricle. These findings imply that treatment of pulmonary hypertension, in addition to reduction of pulmonary vascular resistance, should also aim at reducing right ventricular pressure or by direct effects on the heart limit the organ damaging effects of high pulmonary pressure.

Author Contributions

Conceived and designed the experiments: LHM JDB US MK TFØ. Performed the experiments: JDB LHM CDP UKS. Analyzed the data: LHM JDB CDP UKS NEM JLJ US. Contributed reagents/materials/analysis tools: US JLJ MK TFØ. Wrote the paper: LHM JDB CDP UKS NEM JLJ MK TFØ US.

References

1. Chin KM, Kim NH, Rubin LJ (2005) The right ventricle in pulmonary hypertension. Coron Artery Dis 16: 13–18.
2. Humbert M, Sitbon O, Simonneau G (2004) Treatment of pulmonary arterial hypertension. N Engl J Med 351: 1425–1436.
3. Montalescot G, Drobinski G, Meurin P, Maclouf J, Sotirov I, et al. (1998) Effects of prostacyclin on the pulmonary vascular tone and cardiac contractility of patients with pulmonary hypertension secondary to end-stage heart failure. Am J Cardiol 82: 749–755.
4. Kisch-Wedel H, Kemming G, Meisner F, Flondor M, Kuebler WM, et al. (2003) The prostaglandins epoprostenol and iloprost increase left ventricular contractility in vivo. Intensive Care Med 29: 1574–1583.
5. Mulder P, Richard V, Derumeaux G, Hogie M, Henry JP, et al. (1997) Role of endogenous endothelin in chronic heart failure: effect of long-term treatment with an endothelin antagonist on survival, hemodynamics, and cardiac remodeling. Circulation 96: 1976–1982.
6. Frey N, Olson EN (2003) Cardiac hypertrophy: the good, the bad, and the ugly. Annu Rev Physiol 65: 45–79.
7. Opie LH, Commerford PJ, Gersh BJ, Pfeffer MA (2006) Controversies in ventricular remodelling. Lancet 367: 356–367.
8. Sharma S, Taegtmeyer H, Adrogue J, Razeghi P, Sen S, et al. (2004) Dynamic changes of gene expression in hypoxia-induced right ventricular hypertrophy. Am J Physiol Heart Circ Physiol 286: H1185–H1192.
9. Buermans HP, Redout EM, Schiel AE, Musters RJ, Zuidwijk M, et al. (2005) Microarray analysis reveals pivotal divergent mRNA expression profiles early in the development of either compensated ventricular hypertrophy or heart failure. Physiol Genomics 21: 314–323.
10. Ecarnot-Laubriet A, Assem M, Poirson-Bichat F, Moisant M, Bernard C, et al. (2002) Stage-dependent activation of cell cycle and apoptosis mechanisms in the right ventricle by pressure overload. Biochim Biophys Acta 1586: 233–242.
11. Kogler H, Hartmann O, Leineweber K, Nguyen vP, Schott P, et al. (2003) Mechanical load-dependent regulation of gene expression in monocrotaline-induced right ventricular hypertrophy in the rat. Circ Res 93: 230–237.
12. Hwang DM, Dempsey AA, Lee CY, Liew CC (2000) Identification of differentially expressed genes in cardiac hypertrophy by analysis of expressed sequence tags. Genomics 66: 1–14.
13. Geraci MW, Moore M, Gesell T, Yeager ME, Alger L, et al. (2001) Gene expression patterns in the lungs of patients with primary pulmonary hypertension: a gene microarray analysis. Circ Res 88: 555–562.
14. Bull TM, Coldren CD, Moore M, Sotto-Santiago SM, Pham DV, et al. (2004) Gene microarray analysis of peripheral blood cells in pulmonary arterial hypertension. Am J Respir Crit Care Med 170: 911–919.
15. Gharib SA, Luchtel DL, Madtes DK, Glenny RW (2005) Global gene annotation analysis and transcriptional profiling identify key biological modules in hypoxic pulmonary hypertension. Physiol Genomics 22: 14–23.
16. Bull TM, Coldren CD, Geraci MW, Voelkel NF (2007) Gene expression profiling in pulmonary hypertension. Proc Am Thorac Soc 4: 117–120.
17. Schou UK, Peters CD, Kim SW, Frøkiær J, Nielsen S (2007) Characterization of a rat model of right-sided heart failure induced by pulmonary trunk banding. J Exp Anim Sci 43: 237–254.
18. Lipshutz RJ, Fodor SP, Gingeras TR, Lockhart DJ (1999) High density synthetic oligonucleotide arrays. Nat Genet 21: 20–24.

19. Elmedal B, de Dam MY, Mulvany MJ, Simonsen U (2004) The superoxide dismutase mimetic, tempol, blunts right ventricular hypertrophy in chronic hypoxic rats. Br J Pharmacol 141: 105–113.

20. Gaynor SL, Maniar HS, Bloch JB, Steendijk P, Moon MR (2005) Right atrial and ventricular adaptation to chronic right ventricular pressure overload. Circulation 112: I212–I218.

21. Litz J, Krystal GW (2006) Imatinib inhibits c-Kit-induced hypoxia-inducible factor-1alpha activity and vascular endothelial growth factor expression in small cell lung cancer cells. Mol Cancer Ther 5: 1415–1422. 5/6/1415 [pii];10.1158/1535-7163.MCT-05-0503 [doi].

22. Chang KH, Chan-Ling T, McFarland EL, Afzal A, Pan H, et al. (2007) IGF binding protein-3 regulates hematopoietic stem cell and endothelial precursor cell function during vascular development. Proc Natl Acad Sci U S A 104: 10595–10600.

23. Dupont J, Khan J, Qu BH, Metzler P, Helman L, et al. (2001) Insulin and IGF-1 induce different patterns of gene expression in mouse fibroblast NIH-3T3 cells: identification by cDNA microarray analysis. Endocrinology 142: 4969–4975.

24. Molkentin JD, Dorn GW (2001) Cytoplasmic signaling pathways that regulate cardiac hypertrophy. Annu Rev Physiol 63: 391–426.

25. Sheikh F, Raskin A, Chu PH, Lange S, Domenighetti AA, et al. (2008) An FHL1-containing complex within the cardiomyocyte sarcomere mediates hypertrophic biomechanical stress responses in mice. J Clin Invest 118: 3870–3880.

26. Cheng H, Kimura K, Peter AK, Cui L, Ouyang K, et al. (2010) Loss of enigma homolog protein results in dilated cardiomyopathy. Circ Res 107: 348–356.

27. Essop MF (2007) Cardiac metabolic adaptations in response to chronic hypoxia. J Physiol 584: 715–726.

28. Maeda N, Funahashi T, Hibuse T, Nagasawa A, Kishida K, et al. (2004) Adaptation to fasting by glycerol transport through aquaporin 7 in adipose tissue. Proc Natl Acad Sci U S A 101: 17801–17806.

29. Wakayama Y, Inoue M, Kojima H, Jimi T, Shibuya S, et al. (2004) Expression and localization of aquaporin 7 in normal skeletal myofiber. Cell Tissue Res 316: 123–129.

30. Butler TL, Au CG, Yang B, Egan JR, Tan YM, et al. (2006) Cardiac aquaporin expression in humans, rats, and mice. Am J Physiol Heart Circ Physiol 291: H705–H713.

31. Skowronski MT, Lebeck J, Rojek A, Praetorius J, Fuchtbauer EM, et al. (2007) AQP7 is localized in capillaries of adipose tissue, cardiac and striated muscle: implications in glycerol metabolism. Am J Physiol Renal Physiol 292: F956–F965.

32. Adams JW, Sakata Y, Davis MG, Sah VP, Wang Y, et al. (1998) Enhanced Galphaq signaling: a common pathway mediates cardiac hypertrophy and apoptotic heart failure. Proc Natl Acad Sci U S A 95: 10140–10145.

33. Small K, Feng JF, Lorenz J, Donnelly ET, Yu A, et al. (1999) Cardiac specific overexpression of transglutaminase II (G(h)) results in a unique hypertrophy

34. Chen JS, Mehta K (1999) Tissue transglutaminase: an enzyme with a split personality. Int J Biochem Cell Biol 31: 817–836.

35. Milano CA, Dolber PC, Rockman HA, Bond RA, Venable ME, et al. (1994) Myocardial expression of a constitutively active alpha 1B-adrenergic receptor in transgenic mice induces cardiac hypertrophy. Proc Natl Acad Sci U S A 91: 10109–10113.

36. Faber JE, Szymeczek CL, Salvi SS, Zhang H (2006) Enhanced alpha1-adrenergic trophic activity in pulmonary artery of hypoxic pulmonary hypertensive rats. Am J Physiol Heart Circ Physiol 291: H2272–H2281.

37. Faber JE, Szymeczek CL, Cotecchia S, Thomas SA, Tanoue A, et al. (2007) Alpha1-adrenoceptor-dependent vascular hypertrophy and remodeling in murine hypoxic pulmonary hypertension. Am J Physiol Heart Circ Physiol 292: H2316–H2323.

38. Park HK, Park SJ, Kim CS, Paek YW, Lee JU, et al. (2001) Enhanced gene expression of renin-angiotensin system, TGF-beta1, endothelin-1 and nitric oxide synthase in right-ventricular hypertrophy. Pharmacol Res 43: 265–273.

39. Jiang Y, Dai A, Li Q, Hu R (2007) Hypoxia induces transforming growth factor-beta1 gene expression in the pulmonary artery of rats via hypoxia-inducible factor-1alpha. Acta Biochim Biophys Sin 39: 73–80.

40. Bianchi P, Kunduzova O, Masini E, Cambon C, Bani D, et al. (2005) Oxidative stress by monoamine oxidase mediates receptor-independent cardiomyocyte apoptosis by serotonin and postischemic myocardial injury. Circulation 112: 3297–3305.

41. Bianchi P, Pimentel DR, Murphy MP, Colucci WS, Parini A (2005) A new hypertrophic mechanism of serotonin in cardiac myocytes: receptor-independent ROS generation. FASEB J 19: 641–643.

42. Sivasubramaniam SD, Finch CC, Rodriguez MJ, Mahy N, Billett EE (2003) A comparative study of the expression of monoamine oxidase-A and -B mRNA and protein in non-CNS human tissues. Cell Tissue Res 313: 291–300.

43. Rodriguez MJ, Saura J, Billett EE, Finch CC, Mahy N (2001) Cellular localization of monoamine oxidase A and B in human tissues outside of the central nervous system. Cell Tissue Res 304: 215–220.

44. Redout EM, Wagner MJ, Zuidwijk MJ, Boer C, Musters RJ, et al. (2007) Right-ventricular failure is associated with increased mitochondrial complex II activity and production of reactive oxygen species. Cardiovasc Res 75: 770–781.

45. Iglarz M, Clozel M (2010) At the heart of tissue: endothelin system and end-organ damage. Clin Sci (Lond) 119: 453–463.

46. Balasubramanian S, Mani SK, Kasiganesan H, Baicu CC, Kuppuswamy D (2010) Hypertrophic stimulation increases beta-actin dynamics in adult feline cardiomyocytes. PLoS One 5: e11470.

47. Chen SJ, Chen YF, Meng QC, Durand J, Dicarlo VS, et al. (1995) Endothelin-receptor antagonist bosentan prevents and reverses hypoxic pulmonary hypertension in rats. J Appl Physiol 79: 2122–2131.

phenotype independent of phospholipase C activation. J Biol Chem 274: 21291–21296.

Patients with Congenital Systemic-to-Pulmonary Shunts and Increased Pulmonary Vascular Resistance: What Predicts Postoperative Survival?

Hui-Li Gan*, Jian-Qun Zhang, Qi-Wen Zhou, Lei Feng, Fei Chen, Yi Yang

Department of Cardiac Surgery, Beijing Anzhen Hospital, Capital Medical University, Beijing Institute of Heart, Lung and Blood Vessel Diseases, Beijing, China

Abstract

Background: We carried out a retrospective data review of patients with systemic to pulmonary shunts that underwent surgical repair between February 1990 and February 2012 in order to assess preoperative pulmonary vascular dynamic risk factors for predicting early and late deaths due presumably to pulmonary vascular disease.

Methods and Results: A total of 1024 cases of congenital systemic-to-pulmonary shunt and advanced pulmonary vascular disease beyond infancy and early childhood were closed surgically. The mean follow up duration was 8.5 ± 5.5 (range 0.7 to 20) years. Sixty-one in-hospital deaths (5.96%, 61/1024) occurred after the shunt closure procedure and there were 46 late deaths, yielding 107 total deaths. We analyzed preoperative pulmonary vascular resistance index (PVRI), pulmonary vascular resistance index on pure oxygen challenge (PVRIO), difference between PVRI and PVRIO (PVRID), Qp:Qs, and Rp:Rs as individual risk predictors. The results showed that these individual factors all predicted in-hospital death and total death with PVRIO showing better performance than other risk factors. A multivariable Cox regression model was built,and suggested that PVRID and Qp:Qs were informative factors for predicting survival time from late death and closure of congenital septal defects was safe with a $PVRIO < 10.3$ $WU.m^2$ and $PVRID > 7.3$ $WU.m^2$ on 100% oxygen.

Conclusions: All 4 variables, PVRI, PVRIO, PVRID and Qp:Qs, should be considered in deciding surgical closure of congenital septal defects and a $PVRIO < 10.3$ $WU.m^2$ and $PVRID > 7.3$ $WU.m^2$ on 100% oxygen are associated with a favorable risk benefit profile for the procedure.

Editor: Saeed Dastgiri, Tabriz University of Medical Sciences, Iran (Islamic Republic of)

Funding: This project was supported by of a grant (#81070041) from the China Nature Science Foundation Committee, a grant (#2013-2-002) from the Beijing health system special foundation for building high-level health personnel, and a grant (#Z121107001012067) from the Beijing Science and Technology Project. The funders had no role in study design, data collection and analysis, decision to publish, or preparation of the manuscript.

Competing Interests: The authors have declared that no competing interests exist.

* E-mail: ganhuili@hotmail.com

Introduction

Cardiac defects are among the most common causes of congenital disease with atrial and ventricular intracardiac shunts accounting for a significant proportion of such malformations. Preoperative pulmonary vascular disease is an important risk factor for death or right-heart failure in older patients undergoing palliative surgical repair for intracardiac shunting lesions. Despite many published reports, it remains unclear which preoperative hemodynamic variables best predict a satisfactory surgical outcome, i.e., acceptably low pulmonary vascular resistance (PVR) after operation [1,2]. Previous papers report a relatively small number of patients, a serious limitation given the substantial variation in the pulmonary vascular response to increased pressure and flow. Postoperative follow-up is limited in most previous reports, which becomes a significant issue over time as PVR may increase years after operation. Moreover, few reports have been published that present the results of studies designed to determine the risk factors (using multivariate analysis) affecting the outcome of the surgical procedures to treat intracardiac shunts. This has led to a lack of clear guidelines for all surgical centers, especially those

in parts of the world where surgeons have to deal with a large population of untreated older patients with congenital heart disease (CHD) and elevated PVR.

Surgical interventions for CHD have allowed long-term survival despite incomplete elimination of shunting. However, whether pulmonary vascular hemodynamic parameters could predict in-hospital death or late death in surgical patients with intracardiac shunts remain ill defined. Here, we carried out a retrospective data review of patients with systemic to pulmonary shunts that underwent surgical repair over a 10-year span between February 1990 and February 2012 in order to assess preoperative pulmonary vascular dynamic risk factors for predicting early and late deaths due presumably to pulmonary vascular disease.

Methods

The Ethics Committee of Beijing Anzhen Hospital approved this retrospective study and written informed consent was obtained from each patient or his or her legal surrogate for the operation. Because of the retrospective nature of this study, no patient consent was required; it was specifically waived by the approving IRB.

Patients

We retrospectively reviewed the demographic, clinical and surgical data of patients who underwent surgical repair for congenital intracardiac shunts at Beijing Anzhen Hospital over a 10-year span between February 1990 and February 2012. A patient was excluded from the analysis if 1) he or she also received heart valve repair or replacement, or other cardiac surgical procedures; 2) he or she had a residual heart defect after surgery, which may have impacted the severity of residual pulmonary hypertension; 3) he or she had defects such as branch pulmonary arterial stenosis, or obstruction of isolated pulmonary veins that preclude accurate calculation of PVR, Qp:Qs, and Rp:Rs. To determine surgical operability, all patients were discussed at a multidisciplinary team meeting consisting of pulmonary hypertension specialists, radiologists and cardiac surgeons. Closure of the defect was carried out for patients with PVR<10 Wood units (WU) and/or Qp:Qs>1.50 while medical therapy was recommended for patients with PVR≥20 WU and/or Qp:Qs≤1.0. For those with PVR between 10 and 20 WU and Qp:Qs between 1.0 and 1.5, operability was determined by the cardiac surgical team after a comprehensive evaluation of clinical data, history, physical examination, chest X-ray, arterial blood gas, electrocardiogram (ECG), echocardiography and catheterization data and careful consideration of the wishes of the patient and his or her family.

Cardiac catheterization

Cardiac catheterization was performed in all patients, using conscious sedation with continuous intravenous infusions of propofol and local analgesia, without intubation. Right atrial, pulmonary artery, and pulmonary capillary wedge pressures were measured using fluid-filled catheters. Cardiac output and pulmonary blood flow were measured by Fick's method, using assumed VO_2 and indexed to body surface area (BSA). Assumed VO_2 values were calculated according to the formula of LaFarge-Miettinen as follows:

$$VO_2/BSA = (138.1 - 17.04\ln(age) + 0.378HR)/BSA(mL/min)/m^2$$

For female subjects and

$$VO_2/BSA = (138.1 - 11.49\ln(age) + 0.378HR)/BSA(mL/min)/m^2$$

For male subjects, where age is presented in years and HR is defined as heart rate (in min). PVRI, which is PVR indexed to BSA, was calculated using the following equation:

$$PVRI(WUm^2) = [mPAP]/CI$$

Where CI represents the cardiac index, PCWP represents pulmonary capillary wedge pressure, and WU represents Wood units. Hemodynamic measurements were made with patient breathing room air and repeated while breathing 100% oxygen, 5 to 15 L/min by facemask. PVRIO is PVRI on 100% oxygen challenge, and PVRID is the numerical difference (in Wood units) between PVRI in room air and 100% oxygen.

Therapeutic regimen

All patients were operated under general anesthesia and moderate hypothermic cardiopulmonary bypass with cardiac arrest, and the defect was closed using standard techniques. Long-term management included the use of calcium channel blockers, phosphodiesterase 5 inhibitors (PDE5i), bosentan, cardiotonic glycosides, diuretics and warfarin, which were prescribed, where needed, at the discretion of attending physicians.

Follow-up

Patients were followed up at 12 months postoperatively and at one year interval thereafter. They were evaluated by cardiac surgeons or pulmonologists during each follow up visit for New York Heart Association (NYHA) functional class and by six-min walk test, transthoracic echocardiography (TTE) and ECG. These variables were examined at 12 month intervals at their local pulmonary hypertension specialist centre. Long-term clinical outcome was assessed up to August 2010 by reviewing the medical files of their pulmonologists, cardiologists, and general practitioners. Baseline demographics, procedural data, and perioperative outcomes were recorded. One of the investigators reviewed the medical files of all late deaths. A separate team of research assistants prospectively collected follow-up clinical data by telephone questionnaire after the patient was discharged from the hospital.

Statistical analysis

Basic statistical analyses were performed using the statistical software SPSS 17.0 (SPSS Inc, NUIT, and Evanston, IL, USA). Categorical data were expressed in total numbers and relative frequencies and continuous data were expressed in mean ± standard deviation (SD). The binary logistic regression models [3,4] were chosen to predict in-hospital (early) death and total death (early death plus late death), both of which both had binary outcomes. Receiver operating characteristic (ROC) curves were used to evaluate the corresponding balance between sensitivity and specificity over a range of values for PVRI, PVRIO, PVRID, Qp:Qs, and Rp:Rs, and the best cutoffs of sensitivity and specificity that corresponded to the maximum area under the curve (AUC) score were determined by choosing cutoffs that engendered maximum sensitivity plus specificity. In order to assess and compare the generalization of our predictors, ten-fold cross-validation on all patients were adopted. All patients were separated into ten groups randomly at beginning. For each time, we chose one group for testing and trained a predictive model on the remaining nine-fold data, and repeated this process for ten times. Finally, we obtained ten AUC scores after ten-fold cross validation for each predictive model based on each factor. Then, Student's t test was used for statistical comparison of AUC scores. In addition, multivariable Cox regression was used to build predictive models for evaluating patient survival and the corresponding concordance indices were calculated by the Survcomp package in statistical language R. Hosmer-Lemeshow (H-L) test was performed for "goodness of fit" evaluation. The logistic regression model was expressed as follows:

$$\text{Predicted Risk} = \frac{e^{(\beta_1 x_1 + \cdots + \beta_n x_n)}}{1 + e^{(\beta_1 x_1 + \cdots + \beta_n x_n)}},$$

Where $x_1, x_2, \ldots$ and x_n denote patient preoperative risk factors (e.g., PVRI, PVRIO, and PVRID) and $\beta_1, \beta_2 \ldots$ and β_n denote regression coefficients. The Cox regression (proportional hazards model) was expressed as follows:

$$\text{Hazard rate } h_i(t) = [h_0(t)]e^{b_0 + b_1 x_{i1} + \cdots + b_n x_{in}},$$

Where x_1, x_2, ..., and x_n denote patient preoperative risk factors (e.g., PVRI, PVRIO, and PVRID) and b_0, b_1, ...and b_n denote regression coefficients.

Results

Patient baseline demographic and disease characteristics

The study flow chart is shown in Figure 1. A total of 19451 patients with congenital intracardiac shunts received surgical treatment at our institutions throughout the study period and 1087 (5.59%) of these patients met our criteria for inclusion in this analysis. Twenty-one cases were excluded from the study because they had received heart valve repair or replacement, or other cardiac surgical procedures. Thirty-three cases were excluded because of residual heart defect after surgery, which may have impacted the severity of residual pulmonary hypertension. Nine cases were excluded because of defects such as branch pulmonary arterial stenosis, or obstruction of isolated pulmonary veins that preclude accurate calculation of PVR, Qp:Qs, and Rp:Rs. As a result, a total of 1024 (5.26%, including 5 patients with Down's syndrome) met the study criteria and were included in the analysis. The demographic and disease characteristics of these patients are shown in Table 1. They included 335 (34.7%) females and their mean age was 18.8±8.1 years (range, 2.4 to 44.6 years). They had a mean pulmonary arterial pressure (mPAP) of 70.2±9.2 mmHg and a PVRI of 15.5±2.6 Wood units and Qp:Qs of 2.20±0.87. The age at the diagnosis of the cardiac defect ranged from 29 months to 45 years, and the age of operation was 30 months to 45 years. The interval between age at diagnosis and age at operation was less than three weeks.

Early and late mortality

Three hundred and twenty nine (32.1%) patients experienced pulmonary hypertensive crisis and acute heart failure, and 61 succumbed to the crisis despite therapy with PGE$_1$, iloprost and

Table 1. Baseline Demographic and Disease Characteristics (n = 1024).

Age, mean ± SD(interquartile range), yrs	18.8±8.1(13.2–23.9)
Age older than 18 yrs, n (%)	543(53)
Female, n (%)	335(34.7)
Primary CHD	
ASD, n (%)	126 (12.3)
VSD, n (%)	576 (56.2)
PDA, n (%)	123(12.1)
ASD+VSD, n (%)	74 (7.2)
ASD+PDA, n (%)	23 (2.3)
VSD+PDA, n (%)	71 (7.0)
ASD+VSD+PDA, n (%)	20 (2.0)
APW, n (%)	11 (1.1)
Shunt level	
NYHA functional class ≥III, n (%)	237(23.1)
6MWD (m)	386±116.6
Hemoglobin (g/L)	179±21
LVEF (%)	61.6±7.9
SaO$_2$ (%)	91.3±3.4
Right atrial pressure (mmHg)	10.7±2.7
mPAP (mm Hg)	70.2±9.2
SPAP/SBP	0.99±0.078
PVRI (Wood Units)	15.5±2.6
Qp:Qs, mean ± SD (interquartile range)	2.20±0.87(1.56–2.65)
Rp:Rs, mean + SD (interquartile range)	0.71±0.17(0.59–0.83)

6MWD, 6 min walk distance; APW, aorto-pulmonary windows; ASD, atrial septal defect; CHD, congenital heart disease; LVEF, left ventricular ejection fraction; mPAP, mean pulmonary artery pressure; PDA, patent ductus arteriosus; PVRI, pulmonary vascular resistance, indexed to body surface area; Qp:Qs, pulmonary to systemic flow ratio; Rp:Rs, ratio of pulmonary and systemic vascular resistance; SPAP, systolic pulmonary artery pressure; SPAP/SBP, pulmonary to systemic systolic artery pressure ratio; TTE, transthoracic echocardiography; VSD, ventricular septal defect.

inhaled NO, and mechanical ventilatory support. Thus, the in-hospital surgical mortality was 5.96% (61/1024) and 963 patients, including 5 patients with Down syndrome, were available for follow up. The mean duration of the follow-up period was 8.5±5.5 years (range, 0.7 to 20 years). One hundred sixty-nine patients (17.5%) received medication with calcium channel blockers, 23 (2.4%) with PDE5i, 6 (0.63%) with bosentan, 138 (14.3%) with glycosides, 139 (14.4%) with diuretics, and 15 (1.6%) with warfarin. Forty-six late deaths were reported from chronic right heart failure (23), arrhythmia (8), acute pulmonary hypertension (7), lung infection (4), hemoptysis (3), and brain abscess (1). The late postoperative mortality rate was 4.49%. The Kaplan-Meier survival curve for late death after shunt closure is depicted in Figure 2. The cumulative survival stood at 95.7% at 10 years and 81.7% at 20 years.

Pulmonary vascular hemodynamic parameters predict risks for early and late mortality

We further examined whether survival was associated with any of the demographic or pulmonary hemodynamic characteristics of these patients. We found a statistically significant difference in PVRI, PVRIO, PVRID, Qp:Qs, and Rp:Rs in early survivors and

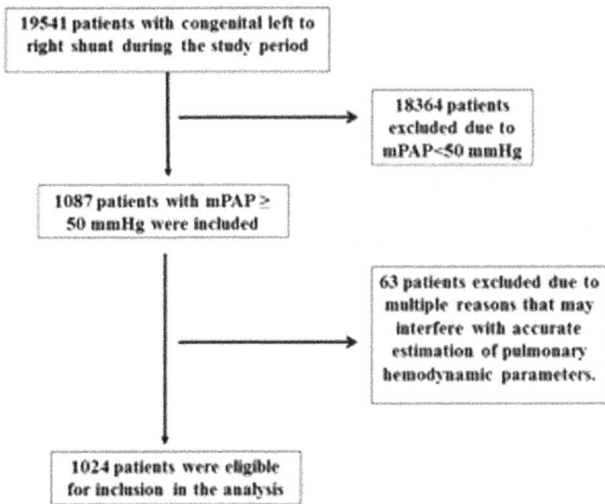

Figure 1. The study flow chart for 1024 patients with intracardiac shunts who had undergone surgical closure of the defects.

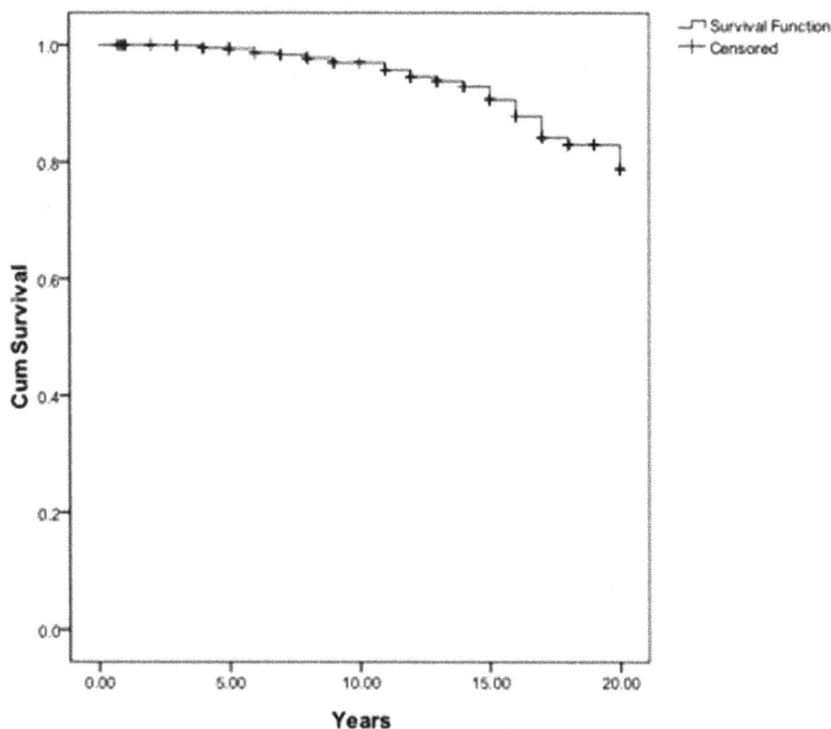

Figure 2. The Kaplan-Meier survival curve after the shunt closure procedure for patients with congenital systemic-to-pulmonary shunts and increased pulmonary vascular resistance.

early non-survivors (P<0.001) (Table 2). ROC curve analysis further revealed that the use of PVRI<18.1 WU.m^2, PVRIO<11.1 WU.m^2, PVRID>7.3 WU.m^2 on 100% oxygen, Qp:Qs<1.34, and Rp:Rs>0.82 as pulmonary hemodynamic criteria for surgical closure of intracardiac shunts provided the optimal positive and negative predictive value, sensitivity, specificity, and accuracy for in-hospital death (see Fig. S1 and Table S1 in File S1). On the other hand, PVRI>17.6 WU.m^2, PVRIO>10.3 WU.m^2, PVRID<7.3 WU.m^2 on 100% oxygen, Qp:Qs<1.55, and Rp:Rs>0.83 provided the optimal positive and negative predictive value, sensitivity, specificity, and accuracy for total death, respectively (see Fig. S2 and Table S2 in File S1). In addition, PVRIO better predicted in-hospital and total death than PVRI, PVRID, Qp:Qs, and Rp:Rs (P<0.000 in all).

The above findings suggested that these individual parameters predicted in-hospital death and total death risk. We were further interested in investigating whether these parameters in combination could predict early and late mortality. We firstly built logistic regression for each factor, and then used binary logistic regression with likelihood ratio-based forward stepwise strategy to predict early death and late death by automatically selecting useful factors from all the factors. The results for each single factor and for the final model for in-hospital death and late death prediction are shown in the supplementary tables (Table S3 and Table S4 in File S1, respectively) with corresponding H-L test for "goodness of fit" evaluation. The results showed that PVRIO and PVRID were the most important risk factors for both in-hospital death and late

Table 2. Pulmonary Vascular Hemodynamic Risk Factors in Early Survivors and Non-survivors of Surgical Patients with Intracardiac Shunts.

	Early Death (n = 61)	Early Survival (n = 963)	P
Age at operation, mean ± SD, yrs, (interquartile range)	19.8±9.1 (11.1–27.7)	18.8±8.1 (13.3–23.8)	0.238
Age at operation, median, yrs	20.9	18.5	
PVRI (WU)	20.25±2.20	15.17±2.25	0.000
PVRIO (WU)	16.63±3.20	7.15±2.58	0.000
PVRID (WU)	3.63±1.83	8.01±1.01	0.000
Rp:Rs	1.02±0.14	0.69±0.15	0.000
Qp:Qs	1.19±0.22	2.26±0.86	0.000

PVRI, pulmonary vascular resistance index; PVRIO, pulmonary vascular resistance index on pure oxygen challenge; PVRID, difference between PVRI and PVRIO; Qp:Qs, pulmonary to systemic flow ratio; Rp:Rs, ratio of pulmonary and systemic vascular resistance; WU, Wood units.

death and Qp:Qs was another important factor for predicting in-hospital death.

Using late death data, we asked how these hemodynamic factors affected the prediction of survival time. Using ROC curves to obtain the optimal thresholds as separate criteria for predicting late death as we did in predicting early death and total death (Figure S1 and S2), we found that PVRIO also better predicted late death than PVRI, PVRID, Qp:Qs, and Rp:Rs ($P<0.000$ in all) (also see Table S5 in File S1). Given the abundance of available survival data, we then used more advanced methods with consideration of censoring information to predict late death. We built Cox regression models based on each individual factor to predict late death and used concordance index [5] to assess their performance. The results show that, of the four parameters, PVRIO displayed the best performance (Table S6 in File S1). We further selected all the variables together to build a forward stepwise Cox regression model (based on likelihood ratio) to predict late death. We found that the final model only included PVRID and Qp:Qs, as shown in the formula: $exp(-0.849 \times PVRID - 1.548 \times Qp:Qs)$, and the corresponding concordance index was equal to 0.796 ± 0.041 with $P<0.000$.

We further analyzed the performance of hemodynamic parameters in predicting survival of patients with intracardiac shunts (see Table S7 in File S1 for detailed characteristics). We built three Cox regression models (with a likelihood ratio-based forward stepwise strategy) separately for patients with pre-tricuspid shunt, post-tricuspid shunt or both. The final model for the ASD subgroup contained only PVRID (with coefficient of -1.284); and the same was true for the VSD subgroup (coefficient of -1.015), while for the ASD and VSD subgroup, the final model contained two hemodynamic parameters PVRID (with coefficient of -0.851) and Qp:Qs (with coefficient of -1.519). The PVRID was thus the most important predictor for survival events no matter which subgroups the patient belongs to, and gender was not a significant factor for any of the subgroups.

Discussion

Pulmonary arterial hypertension (PAH) commonly arises in patients with CHD and its management may involve surgical correction of the cardiac defect and/or treatment of PAH, depending on the underlying cardiac defect and status of disease progression. The timing of intervention in patients with PAH-CHD is important, but the optimum time is sometimes difficult to determine, with limited robust data to support an informed management decision [6]. In patients with congenital intracardiac shunting lesions, once advanced pulmonary vascular occlusive disease is established, closure of the defect may markedly shorten survival relative to leaving the defect open as in Eisenmenger syndrome [7]. This often remains a critical issue for older patients and for children 2 or 3 years of age who have a complete atrioventricular canal or Down syndrome. It is therefore imperative to assess the risk of post-shunt closure pulmonary hypertension in all patients before referring them for operation. Many papers have been published relating various hemodynamic variables to outcome after shunt closure, but considerable uncertainty remains regarding which baseline variables and what values associated with these variables confer a favorable risk-benefit ratio for operation [1,2]. The utility of pulmonary vasodilators in revealing the likelihood of high postoperative PVR is also uncertain. Two studies suggest that PVRI≤7 WU with a vasodilator (tolazoline) conferred suitability for operation [8,9], but a third study found that PVRI (with iNO and 100% O_2) of <5.3 was more suitable [1]. Still others indicate that Rp:Rs with

vasodilators is a better indicator of operative risk [1]. One study found that vasodilation with 100% oxygen did not guarantee low PVR after defect closure [10].

There are multiple reasons for this uncertainty, including considerable biological variability in the response of the pulmonary circulation to intracardiac shunting. Previous papers report different hemodynamic variables (e.g., Rp:Rs vs. PVR, and PVR vs. indexed PVR), in patients of different ages, with different durations of follow-up. How outcomes are reported varies, and it is sometimes unclear whether postoperative death was related to PAH or some other factors. Some papers reflect relatively early experience in the era of open heart surgery before effective management of postoperative PAH was available [11,12]. Finally, available reports include only a relatively small number of patients (<100 patients/report) with septal defects and significantly increased PAP and PVR [1,8–18]. Mean duration of follow-up is often not clearly given, but is usually much less than 10 years [8,11,16,18]. Except the study by Balzer et al., these reports lack a sufficient number of patients and detailed follow-up to permit a formal and thorough statistical analysis of the predictive power of multiple hemodynamic variables to predict outcome after operation.

In this study, we report our retrospective review of clinical and hemodynamic data of a large cohort of patients with intracardiac shunts who had undergone surgical closure of cardiac defects. The longest follow up of these patients is 20 years with a mean duration follow up of 8.5 ± 5.5 years. The abundance of available data from the data set and the length of follow up allowed us to carry out a considerably more extensive analysis of hemodynamic predictors of survival for these patients. Notably, we found that the risk of early or late death was unrelated to patient age. It has been clearly documented that very young patients ($<\sim2$ years old) are much less likely to have persistently increased PVR after VSD repair than older children [13,19]. It appears that beyond the first few years of life, age is not a significant discriminator of outcome (at least in the first ~20 years of life). Our findings support the idea that some adolescents with high pressure shunts can safely undergo repair. Though this is not a new finding, our finding carries more weight given the much larger number of patients in our study than any previous reports [17,18,20].

We further show that PVRIO<10.3 WU.m^2 and PVRID>7.3 WU.m^2 best predicted survival. Perhaps not surprisingly, and consistent with previous reports [1,14], Rp:Rs is different in survivors and non-survivors, with Rp:Rs of <0.83 being associated with a good outcome, although it is not as good a predictor of outcome as PVRIO or PVRID. Qp:Qs is also not as powerful a predictor, although it is notable that the average Qp:Qs in survivors is substantially different from non-survivors. The final model for predicting survival from late death after the shunt closure procedure only includes PVRID and Qp:Qs, suggesting that the combination of informative factors can yield much better performance and the final model could predict the survival time quite well. Since measurement of PVR is fraught with potential error, taking into account all 4 variables, not only PVRIO and PVRID, but also PVRID and Qp:Qs, is important in determining whether to proceed an operation.

The iNO, with or without enhanced inspired oxygen, is usually used for vasodilator testing today [1,21]. When we first commenced this protocol, iNO was not available for such use, for the sake of consistency; we report here only our experience with 100% oxygen. Despite the use of a seemingly sub-optimal vasodilator regimen, we found that PVRID with 100% fiO$_2$ is a sensitive and specific predictor of postoperative mortality. Our finding that a fall in PVRI with a vasodilator of <17.6 Wood units suggesting a low likelihood of postoperative death is consistent with other studies [1,8,9], but not with that by Lock, *et al* [10]. In addition, we found little difference between patients with ASD and those with VSD regarding survival predictors. PVRID is thus the most important predictor for survival events no matter which subgroups (i.e., post-tricuspid shunt, pre-tricuspid shunt and both) the patient belongs to, and gender is not a significant factor for any of the subgroups.

This report has several limitations. As noted, our vasodilator testing protocol no longer reflects the most current practice; it is possible that the addition of iNO may further enhance predictive power of the change in PVR with vasodilation. In addition, we used assumed oxygen consumption, doubtlessly introducing some errors into calculations of pulmonary blood flow and derived variables. Furthermore, we only reported the outcomes of patients who had defect closure; it is likely that some patients who did not undergo operation would have done well with repair. Moreover, our study is only weakly powered to identify patients who develop findings related to progressive PAH very late (>10 years postoperatively).

In summary, we have taken advantage of a very large clinical data set to ask which pulmonary vascular hemodynamic parameters best predict survival in patients with congenital shunting lesions and high preoperative PAP after surgical repair. We found that preoperative PVRI, PVRIO, Qp:Qs, Rp:Rs, and change in PVRI with 100% O_2 can all predict in-hospital death and total death, with PVRIO being the most sensitive and specific predictor. A very similar result was obtained for predicting late death (by evaluating the survival time). Despite the very high degree of sensitivity and specificity of PVRID in predicting postoperative survival, it is important that this only occurs when multiple factors have been taken into account in judging suitability for repair of patients with intracardiac shunting lesions.

Conclusion

In conclusion, our study demonstrates that all 4 pulmonary hemodynamic variables, PVRI, PVRIO, PVRID and Qp:Qs, should be considered in deciding surgical closure of congenital septal defects and a PVRIO<10.3 WU.m^2 and PVRID>7.3 WU.m^2 on 100% oxygen are associated with a favorable risk benefit profile for the procedure and suggests that closure of congenital septal defects can be undertaken with acceptable risk.

Supporting Information

Figure S1 ROC curves for PVRI, PVRIO, PVRID, Rp:Rs, and Qp:Qs as predictors of early death. We chose cutoff points for operability for the 5 variables by inspecting the ROC curves to identify the point where specificity plus sensitivity

was found to be maximal. PVRI, pulmonary vascular resistance index; PVRID, difference between PVRI and PVRIO; PVRIO, pulmonary vascular resistance index on pure oxygen challenge; Qp:Qs, pulmonary to systemic flow ratio; Rp:Rs, ratio of pulmonary and systemic vascular resistance; WU, Wood units.

Figure S2 ROC curves for PVRI, PVRIO, PVRID, Rp:Rs, and Qp:Qs as predictors of total death (early and late death). We picked cutoff points for operability for the 5 variables by inspecting the ROC curves to identify the point where specificity plus sensitivity was found to be maximal. PVRI, pulmonary vascular resistance index; PVRID, difference between PVRI and PVRIO; PVRIO, pulmonary vascular resistance index on pure oxygen challenge; Qp:Qs, pulmonary to systemic flow ratio; Rp:Rs, ratio of pulmonary and systemic vascular resistance; WU, Wood units.

File S1 Table S1 in File S1. ROC Characteristics of Pulmonary Vascular Hemodynamic Parameters as Predictors of Early Mortality in Surgical Patients with Intracardiac Shunts. Table S2 in File S1. ROC characteristics of Pulmonary Vascular Hemodynamic Parameters as Predictors of Total (Early and Late) Mortality in Surgical Patients with Intracardiac Shunts. Table S3 in File S1. Odds Ratios with 95% Confidence Intervals (CI) for Single Factor-based Risk Models. Table S4 in File S1. Multivariate Logistic Regression Model Performance. Table S5 in File S1. ROC characteristics of Pulmonary Vascular Hemodynamic Parameters as Predictors of Late Mortality in Surgical Patients with Intracardiac Shunts. Table S6 in File S1. The Performance of Cox Regression Model for Predicting Late Deaths Built on Different Pulmonary Vascular Hemodynamic Parameters. Table S7 in File S1. Characteristics of Patients with Pre-tricuspid and Post-tricuspid shunts

Acknowledgments

The authors would like to thank Thomas J. Kulik, MD for his assistance in the preparation of this manuscript. We would also like to thank professional biostatisticians from Beijing Preintell Biotechnology Investment Ltd. for their help in data analysis.

Author Contributions

Conceived and designed the experiments: H-LG. Performed the experiments: H-LG J-QZ Q-WZ LF FC YY. Analyzed the data: H-LG. Contributed reagents/materials/analysis tools: H-LG. Carried out the shunt closure surgery: H-LG J-QZ Q-WZ LF FC YY. Designed the study and prepared the manuscript: H-LG. Read and approved the final manuscript: H-LG J-QZ Q-WZ LF FC YY.

References

1. Balzer DT, Kort HW, Day RW, Corneli HM, Kovalchin JP, et al. (2002) Inhaled Nitric Oxide as a Preoperative Test (INOP Test I): the INOP Test Study Group. Circulation 106:I76–I81.

2. Giglia TM, Humpl T (2010) Preoperative pulmonary hemodynamics and assessment of operability: is there a pulmonary vascular resistance that precludes cardiac operation? Pediatric Critical Care Medicine: A Journal Of The Society Of Critical Care Medicine And The World Federation Of Pediatric Intensive And Critical Care Societies 11:S57–S69.

3. Shahian DM, O'Brien SM, Filardo G, Ferraris VA, Haan CK, et al. (2009) Society of Thoracic Surgeons Quality Measurement Task Force. The Society of Thoracic Surgeons 2008 cardiac surgery risk models: part 1–coronary artery bypass grafting surgery. Ann Thorac Surg 88:S2–22.

4. Shroyer AL, Coombs LP, Peterson ED, Eiken MC, DeLong ER, et al. (2003) Society of Thoracic Surgeons. The Society of Thoracic Surgeons: 30-day operative mortality and morbidity risk models. Ann Thorac Surg 75:1856–1865.

5. Schröder MS, Culhane AC, Quackenbush J, Haibe-Kains B (2011) Survcomp: an R/Bioconductor package for performance assessment and comparison of survival models. Bioinformatics 27:3206–3208.

6. Gatzoulis MA, Alonso-Gonzalez R, Beghetti M (2009) Pulmonary arterial hypertension in paediatric and adult patients with congenital heart disease. Eur Respir Rev 18:154–161.

7. Beghetti M, Galiè N, Bonnet D (2012) Can "inoperable" congenital heart defects becomeoperable in patients with pulmonary arterial hypertension? Dream or reality? Congenital Heart Disease 7:3–11.

8. Neutze JM, Ishikawa T, Clarkson PM, Calder AL, Barratt-Boyes BG, et al. (1989) Assessment and follow-up of patients with ventricular septal defect and elevated pulmonary vascular resistance. The American Journal of Cardiology 63:327–331.

9. Momma K, Takao A, Ando M, Nakazawa M, Takamizawa K (1981) Natural and post-operative history of pulmonary vascular obstruction associated with ventricular septal defect. Japanese Circulation Journal 45:230–237.

10. Lock JE, Einzig S, Bass JL, Moller JH (1982) The pulmonary vascular response to oxygen and its influence on operative results in children with ventricular septal defect. Pediatric Cardiology 3:41–46.
11. Hallidie-Smith KA, Hollman A, Cleland WP, Bentall HH, Goodwin JF (1969) Effects of surgical closure of ventricular septal defects upon pulmonary vascular disease. British Heart Journal 31:246–260.
12. Cartmill TB, DuShane JW, McGoon DC, Kirklin JW (1966) Results of repair of ventricular septal defect. J Thorac Cardiovasc Surg 52:486–501.
13. Castaneda AR, Zamora R, Nicoloff DM, Moller JH, Hunt CE, et al. (1971) High-pressure, high-resistance ventricular septal defect. Surgical results of closure through right atrium. Ann Thorac Surg 12:29–38.
14. Friedli B, Kidd BS, Mustard WT, Keith JD (1974) Ventricular septal defect with increased pulmonary vascular resistance. Late results of surgical closure. The American Journal of Cardiology 33:403–409.
15. Blackstone EH, Kirklin JW, Bradley EL, DuShane JW, Appelbaum A (1976) Opitmal age and results in repair of large ventricular septal defects. J Thorac Cardiovasc Surg 72:661–679.
16. John S, Korula R, Jairaj PS, Muralidharan S, Ravikumar E, et al. (1983) Results of surgical treatment of ventricular septal defects with pulmonary hypertension. Thorax 38:279–283.
17. Ikawa S, Shimazaki Y, Nakano S, Kobayashi J, Matsuda H, et al. (1995) Pulmonary vascular resistance during exercise late after repair of large ventricular septal defects. Relation to age at the time of repair. J Thorac Cardiovasc Surg 109:1218–1224.
18. Kannan BRJ, Sivasankaran S, Tharakan JA, Titus T, Ajith Kumar VK, et al. (2003) Long-term outcome of patients operated for large ventricular septal defects with increased pulmonary vascular resistance. Indian Heart Journal 55:161–166.
19. DuShane JW, Krongrad E, Ritter DG, McGoon DC (1976) The Fate of Raised Pulmonary Vascular Resistance After Surgery in Ventricular Septal Defect. In: Kidd BS, Rowe RD, editors. The Child With Congenital Heart Disease After Surgery. Mount Kisco, NY: Futura Publishing Company, Inc. p. 299–312.
20. Braunwald NS, Braunwald E, Morrow A (1962) The effects of surgical abolition of left-to-right shunts on the pulmonary vascular dynamics of patients with pulmonary hypertension. Circulation 26:1270–1278.
21. Berner M, Beghetti M, Spahr-Schopfer I, Oberhansli I, Friedli B (1996) Inhaled nitric oxide to test the vasodilator capacity of the pulmonary vascular bed in children with long-standing pulmonary hypertension and congenital heart disease. The American Journal of Cardiology 77:532–535.

17

Supplementing Exposure to Hypoxia with a Copper Depleted Diet Does Not Exacerbate Right Ventricular Remodeling in Mice

Ella M. Poels[1], Nicole Bitsch[1], Jos M. Slenter[2], M. Eline Kooi[2], Chiel C. de Theije[3], Leon J. de Windt[1], Vanessa P. M. van Empel[4,9], Paula A. da Costa Martins[1*,9]

1 Department of Cardiology, CARIM School for Cardiovascular Diseases, Faculty of Health, Medicine and Life Sciences, Maastricht University, Maastricht, The Netherlands, 2 Department of Radiology, CARIM School for Cardiovascular Diseases, Maastricht University Medical Centre, Maastricht, The Netherlands, 3 Department of Respiratory Medicine, NUTRIM School Nutrition, Toxicology and Metabolism, Maastricht University Medical Centre, Maastricht, The Netherlands, 4 Department of Cardiology, Heart Vessel Center, Maastricht University Medical Centre, Maastricht, The Netherlands

Abstract

Background: Pulmonary hypertension and subsequent right ventricular (RV) failure are associated with high morbidity and mortality. Prognosis is determined by occurrence of RV failure. Currently, adequate treatment for RV failure is lacking. Further research into the molecular basis for the development of RV failure as well as the development of better murine models of RV failure are therefore imperative. We hypothesize that adding a low-copper diet to chronic hypoxia in mice reinforces their individual effect and that the combination of mild pulmonary vascular remodeling and capillary rarefaction, induces RV failure.

Methods: Six week old mice were subjected to normoxia (N; 21% O_2) or hypoxia (H; 10% O_2) during a period of 8 weeks and received either a normal diet (Cu+) or a copper depleted diet (Cu-). Cardiac function was assessed by echocardiography and MRI analysis.

Results and Conclusion: Here, we characterized a mouse model of chronic hypoxia combined with a copper depleted diet and demonstrate that eight weeks of chronic hypoxia (10%) is sufficient to induce RV hypertrophy and subsequent RV failure. Addition of a low copper diet to hypoxia did not have any further deleterious effects on right ventricular remodeling.

Editor: James West, Vanderbilt University Medical Center, United States of America

Funding: EP was supported by a grant from Stichting Sint Annadal and PCM was supported by a Leducq Career Development Award and the Dutch Heart Foundation grant NHS2010B261. The funders had no role in study design, data collection and analysis, decision to publish or preparation of the manuscript.

* E-mail: p.dacostamartins@maastrichtuniversity.nl

9 These authors contributed equally to this work.

Introduction

Pulmonary hypertension (PH) and subsequent right ventricular (RV) failure are associated with high morbidity and mortality. Prognosis is mainly determined by the ability of the RV to adapt to increased afterload, a key characteristic of PH. [1–5] Little is known about the mechanisms underlying the development of RV failure, and transition of RV hypertrophy to RV failure.

There are several animal models available to study RV failure. The most frequently used models are rodent-models, where exposure to either monocrotaline or hypoxia induces RV remodeling and failure. [6,7] Chronic hypoxia induces both vasoconstriction and remodeling of the pulmonary vascular bed resulting in increased pulmonary pressure, leading to RV failure. [8,9] This model was predominantly studied in rats, but recent studies demonstrated that mice exhibit a less severe pulmonary vascular remodeling when exposed to chronic hypoxia compared to rats. [9] In mice, chronic hypoxia induced RV hypertrophy and increased right ventricular systolic pressure (RVSP). [10–22] Although the effect of hypoxia on RV function remains largely unstudied, the few studies that did look at fractional shortening or RV cardiac output failed to show a decrease. [23,24] However, one must note that this included only short-term exposure to hypoxia.

Other rodent models of pulmonary hypertension mostly involve multiple insults, including the combination of chronic hypoxia with VEGFR inhibition (SuHx) and monocrotalin treatment with pneumonectomy, to induce not only pulmonary vascular remodeling but also subsequent RV failure. [14,25–27] In mice, SuHx is the only double-insult model previously described to induce RV failure [14].

Bogaard et al. showed that addition of a copper-depleted diet to pulmonary artery banding (PAB) in rats led to increased RV fibrosis and RV dilation as well as capillary rarefaction. [26] Low-copper diet interferes with HIF-1α protein stabilization, which is necessary for vascular endothelial growth factor (VEGF) expression, and therefore subsequently affects angiogenesis. [26,28] Under hypoxic conditions, myofiber area increases two-fold, leading to a reduction in capillary density, however a small increase in capillary: fiber ratio is seen as a result of modest proliferation of capillaries secondary to RV hypertrophy. [29] It is known that maintaining cardiac function during hypertrophy is in part, angiogenesis-dependent, and that lack of VEGF expression contributes to the progression from adaptive cardiac hypertrophy to heart failure [30,31].

In contrast, a copper-depleted diet prevented the development of severe experimental pulmonary hypertension in the rat model, which included VEGF receptor blockade with chronic hypoxia (SuHx model), by reducing obliteration of the small pulmonary vessels [32].

In recent years, the possibilities for genetic engineering in mice have significantly evolved, making the use of mice as an animal model highly attractive. It would therefore be beneficial to have murine models of right ventricular failure. We hypothesize that a low-copper diet added to chronic hypoxia in mice reinforces their individual effects and the combination of mild pulmonary vascular remodeling, with RV capillary rarefaction, induces RV failure. Therefore we propose to investigate the effect of a low copper diet in a murine model of chronic hypoxia on right ventricular function.

Materials and Methods

Animals

All animal handling and procedures were approved by the ethics committee of animal welfare at Maastricht University, and were in accordance with governmental guidelines.

A total of 48 C57BL/6 male mice were used at 6 weeks of age at the start of the experiment. Mice were housed at room temperature ($20°C$) and placed in a 12-hour light-dark cycle. Food and water were accessible ad libitum; food consumption was monitored and was similar for all four experimental groups, hence pair-feeding was deemed unnecessary throughout the experiment. Mice received either a copper depleted diet (Harlan Teklad, TD 80388) or a normal chow diet (Harlan Teklad LM-485).

For hypoxia, the animals were placed in a sealed chamber (n = 12 per experimental group); a fan circulated air within the chamber. O_2 concentration was maintained at 10% by controlling the inflow rate of N_2. Prior to keeping mice at 10% O_2, they were allowed to adjust to their surroundings for 24 hours to minimize stress, and O_2 levels were gradually decreased to 10% over an additional period of 72 hours. Littermates served as controls in the normoxia group and were kept in room air (21% O_2); a fan ensured proper air circulation within the chamber. Chambers were unsealed for less than 15 minutes per day in order to replenish food, clean cages and check ventilators.

Echocardiography

Mice were anaesthetized with isoflurane (mean 1.5% in oxygen), shaved and allowed to breathe spontaneously through a nasal cone. Non-invasive, echocardiographic parameters were measured using a digital cardiac ultrasound platform (Vevo 2100, Visual-Sonics); for cardiac parameters, the transducer was applied parasternally to the shaved chest wall, and measurements were performed as previously described [33].

MRI

Mice were anaesthetized using isoflurane. Body temperature was monitored using a rectal temperature probe and mice were placed under a warm-water blanket. Additionally, respiratory rate

was monitored continuously. MRI was performed using a 7 Tesla Bruker Biospec 70/30 USR (Bruker Biospin, Ettlingen, Germany).

The right ventricle was measured using an Intragate sequence, with a field of view of 25.6×25.6 mm, matrix was 256×256, TE 3 ms, TR, 60 ms, 7 slices. The cine calculated out of the Intragate sequence consists of 15 frames. All images were analyzed in OsiriX (Dicom viewer, version 3.5, Pixmeo, Geneva, Switzerland). The RV end-diastolic and RV end-systolic volumes were analysed using multi-slice short axis cine-images of the complete right ventricle. RV ejection fraction was calculated as (RVEDV-RVESV)/RVEDV *100.

Assessment of RV Hypertrophy

The heart was dissected and both atria, the aorta, and the pulmonary trunk were removed. The right ventricle was separated from the left ventricle and the ventricular septum. Right ventricular hypertrophy was expressed using the Fulton index; the ratio of the weight of the right ventricular wall to the left ventricular wall and ventricular septum (RV/LV+S).

Histology, Immunohistochemistry and Immunofluorescence

Heart- and lung specimens were fixed and cleared of blood by perfusion with 3.8% paraformaldehyde and subsequently embedded in paraffin. Tissue sections (4 µm) were stained with hematoxylin and eosin (H&E) for routine histological anaylsis, or with picro-Sirius red for visualization of collagen deposition. Additionally, FITC-labeled wheat-germ-agglutinin (WGA) was used to visualize and quantify cross-sectional cell area; capillary density was visualized and quantified using a Griffonia simplicifolia agglutin-I (GS-I) lectin stain.

Slides were visualized and imaged using a Zeiss Axioskop 2Plus with an AxioCamHRc.

Fulton-index was used as an index for RV hypertrophy and calculated as the ratio of the RV free wall weight over the septum plus left ventricular free wall weight.

Real-time PCR

Primers were designed to detect transcripts for *nppa* (NM_008725, 5'-TCTTCCTCGTCTTGGCCTTT, 5'-CCAGGTGGTCTAGCAGGTTC), *nppb* (NM_008726, 5'-TGGGAGGTCACTCCTATCCT, 5'-GGCCATTTCCTCC-GACTTT), *acta1* (NM_009606, 5'-CCGGGAGAAGATGACT-CAAA, 5'-GTAGTACGGCC GGAAGCATA), *myh7* (NM_080728, 5'-CGGACCTTGGAAGACCAGAT, 5'-GA-CAGC TCCCCATTCTCTGT) and *rcan1.4* (NM_019466, 5'-GCTTGACTGAGAGAGCGAGTC, 5'-CCACACAAGCAAT-CAGGGAGC).

RNA was isolated from tissue using TRIzol reagent (Invitrogen) RNA (1 µg) from right ventricular mouse heart tissue was reverse-transcribed using Superscript II reverse transcriptase (Invitrogen). Real-time PCR was performed on a BioRad iCycler (Biorad) using SYBR Green. Transcript quantities were compared using the relative Ct method, which normalizes the amount of target to the amount of endogenous control (L7) relative to the control sample, and are given by 2−ΔΔCt.

Statistical Analysis

The results are presented as mean ± standard error of the mean (s.e.m.). Statistical analyses were performed using Prism software (GraphPad Software), and consisted of ANOVA followed by Tukey's post-test when group differences were detected at the 5%

significance level, or Student's t-test when comparing two groups. Differences were considered significant when P<0.05.

Results

Chronic Hypoxia Induces RV Hypertrophy

In order to study the effect of a low copper diet on right ventricular function in a murine model of chronic hypoxia we used four different wildtype mice groups subjected to different conditions as depicted in Figure 1a. The animals were followed for 8 weeks, during which cardiac function was analyzed every two weeks by echocardiography and complemented with MRI analysis at week 4 and 8 (Figure 1b). Pictures of whole hearts and HE stains, after 8 weeks of hypoxia, showed normal tissue morphology and absence of inflammatory cell infiltration for all groups. Additionally, there was no significant increase in fibrosis, assessed using Sirius Red staining, in hypoxia groups when compared to normoxia (Figure 1c). Moreover, the difference in mean heart weight corrected for body weight between normoxia/Cu+ (4.1±0.1 g/g), normoxia/Cu- (4.2±0.1 g/g), hypoxia/Cu+ (4.5±0.1 g/g), hypoxia/Cu- (4.1±0.1 g/g) did not differ (Figure 1d). Right ventricular weight, expressed using Fulton index (RV: (LV+septum)), was increased in hypoxia/Cu+ mice (0.39±0.02) compared to normoxia/Cu+ mice (0.23±0.01; p=0.033; Figure 1e), indicating that hypoxia was sufficient to induce hypertrophic growth of the right ventricle. There was no further increase in Fulton index after adding a copper deficient diet to hypoxia treatment (hypoxia/Cu- 0.40±0.0.06, p=0.988), indicating no additional effect of a copper deficient diet on RV hypertrophy. Cell surface area demonstrated a trend towards an increase when comparing hypoxia to normoxia groups (Figure 1i, j). Mice showed no clinical signs of overt heart failure, e.g. no peripheral edema. Liver- and lung weights were normal and showed no significant differences between groups (p=0.337, p=0.223 respectively) (Figure 1f, g). This data correlates with the observed heart weights in Figure 1d. Furthermore, mice showed no drop in body weight after the introduction of hypoxia (normoxia/Cu+: 26.0±1.6 g, hypoxia/Cu+: 23.3±1.2 g, p=0.528; Figure 1h).

Combination of Low-copper Diet with Hypoxia does not Exacerbate RV Failure

RV ejection fraction was decreased after 8 weeks in hypoxia/Cu+ mice (58.8±3.3) compared to normoxia/Cu+ mice (71.7±2.6%, p=0.05), demonstrating that hypoxia lead to RV failure (Figure 2a). However combination of low-copper diet with hypoxia did not have an additional detrimental effect with regard to RV failure. Interestingly, the RV end-systolic and end-diastolic volumes remained unchanged between all four groups at both 4 and 8 weeks (Figure 2b, c).

Hypoxia nor Low-copper Diet Affected Capillary Density

Capillary density was determined by a GS-1 stain, showing no differences between hypoxia/Cu-, hypoxia/Cu+, nor normoxia/Cu- and normoxia/Cu+ mice (Figure 2d, e).

Stress Markers

Real-time PCR was performed to determine the expression levels of cardiac stress markers in the right ventricle (Figure 2f). There were no significant changes in cardiac stress marker expression when comparing all experimental conditions. We have also assessed Calcineurin-NFAT signaling activity by determining rcan1.4 expression at the mRNA level. Although there seems to be a trend for increased expression under a copper-deficient diet, this

effect was not statistical significant. Furthermore, no differences were observed when comparing all 4 groups.

Discussion

This study demonstrates that exposing mice to 8 weeks of hypoxia induces RV failure. The addition of a copper depleted diet to hypoxia did not have an additional deleterious effect on RV function. Furthermore copper depletion alone did not have an effect on RV hypertrophy or RV function.

Dempsey at al. showed that susceptibility to chronic hypoxia varies between species and murine susceptibility strongly depends on genetic background. [9,34] Response to hypoxia was also significantly affected by the age of the animal; 'infant' rats of 8 days old with maturing lungs were more susceptible to a hypoxic trigger compared to older, adult animals. [8] [35] We used C57BL/6 mice and started the experiment at an adult age with 6 weeks-old mice, however it is possible that using a different strain of mice and/or starting the experiment at a younger age elicits a different response to hypoxia. Vascular remodeling after exposure to hypoxia was less significant in mice compared to rats. [36] Even when VEGF blocker was added to hypoxia in mice this did not lead to the typical plexiform lesions described in rats. [14] Several studies have previously shown that 3 weeks of hypoxia (10% O_2) in mice leads to an increase in RV hypertrophy, and our data indicate that prolonged hypoxia exposure also results in a larger increase in Fulton index. [14,24,37] Although RV dilation was shown previously, our model demonstrates that chronic hypoxia for 8 weeks induces RV failure.

Our study demonstrated that copper depleted diet combined with exposure to hypoxia did not influence RV hypertrophy. During sustained pressure overload, cardiac copper and VEGF levels decreased, coinciding with a suppression of myocardial angiogenesis. [28] Previous studies demonstrated that copper supplementation reverses hypertrophy by copper stimulation of VEGF production through activation of HIF1a. [38,39] This is in accordance with the fact that copper depleted diet interfered with angiogenesis, which is needed to sustain RV hypertrophy. Additionally, it has been shown that copper depletion itself, in the absence of other forms of stress on the ventricle, can induce ventricular hypertrophy, mainly through an increase in mitochondrial volume density as well as in increase in mitochondria. [40] Furthermore, lack of cardiac copper promoted cardiac electrical conduction abnormalities, including ventricular fibrillation and heart block, which could be abrogated by adequate copper supplementation. [40–42] We, however, did not observe any dropout in our animal groups on copper depleted diet, suggesting that there were no lethal cardiac conduction disturbances. Perhaps prolonging the study duration beyond 8 weeks would increase the risk and induction of arrhythmias, although it is known that mice and rats are more resistant to the development of cardiac conduction abnormalities than other species.

Copper is needed in the development of severe pulmonary hypertension and the formation of angioproliferative lesions in the SuHx model. [32] Although these lesions resemble plexiform lesions typical for pulmonary artery hypertension, patients with pulmonary hypertension due to left heart disease and/or lung disease, which represent the majority of PH patients do not present with plexiform lesions. [43] Furthermore, copper depletion did not influence the degree of pulmonary artery media thickness in the SuHx rat model, or influence pulmonary pressures, RV hypertrophy or media thickness. We did not see an influence of copper in the development of RV hypertrophy or the development of RV failure in our hypoxia mice model.

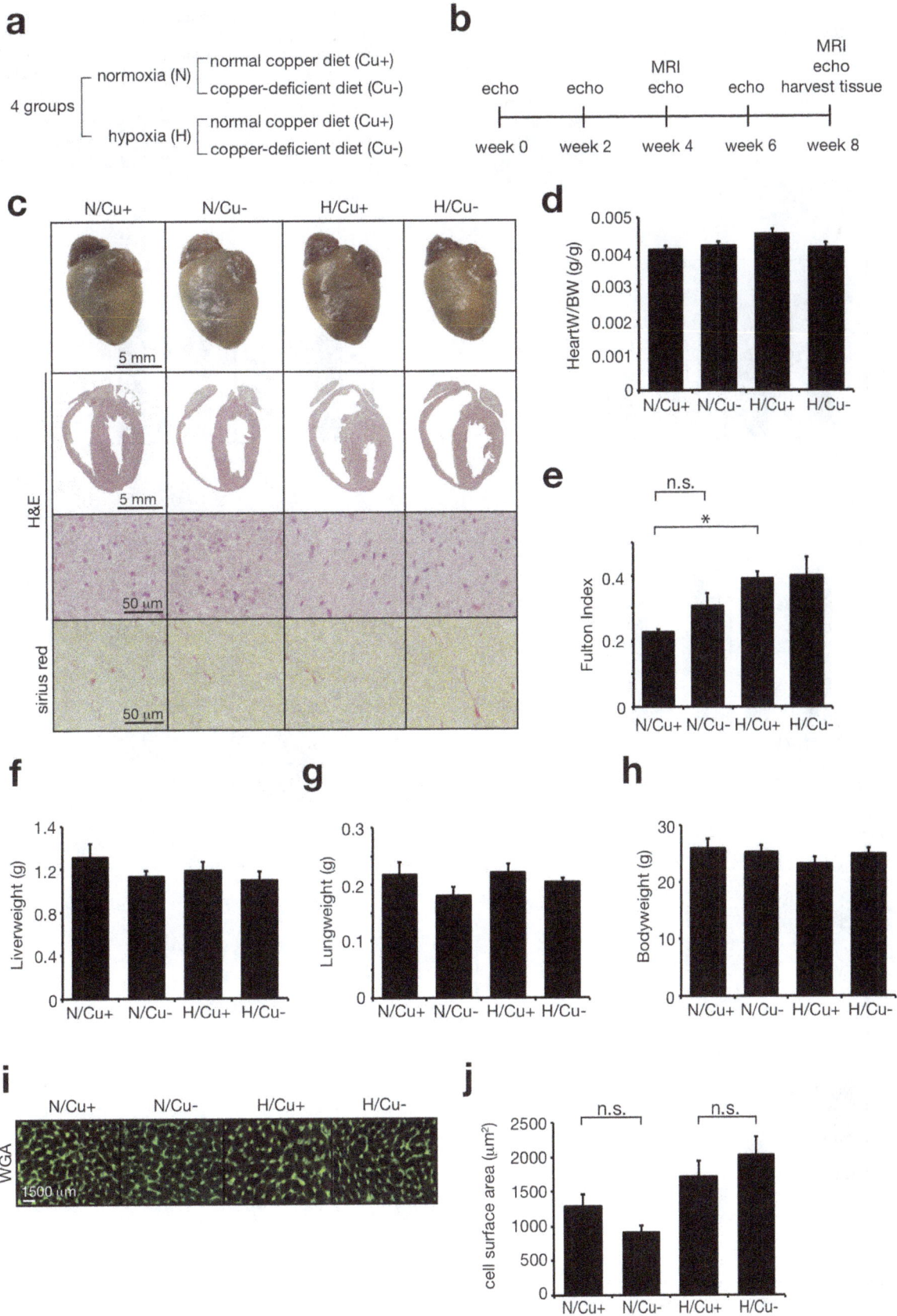

Figure 1. Chronic hypoxia leads to an increase in Fulton index. (a) Experimental groups. (b) Study design. (c) Representative images of whole hearts (upper panels), haematoxylin & eosin (H&E) stained 4-chamber paraffin sections (second panels), high magnification H&E stained free right ventricular wall histological sections (third panels), high magnification sirius red stained free right ventricular wall sections (lower panels. The

following groups are compared: normoxia on normal chow diet (N/Cu+), normoxia on copper depleted diet (N/Cu-), hypoxia on normal chow diet (H/Cu+) and hypoxia on copper depleted diet (H/Cu-). (d) Heartweight corrected for bodyweight in grams per gram. (n = 9) *P<0.05. (e) Fulton index calculated as ratio of RV free wall weight over septum plus LV free wall weight. (f) Liverweight in grams. (g) Lungweight in grams. (h) Bodyweight in grams. (i) Representative images of wheat germ agglutinin (WGA) stained sections. (j) Quantification of average cell surface area using WGA stained sections. (n≥610) *P<0.05 (mean ± s.e.m.).

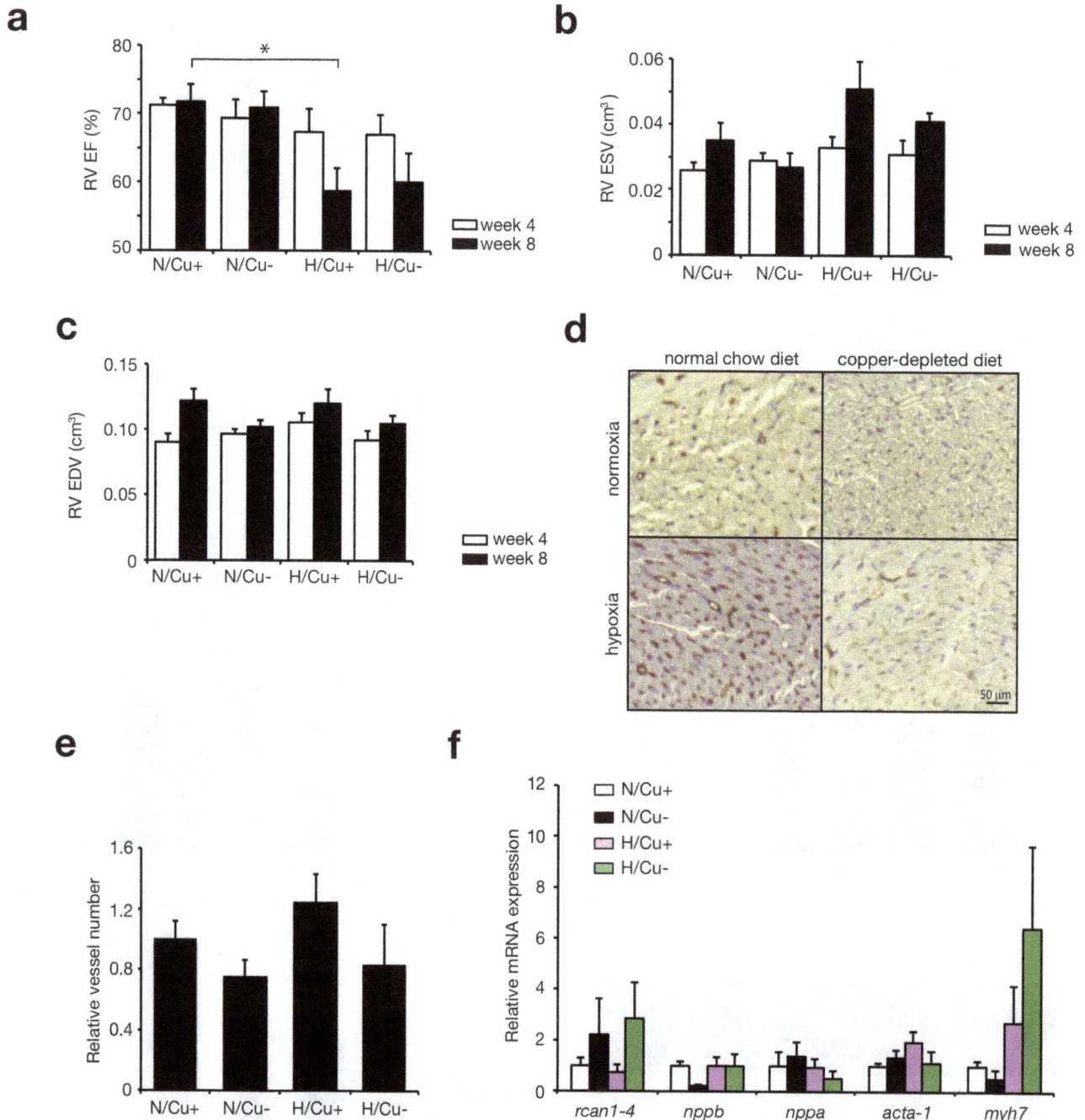

Figure 2. Chronic hypoxia induces a decrease in right ventricular ejection fraction. Right ventricular ejection fraction (EF) measured by MRI at 4 and 8 weeks. The following groups are compared: normoxia on normal chow diet (N/Cu+), normoxia on copper depleted diet (N/Cu), hypoxia on normal chow diet (H/Cu+) and hypoxia on copper depleted diet (H/Cu-). (b) Right ventricular end systolic volumes in cm^3 and (c) right ventricular end diastolic volumes in cm^3. (n = 6) (d) Griffonia simplicifolia 1 (GS-1)-stain on representative right ventricular free wall paraffin sections. (e) Quantification of GS-1 stain, expressed as relative vessel number. (f) Real-time PCR analysis of transcript abundance for cardiac stress marker genes in right ventricles at 8 weeks. (n = 3) *P<0.05 (mean ± s.e.m.).

During hypertrophy, the ventricle reaches a critical point where the amount of capillaries can no longer sustain the amount of ventricular tissue and the ventricle will rapidly start to fail.

We are aware that our results may be the consequence of the timeframe of our experimental setup (8 weeks under hypoxic conditions) and it is likely that increasing the period of hypoxia will strengthen the effect of adding copper depleted diet to chronic hypoxia. Nevertheless, eight weeks of hypoxia was sufficient to induce RV failure in mice.

The fact that cardiac stress markers are not increased in hypoxia could be explained by differences in stress response between the right and left ventricles. Accordingly, it is known that the right ventricle reacts differently to stress by activating different mechanisms and pathways. [44,45] Therefore, it is reasonable to think that under chronic stress conditions, different markers are induced in the right ventricle compared to the left ventricle. On the other hand, the degree of RV hypertrophy and failure caused by 8 weeks of exposure to 10% hypoxia may be insufficient to induce increased expression levels of the tested cardiac stress markers. A recent study has implicated NFAT activation as a requirement for chronic hypoxia-induced pulmonary hypertension. [46] Since activation of NFAT signaling is a direct modulator of the left ventricle response to cardiac stress [47] leading to left

ventricle hypertrophic growth and eventually heart failure, we investigated whether chronic hypoxia leads to RV hypertrophy through direct activation of NFAT transcription factors. RCAN1.4 gene expression, a target gene of the calcineurin/NFAT pathway, responsive to NFAT activation, did not significantly change between all groups. Although a trend for increased RCAN1.4 expression under a low-copper diet was observed, suggesting that copper-deficiency induced cardiac stress may lead to calcineurin/NFAT signaling activation, more investigation is needed to clarify this matter.

In conclusion, we demonstrate that prolonged exposure to hypoxia induces RV failure. Prolonged exposure to hypoxia leads to more pronounced RV hypertrophy, compared to short-term exposure. [10–22] Finally, dietary copper deficiency did not have any further deleterious effects on RV function.

Author Contributions

Conceived and designed the experiments: VPME PCM. Performed the experiments: EMP NB JS CCT. Analyzed the data: EMP MEK LJW VPME PCM. Contributed reagents/materials/analysis tools: CCT MEK LJW PCM. Wrote the paper: EMP VPME PCM.

References

1. Chin KM, Kim NH, Rubin LJ (2005) The right ventricle in pulmonary hypertension. Coron Artery Dis 16: 13–18.
2. Chin KM, Rubin LJ (2008) Pulmonary arterial hypertension. J Am Coll Cardiol 51: 1527–1538.
3. Galie N, Hoeper MM, Humbert M, Torbicki A, Vachiery JL, et al. (2009) Guidelines for the diagnosis and treatment of pulmonary hypertension: the Task Force for the Diagnosis and Treatment of Pulmonary Hypertension of the European Society of Cardiology (ESC) and the European Respiratory Society (ERS), endorsed by the International Society of Heart and Lung Transplantation (ISHLT). Eur Heart J 30: 2493–2537.
4. Howard LS (2011) Prognostic factors in pulmonary arterial hypertension: assessing the course of the disease. Eur Respir Rev 20: 236–242.
5. Rubin LJ (1997) Primary pulmonary hypertension. N Engl J Med 336: 111–117.
6. Brown L, Miller J, Dagger A, Sernia C (1998) Cardiac and vascular responses after monocrotaline-induced hypertrophy in rats. Journal of cardiovascular pharmacology 31: 108–115.
7. Pelouch V, Kolar F, Ost'adal B, Milerova M, Cihak R, et al. (1997) Regression of chronic hypoxia-induced pulmonary hypertension, right ventricular hypertrophy, and fibrosis: effect of enalapril. Cardiovascular drugs and therapy/sponsored by the International Society of Cardiovascular Pharmacotherapy 11: 177–185.
8. Stenmark KR, Fagan KA, Frid MG (2006) Hypoxia-induced pulmonary vascular remodeling: cellular and molecular mechanisms. Circulation research 99: 675–691.
9. Stenmark KR, Meyrick B, Galie N, Mooi WJ, McMurtry IF (2009) Animal models of pulmonary arterial hypertension: the hope for etiological discovery and pharmacological cure. American journal of physiology Lung cellular and molecular physiology 297: L1013–1032.
10. Bauer EM, Zheng H, Comhair S, Erzurum S, Billiar TR, et al. (2011) Complement C3 deficiency attenuates chronic hypoxia-induced pulmonary hypertension in mice. PloS one 6: e28578.
11. Brusselmans K, Compernolle V, Tjwa M, Wiesener MS, Maxwell PH, et al. (2003) Heterozygous deficiency of hypoxia-inducible factor-2alpha protects mice against pulmonary hypertension and right ventricular dysfunction during prolonged hypoxia. The Journal of clinical investigation 111: 1519–1527.
12. Calmettes G, Deschodt-Arsac V, Gouspillou G, Miraux S, Muller B, et al. (2010) Improved energy supply regulation in chronic hypoxic mouse counteracts hypoxia-induced altered cardiac energetics. PloS one 5: e9306.
13. Caruso P, Dempsie Y, Stevens HC, McDonald RA, Long L, et al. (2012) A role for miR-145 in pulmonary arterial hypertension: evidence from mouse models and patient samples. Circulation research 111: 290–300.
14. Ciuclan L, Bonneau O, Hussey M, Duggan N, Holmes AM, et al. (2011) A novel murine model of severe pulmonary arterial hypertension. American journal of respiratory and critical care medicine 184: 1171–1182.
15. Paddenberg R, Stieger P, von Lilien AL, Faulhammer P, Goldenberg A, et al. (2007) Rapamycin attenuates hypoxia-induced pulmonary vascular remodeling and right ventricular hypertrophy in mice. Respiratory research 8: 15.
16. Scherrer-Crosbie M, Steudel W, Hunziker PR, Foster GP, Garrido L, et al. (1998) Determination of right ventricular structure and function in normoxic

and hypoxic mice: a transesophageal echocardiographic study. Circulation 98: 1015–1021.
17. Steudel W, Scherrer-Crosbie M, Bloch KD, Weimann J, Huang PL, et al. (1998) Sustained pulmonary hypertension and right ventricular hypertrophy after chronic hypoxia in mice with congenital deficiency of nitric oxide synthase 3. The Journal of clinical investigation 101: 2468–2477.
18. van Suylen RJ, Aartsen WM, Smits JF, Daemen MJ (2001) Dissociation of pulmonary vascular remodeling and right ventricular pressure in tissue angiotensin-converting enzyme-deficient mice under conditions of chronic alveolar hypoxia. American journal of respiratory and critical care medicine 163: 1241–1245.
19. Vanderpool RR, El-Bizri N, Rabinovitch M, Chesler NC (2013) Patchy deletion of Bmpr1a potentiates proximal pulmonary artery remodeling in mice exposed to chronic hypoxia. Biomechanics and modeling in mechanobiology 12: 33–42.
20. Yoshikawa N, Shimizu N, Maruyama T, Sano M, Matsuhashi T, et al. (2012) Cardiomyocyte-specific overexpression of HEXIM1 prevents right ventricular hypertrophy in hypoxia-induced pulmonary hypertension in mice. PloS one 7: e52522.
21. Yu AY, Shimoda LA, Iyer NV, Huso DL, Sun X, et al. (1999) Impaired physiological responses to chronic hypoxia in mice partially deficient for hypoxia-inducible factor 1alpha. The Journal of clinical investigation 103: 691–696.
22. Zhang Y, Talwar A, Tsang D, Bruchfeld A, Sadoughi A, et al. (2012) Macrophage migration inhibitory factor mediates hypoxia-induced pulmonary hypertension. Molecular medicine 18: 215–223.
23. Brown RD, Ambler SK, Li M, Sullivan TM, Henry LN, et al. (2013) MAP kinase kinase kinase-2 (MEKK2) regulates hypertrophic remodeling of the right ventricle in hypoxia-induced pulmonary hypertension. American journal of physiology Heart and circulatory physiology 304: H269–281.
24. Cruz JA, Bauer EM, Rodriguez AI, Gangopadhyay A, Zeineh NS, et al. (2012) Chronic hypoxia induces right heart failure in caveolin-1−/− mice. American journal of physiology Heart and circulatory physiology 302: H2518–2527.
25. Sakao S, Taraseviciene-Stewart L, Lee JD, Wood K, Cool CD, et al. (2005) Initial apoptosis is followed by increased proliferation of apoptosis-resistant endothelial cells. FASEB journal : official publication of the Federation of American Societies for Experimental Biology 19: 1178–1180.
26. Bogaard HJ, Natarajan R, Henderson SC, Long CS, Kraskauskas D, et al. (2009) Chronic pulmonary artery pressure elevation is insufficient to explain right heart failure. Circulation 120: 1951–1960.
27. Okada K, Tanaka Y, Bernstein M, Zhang W, Patterson GA, et al. (1997) Pulmonary hemodynamics modify the rat pulmonary artery response to injury. A neointimal model of pulmonary hypertension. The American journal of pathology 151: 1019–1025.
28. Jiang Y, Reynolds C, Xiao C, Feng W, Zhou Z, et al. (2007) Dietary copper supplementation reverses hypertrophic cardiomyopathy induced by chronic pressure overload in mice. The Journal of experimental medicine 204: 657–666.
29. Clark DR, Smith P (1978) Capillary density and muscle fibre size in the hearts of rats subjected to stimulated high altitude. Cardiovascular research 12: 578–584.

30. Shiojima I, Sato K, Izumiya Y, Schiekofer S, Ito M, et al. (2005) Disruption of coordinated cardiac hypertrophy and angiogenesis contributes to the transition to heart failure. The Journal of clinical investigation 115: 2108–2118.

31. Izumiya Y, Shiojima I, Sato K, Sawyer DB, Colucci WS, et al. (2006) Vascular endothelial growth factor blockade promotes the transition from compensatory cardiac hypertrophy to failure in response to pressure overload. Hypertension 47: 887–893.

32. Bogaard HJ, Mizuno S, Guignabert C, Al Hussaini AA, Farkas D, et al. (2012) Copper dependence of angioproliferation in pulmonary arterial hypertension in rats and humans. American journal of respiratory cell and molecular biology 46: 582–591.

33. da Costa Martins PA, Bourajjaj M, Gladka M, Kortland M, van Oort RJ, et al. (2008) Conditional dicer gene deletion in the postnatal myocardium provokes spontaneous cardiac remodeling. Circulation 118: 1567–1576.

34. Dempsey EC, Wick MJ, Karoor V, Barr EJ, Tallman DW, et al. (2009) Neprilysin null mice develop exaggerated pulmonary vascular remodeling in response to chronic hypoxia. The American journal of pathology 174: 782–796.

35. Rabinovitch M, Gamble WJ, Miettinen OS, Reid L (1981) Age and sex influence on pulmonary hypertension of chronic hypoxia and on recovery. The American journal of physiology 240: H62–72.

36. Yet SF, Perrella MA, Layne MD, Hsieh CM, Maemura K, et al. (1999) Hypoxia induces severe right ventricular dilatation and infarction in heme oxygenase-1 null mice. The Journal of clinical investigation 103: R23–29.

37. Steiner MK, Syrkina OL, Kolliputi N, Mark EJ, Hales CA, et al. (2009) Interleukin-6 overexpression induces pulmonary hypertension. Circulation research 104: 236–244, 228p following 244.

38. Zhou Y, Bourcy K, Kang YJ (2009) Copper-induced regression of cardiomyocyte hypertrophy is associated with enhanced vascular endothelial growth factor receptor-1 signalling pathway. Cardiovascular research 84: 54–63.

39. Hughes WM, Jr., Rodriguez WE, Rosenberger D, Chen J, Sen U, et al. (2008) Role of copper and homocysteine in pressure overload heart failure. Cardiovascular toxicology 8: 137–144.

40. Wildman RE, Medeiros DM, Hamlin RL, Stills H, Jones DA, et al. (1996) Aspects of cardiomyopathy in copper-deficient pigs. Electrocardiography, echocardiography, and ultrastructural findings. Biological trace element research 55: 55–70.

41. Klevay LM (2000) Cardiovascular disease from copper deficiency–a history. The Journal of nutrition 130: 489S–492S.

42. Klevay LM, Viestenz KE (1981) Abnormal electrocardiograms in rats deficient in copper. The American journal of physiology 240: H185–189.

43. Moraes DL, Colucci WS, Givertz MM (2000) Secondary pulmonary hypertension in chronic heart failure: the role of the endothelium in pathophysiology and management. Circulation 102: 1718–1723.

44. Bartelds B, Borgdorff MA, Smit-van Oosten A, Takens J, Boersma B, et al. (2011) Differential responses of the right ventricle to abnormal loading conditions in mice: pressure vs. volume load. European journal of heart failure 13: 1275–1282.

45. Walker LA, Buttrick PM (2009) The right ventricle: biologic insights and response to disease. Current cardiology reviews 5: 22–28.

46. Ramiro-Diaz JM, Nitta CH, Maston LD, Codianni S, Giermakowska W, et al. (2013) NFAT is required for spontaneous pulmonary hypertension in superoxide dismutase 1 knockout mice. American journal of physiology Lung cellular and molecular physiology 304: L613–625.

47. Wilkins BJ, Dai YS, Bueno OF, Parsons SA, Xu J, et al. (2004) Calcineurin/NFAT coupling participates in pathological, but not physiological, cardiac hypertrophy. Circulation research 94: 110–118.

18

Quantification of Tortuosity and Fractal Dimension of the Lung Vessels in Pulmonary Hypertension Patients

Michael Helmberger[1,2⑨], Michael Pienn[1⑨], Martin Urschler[2,3], Peter Kullnig[4], Rudolf Stollberger[5], Gabor Kovacs[1,6], Andrea Olschewski[1,7], Horst Olschewski[1,6], Zoltán Bálint[1]*

1 Ludwig Boltzmann Institute for Lung Vascular Research, Graz, Austria, 2 Institute for Computer Graphics and Vision, Graz University of Technology, Graz, Austria, 3 Ludwig Boltzmann Institute for Clinical Forensic Imaging, Graz, Austria, 4 DiagnostikZentrum Graz, Graz, Austria, 5 Institute for Medical Engineering, Graz University of Technology, Graz, Austria, 6 Division of Pulmonology, Department of Internal Medicine, Medical University of Graz, Graz, Austria, 7 Experimental Anesthesiology, Department of Anesthesia and Intensive Care Medicine, Medical University of Graz, Graz, Austria

Abstract

Pulmonary hypertension (PH) can result in vascular pruning and increased tortuosity of the blood vessels. In this study we examined whether automatic extraction of lung vessels from contrast-enhanced thoracic computed tomography (CT) scans and calculation of tortuosity as well as 3D fractal dimension of the segmented lung vessels results in measures associated with PH. In this pilot study, 24 patients (18 with and 6 without PH) were examined with thorax CT following their diagnostic or follow-up right-sided heart catheterisation (RHC). Images of the whole thorax were acquired with a 128-slice dual-energy CT scanner. After lung identification, a vessel enhancement filter was used to estimate the lung vessel centerlines. From these, the vascular trees were generated. For each vessel segment the tortuosity was calculated using distance metric. Fractal dimension was computed using 3D box counting. Hemodynamic data from RHC was used for correlation analysis. Distance metric, the readout of vessel tortuosity, correlated with mean pulmonary arterial pressure (Spearman correlation coefficient: $\rho = 0.60$) and other relevant parameters, like pulmonary vascular resistance ($\rho = 0.59$), arterio-venous difference in oxygen ($\rho = 0.54$), arterial ($\rho = -0.54$) and venous oxygen saturation ($\rho = -0.68$). Moreover, distance metric increased with increase of WHO functional class. In contrast, 3D fractal dimension was only significantly correlated with arterial oxygen saturation ($\rho = 0.47$). Automatic detection of the lung vascular tree can provide clinically relevant measures of blood vessel morphology. Non-invasive quantification of pulmonary vessel tortuosity may provide a tool to evaluate the severity of pulmonary hypertension.

Editor: Giacomo Frati, Sapienza University of Rome, Italy

Funding: This study was funded by the Ludwig Boltzmann Institute for Lung Vascular Research. The funders had no role in study design, data collection and analysis, decision to publish, or preparation of the manuscript.

Competing Interests: G. Kovacs reports personal fees from Glaxo Smithkline, personal fees from Actelion, personal fees from Pfizer, personal fees from Boehringer Ingelheim, personal fees from Astra Zeneca, personal fees from Nycomed-Takeda, personal fees from Bayer, personal fees from Chiesi, outside the submitted work. H. Olschewski reports personal fees from Ludwig Boltzmann Institute for Lung Vascular Research, during the conduct of the study; grants and personal fees from Actelion, grants and personal fees from Bayer, personal fees from Chiesi, personal fees from Gilead, personal fees from Lilly, personal fees from Boehringer, personal fees from Almirall, personal fees from Pfizer, grants and personal fees from GSK, personal fees from Astra Zeneca, personal fees from Novartis, personal fees from Takeda, outside the submitted work. PK is radiologist in the private practice of radiologists, DiagnostikZentrum Graz.

* E-mail: zoltan.balint@lvr.lbg.ac.at

⑨ These authors contributed equally to this work.

Introduction

Pulmonary hypertension (PH) is a chronic disorder of the pulmonary circulation, marked by an elevated vascular resistance and pressure. This results in functional limitations, increased load on the right heart and may subsequently lead to right-heart failure [1]. PH is defined as a mean pulmonary arterial pressure (mPAP) ≥ 25 mmHg, which is determined during invasive right heart catheterisation (RHC) [1,2]. Despite the low risk of adverse events of this invasive investigation, there is a need for non-invasive procedures to support the indication for an RHC investigation or to replace an invasive procedure in the follow-up of patients [3,4].

Radiological features of PH are vascular pruning due to vascular remodelling and loss of arterial branching [5]. Recently,

a non-invasive, thoracic computed tomography derived, lung vessel based diagnostic method for chronic obstructive lung diseases (COPD) was presented [6]. The authors characterize smoking-related COPD by the magnitude of distal pruning measured from automatically identified and segmented lung vessels. Application of parallel computing algorithms on general purpose graphic processor units can lead to proper vessel segmentation through automatic processing of 3D volumetric CT data within a reasonable time [7,8]. This is a crucial step for the quantification of vascular measures in order to aid the diagnosis of vascular diseases [9,10].

Tortuosity is a measure of twistedness of blood vessels and can increase due to hypertension or vasculopathies [11–13]. Tortuosity is also applied in clinical settings to differentiate between benign and malignant tumours [14,15] or to characterize retinal vascular changes [16]. The most common metric of vascular tortuosity is the "distance metric", which provides a ratio of the actual vessel path length to the linear distance between its endpoints [17,18]. This metric has been used to characterize tortuosity of tumors using 3D animal microCT [19,20]. Another parameter to measure the complexity of the lung vascular tree is the fractal dimension. A fractal is a self-similar object over different scales [21]. The complexity of a fractal object can be measured by the fractal dimension (FD) which is a measure of space filling [22–24]. This parameter has been used for characterization of the human retina [16,25] or different tumour entities [26,27]. Two studies evaluated the fractal dimension of 2D projections of the lung vascular system in patients with PH [28,29]. Moledina et al. showed that the 2D FD of children suffering from PH negatively correlated with the pulmonary vascular resistance, WHO functional class and 6-min walk distance. Moreover, in their study, decreased FD was associated with poor survival. In the other study [29] an increased 2D FD of the projected pulmonary arteries in PH patients was associated with an increased mPAP.

The purpose of this study was to automatically detect the lung vessels from contrast-enhanced chest CT scans in 3D and quantify their tortuosity and 3D fractal dimension. These measures were compared to patient clinical parameters derived from RHC.

Patients and Methods

Ethics statement
The study was approved by the Institutional Review Board of the Medical University of Graz under the number *23–356 ex 10/11* and written informed consent was obtained from all patients.

Patient population
All patients undergoing diagnostic or follow-up RHC at the Division of Pulmonology between June 2011 and January 2013 with indication for diagnostic contrast-enhanced thoracic CT were included (Figure 1). Both, patients with and without PH were included. Exclusion criteria were renal failure (creatinin > 1.3 mg/dl), known adverse reactions against iodinated CM, a recent diagnostic CT, more than 1 month between RHC and CT examination, pregnancy and missing written informed consent.

Examinations
RHC was performed on all patients for diagnostic or follow-up reasons by the same medical personal with 8 years of experience. A 7-F quadruple-lumen, balloon-tipped, flow-directed Swan-Ganz catheter (Baxter Healthcare, Irvine, California) was used in a transjugular approach without transparency.

The thoracic CT examination was performed with a 128-slice dual-energy CT scanner (Somatom Definition Flash, Siemens, Forchheim, Germany). X-ray tube A was set to an acceleration voltage of 100 kV with a reference current time product of 91 mAs$_{ref}$ and tube B to 140 kV with 77 mAs$_{ref}$ together with a 0.4 mm tin filter. Pitch was set to 1.0 and an automatic exposure control was used to reduce the X-ray dose. 40 ml of non-ionic contrast material (Ultravist 370 mg/ml iodine, Bayer Schering Pharma Diagnostic Imaging, Leverkusen, Germany) were injected into an arm vein at 5 ml/s with an automatic power injector (CT-Injector Ohio Tandem, Ulrich, Ulm, Germany). This was followed by a 21 ml saline chaser injected at the same rate. For timing of the scan a test bolus was used. The CT examination protocol was set before the first examination. The results of the RHC were known at the CT examination in order to set time intervals for the test bolus examination [30]. The images were

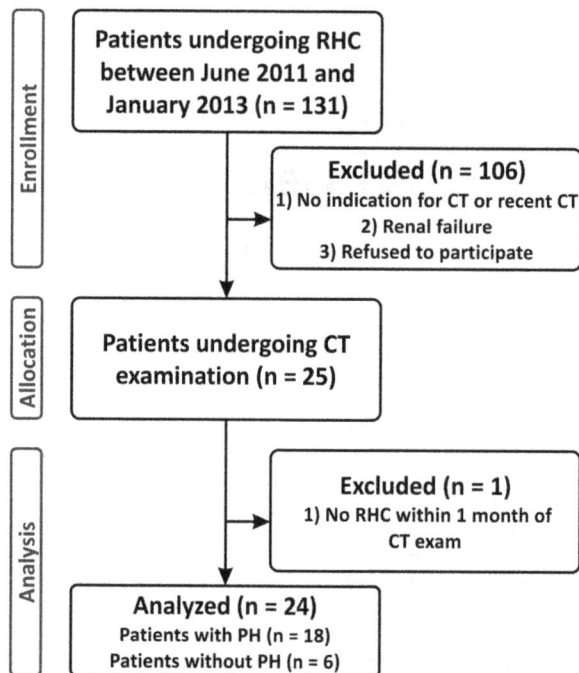

Figure 1. Flowchart of patient recruitment. RHC = right-sided heart catheterization, CT = computed tomography, PH = pulmonary hypertension

reconstructed with 0.6 mm slice thickness using a medium-soft kernel (D30f), anonymised and transferred to an independent workstation. Dual-energy CT was used to determine the blood flow in the lung parenchyma but is not evaluated in this study. Therefore, for the analysis the mixed images from both detectors with a mixture of tube A/tube B of 60%/40% were used, thus resembling typical appearance of a single 120 kV scan.

Data processing and analysis
Vessel segmentation algorithm. The lung vessels were segmented fully automatically with a validated algorithm developed in-house [31]. The flowchart of the algorithm is shown on Figure 2. The inputs for the algorithm were contrast enhanced thoracic CT scans. In a preprocessing step the CT image was smoothed using an edge preserving total variation based denoising filter [32]. The lung was then segmented by grey-level thresholding [33] followed by morphological closing operations. The bronchi were segmented automatically by detecting a point inside the trachea, applying an iterative 3D-region growing algorithm and splitting the result at the carina. Bronchi segmentation was used to separate the lung segmentation into left and right lung and to remove the bronchial walls from the target processing region. This was necessary since the intensity contrast between the airway border and the vessels is low, therefore, incorrect detection of the blood vessels could occur.

The vessel-enhancement filter (VEF) was using the eigenvectors and eigenvalues of a Hessian matrix, which give information about the local image structure, to detect tubular structures. To improve accuracy and robustness, at each position an offset-medialness boundary measure perpendicular to the estimated vessel direction was evaluated [34] and combined with the gradient magnitude at the current position [35]. This led to the final VEF response (Figure 2). After non-maxima suppression of the VEF response, centerlines of the vessels were detected and connected by applying

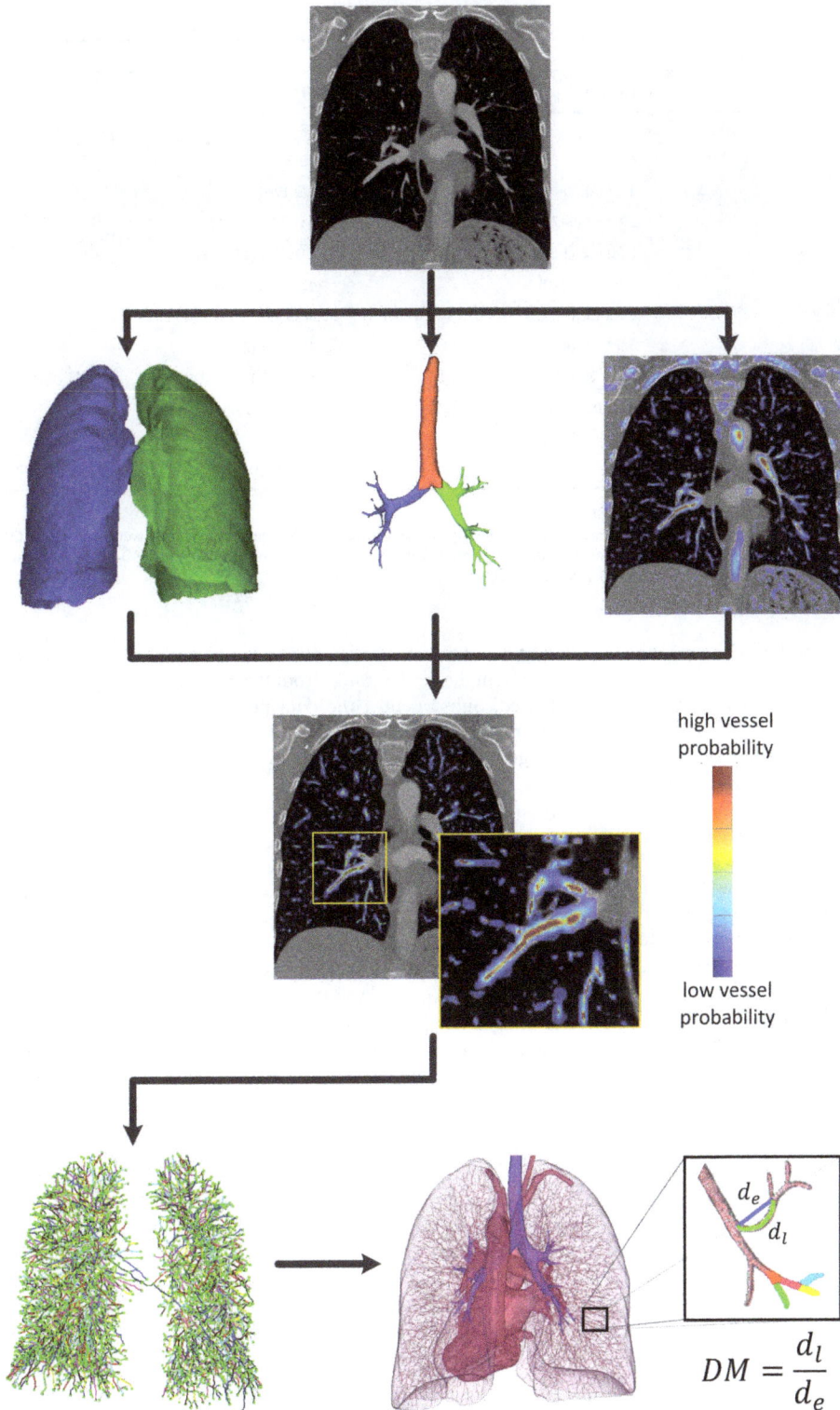

$$DM = \frac{d_l}{d_e}$$

Figure 2. Flowchart of the automatic vessel extraction algorithm. (top) Sample CT image, (2nd row) lung, airway segmentation and the vessel enhancement filter response superimposed on the CT image, (3rd row) vessel enhancement filter response restricted to the region of interest, (bottom row, left) connected centerlines, (bottom row, right) 3D rendering of the lung vessel centerlines. Inset shows the computation of distance metric (DM). The sum of distances along the 3D points of the vessel is divided by the length of the straight path between the two endpoints (first and last 3D point of the vessel segment).

Table 1. Patient characteristics.

Patient characteristics	All patients	No PH	PH
Number of patients	24	6	18
Female/male	14/10	4/2	10/8
WHO class (I/II/III/IV)	2/14/8/0	1/5/0/0	1/9/8/0
Age [years]	60±13 (27–76)	59±8 (50–71)	61±15 (27–76)
BSA [m²]	2.0±0.3 (1.6–2.9)	2.0±0.2 (1.8–2.3)	2.0±0.3 (1.6–2.9)
mPAP [mmHg]	36±15 (14–66)	17±2 (14–20)	43±12 (26–66)
PAWP [mmHg]	9±3 (3–15)	8±2 (5–11)	9±3 (3–15)
CO [l/min]	4.5±1.2 (2.9–7.8)	5.5±1.5 (4.3–7.8)	4.2±0.9 (2.9–5.7) *
PVR [dynscm^{-5}]	540±370 (80–1420)	110±20 (80–130)	680±320 (230–1420) ***
AVDO₂ [vol%]	4.9±1.0 (2.4–6.4)	4.0±0.5 (3.3–4.7)	5.2±1.0 (2.4–6.4) **
art SO₂ [%]	94±2 (89–98)	96±1 (95–98)	93±2 (89–98) **
ven SO₂ [%]	68±7 (50–84)	74±2 (71–76)	66±7 (50–84)*

Data are presented as mean ± SD (range). The significance was tested with t-test.
PH: pulmonary hypertension, BSA: body surface area after Dubois and Dubois, mPAP: mean pulmonary arterial pressure, PAWP: pulmonary artery wedge pressure, CO: cardiac output, PVR: pulmonary vascular resistance, AVDO₂: arterial-venous difference in oxygen content, art SO₂: arterial oxygen saturation, ven SO₂: venous oxygen saturation, */**/***: significant difference between PH and non-PH patients (p<0.05/0.01/0.001).

a shortest path algorithm [36]. The 3D rendering of the resulting centerlines is presented in the bottom part of Figure 2. Therefore, we obtained vessel segments for arteries and veins combined which were counted and used for analysis.

Calculation of vessel tortuosity. A measure of vascular tortuosity is the "distance metric", which provides a ratio of the actual vessel path length to the linear distance between its endpoints. We identified all vessel segments inside the lung, where a vessel segment is defined as the path between either two branching points or between a branching point and an end point. For each segment we computed the 3D length of it and divided it by the Euclidean distance between its endpoints (Figure 2, bottom row inset). The result is a dimensionless number reflecting the bending of the vessel segment. The mean value of the distance metric from all vessel segments was used for analysis.

Calculation of 3D FD with the box counting method. The fractal dimension of the connected vessel centerlines was computed by applying a 3D extension of the well-validated box counting method [37]. Box counting consists of dividing the image volume with the vessel centerlines into a grid of equal cubes with size δ, and counting the number of cubes containing part of the vessel centerlines. This process was repeated for different cube sizes (from one pixel up to 100 pixel side length). The number of cubes containing vessels is plotted against the cube size (δ) in a double logarithmic plot (Figure S1). The fractal dimension is equivalent to the slope of the fitted line. To account for limitations in resolution, only the linear part (Figure S1, red dots) was used for

line fitting. This was carried out by iteratively discarding the data points from the small δ range from the linear fit until a good fit was achieved. Subsequently, the data points from the large δ range were discarded while still keeping the good correlation. On average 30 points were used for the fit.

Statistical analysis

Statistical analysis was performed in GraphPad Prism (Version 5.04, La Jolla, California). Correlations between CT and RHC derived parameters were calculated with linear regression and Spearman correlation. Differences between PH and non-PH patients were determined with t-test, whereas differences between patients' WHO functional classes were assessed by non-parametric analysis of variances (ANOVA, Kruskal-Wallis test). Receiver-operating analysis was used to assess the conclusiveness of the parameters to determine the presence of PH and to calculate optimal cut-off values. P-values (p) ≤0.05 were considered as significant.

Results

Twenty-four consecutive patients (female:male = 14:10) were included in this study (Figure 1). Patient characteristics are summarized in Table 1. The patient group consisted of 18 patients with PH ($n = 4$ with idiopathic pulmonary arterial hypertension (IPAH), $n = 5$ with associated pulmonary arterial hypertension (APAH), $n = 2$ with PH associated with lung disease,

Table 2. Values of distance metric, fractal dimension and number of vessel segments.

	All patients (n = 24)	No PH (n = 6)	PH (n = 18)
Distance metric	1.224±0.019 (1.199–1.273)	1.208±0.009 (1.199–1.223)	1.230±0.019 * (1.202–1.273)
Fractal dimension	2.35±0.06 (2.21–2.44)	2.37±0.08 (2.21–2.43)	2.34±0.05 (2.27–2.44)
Nr. vessel segments	12427±3508 (5922–20434)	11719±3041 (5922–14642)	12392±3616 (7815–20434)

Data are presented as mean ± SD (range). The significance was tested with t-test.
PH: pulmonary hypertension, *: significant difference between PH and non-PH patients (p<0.05).

Table 3. Correlations with clinical parameters (Spearman r and p-value) for n = 24 patients.

r (p)	Distance metric	Fractal dimension	No. vessel segments
mPAP	**0.60** (0.002)	**−0.30** (0.15)	**0.01** (0.97)
PVR	**0.59** (0.002)	**−0.34** (0.10)	**−0.11** (0.61)
AVDO$_2$	**0.54** (0.007)	**−0.37** (0.07)	**0.08** (0.68)
art SO$_2$	**−0.54** (0.006)	**0.47** (0.02)	**0.15** (0.48)
ven SO$_2$	**−0.68** (0.0002)	**0.38** (0.07)	**−0.06** (0.77)
Age	**−0.12** (0.57)	**−0.24** (0.24)	**−0.37** (0.07)
BSA	**−0.04** (0.83)	**0.03** (0.89)	**0.08** (0.68)

mPAP: mean pulmonary arterial pressure, PVR: pulmonary vascular resistance, AVDO$_2$: arterial-venous difference in oxygen content, art SO$_2$: arterial oxygen saturation, ven SO$_2$: venous oxygen saturation, BSA: body surface area after Dubois and Dubois.

$n = 7$ with chronic thromboembolic pulmonary hypertension) and 6 patients without PH ($n = 4$ with systemic sclerosis, $n = 1$ with interstitial lung disease and $n = 1$ patient, who presented without PH after pulmonary endarterectomy). The CT examinations were indicated to exclude relevant lung parenchymal diseases ($n = 17$ patients), to control lung fibrosis ($n = 4$) and because of a suspected progression of scleroderma lung disease ($n = 3$). The CT examination was carried out within a median of 1 day (range 1–18 days) from a diagnostic or follow-up RHC. No change in therapy occurred during this time. There were no complications during RHC or during CT examination. The average effective dose of the thoracic CT scan according to ICRP 103 guidelines was 3.6 ± 1.4 mSv (dose length product: 180 ± 70 mGycm) [38,39].

The automatic vessel segmentation algorithm was successful in identifying right and left lung lobes, trachea and bronchi in all cases. The number of vessel segments was on average 12427 ± 3508 (range 5922–20434) and was not correlated with the disease, age, body surface area (BSA) or the hemodynamic parameters (Table 2 and 3; Figure S2).

There was a significant difference between the distance metric of patients with and without PH (1.230 ± 0.019 vs 1.208 ± 0.009,

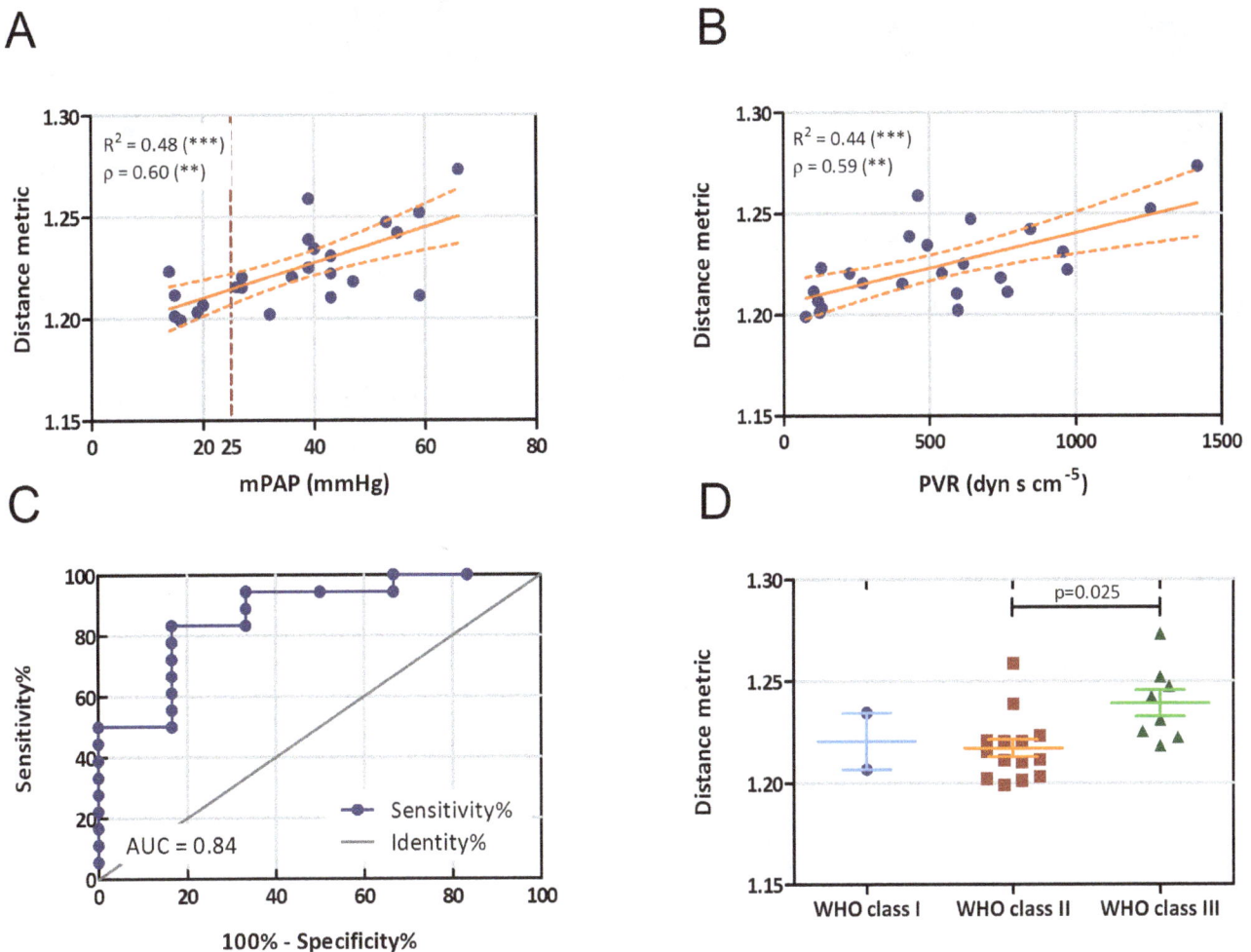

Figure 3. Correlation of distance metric with patient clinical parameters. Correlation of distance metric with (A) mean pulmonary arterial pressure (mPAP), and (B) pulmonary vascular resistance (PVR; R = linear correlation coefficient, r = Spearman correlation coefficient, ** p<0.01, *** p<0.001). (C) Receiver-operating curve for DM determining mPAP >25 mmHg (AUC: area under the curve). (D) Distribution of distance metric according to the WHO classification of the patients. (solid lines represent mean and standard error of mean; p value shows significant difference between WHO class II and III).

A

B

C

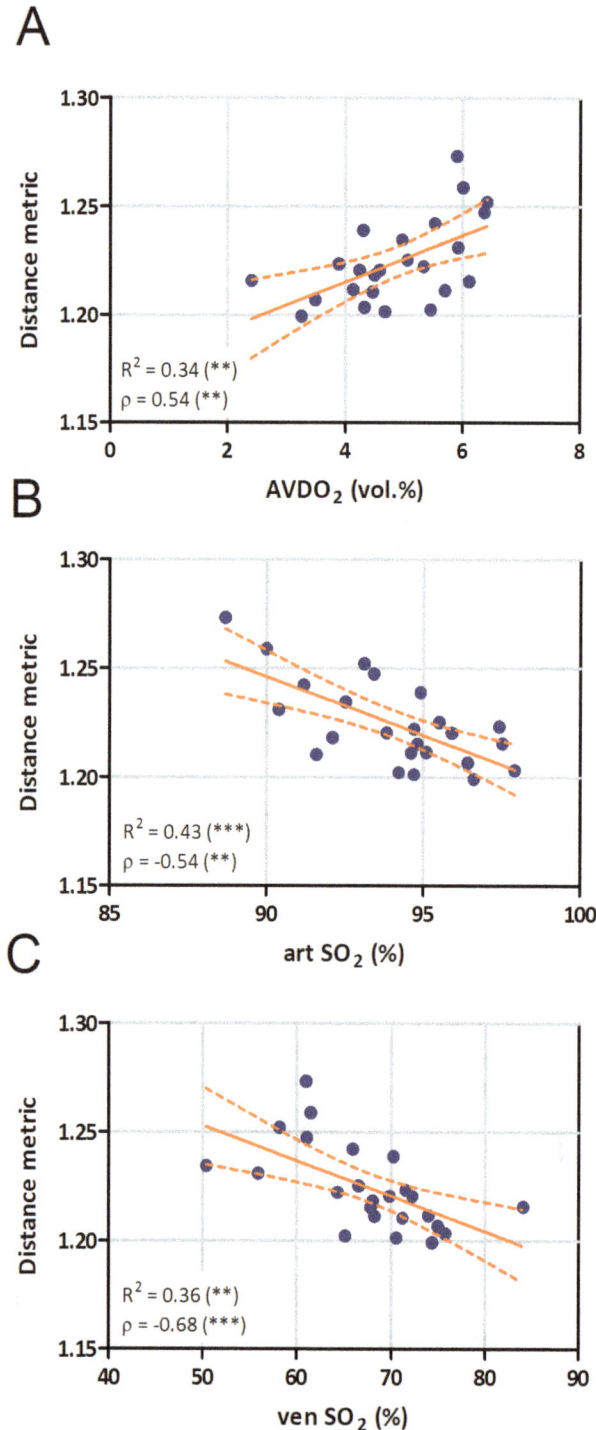

Figure 4. Correlation of distance metric with oxygen exchange parameters. Correlation of distance metric with arterio-venous difference in oxygen content ($AVDO_2$, A), arterial (art SO_2, B) and venous (ven SO_2, C) oxygen saturation (R = linear correlation coefficient, ρ = Spearman correlation coefficient, ** $p<0.01$, *** $p<0.001$).

A

B

Figure 5. Correlation of fractal dimension with clinical parameters. Correlation of 3D fractal dimension (FD) with (A) mean pulmonary arterial pressure (mPAP), and (B) pulmonary vascular resistance (PVR; R = linear correlation coefficient, ρ = Spearman correlation coefficient, ns - not significant).

this parameter. The area under the curve (AUC) was 0.84 (sens/spec 83%/83%, for a distance metric > 1.213; Figure 3c). Moreover, there was a significant association of distance metric with WHO functional class ($p = 0.025$ between WHO class II and III, Figure 3d).

Besides the main diagnostic parameters, distance metric significantly correlated with other hemodynamic parameters, like the difference between arterial and venous oxygen content ($AVDO_2$, $\rho = 0.54$, Figure 4a) or arterial (artSO_2, $\rho = -0.54$, Figure 4b) or venous (venSO_2, $\rho = -0.68$, Figure 4c) oxygen saturation. In order to show the specificity of this tortuosity parameter, we correlated the distance metric with age and BSA. None of these parameters showed a significant correlation (Table 3).

The mean value of the 3D fractal dimension in our patient cohort was 2.35 (range 2.21–2.44, Table 2), which is in good agreement with previously reported values from similar studies [27]. In contrast, there was no significant correlation of 3D FD either with mPAP or with PVR (Figure 5a, b). 3D fractal dimension was negatively correlated with $AVDO_2$ ($\rho = -0.37$), and positively with artSO_2 ($\rho = 0.47$) and venSO_2 ($\rho = 0.38$), but

Table 2). Moreover, we found a correlation between mean pulmonary arterial pressure (mPAP) and the distance metric of $\rho = 0.60$ (Figure 3a). Further, there was a significant correlation with the pulmonary vascular resistance (PVR; $\rho = 0.59$, Figure 3b). The receiver operating curves showed a discriminative power of

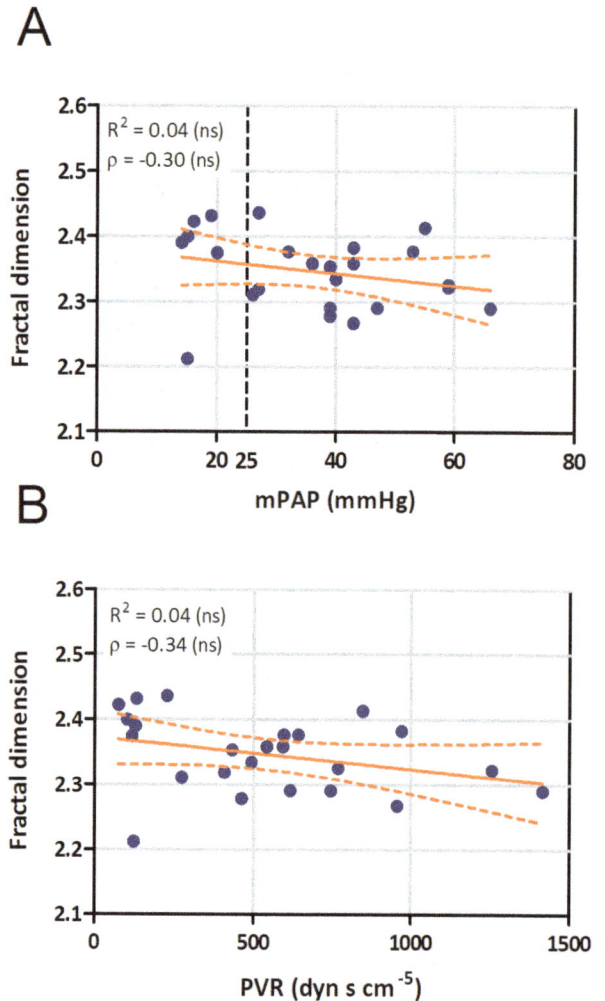

A

B

C

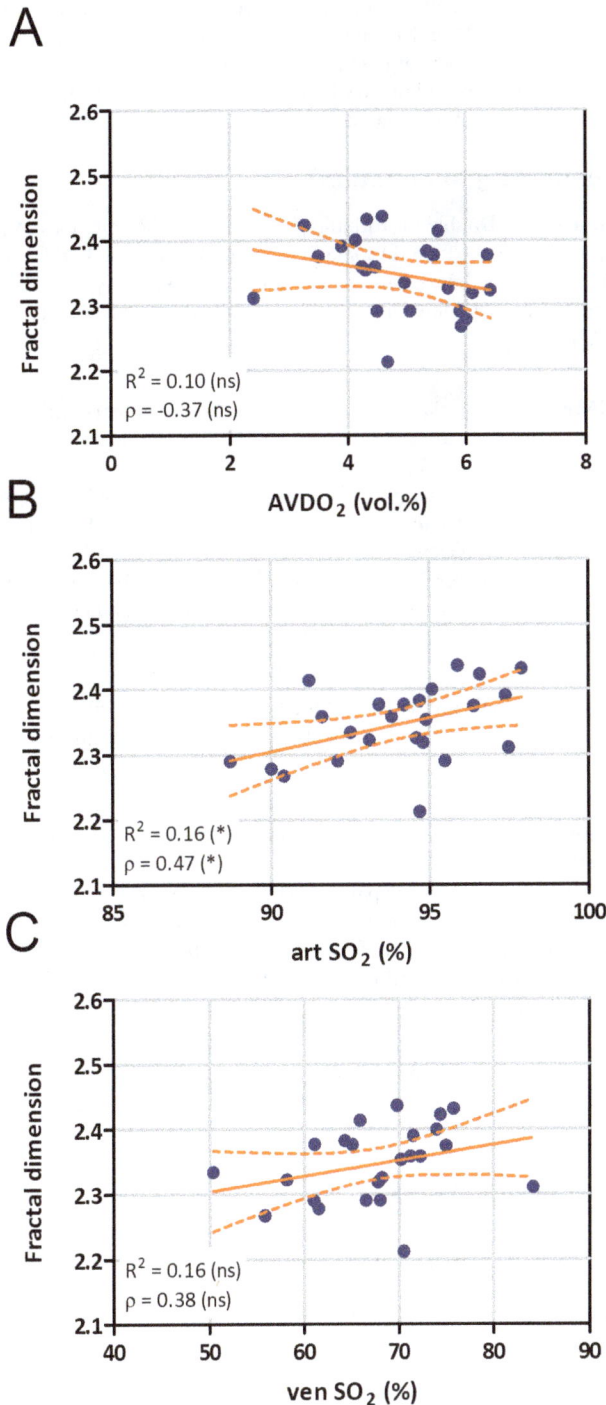

Figure 6. Correlation of fractal dimension with oxygen exchange parameters. Correlation of 3D fractal dimension with arterio-venous difference in oxygen content (AVDO$_2$, A), arterial (art SO$_2$, B) and venous (ven SO$_2$, C) oxygen saturation (R= linear correlation coefficient, ρ = Spearman correlation coefficient, * p<0.05, ns - not significant).

these correlations were weak and significant only for artSO$_2$ (Figure 6). 3D fractal dimension was not associated with WHO functional class (Figure S3).

Neither the distance metric, nor the 3D fractal dimension showed significant differences between different forms of pulmonary hypertension (Figure S4).

Discussion

In this pilot study we showed that vessel tortuosity, determined by our automatic vessel extraction algorithm using routine contrast enhanced thoracic CT scans, is correlated with mean pulmonary arterial pressure, pulmonary vascular resistance as well as measures of pulmonary gas exchange. There was a significant increase of the mean distance metric (tortuosity readout) of patients with PH as compared to patients at risk for PH with mPAP<25mmHg, suggesting that this measure could be suitable for PH screening. In contrast, we did not observe correlations of 3D fractal dimension with pulmonary hemodynamics or gas exchange of these patients.

The automatic vessel detection algorithm allows physical characterization of the pulmonary vessel structure. The total number of vessel segments detected by our algorithm is in the range of ten thousands. The number of vessel segments extracted from the CT dataset did not correlate with any relevant clinical parameter (mPAP, PVR, AVDO$_2$, artSO$_2$ or venSO$_2$), suggesting that pruning of pulmonary vessels either affects only smaller vessels or this phenomenon was not relevant for our patient cohort. Moreover, the absence of correlation shows the robustness of the vessel detection algorithm, and that the other readouts are not influenced by the number of detected vessels.

We applied an advanced 3D method to analyse fractal dimension of the lung vascular tree. This technique gives a quantification of the space filling, providing direct readout for 3 dimensional branching of the tree. We did not find any significant correlation of 3D fractal dimension with the hemodynamic parameters and just a moderate positive correlation with arterial oxygen saturation. This is in contrast to a recent investigation, where fractal dimensions were correlated with PVR index, WHO functional class and 6-min walk distance [28]. However, in that study, very young patients (mainly children) were investigated. Pulmonary hypertension could have a different effect on the vascular anatomy when it develops at a very young age, as if it would develop during adulthood, like in our patients. Additionally, for the pulmonary vessel extraction, that study applied a threshold-based region-growing algorithm followed by skeletonization of the vessels, whereas we used a vessel enhancement filter based automatic extraction algorithm, which allows the detection of smaller vessels with lower contrast without the risk of wrongly segmenting parts of the lung parenchyma with higher density. Another study reported increased FD of PH patients [29]. However, their results might be influenced by the 2 dimensional maximum intensity projections used. As we did not observe any correlations of 3D fractal dimension with the main hemodynamic parameters in our patient cohort, we concluded that this measure may not be suitable for detection or explanation of PH in adult patients.

In the systemic circulation it is a well-established fact that systemic arterial hypertension is associated with tortuous systemic arteries [40,41]. Vascular morphology has been used as diagnostic parameter and for quantification of disease severity in several studies. It was shown that calculating the tortuosity of the brain vessels allows for a distinction between malignant and benign brain tumors [42]. Similarly, the tortuosity of retina vessels was a good measure for vascular malformations in Fabry disease [16]. Although, the presence of tortuous vessels in the lung is considered as a frequent finding in PH [5,43–45], a comprehensive quantification of pulmonary vessel tortuosity, particularly using an automated method, was not presented so far. In pediatric PH patients a significant correlation of the vessel tortuosity (measured as a 3 scale radiological score) with mPAP and PVR was reported [5]. We observed a significant correlation of distance metric with mean pulmonary arterial pressure, pulmonary vascular resistance and measures of gas exchange. Furthermore, there was a significant association of distance metric with WHO functional class, suggesting an increase in tortuosity with increase in disease severity. Moreover, in our adult patient cohort, distance metric, as a measure of tortuosity, showed a good discriminative power between patients with and without PH. The area under the curve of the ROC analysis of 0.84 is similar to the value of 0.86 reported by Janda et al. in their meta-analysis on the diagnostic accuracy of echocardiography [46]. However, a meaningful comparison of the diagnostic accuracy of these two non-invasive methods would require a head-to-head comparison in a larger patient cohort.

Altogether, these results suggest that a non-invasive thoracic CT examination can provide estimates of important parameters derived from an invasive right-sided heart catheterisation. Since there is no user intervention necessary, our algorithm can be run on every thoracic CT scan of patients with an unknown lung disease without additional workload for the radiologist or technician. This might help to non-invasively identify patients with manifest pulmonary hypertension. Additionally, this method could be applied to characterize and better understand gas exchange abnormalities in patients with known pulmonary hypertension.

Limitations

One of the limitations of this pilot study is the small number of patients, allowing only a preliminary conclusion, despite considering a wide range of diseases. An adequately powered prospective study is currently under way to determine the benefits and drawbacks of this method. Another limitation is the number of vessels accessible by CT imaging. The human lung includes hundreds of thousands of vessels. Huang et al. found a total of 15 generations of vessels between the main pulmonary artery and the capillaries, with diameters from 15 mm down to 0.02 mm [47]. In our CT images we could only detect vessels down to a diameter of approximately 2 mm; smaller vessels cannot be detected due to scanner resolution and the partial volume effect. Our algorithm detects vessel segments regardless of whether they are arteries or veins. Since the increased pressure is confined to the arterial vasculature in patients with pulmonary arterial hypertension, we expect that discrimination between arteries and veins would further improve the diagnostic value of our measures. Such an algorithm, capable of distinguishing arteries and veins, was recently published e.g. by Park et al. [48]. As a further limitation, due to radiation exposure, we could not test the repeatability of the method. This would have been necessary to determine the robustness of the results. However, the correlations with many important parameters of pulmonary blood flow and gas exchange suggest a high degree of reliability of the measurements.

Conclusion

Vessel tortuosity derived from thoracic CT by automatic 3D extraction of the pulmonary vessels is correlated with pulmonary

arterial hemodynamics and gas exchange. This non-invasive method may help understanding the impact of pulmonary vascular changes for hemodynamics and gas exchange, and may provide a screening tool for pulmonary hypertension. Prospective validation of our method in a larger patient cohort is warranted.

Supporting Information

Figure S1 Double logarithmic plot of the number of cubes (N_δ) against the cube size (δ) for a representative patient. For linear fitting only the linear part of the data (red crosses) was used. The slope of the fitted line (green) corresponds to the fractal dimension (FD).

Figure S2 Correlation of number of vessel segments with (A) mean pulmonary arterial pressure (mPAP), (B) pulmonary vascular resistance (PVR), (C) arterio-venous difference in oxygen content ($AVDO_2$), (D) arterial (art SO_2) and (E) venous (ven SO_2) oxygen saturation (R = linear correlation coefficient, r = Spearman correlation coefficient, ns - not significant). (F) Distribution of the number of vessel segments according to the WHO classification of the patients (solid lines represent mean and standard error of mean).

Figure S3 Distribution of 3D fractal dimension according to the WHO classification of the patients (solid lines represent mean and standard error of mean).

Figure S4 Distribution of (A) distance metric (DM) and (B) fractal dimension based on disease subtype (PH: pulmonary hypertension, IPAH: idiopathic pulmonary arterial hypertension, APAH: pulmonary arterial hypertension associated with risk factors or conditions, PH-LD: pulmonary hypertension associated with lung disease, CTEPH: chronic thromboembolic pulmonary hypertension).

Checklist S1 STARD checklist for reporting of studies of diagnostic accuracy.

Acknowledgments

The authors would like to thank Wolfgang Loidl for his help in setting up the examination protocol, Dr. Daniela Kleinschek for her help with retrieval of the patients' clinical data, Dr. Alexander Avian for his assistance with the statistical analysis and Dr. Vasile Foris for fruitful discussions.

Author Contributions

Conceived and designed the experiments: MH MP MU ZB. Performed the experiments: MH MP MU PK GK ZB. Analyzed the data: MH MP RS AO HO ZB. Contributed reagents/materials/analysis tools: MU PK AO HO. Wrote the paper: MH MP ZB. Critically revised the manuscript: MU PK RS GK AO HO. Approved the final version to be published: MH MP MU PK RS GK AO HO ZB.

References

1. Galie N, Hoeper MM, Humbert M, Torbicki A, Vachiery J, et al (2009) Guidelines for the diagnosis and treatment of pulmonary hypertension. Eur Resp J 34: 1219–1263.

2. Simonneau G, Robbins IM, Beghetti M, Channick RN, Delcroix M, et al (2009) Updated clinical classification of pulmonary hypertension. J Am Coll Cardiol 54: S43–S54.

3. Okajima Y, Ohno Y, Washko GR, Hatabu H (2011) Assessment of pulmonary hypertension: What CT and MRI can provide. Acad Radiol 18: 437–453.

4. Stevens GR, Fida N, Sanz J (2012) Computed tomography and cardiac magnetic resonance imaging in pulmonary hypertension. Prog Cardiovasc Dis 55: 161–171.

5. Kulik TJ, Clark RL, Hasan BS, Keane JF, Springmuller D, et al (2011) Pulmonary arterial hypertension: What the large pulmonary arteries tell us. Pediatr Cardiol 32: 759–765.

6. Estepar RS, Kinney GL, Black-Shinn JL, Bowler RP, Kindlmann GL, et al (2013) Computed tomographic measures of pulmonary vascular morphology in smokers and their clinical implications. Am J Respir Crit Care Med 188: 231–239.

7. Bauer C, Pock T, Sorantin E, Bischof H, Beichel R (2010) Segmentation of interwoven 3d tubular tree structures utilizing shape priors and graph cuts. Med Image Anal 14: 172–184.

8. Urschler M, Bornik A, Scheurer E, Yen K, Bischof H, et al (2012) Forensic-case analysis: From 3D imaging to interactive visualization. IEEE Comput Graphics Appl 32: 79–87.

9. Chen B, Kitasaka T, Honma H, Takabatake H, Mori M, et al (2012) Automatic segmentation of pulmonary blood vessels and nodules based on local intensity structure analysis and surface propagation in 3D chest CT images. Int J CARS 7: 465–482.

10. Shikata H, McLennan G, Hoffman EA, Sonka M (2009) Segmentation of pulmonary vascular trees from thoracic 3D CT images. Int J Biomed Imaging 2009: 636240.

11. Han H (2012) Twisted blood vessels: Symptoms, etiology and biomechanical mechanisms. J Vasc Res 49: 185–197.

12. Spangler KM, Challa VR, Moody DM, Bell MA (1994) Arteriolar tortuosity of the white-matter in aging and hypertension - a microradiographic study. J Neuropathol Exp Neurol 53: 22–26.

13. Diedrich KT, Roberts JA, Schmidt RH, Kang C, Cho Z, et al (2011) Validation of an arterial tortuosity measure with application to hypertension collection of clinical hypertensive patients. BMC Bioinformatics 12: S15.

14. Bullitt E, Zeng D, Gerig G, Aylward S, Joshi S, et al (2005) Vessel tortuosity and brain tumor malignancy: A blinded study. Acad Radiol 12: 1232–1240.

15. Jain R (2001) Normalizing tumor vasculature with anti-angiogenic therapy: A new paradigm for combination therapy. Nat Med 7: 987–989.

16. Sodi A, Guarducci M, Vauthier L, Ioannidis AS, Pitz S, et al (2013) Computer assisted evaluation of retinal vessels tortuosity in fabry disease. Acta Ophthalmol 91: e113–e119.

17. Smedby Ö, Högman N, Nilsson S, Erikson U, Olsson AG, et al (1993) 2-dimensional tortuosity of the superficial femoral-artery in early atherosclerosis. J Vasc Res 30: 181–191.

18. Hart W, Goldbaum M, Cote B, Kube P, Nelson M (1999) Measurement and classification of retinal vascular tortuosity. Int J Med Inf 53: 239–252.

19. Folarin AA, Konerding MA, Timonen J, Nagl S, Pedley RB (2010) Three-dimensional analysis of tumour vascular corrosion casts using stereoimaging and micro-computed tomography. Microvasc Res 80: 89–98.

20. Kim E, Zhang J, Hong K, Benoit NE, Pathak AP (2011) Vascular phenotyping of brain tumors using magnetic resonance microscopy (mu MRI). J Cereb Blood Flow Metab 31: 1623–1636.

21. Mandelbrot B (1967) How long is coast of britain - statistical self-similarity and fractional dimension. Science 156: 636–638.

22. Mandelbrot BB, Van Ness JW (1968) Fractional brownian motions fractional noises and applications. SIAM Rev 10: 422–437.

23. Kalda J (1999) On the fractality of the biological tree-like structures. Discret Dyn Nat Soc 3: 297–306.

24. Huo Y, Kassab GS (2012) Intraspecific scaling laws of vascular trees. J R Soc Interface 9: 190–200.

25. Masters BR (2004) Fractal analysis of the vascular tree in the human retina. Annu Rev Biomed Eng 6: 427–452.

26. Goh V, Sanghera B, Wellsted DM, Sundin J, Halligan S (2009) Assessment of the spatial pattern of colorectal tumour perfusion estimated at perfusion CT using two-dimensional fractal analysis. Eur Radiol 19: 1358–1365.

27. Lang S, Mueller B, Dominietto MD, Cattin PC, Zanette I, et al (2012) Three-dimensional quantification of capillary networks in healthy and cancerous tissues of two mice. Microvasc Res 84: 314–322.

28. Moledina S, de Bruyn A, Schievano S, Owens CM, Young C, et al (2011) Fractal branching quantifies vascular changes and predicts survival in pulmonary hypertension: A proof of principle study. Heart 97: 1245–1249.

29. Haitao S, Ning L, Lijun G, Fei G, Cheng L (2011) Fractal dimension analysis of MDCT images for quantifying the morphological changes of the pulmonary artery tree in patients with pulmonary hypertension. Korean J Radiol 12: 289–296.

30. Pienn M, Kovacs G, Tscherner M, Johnson T, Kullnig P, et al (2013) Determination of cardiac output with dynamic contrast-enhanced computed tomography. Int J Cardiovasc Imaging 29: 1781–1788.

31. Helmberger M, Urschler M, Pienn M, Bálint Z, Olschewski A, et al (2013) Pulmonary vascular tree segmentation from contrast-enhanced CTImages. Proceedings of the 37th Annual Workshop of the Austrian Association for Pattern Recognition (ÖAGM/AAPR).

32. Rudin LI, Osher S, Fatemi E (1992) Nonlinear total variation based noise removal algorithms. Physica D 60: 259–268.

33. Otsu N (1979) A threshold selection method from gray-level histograms. IEEE Trans Syst, Man, Cybern 9: 62–66.

34. Krissian K, Malandain G, Ayache N, Vaillant R, Trousset Y (2000) Model-based detection of tubular structures in 3D images. Comput Vision Image Understand 80: 130–171.

35. Pock T, Beichel R, Bischof H (2005) A novel robust tube detection filter for 3D centerline extraction. Image Analysis, Proceedings 3540: 481–490.

36. Dijkstra E (1959) A note on two problems in connexion with graphs. Num Math 1: 269–271.

37. Ge Meiling, Lin Qizhong, Lu Wang (2006) Realizing the box-counting method for calculating fractal dimension of urban form based on remote sensing image. Geoscience and Remote Sensing Symposium, 2006 IGARSS 2006 IEEE International Conference on: 1423–1426.

38. International Commission on Radiological Protection ICRP (2007) The 2007 recommendations of the international commission on radiological protection. ICRP publication 103. Ann ICRP 37: 1–332.

39. Huda W, Magill D, He W (2011) CT effective dose per dose length product using ICRP 103 weighting factors. Med Phys 38: 1261–1265.

40. Hiroki M, Miyashita K, Oda M (2002) Tortuosity of the white matter medullary arterioles is related to the severity of hypertension. Cerebrovasc Dis 13: 242–250.

41. Pancera P, Ribul M, Presciuttini B, Lechi A (2000) Prevalence of carotid artery kinking in 590 consecutive subjects evaluated by echocolordoppler. is there a correlation with arterial hypertension? J Intern Med 248: 7–12.

42. Bullitt E, Gerig G, Pizer S, Lin W, Aylward S (2003) Measuring tortuosity of the intracerebral vasculature from MRA images. IEEE Trans Med Imaging 22: 1163–1171.

43. Nikolaou K, Schoenberg S, Attenberger U, Scheidler J, Dietrich O, et al (2005) Pulmonary arterial hypertension: Diagnosis with fast perfusion MR imaging and high-spatial-resolution MR angiography - preliminary experience. Radiology 236: 694–703.

44. Sheehan R, Perloff J, Fishbein M, Gjertson D, Aberle D (2005) Pulmonary neovascularity - A distinctive radiographic finding in eisenmenger syndrome. Circulation 112: 2778–2785.

45. Rothman A, Wiencek RG, Davidson S, Evans WN, Restrepo H, et al (2011) Hemodynamic and histologic characterization of a swine (sus scrofa domestica) model of chronic pulmonary arterial hypertension. Comp Med 61: 258–262.

46. Janda S, Shahidi N, Gin K, Swiston J (2011) Diagnostic accuracy of echocardiography for pulmonary hypertension: A systematic review and meta-analysis. Heart 97: 612–622.

47. Huang W, Yen R, McLaurine M, Bledsoe G (1996) Morphometry of the human pulmonary vasculature. J Appl Physiol 81: 2123–2133.

48. Park S, Lee SM, Kim N, Seo JB, Shin H (2013) Automatic reconstruction of the arterial and venous trees on volumetric chest CT. Med Phys 40: 071906.

19

CXCR4 Inhibition Ameliorates Severe Obliterative Pulmonary Hypertension and Accumulation of C-Kit$^+$ Cells in Rats

Daniela Farkas[1,9], Donatas Kraskauskas[1,9], Jennifer I. Drake[1], Aysar A. Alhussaini[1], Vita Kraskauskiene[1], Harm J. Bogaard[2], Carlyne D. Cool[3], Norbert F. Voelkel[1], Laszlo Farkas[1]*

1 Victoria Johnson Center for Obstructive Lung Research, Department of Internal Medicine, Division of Respiratory Disease and Critical Care Medicine, Virginia Commonwealth University, Richmond, Virginia, United States of America, 2 Department of Pulmonary Medicine, VU University Medical Center, Amsterdam, The Netherlands, 3 Department of Pathology, University of Colorado at Denver and Health Sciences Center, Denver, Colorado, United States of America

Abstract

Successful curative treatment of severe pulmonary arterial hypertension with luminal obliteration will require a thorough understanding of the mechanism underlying the development and progression of pulmonary vascular lesions. But the cells that obliterate the pulmonary arterial lumen in severe pulmonary arterial hypertension are incompletely characterized. The goal of our study was to evaluate whether inhibition of CXC chemokine receptor 4 will prevent the accumulation of c-kit$^+$ cells and severe pulmonary arterial hypertension. We detected c-kit^{+-} cells expressing endothelial (von Willebrand Factor) or smooth muscle cell/myofibroblast (α-smooth muscle actin) markers in pulmonary arterial lesions of SU5416/chronic hypoxia rats. We found increased expression of CXC chemokine ligand 12 in the lung tissue of SU5416/chronic hypoxia rats. In our prevention study, AMD3100, an inhibitor of the CXC chemokine ligand 12 receptor, CXC chemokine receptor 4, only moderately decreased pulmonary arterial obliteration and pulmonary hypertension in SU5416/chronic hypoxia animals. AMD3100 treatment reduced the number of proliferating c-kit$^+$ α-smooth muscle actin$^+$ cells and pulmonary arterial muscularization and did not affect c-kit$^+$ von Willebrand Factor$^+$ cell numbers. Both c-kit$^+$ cell types expressed CXC chemokine receptor 4. In conclusion, our data demonstrate that in the SU5416/chronic hypoxia model of severe pulmonary hypertension, the CXC chemokine receptor 4-expressing c-kit$^+$ α-smooth muscle actin$^+$ cells contribute to pulmonary arterial muscularization. In contrast, vascular lumen obliteration by c-kit$^+$ von Willebrand Factor$^+$ cells is largely independent of CXC chemokine receptor 4.

Editor: Wei Shi, Children's Hospital Los Angeles, United States of America

Funding: The study was supported by the NIH/NHLBI grant HL109918 and the Victoria Johnson Center for Obstructive Lung Disease Funds (VCU). Confocal microscopy was performed at the VCU Department of Anatomy and Neurobiology Microscope Facility, supported, in part, with funding from NIH-National Institute of Neurological Disorders and Stroke Center core grant (5P30NS047463-02). The funders had no role in study design, data collection and analysis, decision to publish, or preparation of the manuscript.

Competing Interests: The authors have declared that no competing interests exist.

* E-mail: lfarkas@vcu.edu

9 These authors contributed equally to this work.

Introduction

Severe pulmonary arterial hypertension (PAH) is characterized by a lumen-obliterating pulmonary microvasculopathy and complex, multicellular plexiform lesions [1]. These vascular lesions and abnormal vessel tone lead to increased pulmonary vascular resistance and right heart failure [2]. Endothelial cell (EC) apoptosis-dependent compensatory cell overgrowth appears to be an important confounding cause of lumen obliteration in severe PAH [3,4]. Additional factors that are likely pathobiologically relevant, are mutations in the bone morphogenic protein receptor 2 and inflammation [5]._ENREF_6 However, the nature and the origin of the phenotypically altered and proliferating cells that occlude the pulmonary vascular lumen are incompletely understood.

Progenitor cells are non-terminally differentiated cells with the potential to undergo proliferation and terminal differentiation [6,7]. Bone marrow (BM)-derived endothelial progenitor cells

(EPCs) may contribute to neoangiogenesis [8]. Stem- and progenitor cell niches, harboring EPCs, hematopoietic progenitor cells and mesenchymal stem cells have been identified in the vessel wall of the systemic circulation [9]. One way to identify progenitor cells in addition to their proliferative capacity is the use of cellular markers that are not expressed by terminally differentiated cells, such as c-kit, a tyrosine kinase receptor for stem cell factor. c-kit has been originally detected on the surface of embryonic stem cells, primitive hematopoietic cells and mast cells, and signaling *via* c-kit is important for hematopoiesis and vascular development [10,11]. In the human lung, c-kit$^+$ stem cells can repopulate airways and vessels [12] and a recent study has identified that mouse lung ECs contain a c-kit$^+$ population of rare vascular endothelial stem cells that can generate functional blood vessels [13].

The accumulation of stem and progenitor cells at sites of injury requires CXC chemokine receptor 4 (CXCR4), a G-protein coupled receptor for CXC chemokine ligand 12 (CXCL12). CXCR4 is expressed on progenitor and stem cells, phagocytic cells of the innate immune system and tumor cells [14]. Signaling *via* CXCR4 is important for migration of circulating and resident cells towards a CXCL12 gradient, as well as for cell survival and proliferation [14]. Activation of the CXCL12/CXCR4 axis contributes to the repair of the ischemic myocardium [15]. CXCR4 and its ligand CXCL12 have been identified in plexiform lesions of patients with advanced PAH [15,16]._ENREF_17 However, the potential relevance of this signaling pathway for the development of lumen-obliterating pulmonary arterial lesions remains unclear.

Inhibition of CXCR4 in chronically hypoxic mice prevents the accumulation of c-kit$^+$ putative HPCs in pulmonary arteries and the development of pulmonary hypertension [17,18]. We hypothesized that c-kit$^+$ cells, including c-kit$^+$ progenitor cells, accumulate in and around the lumen-occluding lesions of pulmonary arteries in severe PAH and that severe PAH and accumulation of c-kit$^+$ cells depends on CXCR4.

In our study, we show the spatiotemporal localization of c-kit$^+$ cells in the pulmonary vascular lesions from rats with SU5416/ chronic hypoxia (SuHx)-induced angioobliterative PAH [4]. Our work extends previous experimental studies by demonstrating that some c-kit$^+$ cells in the pulmonary arteries express endothelial and vascular smooth muscle cell (VSMC)/myofibroblast markers. Having found elevated CXCL12 protein levels in the lungs of SuHx animals, we examined the effects of the CXCR4 inhibitor AMD3100 in the SuHx model. We demonstrate that AMD3100 treatment prevented pulmonary arterial muscularization, but only partially reduced the pulmonary arterial obliteration. The overall result was a moderate reduction in pulmonary hypertension. CXCR4 blockade reduced the total number of c-kit$^+$ cells and CXCR4$^+$ cells, in particular the number of c-kit$^+$ α-smooth muscle actin (α-SMA)$^+$ cells, CXCR4$^+$ α-SMA$^+$ and proliferating c-kit$^+$ α-SMA$^+$ cells.

Materials and Methods

Animal experiments

All animal experiments were approved by the institutional animal care and utilization committee of Virginia Commonwealth University, Richmond, VA (Protocol number AM10157). This study was carried out in strict accordance with the recommendations in the Guide for the Care and Use of Laboratory Animals of the National Institutes of Health. All surgery was performed under Ketamine/Xylazine anesthesia, and all efforts were made to minimize suffering. SuHx-induced severe angioobliterative PAH was established by a single subcutaneous injection of 20 mg·kg^{-1} SU5416 at day 0 and exposure to chronic hypoxia for up to 28 days, followed by housing under normoxic conditions for experiments with a total duration of 42 days [4,19,20]. The animals were euthanized at the given time points by exsanguination following hemodynamic measurements [19] and blood sampling. Lung and heart were removed *en bloc*, and the right lung was snap frozen for molecular biology studies. The left lung was inflated with 0.5% low-melting agarose (20 cmH$_2$O) and formalin-fixed (48 h), then paraffin-embedded for Elastica van Gieson (EvG) staining, immunohistochemistry (IHC) and immunofluorescence (IF) staining, as well as *in situ* hybridization. Naïve control animals were housed at room air. SuHx animals received 5 mg·kg^{-1}·day^{-1} AMD3100 (Tocris Bioscience, Ellisville, MI) or vehicle (PBS) intraperitoneally from day 1–21. At day 21, the animals were euthanized for tissue harvest.

Histology

Paraffin-embedded and formalin-fixed lung tissue was sectioned at a thickness of 3 µm. EvG staining was performed as published previously [21]. For vascular histomorphometry, images of EvG-stained sections were randomly taken with an AXIO imager.A1 microscope, Axiocam HRc camera and Axiovision software (all Zeiss, Jena, Germany) at 100× magnification. Each animal received a numeric code to ensure objectivity. Media thickness (MT) and external diameter (ED) were measured by an investigator blinded to the treatment groups as published before and media wall thickness (MWT) was calculated according to the formula: MWT (%) = $[2 \times (MT \cdot ED^{-1})] \times 100\%$ [21]. Pulmonary arteries were categorized according to their size as follows: small: 25 µm<ED<50 µm, medium size: 50 µm ≤ ED<100 µm. For each animal, 30–40 pulmonary arteries were measured in two orthogonal directions using ImageJ [22].

For vWF IHC, 3 µm sections were rehydrated, followed by antigen retrieval using enzymatic digestion (proteinase K, 1:50, DAKO, Carpinteria, CA) for 6 min in PBS. Then, endogenous peroxidase (3% H$_2$O$_2$ in PBS) was blocked for 5 min and unspecific interactions were inhibited with 1% normal swine serum (NSS) for 15 min. The sections were incubated with the primary antibody (anti-vWF A008202, DAKO, dilution 1:5000,) in 1% NSS/PBS overnight at 4°C and with the secondary, biotin-conjugated antibody (AP132B, Millipore, Billierica, MA, dilution 1:1500) in 1%NSS/PBS for 1 h at room temperature. This was followed by 45 min incubation with HRP-conjugated Streptavidin in 1%NSS/PBS (dilution 1:200, Vector Laboratories, Burlingame, CA), counterstaining with Mayer's Hematoxylin, dehydration and mounting.

For IF stainings, 3 µm sections were rehydrated, followed by antigen retrieval with heat in citrate buffer pH 6.0 for 20 min. Then, sections were blocked with 1% NSS/PBS for 15 min and incubated with primary antibody #1 in 1% NSS in PBS overnight at 4 °C. Sections were then incubated with the secondary antibody #1 in PBS for 4 h. For double and triple IF stainings, additional sequential incubations were performed with primary and secondary antibody #2 (and #3 for triple IF) similar to #1. Finally, the sections were counterstained with 4',6-diamidino-2-phenylindole (DAPI) 1:20000 for 5 min and mounted in Slow Fade Gold (both Life Technologies/Invitrogen, Carlsbad, CA). The following primary antibodies were used: α-SMA (C6198, Sigma-Aldrich, St. Louis, MO, dilution 1:200, no secondary antibody as this antibody is directly Cy3-conjugated) or (M0851, DAKO, dilution 1:200, no label), c-kit (LS-C78828, LifeSpan Biosciences, Seattle, WA, dilution 1:50), CXCR4 #1 (ab2074, Abcam, Cambridge, MA, dilution 1:50), CXCR4 #2 (ab1671, Abcam, dilution 1:25), mast cell tryptase (IMG-80250, Imgenex, San Diego, CA, dilution 1:20), PCNA (#2586, Cell Signaling Technology, Danvers, MA, dilution 1:100), vWF (A008202, DAKO, dilution 1:50). The following secondary antibodies were used: A11058 (Life Technologies/Invitrogen, dilution 1:50), A21202 (Life Technologies/Invitrogen, dilution 1:100), A21203 (Life Technologies/Invitrogen, dilution 1:100), A21121 (Life Technologies/Invitrogen, dilution 1:50), A21131 (Life Technologies/Invitrogen, dilution 1:50), A21442 (Life Technologies/Invitrogen, dilution 1:100), A21443 (Life Technologies/Invitrogen, dilution 1:50). For all IHC and IF stainings, controls with unspecific IgG were run in parallel with each staining batch and treatment group.

In situ hybridization

5 µm thick formalin-fixed, paraffin-embedded lung tissue sections were used for *in situ* hybridization with the QuantiGene ViewRNA ISH Tissue Assay kit (Affymetrix, Cleveland, OH)

according to the manufacturer's instructions. Custom TYPE1 QuantiGene View RNA probes were obtained from Affymetrix for rat *Kit* (Gen Bank Accession number NM_022264, region 501–1476 covered by probeset). Pretreatment was performed for 10 min at 95°C and protease digestion for 20 min at 40°C. TYPE1 probes were stained with Fast red and counterstained with Gill's Hematoxylin. A negative control (probe omitted) was run in parallel (Figure S1). Images were taken with AXIO imager.A1 microscope, Axiocam HRc camera and Axiovision software (all Zeiss)

Quantification of IHC and IF stainings

For the quantification of vascular obliteration in vWF-stained sections, 15 images were randomly acquired for each animal from 2 transversal sections through the left lung (one at the level of the hilum, one at least 200 μm caudal of the hilum) at a magnification of 100×, containing >80 pulmonary arteries of different calibers. The images were obtained with an AXIO imager.A1 microscope, Axiocam HRc camera and Axiovision software. Each animal received a number code to ensure objectivity. For each pulmonary artery, an investigator blinded to the treatment groups classified

the degree of occlusion as none, partial or complete, and measured the ED.

For quantification of double IF stainings, red, green and blue fluorescence channel images were acquired of 10–15 randomly selected pulmonary arteries from 2 transversal sections through the left lung (one at the level of the hilum, one at least 200 μm caudal of the hilum) for each animal at a magnification of 400× with an IX70 fluorescence microscope, XM10 camera and Cellsens software (all Olympus). For triple IF stainings, 10 randomly selected pulmonary arteries from 2 transversal sections through the left lung were acquired at a magnification of 630× with a laser scanning confocal microscope using specific filters for DAPI, AlexaFluor 488, 594 and 647 (see below). The images of each animal received a unique numeric code to ensure objectivity. The number of c-kit$^+$, CXCR4$^+$, vWF$^+$ c-kit$^+$, vWF$^+$ CXCR4$^+$, α-SMA$^+$ c-kit$^+$, α-SMA$^+$ CXCR4$^+$, PCNA$^+$ c-kit$^+$, PCNA$^+$ c-kit$^+$ vWF$^+$ and PCNA$^+$ c-kit$^+$ α-SMA$^+$ cells per pulmonary artery (lumen/lumen-occluding cells, cells in intima, media, adventitia and perivascular infiltrate) was counted in the assembled multichannel image using the cell counter plugin of ImageJ by an investigator blinded to the treatment groups.

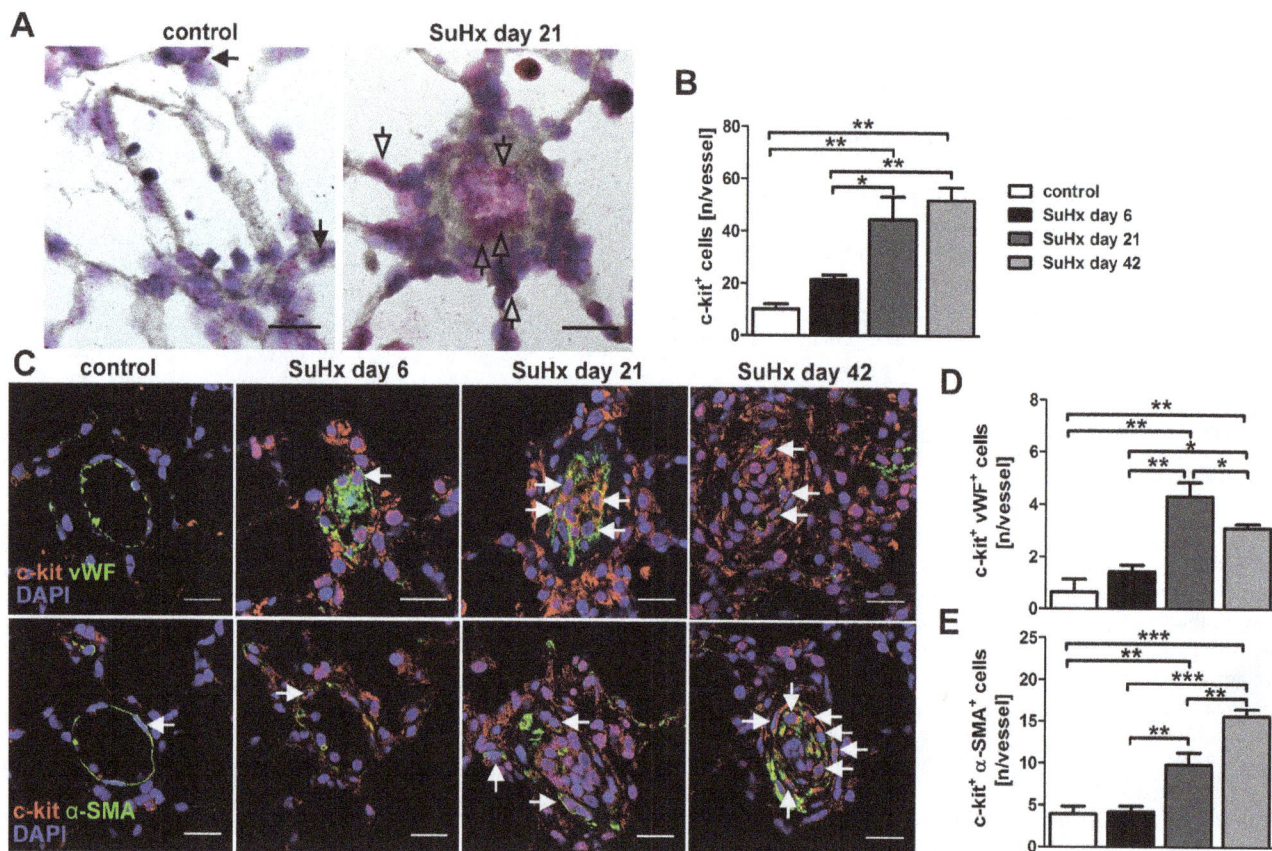

Figure 1. Accumulation of c-kit$^+$ cells in the SU5416/chronic hypoxia (SuHx) model. (**A**) Representative images of *in situ* hybridization images demonstrating *Kit* mRNA expression. In naïve control animals, occasional low *Kit* expression was found in cells of vessels and alveolar walls, whereas multiple cells in lumen-obliterating regions and vessel wall/perivascular region expressed *Kit* (granular staining pattern) in the lung of a SuHx animal. The open arrows indicate cells with strong *Kit* expression. Counterstaining with Gill's Hematoxylin. Magnification: 400×. Scale bar: 20 μm. (**B**) Quantification of the number of c-kit$^+$ cells/vessel over time. n = 3 animals per group. * $P<0.05$, ** $P<0.01$. (**C**) Images demonstrate representative optical sections (confocal microscopy). c-kit$^+$, c-kit$^+$ von Willebrand Factor$^+$ (vWF$^+$) and c-kit$^+$ α-smooth muscle actin$^+$ (α-SMA$^+$) cells were occasionally found in alveolar walls and vessel walls of naïve control animals. c-kit$^+$ and c-kit$^+$ α-SMA$^+$ cells accumulated in and around the pulmonary arteries of SuHx animals over time. The number of c-kit$^+$ vWF$^+$ cells also increased until day 21 in and around the pulmonary arteries of SuHx animals and started to decline thereafter. Arrows indicate c-kit$^+$ vWF$^+$ or c-kit$^+$ α-SMA$^+$ cells. Nuclear counterstaining with 4′,6-diamidino-2-phenylindole (DAPI). Magnification: 630×. Scale bar: 20 μm. (**D-E**) Quantification of the number of c-kit$^+$ vWF$^+$ (D) and c-kit$^+$ α-SMA$^+$ (E) cells per vessel. n = 3 animals per group. * $P<0.05$, ** $P<0.01$ and *** $P<0.0001$.

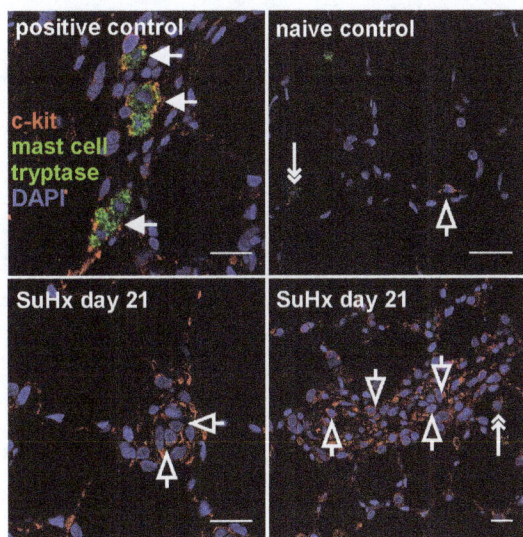

Figure 2. c-kit$^+$ cells in the angioobliterative lesions were not mast cells. Representative optical section obtained by confocal microscopy demonstrates the presence of mast cells (c-kit$^+$ mast cell tryptase$^+$, arrows) around the airway mucosa of SU5416/chronic hypoxia (SuHx) animal at day 21 (positive control). In a naïve control lung, only one isolated c-kit$^+$ mast cell tryptase$^-$ cell was present in the pulmonary artery (open arrow). One cell with faint granular green autofluorescence (likely a macrophage) was present in the alveolar space (double-headed arrow). No mast cells were seen in the lumen-obliterating lesions of SuHx animals at day 21, only c-kit$^+$ mast cell tryptase$^-$ cells (open arrows). A single cell with faint granular green autofluorescence was seen in the alveolar space, likely a macrophage (double-headed arrow). Nuclear counterstaining: 4′,6-diamidino-2-phenylindole (DAPI). Magnification: 630×. Scale bar: 20 μm.

Confocal microscopy

Confocal microscopy was performed with a Leica TCS SP2 laser scanning confocal microscopy system or a Zeiss LSM 700 laser scanning confocal microscope system housed in the VCU Department of Anatomy and Neurobiology Microscope Facility. If confocal imaging was done in addition to widefield microscopy, the sections used for confocal microscopy were serial sections of the ones used for widefield microscopy and quantification.

Protein lysate preparation and Western blot

One whole right lobe was homogenized in radioimmunoprecipitation assay (RIPA) buffer (tissue to buffer ratio: $0.3 \text{ g} \cdot \text{ml}^{-1}$) (Sigma Aldrich) supplemented with protease- and phosphatase-inhibitors (Roche Diagnostics, Indianapolis, IN; Sigma Aldrich; New England Biolabs, Ipswich, MA). After 30 min of incubation in RIPA buffer, lung protein lysate was centrifuged at $13,000 \times g$ for 10 min and the supernatant stored at $-80°C$. Protein concentration was determined by Bio-Rad Protein Assay (Bio-Rad). The protein lysate was incubated for 10 min at 70°C in SDS loading buffer (Santa Cruz Biotechnology) and 50 μg protein was loaded into each well for SDS-PAGE. After electrophoresis, proteins were blotted onto a PVDF membrane (Bio-Rad), blocked for 1 h in 5% dry milk-PBS-0.1% Tween 20 (blocking buffer) and incubated with the respective primary antibodies overnight at 4°C in blocking buffer: cleaved caspase-3 (#9661, Cell Signaling Technologies, dilution 1:1000), CXCL12 (sc-28876, Santa Cruz, dilution 1:200), PCNA (#2586, Cell Signaling Technologies, dilution 1:1000), β-actin (A5441, Sigma-Aldrich, dilution 1::00). Secondary HRP-conjugated antibodies were applied for 1 h at room temperature in blocking buffer. The blots were developed with ECL reagent (PerkinElmer, Waltham, MA) on Genemate X-ray films (BioExpress, Kaysville, UT).

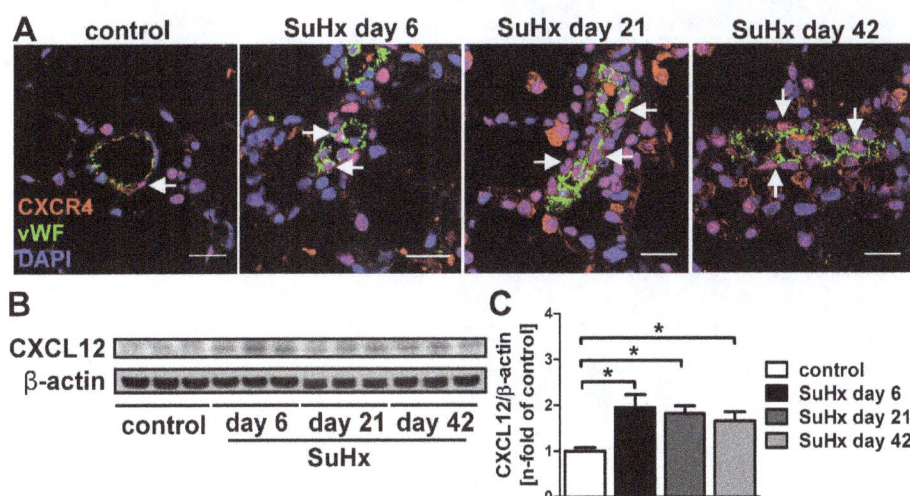

Figure 3. CXC chemokine receptor 4 (CXCR4) and CXC chemokine ligand 12 (CXCL12) expression. (**A**) Representative immunofluorescence stainings for CXCR4 and von Willebrand Factor (vWF) showing that while CXCR4 was found on vWF$^+$ endothelial cells (arrow), perivascular cells and cells in the alveolar walls in the lungs of control animals, there was an increase in CXCR4 expression in luminal, vessel wall and perivascular cells with multiple CXCR4$^+$ vWF$^+$ cells (arrows) in the lumen of the pulmonary artery in the lungs of SuHx animals. Please note that the vessel shown in the image of SuHx day 6 was sectioned transversally, whereas the vessels in the images of SuHx day 21 and 42 were sectioned in a more longitudinal manner. Nuclear staining with 4′,6-diamidino-2-phenylindole (DAPI). Magnification: 630×. Scale bar: 20 μm. (**B**) Representative Western blot analysis indicates that the protein expression of the CXCR4 ligand CXCL12 was increased in SuHx lung tissue protein lysate as compared to naïve control animals. β-actin was used as loading control. (**C**) Densitometry of the Western blot in (B). Densitometric values were normalized vs. β-actin and expressed as n-fold of naïve controls. n = 3 animals per group. * $P < 0.05$.

Statistical analysis

Data are presented as mean ± SEM. The groups were compared with 2-tailed unpaired Student's t test (2 groups) or 1-way ANOVA followed by a multiple comparison test according to Newman-Keuls (>2 groups). Statistics and graphs were done with GraphPad Prism 5.0 (GraphPad Software). $P<0.05$ was considered significant.

Results

c-kit$^+$ cells accumulated in experimental angioobliterative PAH

First, the spatiotemporal distribution of cells expressing c-kit was examined in the lung of control and SuHx animals by *in situ* hybridization and IF staining. Then, it was investigated whether these c-kit$^+$ cells express the EC marker vWF and the VSMC/myofibroblast marker α-SMA. *In-situ* hybridization and IF staining revealed that rare c-kit$^+$ cells were localized in the alveolar walls and pulmonary arteries, in particular in the intima, media and adventitia layers of naïve control rats, and that some of these c-kit$^+$ cells also expressed either the EC marker vWF or the VSMC/myofibroblast marker α-SMA (Figure 1). In the lungs of SuHx animals, an accumulation of c-kit$^+$ cells was detected as early as day 6 and the vascular aggregates of c-kit$^+$ cells were most

extensive at day 21 and 42 (Figure 1). There was a progressive accumulation of c-kit$^+$ vWF$^+$ cells until day 21 and of c-kit$^+$ α-SMA$^+$ cells until day 42 (Figure 1C-E). Co-staining of c-kit with mast cell tryptase was used to investigate whether the lung vascular lesion c-kit$^+$ cells were mast cells [17]. c-kit$^+$ mast cell tryptase$^+$ cells were not detected in and around the obliterated pulmonary arteries of SuHx animals (Figure 2).

Lung tissue expression of CXCR4 and lung protein levels of CXCL12 in SuHx animals

In naïve control animals, CXCR4$^+$ vWF$^+$ ECs and CXCR4$^+$ cells were identified in the pulmonary artery wall and perivascular region, as well as in the alveolar walls (Figure 3A). In SuHx animals, CXCR4$^+$ cells accumulated in the lumen, pulmonary artery wall and perivascular region over time (Figure 3A). The protein expression of the CXCR4 ligand CXCL12 was increased at day 6, 21 and 42 in the lung tissue protein lysate of SuHx animals (Figure 3B-C).

Expression of CXCR4, vWF and α-SMA in c-kit$^+$ cells in SuHx animals

In order to investigate whether various c-kit$^+$ cells express CXCR4 and may therefore be a valid target for CXCR4 inhibition, the expression profile of CXCR4, vWF and α-SMA

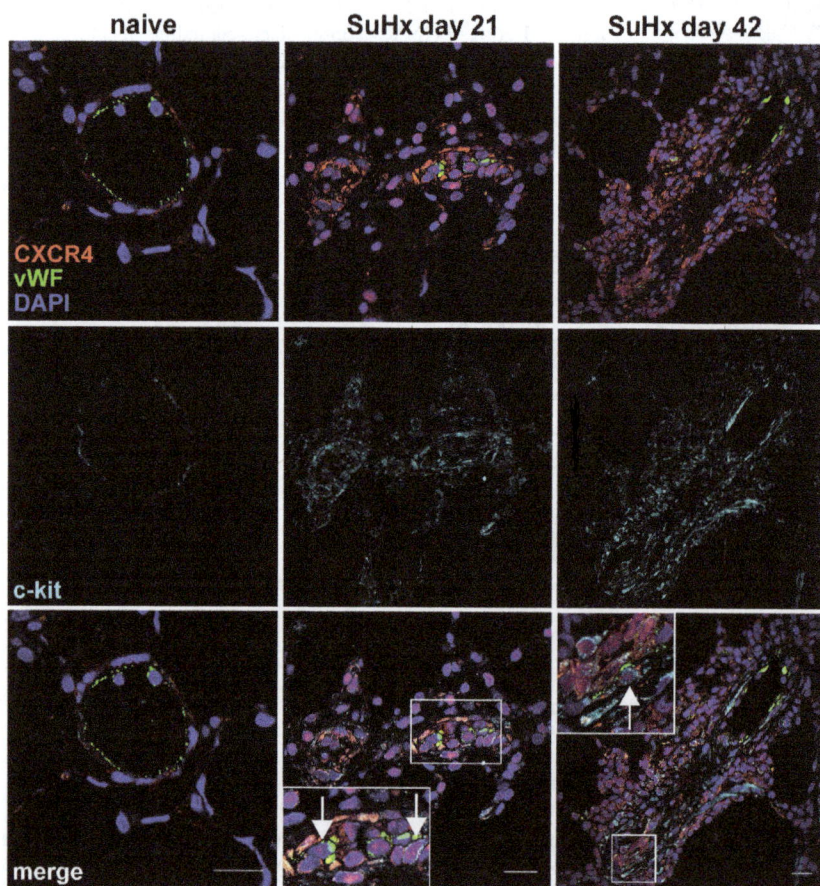

Figure 4. Expression of CXC chemokine receptor 4 (CXCR4) and von Willebrand Factor (vWF) in c-kit$^+$ cells. Representative optical sections obtained by confocal microscopy demonstrating the co-expression of CXCR4, vWF and c-kit in the pulmonary artery wall of a naïve animal and in pulmonary vascular lesion cells of animals with SU541/chronic hypoxia (SuHx) induced severe PAH. The inserts show the area outlined by a box in more detail. Arrows indicate triple positive cells in the inserts. Nuclear counterstaining: 4'-6-diamidino-2-phenylindole (DAPI). Magnification: 400×. Scale bar: 20 μm.

was determined in c-kit$^+$ cells by triple IF stainings and confocal microscopy. The concomitant expression of CXCR4, vWF and c-kit was not detected in pulmonary arteries of naïve animals (Figure 4). In SuHx animals, multiple CXCR4$^+$ vWF$^+$ c-kit$^+$ cells were found in pulmonary arterial lesions of SuHx animals at day 21 and 42 (Figure 4). Co-expression of the three markers CXCR4, α-SMA and c-kit was also not identified in pulmonary arteries of naïve animals (Figure 5). In contrast, multiple CXCR4$^+$ α-SMA$^+$ c-kit$^+$ cells were detected in the obliterated pulmonary arteries of SuHx animals at day 21 and 42 (Figure 5).

CXCR4 inhibition prevented the increased muscularization and partially the obliteration of pulmonary arteries in the SuHx model

To address the question whether CXCR4 signaling contributes to the lung vascular lesion formation, SuHx rats were treated with the CXCR4 inhibitor AMD3100. AMD3100 treatment moderately reduced the right ventricular (RV) systolic pressure (RVSP) and RV hypertrophy. AMD3100 treatment further completely prevented the increase in average pulmonary artery MWT, a measure of pulmonary arterial muscularization (Figure 6). CXCR4 inhibition only partially prevented the obliteration of small and medium-sized pulmonary arteries as assessed by vWF IHC (Figure 6).

CXCR4 inhibition reduced lung cell proliferation and decreased the presence of c-kit$^+$ cells

AMD3100 treatment significantly reduced the protein expression of PCNA and cleaved caspase-3 in the lung tissue protein lysate of SuHx animals (Figure 7A-C). These findings were associated with the decreased presence of c-kit$^+$ cells and c-kit$^+$ α-SMA$^+$ cells in and around pulmonary arteries, but not with a reduction in the number of c-kit$^+$ vWF$^+$ cells in pulmonary arteries (Figure 8A-B). Less PCNA$^+$ cells, c-kit$^+$ PCNA$^+$ cells and c-kit$^+$ α-SMA$^+$ PCNA$^+$ were found in and around pulmonary arteries following AMD3100 treatment, but a significant reduction in the number of c-kit$^+$ vWF$^+$ PCNA$^+$ cells was not detected (Figure 8A, C). These results indicate that the number and the proliferation of these c-kit$^+$ vWF$^+$ cells were not affected by CXCR4 inhibition. Hence, the reduced proliferation of primitive α-SMA$^+$ c-kit$^+$ cells after AMD3100 treatment correlated with the prevention of increased muscularization in pulmonary arteries.

The accumulation of vWF$^+$ CXCR4$^+$ cells was not significantly reduced by AMD3100

AMD3100 treatment reduced the total number of CXCR4$^+$ cells and CXCR4$^+$ α-SMA$^+$ per vessel in the pulmonary arteries of SuHx animals, but there was only a small trend towards reduced

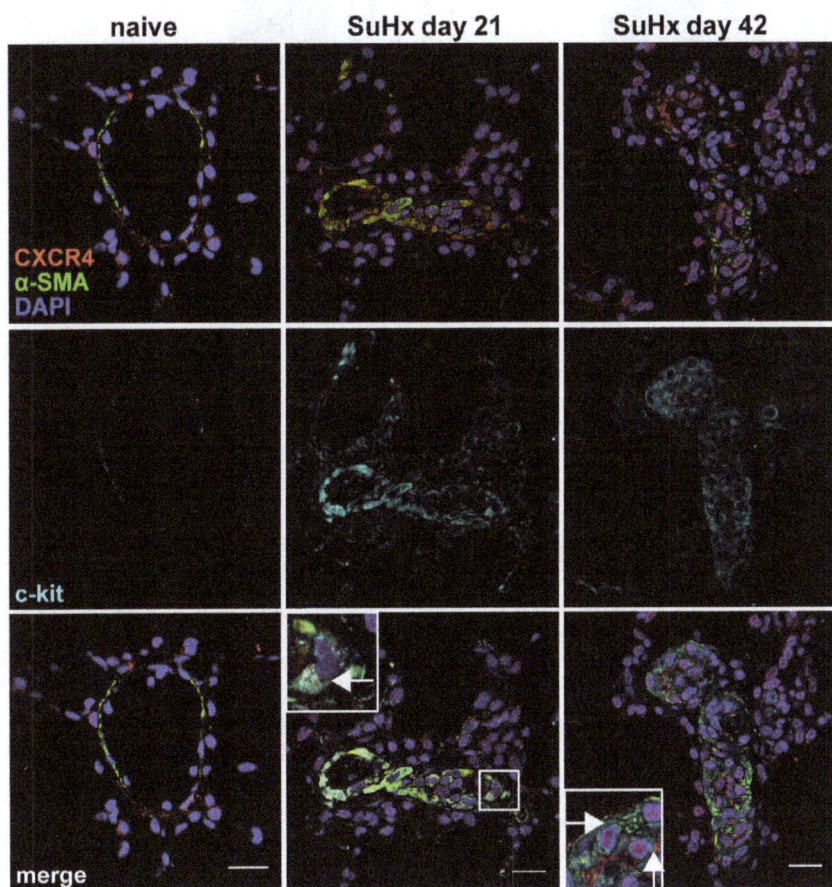

Figure 5. Expression of CXC chemokine receptor 4 (CXCR4) and α-smooth muscle actin (α-SMA) in c-kit$^+$ cells. Representative optical sections obtained by confocal microscopy demonstrating the co-expression of CXCR4, α-SMA and c-kit in the pulmonary artery of a naïve animal and in pulmonary vascular lesion cells of animals with SU5416/chronic hypoxia (SuHx) induced severe PAH. The inserts show the area outlined by a box in more detail. Arrows indicate triple positive cells in the inserts. Nuclear counterstaining: 4′-6-diamidino-2-phenylindole (DAPI). Magnification: 400×. Scale bar: 20 μm.

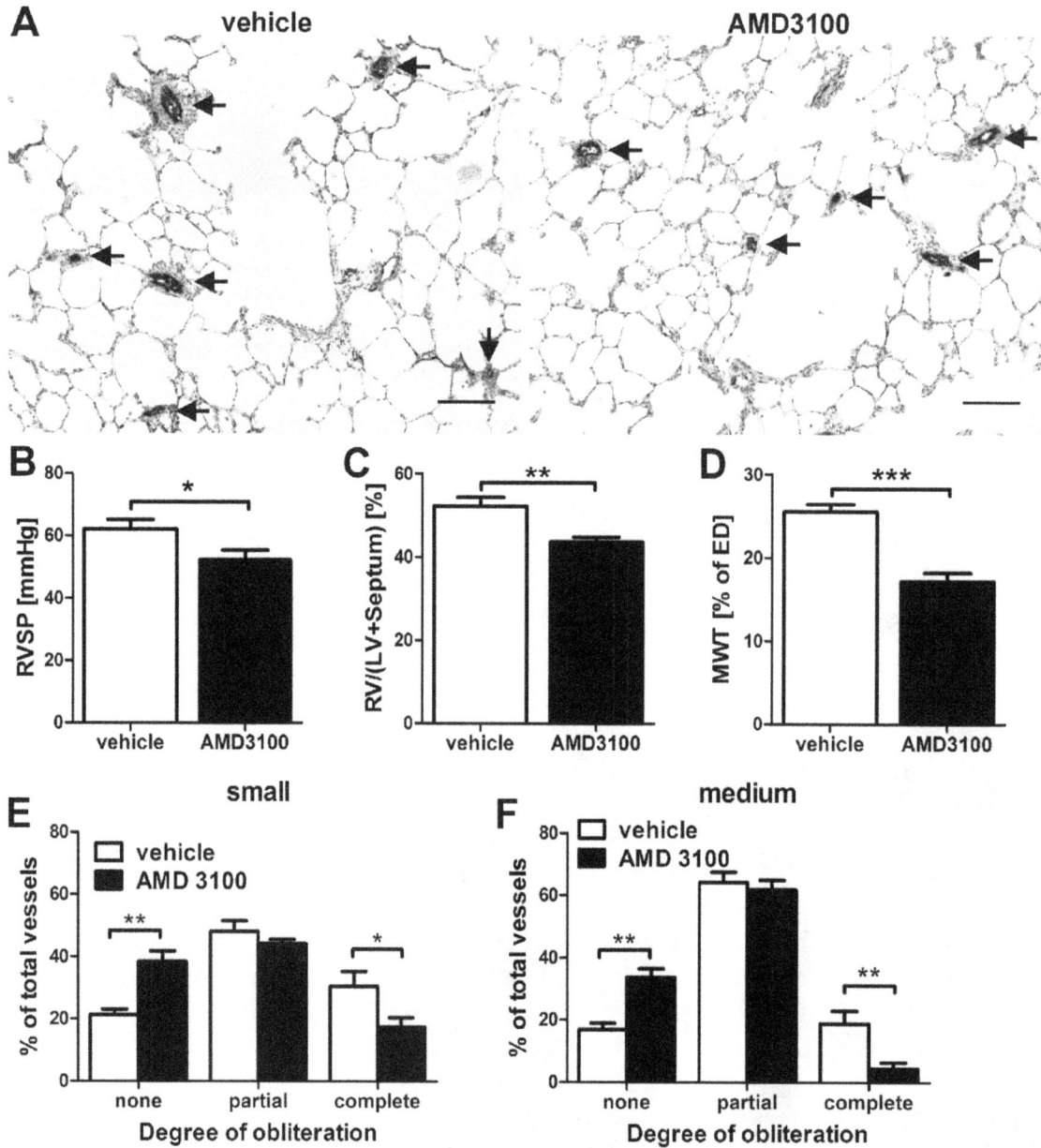

Figure 6. AMD3100 prevented severe pulmonary arterial hypertension (PAH) in the SU5416/chronic hypoxia (SuHx) model. (A) Representative von Willebrand Factor (vWF) immunohistochemistry indicates the occlusion of pulmonary arteries (arrows). These images demonstrate that treatment with the CXC chemokine receptor 4 inhibitor AMD3100 only partially prevented the obliteration of pulmonary arteries. Counterstaining: Mayer's Hematoxylin. Magnification: 100×. Scale bar: 100 μm. (B) Reduced right ventricular systolic pressure (RVSP) and (C) decreased right ventricle (RV)/(left ventricle [LV]+Septum) ratio. (D) Reduced pulmonary arterial muscularization (external diameter [ED] <100 μm) was detected after AMD3100 treatment. (E-F) The degree of obliteration of pulmonary arteries in AMD3100-treated SuHx animals was partially reduced for small (E) (25 μm<ED<50 μm) and for medium-sized (F) (50 μm ≤ ED<100 μm) pulmonary arteries. (B-F): n = 6 animals per group. * $P<0.05$, ** $P<0.01$, *** $P<0.0001$.

number of CXCR4+ vWF+ cells after AMD3100 treatment (Figure 9A-C).

Discussion

The pathophysiology of severe PAH has been traditionally explained largely as a consequence of chronic hemodynamic stress, such as pulmonary vasoconstriction and elevated shear stress [23]. The increase in the pulmonary vascular resistance is now also attributed to the structural alterations of the pulmonary arteries and reversal of these structural changes has become a treatment goal [2]. Successful and permanent reversal of the pulmonary arterial remodeling will likely require a detailed knowledge of the altered microenvironment of the remodeled pulmonary artery [2]. The early phase of lung vessel disease development in human PAH remains unexamined and it is not feasible to serially study diseased human lungs. Hence, we investigated the development of vascular obliteration in an animal model of severe PAH that predictably generates obliterative

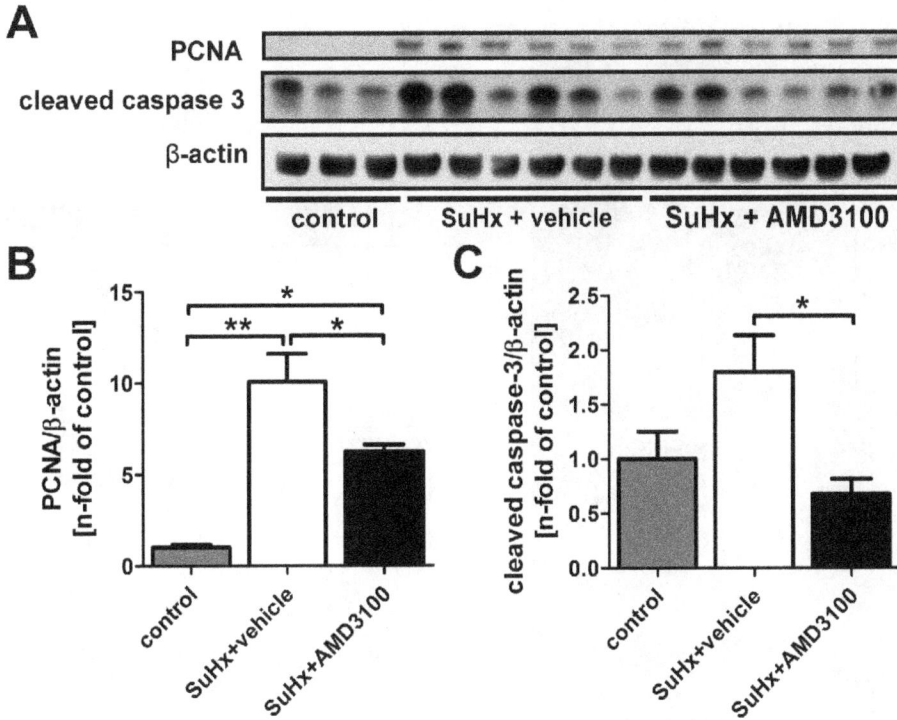

Figure 7. Proliferation and apoptosis in the lungs of AMD3100-treated SU5416/chronic hypoxia (SuHx) animals. (A) Representative Western blot for proliferating cell nuclear antigen (PCNA) and cleaved caspase-3 in the lung tissue protein lysate of naïve control animals (n = 3), SuHx + vehicle (n = 6) and SuHx + AMD3100 treated rats (n = 6). β-actin was used as loading control. **(B-C)** Densitometric analysis indicates increased PCNA (B) and cleaved caspase-3 (C) protein levels in the lungs of SuHx + vehicle animals vs. controls, and that AMD3100 treatment significantly reduced PCNA and cleaved caspase-3 protein levels in the lungs of SuHx animals. Densitometric values were normalized vs. β-actin and expressed as n-fold of naïve controls. n = 3 animals per group for controls and n = 6 animals per group for SuHx + vehicle and SuHx + AMD3100 groups. * $P<0.05$ and ** $P<0.01$.

pulmonary arterial lesions resembling those observed in the lungs of patients with severe PAH [4,24].

The pulmonary vascular lesions in severe PAH are complex and multicellular, and it has been suggested that the lesions contain primitive angiogenic cells that express endothelial markers [25]. Indeed, a variety of stem and progenitor cell markers has been detected in vascular lesions of patients with severe PAH [16,17,26]. BM-derived progenitors from PAH patients can induce vascular remodeling, including *in situ* thrombi, in the pulmonary arteries of mice [27]._ENREF_15_ENREF_30 In the present study, we concentrated on the role of cells expressing the tyrosine kinase receptor c-kit: c-kit is a common marker of primitive progenitor and stem cells, including the recently described lung stem cells [12] and rare vascular endothelial stem cells [13]. c-kit+ mast cells and c-kit+ progenitor cells have also been identified in pulmonary vascular lesions of patients with severe PAH [17,26] and around pulmonary arteries of chronic hypoxic mice [18].

The main findings of our experimental studies are: 1) c-kit+ cells accumulate in and around the pulmonary artery lesions in the SuHx model of severe obliterative PAH. 2) Some c-kit+ cells express endothelial and mesenchymal markers. 3) CXCR4+ cells accumulate in the pulmonary vascular lesions of SuHx animals and the CXCR4 ligand CXCL12 is found at elevated protein levels in the lung tissue of SuHx animals. 4) c-kit+ cells in the pulmonary vascular lesions frequently express CXCR4. 5) CXCR4 blockade affects c-kit+ cell participation, in particular the proliferation of α-SMA+ c-kit+ cells, and pulmonary arterial muscularization. 6) Occlusion of pulmonary arteries and severe

PAH were only partially prevented by CXCR4 blockade. 7) CXCR4+ α-SMA+ cells, but not CXCR4+ vWF+ cells, were reactive to AMD3100 treatment.

Similar to human PAH [17,26], we identified in our study in the lungs of the animals with severe SuHx-induced PAH c-kit+ cells within the lumen-occluding cells and in the perivascular cellular aggregates. We extend the current knowledge of the presence of c-kit+ cells in pulmonary vascular lesions by demonstrating that the c-kit+ cells found in the pulmonary vascular lesions are not a uniform population: Some c-kit+ cells in the pulmonary arterial wall expressed the endothelial marker vWF or the VSMC/myofibroblast marker α-SMA. c-kit expression has been demonstrated on a variety of cell types, including mast cells, dendritic cells, pre-T and pre-B lymphocytes, hematopoietic progenitor and stem cells, as well as various forms of tissue-derived progenitor and stem cells [12,13,17,28]. As expected, a small number of c-kit+ cells were also detected in the pulmonary arteries and alveolar walls from control animals. The population of c-kit+ cells, and in particular the pool of c-kit+ vWF+ and c-kit+ α-SMA+ cells, was vastly expanded in and around the pulmonary arterial lesions of SuHx animals. It is interesting that the presence of c-kit+ vWF+ cells started to decline after day 21 in the SuHx model. At the same time, c-kit+ α-SMA+ cell continued to accumulate in the remodeled pulmonary arteries and were also increasingly found among lumen-obliterating cells. One possible explanation is the transdifferentiation of c-kit+ EPCs into α-SMA expressing VSMC or myofibroblast precursors in more mature lesions, a process that has been already suggested *in vitro* [29-31]. Because α-SMA expression is also frequently found in activated myofibroblasts in

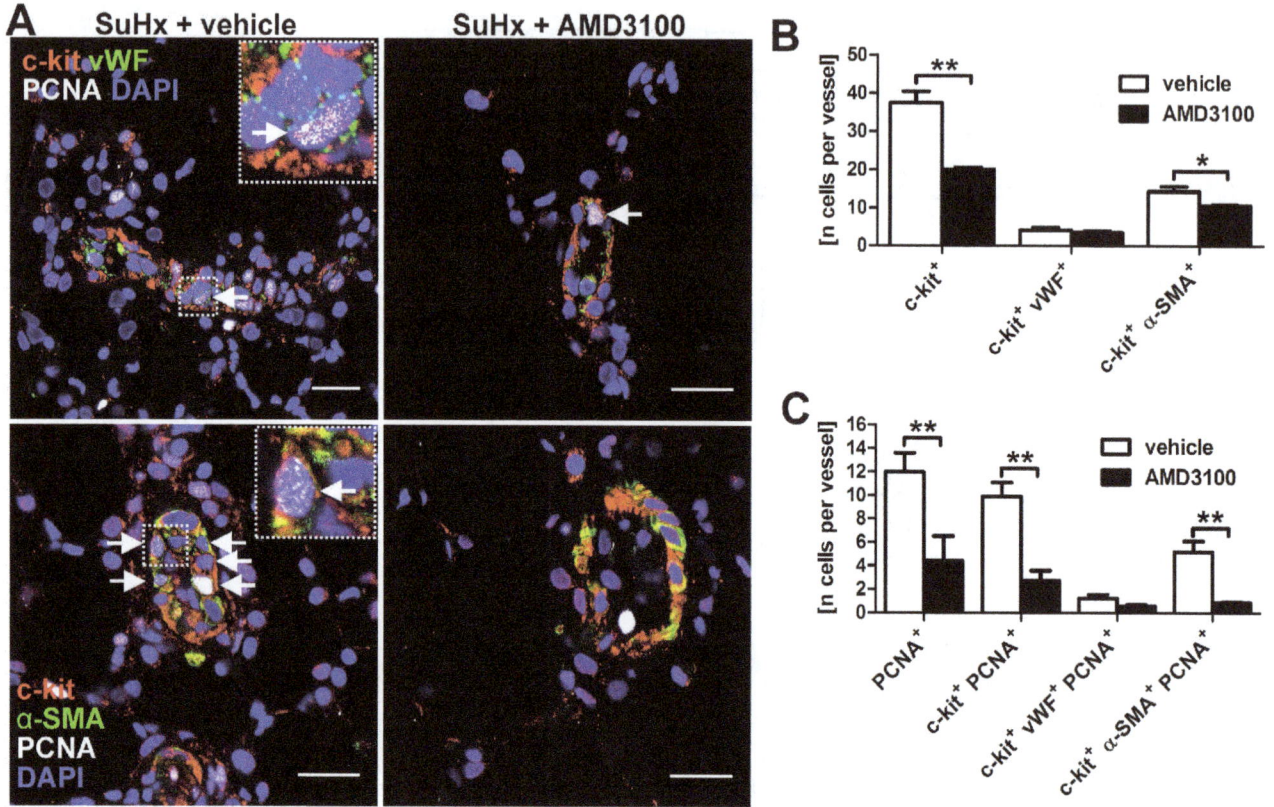

Figure 8. Proliferation of c-kit+ cells in the lungs of AMD3100-treated SU5416/chronic hypoxia (SuHx) animals. (**A**) Representative optical sections (confocal microscopy) demonstrate c-kit+ von Willebrand Factor+ (vWF+) proliferating cell nuclear antigen+ (PCNA+) cells (upper row) or c-kit+ α-smooth muscle actin+ (α-SMA+) PCNA+ cells (lower row) in pulmonary arteries of SuHx + vehicle and SuHx + AMD3100 treated animals. The inserts show a triple positive cell (arrow) in more detail. Please note that the bright white stained dots indicate cells with very strong PCNA staining. Nuclear counterstaining: 4′,6-diamidino-2-phenylindole (DAPI). Magnification: 630×. Scale bar: 20 μm. (**B-C**) Quantification of the number of c-kit+, c-kit+ vWF+ and c-kit+ α-SMA+, as well as PCNA+, c-kit+ PCNA+, c-kit+ vWF+ PCNA+ and c-kit+ α-SMA+ PCNA+ cells in and around the pulmonary arteries of SuHx + vehicle and SuHx + AMD3100 animals. n = 3 animals per group. * $P < 0.05$ and ** $P < 0.01$.

scar tissue, the c-kit+ α-SMA+ may also represent myofibroblast precursors [32,33] that accumulate in the obliterated pulmonary arteries during a process of intravascular scar formation. Fibrocytes, which are characterized as cells expressing hematopoietic and mesenchymal markers, have been identified as an important source of myofibroblasts in the context of lung fibrosis

[34-36]. Because fibrocytes express markers of immature hematopoietic cells, such as CD34, it is possible that at least a fraction of the c-kit+ cells, the c-kit+ α-SMA+ cells, represents fibrocytes [34,35]. Fibrocytes have been suggested to contribute to pulmonary vascular remodeling in mice, rats and calves under conditions

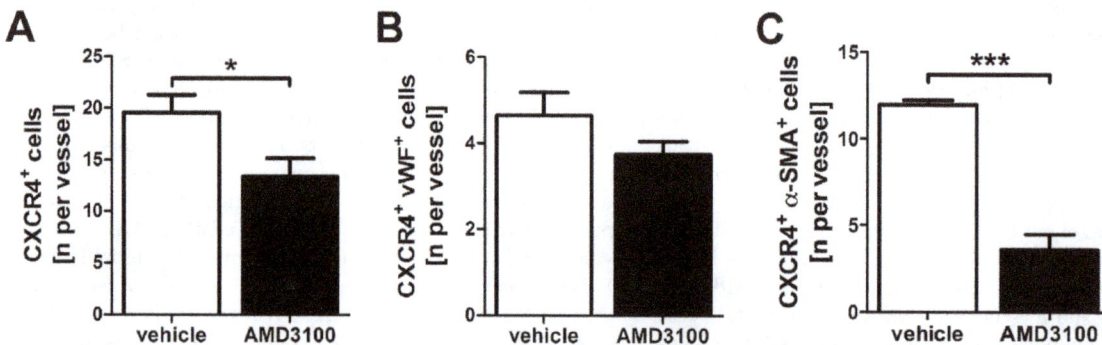

Figure 9. Effect of AMD3100 treatment on CXC chemokine receptor 4+ (CXCR4+) cells. Quantification of the number of total CXCR4+ cells (**A**), CXCR4+ von Willebrand Factor+ (vWF+) cells (**B**) and CXCR4+ α-smooth muscle actin+ (α-SMA+) cells (**C**) per vessel in pulmonary arteries of SuHx animals treated with vehicle or AMD3100. The data indicate that while the number of total CXCR4+ cells and CXCR4+ α-SMA+ cells per vessel was significantly reduced by AMD3100 treatment, there was only a small trend towards decreased number of CXCR4+ vWF+ cells per vessel in AMD3100 treated SuHx animals. n = 4 animals/group. * $P < 0.05$, *** $P < 0.0001$.

of chronic hypoxia [33,37] and fibrocytes may also contribute to pulmonary vascular remodeling in severe obliterative PAH.

The receptor for CXCL12, CXCR4, is important for the homing of stem and progenitor cells to sites of tissue injury [38]. CXCR4 is expressed in the lung vascular lesions of patients with severe PAH [16,26]. Therefore, we investigated the expression of CXCR4 and CXCL12 in the lungs of SuHx animals. We found CXCR4 expression in the cells that accumulated over time in the lumen, pulmonary artery wall and perivascular region of SuHx animals. CXCR4 expression was also frequently detected in c-kit$^+$ cells, including the c-kit$^+$ vWF$^+$ and c-kit$^+$ α-SMA$^+$ cells that clustered in and around the remodeled pulmonary arteries of SuHx animals. Because the accumulation of CXCR4$^+$ cells is directed by the tissue expression of its ligand CXCL12 [39], it is not surprising that the expression of the CXCR4 ligand CXCL12 was significantly increased in the lung tissue of SuHx animals. The expression of CXCL12 is extensively regulated by tissue hypoxia and by local tissue injury [36,40]. We suggest that the upregulation of CXCL12 in the lungs of SuHx animals is likely dependent on chronic hypoxia, as demonstrated in chronic hypoxic mice [18,41], and the ongoing vascular injury originally initiated by injection of SU5416 [3,29]. The increased expression of CXCL12, the accumulation of CXCR4$^+$ cells and the expression of CXCR4 in the c-kit$^+$ cells in the lung vascular lesions provided the rationale to investigate whether the formation of lesions in the pulmonary arteries was dependent on CXCL12/CXCR4.

CXCR4 inhibition with AMD3100 reduced the accumulation and proliferation of c-kit$^+$ cells and the muscularization of the remodeled pulmonary arteries from SuHx animals. The main effect was decreased proliferation of c-kit$^+$ α-SMA$^+$ cells, a finding that provides a cellular correlate to the morphologically reduced muscularization of pulmonary arteries. Our findings in a rat model of severe, obliterative PAH complement recent work in chronic hypoxic mice indicating that c-kit$^+$ cells may contribute to pulmonary arterial muscularization in a CXCR4-dependent manner [18]. The findings that c-kit$^+$ α-SMA$^+$ cells express CXCR4 and accumulate in a CXCR4-dependent manner in the remodeled pulmonary arteries further support the concept that these c-kit$^+$ α-SMA$^+$ CXCR4$^+$ cells may be fibrocytes that contribute to pulmonary vascular remodeling. Various studies have shown that CXCR4 inhibition reduces lung fibrosis *via* reduced fibrocyte migration [36,42,43]. However, in SuHx animals, CXCR4 inhibition only caused a modest reduction in PAH and did not significantly decrease the number of c-kit$^+$ vWF$^+$ or proliferating c-kit$^+$ vWF$^+$ cells in pulmonary arteries. Our data also indicate that the accumulation of CXCR4$^+$ vWF$^+$ ECs/EPCs is largely independent of CXCR4, in contrast to the accumulation of CXCR4$^+$ cells and CXCR4$^+$ α-SMA$^+$ cells. We propose that the cells retained in the obliterated pulmonary arteries may represent a c-kit$^+$ EPC pool, that was largely unaffected by AMD3100. We base our assumption on the localization of the cells in the lumen obliterating lesions and the co-expression of the EC marker vWF with c-kit in these cells [13]. It is possible that

CXCR4 inhibition may not only decrease homing of circulating cells, but may also reduce migration of lung resident cells or impact the function of stem/progenitor cells [44,45]._ENREF_56 Because AMD3100 does not affect the c-kit$^+$ vWF$^+$ cells, we propose that these c-kit$^+$ vWF$^+$ cells are likely lung resident EPCs and/or that their migration and homing is not critically dependent on CXCR4 [13,18,29,36,46]. Our data indicate that lumen obliteration by vWF$^+$ cells may be promoted by mechanisms in addition to CXCL12/CXCR4 signaling. One example of such an additional mechanism may be the increased expression of the pro-angiogenic factor fibroblast growth factor 2. Fibroblast growth factor 2 has been shown to be elevated in pulmonary arterial lesions of PAH patients and animals with SuHx-induced severe PAH [47,48].

The reduction in RVSP following CXCR4 inhibition was only moderate in SuHx rats – in contrast to the studies conducted in the chronic hypoxic model of PAH. Our data suggest that the persistent RVSP elevation can be explained, similar to concepts in human severe PAH, by the residual obliteration of pulmonary arteries that was only partially prevented by CXCR4 blockade [2]. The data further indicate that the arteriolar occlusion is due to a different set of c-kit$^+$ cells, likely EPCs, that seem to be largely unaffected by AMD3100 treatment.

In conclusion, our data indicate that c-kit$^+$ progenitor cells accumulate in and around the lung vascular lesions of SuHx rats. Our data also suggest that in severe experimental PAH, lung vascular obliteration and the accumulation of c-kit$^+$ cells only partially depend on CXCR4 activity. In contrast, CXCR4 signaling is required for pulmonary arterial muscularization. c-kit$^+$ α-SMA$^+$ cells appear to contribute to pulmonary arterial muscularization in a CXCR4-dependent manner. A different subset of c-kit$^+$ cells with endothelial markers seems to contribute to pulmonary arterial obliteration in a largely CXCR4-independent fashion. Whether c-kit$^+$ progenitor cell populations are sufficient to cause obliterative pulmonary vascular disease or whether additional factors are required will have to be examined by cell transfer experiments.

Supporting Information

Figure S1 Negative control for *in situ* hybridization. Negative control (SU5416/chronic hypoxia angioobliterative lesion at day 21) was generated by omitting the hybridization probe. Counterstaining with Gill's Hematoxylin. Magnification: 400×. Scale bar: 20 μm.

Author Contributions

Conceived and designed the experiments: DF DK HJB CDC NFV LF. Performed the experiments: DF DK JID AAA VK LF. Analyzed the data: DF DK JID AAA VK LF. Contributed reagents/materials/analysis tools: CDC NFV LF. Wrote the paper: DF DK JID AAA VK HJB CDC NFV LF.

References

1. Simonneau G, Robbins IM, Beghetti M, Channick RN, Delcroix M, et al. (2009) Updated Clinical Classification of Pulmonary Hypertension. Journal of the American College of Cardiology 54: S43–S54.
2. Erzurum S, Rounds SI, Stevens T, Aldred M, Aliotta J, et al. (2010) Strategic Plan for Lung Vascular Research: An NHLBI-ORDR Workshop Report. Am J Respir Crit Care Med 182: 1554–1562.
3. Sakao S, Taraseviciene-Stewart L, Lee JD, Wood K, Cool CD, et al. (2005) Initial apoptosis is followed by increased proliferation of apoptosis-resistant endothelial cells. Faseb J 19: 1178–1180.
4. Taraseviciene-Stewart L, Kasahara Y, Alger L, Hirth P, Mc Mahon G, et al. (2001) Inhibition of the VEGF receptor 2 combined with chronic hypoxia causes

cell death-dependent pulmonary endothelial cell proliferation and severe pulmonary hypertension. Faseb J 15: 427–438.
5. Rabinovitch M (2012) Molecular pathogenesis of pulmonary arterial hypertension. The Journal of Clinical Investigation 122: 4306–4313.
6. Weiss DJ, Bertoncello I, Borok Z, Kim C, Panoskaltsis-Mortari A, et al. (2011) Stem Cells and Cell Therapies in Lung Biology and Lung Diseases. Proc Am Thorac Soc 8: 223–272.
7. Simons Benjamin D and Clevers H (2011) Strategies for Homeostatic Stem Cell Self-Renewal in Adult Tissues. Cell 145: 851–862.
8. Yoder MC and Ingram DA (2009) The definition of EPCs and other bone marrow cells contributing to neoangiogenesis and tumor growth: is there

common ground for understanding the roles of numerous marrow-derived cells in the neoangiogenic process? Biochim Biophys Acta 1796: 50–54.

9. Zengin E, Chalajour F, Gehling UM, Ito WD, Treede H, et al. (2006) Vascular wall resident progenitor cells: a source for postnatal vasculogenesis. Development 133: 1543–1551.

10. Roskoski Jr R (2005) Signaling by Kit protein-tyrosine kinase—The stem cell factor receptor. Biochemical and Biophysical Research Communications 337: 1–13.

11. Heissig B, Werb Z, Rafii S and Hattori K (2003) Role of c-kit/Kit ligand signaling in regulating vasculogenesis. Thromb Haemost 90: 570–576.

12. Kajstura J, Rota M, Hall SR, Hosoda T, D'Amario D, et al. (2011) Evidence for Human Lung Stem Cells. New England Journal of Medicine 364: 1795–1806.

13. Fang S, Wei J, Pentinmikko N, Leinonen H and Salven P (2012) Generation of Functional Blood Vessels from a Single c-kit+ Adult Vascular Endothelial Stem Cell. PLoS Biol 10: e1001407.

14. Domanska UM, Kruizinga RC, Nagengast WB, Timmer-Bosscha H, Huls G, et al. (2013) A review on CXCR4/CXCL12 axis in oncology: No place to hide. European Journal of Cancer 49: 219–230.

15. Askari AT, Unzek S, Popovic ZB, Goldman CK, Forudi F, et al. (2003) Effect of stromal-cell-derived factor 1 on stem-cell homing and tissue regeneration in ischaemic cardiomyopathy. The Lancet 362: 697–703.

16. Toshner M, Voswinckel R, Southwood M, Al-Lamki R, Howard LSG, et al. (2009) Evidence of Dysfunction of Endothelial Progenitors in Pulmonary Arterial Hypertension. Am J Respir Crit Care Med 180: 780–787.

17. Montani D, Perros F, Gambaryan N, Girerd B, Dorfmuller P, et al. (2011) C-Kit-Positive Cells Accumulate in Remodeled Vessels of Idiopathic Pulmonary Arterial Hypertension. Am J Respir Crit Care Med 184: 116–123.

18. Gambaryan N, Perros F, Montani D, Cohen-Kaminsky S, Mazmanian M, et al. (2011) Targeting of c-kit+ haematopoietic progenitor cells prevents hypoxic pulmonary hypertension. European Respiratory Journal 37: 1392–1399.

19. Bogaard HJ, Natarajan R, Henderson SC, Long CS, Kraskauskas D, et al. (2009) Chronic pulmonary artery pressure elevation is insufficient to explain right heart failure. Circulation 120: 1951–1960.

20. Nicolls MR, Mizuno S, Taraseviciene-Stewart L, Farkas L, Drake JI, et al. (2012) New models of pulmonary hypertension based on VEGF receptor blockade-induced endothelial cell apoptosis. Pulm Circ 2: 434–442.

21. Farkas L, Farkas D, Ask K, Möller A, Gauldie J, et al. (2009) VEGF ameliorates pulmonary hypertension through inhibition of endothelial apoptosis in experimental lung fibrosis in rats. The Journal of Clinical Investigation 119: 1298–1311.

22. Abramoff MD, Magelhaes PJ and Ram SJ (2004) Image Processing with ImageJ. Biophotonics International 11: 36–42.

23. Sakao S, Tatsumi K and Voelkel NF (2010) Reversible or irreversible remodeling in pulmonary arterial hypertension. Am J Respir Cell Mol Biol 43: 629–634.

24. Abe K, Toba M, Alzoubi A, Ito M, Fagan KA, et al. (2010) Formation of plexiform lesions in experimental severe pulmonary arterial hypertension. Circulation 121: 2747–2754.

25. Tuder RM, Groves B, Badesch DB and Voelkel NF (1994) Exuberant endothelial cell growth and elements of inflammation are present in plexiform lesions of pulmonary hypertension. Am J Pathol 144: 275–285.

26. Rai PR, Cool CD, King JAC, Stevens T, Burns N, et al. (2008) The Cancer Paradigm of Severe Pulmonary Arterial Hypertension. Am J Respir Crit Care Med 178: 558–564.

27. Asosingh K, Farha S, Lichtin A, Graham B, George D, et al. (2012) Pulmonary vascular disease in mice xenografted with human BM progenitors from patients with pulmonary arterial hypertension. Blood 120: 1218–1227.

28. Ray P, Krishnamoorthy N and Ray A (2008) Emerging functions of c-kit and its ligand stem cell factor in dendritic cells. Cell Cycle 7: 2826–2832.

29. Sakao S, Taraseviciene-Stewart L, Cool CD, Tada Y, Kasahara Y, et al. (2007) VEGF-R blockade causes endothelial cell apoptosis, expansion of surviving CD34+ precursor cells and transdifferentiation to smooth muscle-like and neuronal-like cells. Faseb J 21: 3640–3652.

30. Arciniegas E, Frid MG, Douglas IS and Stenmark KR (2007) Perspectives on endothelial-to-mesenchymal transition: potential contribution to vascular

remodeling in chronic pulmonary hypertension. Am J Physiol Lung Cell Mol Physiol 293: L1–8.

31. Frid MG, Kale VA and Stenmark KR (2002) Mature vascular endothelium can give rise to smooth muscle cells via endothelial-mesenchymal transdifferentiation: in vitro analysis. Circ Res 90: 1189–1196.

32. Burke DL, Frid MG, Kunrath CL, Karoor V, Anwar A, et al. (2009) Sustained hypoxia promotes the development of a pulmonary artery-specific chronic inflammatory microenvironment. American Journal of Physiology - Lung Cellular and Molecular Physiology 297: L238–L250.

33. Frid MG, Brunetti JA, Burke DL, Carpenter TC, Davie NJ, et al. (2006) Hypoxia-Induced Pulmonary Vascular Remodeling Requires Recruitment of Circulating Mesenchymal Precursors of a Monocyte/Macrophage Lineage. Am J Pathol 168: 659–669.

34. Mehrad B, Burdick MD, Zisman DA, Keane MP, Belperio JA, et al. (2007) Circulating peripheral blood fibrocytes in human fibrotic interstitial lung disease. Biochemical and Biophysical Research Communications 353: 104–108.

35. Moeller A, Gilpin SE, Ask K, Cox G, Cook D, et al. (2009) Circulating fibrocytes are an indicator of poor prognosis in idiopathic pulmonary fibrosis. Am J Respir Crit Care Med 179: 588–594.

36. Phillips RJ, Burdick MD, Hong K, Lutz MA, Murray LA, et al. (2004) Circulating fibrocytes traffic to the lungs in response to CXCL12 and mediate fibrosis. J Clin Invest 114: 438–446.

37. Nikam VS, Schermuly RT, Dumitrascu R, Weissmann N, Kwapiszewska G, et al. (2010) Treprostinil inhibits the recruitment of bone marrow-derived circulating fibrocytes in chronic hypoxic pulmonary hypertension. European Respiratory Journal 36: 1302–1314.

38. Zernecke A, Schober A, Bot I, von Hundelshausen P, Liehn EA, et al. (2005) SDF-1{alpha}/CXCR4 Axis Is Instrumental in Neointimal Hyperplasia and Recruitment of Smooth Muscle Progenitor Cells. Circ Res 96: 784–791.

39. Levesque JP, Hendy J, Takamatsu Y, Simmons PJ and Bendall LJ (2003) Disruption of the CXCR4/CXCL12 chemotactic interaction during hemato-poietic stem cell mobilization induced by GCSF or cyclophosphamide. J Clin Invest 111: 187–196.

40. Ceradini DJ, Kulkarni AR, Callaghan MJ, Tepper OM, Bastidas N, et al. (2004) Progenitor cell trafficking is regulated by hypoxic gradients through HIF-1 induction of SDF-1. Nat Med 10: 858–864.

41. Yu L and Hales C (2011) Effect of chemokine receptor CXCR4 on hypoxia-induced pulmonary hypertension and vascular remodeling in rats. Respiratory Research 12: 21.

42. Song JS, Kang CM, Kang HH, Yoon HK, Kim YK, et al. (2010) Inhibitory effect of CXC chemokine receptor 4 antagonist AMD3100 on bleomycin induced murine pulmonary fibrosis. Exp Mol Med 42: 465–472.

43. Makino H, Aono Y, Azuma M, Kishi M, Yokota Y, et al. (2013) Antifibrotic effects of CXCR4 antagonist in bleomycin-induced pulmonary fibrosis in mice. The journal of medical investigation : JMI 60: 127–137.

44. Yu X, Chen D, Zhang Y, Wu X, Huang Z, et al. (2012) Overexpression of CXCR4 in mesenchymal stem cells promotes migration, neuroprotection and angiogenesis in a rat model of stroke. Journal of the Neurological Sciences 316: 141–149.

45. Cheng M, Zhou J, Wu M, Boriboun C, Thorne T, et al. (2010) CXCR4-Mediated Bone Marrow Progenitor Cell Maintenance and Mobilization Are Modulated by c-kit Activity / Novelty and Significance. Circulation Research 107: 1083–1093.

46. Alvarez DF, Huang L, King JA, ElZarrad MK, Yoder MC, et al. (2008) Lung microvascular endothelium is enriched with progenitor cells that exhibit vasculogenic capacity. American Journal of Physiology - Lung Cellular and Molecular Physiology 294: L419–L430.

47. Izikki M (2009) Endothelial-derived FGF2 contributes to the progression of pulmonary hypertension in humans and rodents. The Journal of Clinical Investigation 119: 512–523.

48. Al Husseini A, Bagnato G, Farkas L, Gomez-Arroyo J, Farkas D, et al. (2013) Thyroid hormone is highly permissive in angioproliferative pulmonary hypertension in rats. European Respiratory Journal 41: 104–114.

20

Recipient-Related Clinical Risk Factors for Primary Graft Dysfunction after Lung Transplantation: A Systematic Review and Meta-Analysis

Yao Liu, Yi Liu, Lili Su, Shu-juan Jiang*

Department of Respiratory Medicine, Provincial Hospital Affiliated to Shandong University, Jinan, Shandong, China

Abstract

Background: Primary graft dysfunction (PGD) is the main cause of early morbidity and mortality after lung transplantation. Previous studies have yielded conflicting results for PGD risk factors. Herein, we carried out a systematic review and meta-analysis of published literature to identify recipient-related clinical risk factors associated with PGD development.

Method: A systematic search of electronic databases (PubMed, Embase, Web of Science, Cochrane CENTRAL, and Scopus) for studies published from 1970 to 2013 was performed. Cohort, case-control, or cross-sectional studies that examined recipient-related risk factors of PGD were included. The odds ratios (ORs) or mean differences (MDs) were calculated using random-effects models

Result: Thirteen studies involving 10042 recipients met final inclusion criteria. From the pooled analyses, female gender (OR 1.38, 95% CI 1.09 to 1.75), African American (OR 1.82, 95%CI 1.36 to 2.45), idiopathic pulmonary fibrosis (IPF) (OR 1.78, 95% CI 1.49 to 2.13), sarcoidosis (OR 4.25, 95% CI 1.09 to 16.52), primary pulmonary hypertension (PPH) (OR 3.73, 95%CI 2.16 to 6.46), elevated BMI (BMI$\geq$25 kg/m^2) (OR 1.83, 95% CI 1.26 to 2.64), and use of cardiopulmonary bypass (CPB) (OR 2.29, 95%CI 1.43 to 3.65) were significantly associated with increased risk of PGD. Age, cystic fibrosis, secondary pulmonary hypertension (SPH), intra-operative inhaled nitric oxide (NO), or lung transplant type (single or bilateral) were not significantly associated with PGD development (all $P>0.05$). Moreover, a nearly 4 fold increased risk of short-term mortality was observed in patients with PGD (OR 3.95, 95% CI 2.80 to 5.57).

Conclusions: Our analysis identified several recipient related risk factors for development of PGD. The identification of higher-risk recipients and further research into the underlying mechanisms may lead to selective therapies aimed at reducing this reperfusion injury.

Editor: Mauricio Rojas, University of Pittsburgh, United States of America

Funding: This work was supported by the research grant from National Natural Science Foundation of China (No. 81301790). The funders had no role in study design, data collection and analysis, decision to publish, or preparation of the manuscript.

Competing Interests: The authors have declared that no competing interests exist.

* E-mail: doctorliuyao@126.com

Introduction

Although lung transplantation has become an increasingly common procedure in recent years, it has consistently lagged behind other organs in survival rates [1], and early postoperative allograft dysfunction remains a significant cause of post-transplantation morbidity and mortality [2]. Primary graft dysfunction (PGD) is a severe form of acute lung injury induced by ischemia-reperfusion injury that occurs in approximately 10–25% of lung graft recipients [2,3]. Reported 30-day mortality rates of patients with severe PGD are nearly 8 times as high as those for patients without PGD [4]. PGD leads to increased duration of mechanical ventilation and intensive care unit stay, poor functional outcomes, and increase rates of perioperative complications [5].

A number of previous studies have been designed to identify the clinical risk factors associated with PGD [6–23]. This field is of great clinical interest, since better understanding those transplant recipients most at risk might revolve around a concept of earlier detection for targeted therapy and aggressive support. In this regard, a number of clinical risk factors have been identified, including both organ donor and recipient characteristics. Donor characteristics previously identified include female gender, African American race, heavy smokers, older (>45 yr) or younger (<21 yr) donor age, and closed head injury as a cause of death [9,10,18,19,20]. Recipient characteristics previously linked to PGD include a diagnosis of primary pulmonary hypertension (PPH) [6,10,13,19], and elevated pulmonary artery pressures (PAP) [6,19]. In spite of this, there are several recipient-related risk factors that have been inconsistently reported in the literature.

Considering a single study may lack the power of providing a reliable conclusion, we carried out a rigorous systematic review and meta-analysis of published literature to gain more precise and quantitative estimates of recipient-related risk factors associated with development of PGD.

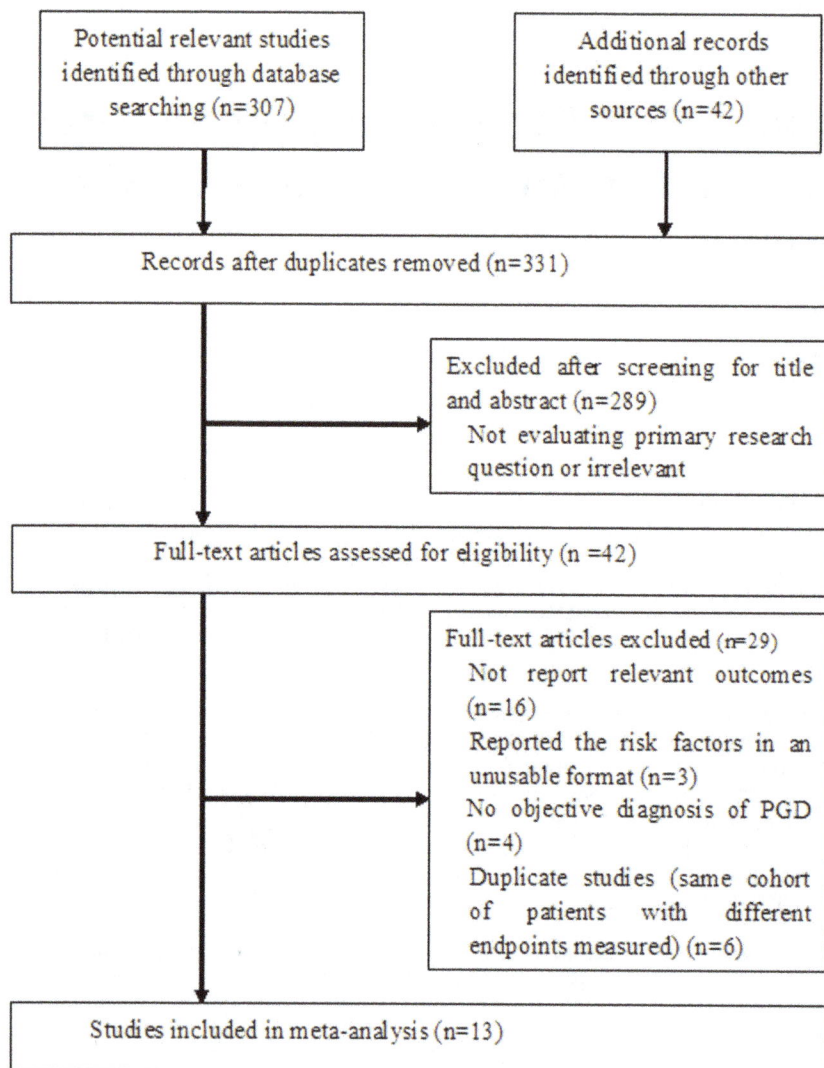

Figure 1. Flow of study identification, inclusion, and exclusion.

Methods

This meta-analysis followed the Meta-analysis of Observational Studies in Epidemiology (MOOSE) guidelines [24].

Search Strategy

Two reviewers (YL and SJJ) systematically searched PubMed, Embase, ISI Web of Science, Cochrane CENTRAL, and Scopus for articles published until October 2013. The following keywords were used in searching: "primary graft dysfunction" or "primary graft failure" or "ischemia-reperfusion injury" or "acute lung injury" or "early graft failure", combined with "lung transplantation". Language restrictions were not applied. From the title, abstract or descriptors, the literature search was reviewed independently to identify potentially relevant trials for full review. The "related articles" function was used to broaden the search. In addition, a manual review of references from primary or review articles was performed to identify any additional relevant studies.

Study selection

Cohort, case-control, and cross-sectional studies were included if they investigated which recipient-related factors directly influencing the development of PGD after lung transplantation. The potential variables assessed could be recipient demographics, co-morbidities, laboratory test, operative data, and postoperative complications. We did not address molecular or genetic markers as these require access to laboratory resources and genetic expertise. After obtaining full reports of candidate studies, the same reviewers independently assessed eligibility. Differences in data between the two reviewers were resolved by reviewing corresponding articles, and the final set was agreed on by consensus. When multiple articles for a single study had been published, we used the latest publication and supplemented it, if necessary, with data from the earlier publications. Attempts were also made to contact investigators for unpublished data.

Data Extraction

Two investigators (YL and SJJ) independently summarized the studies meeting the inclusion criteria, and performed data extraction using a standard data sheet [25]. Disagreement was

Recipient-Related Clinical Risk Factors for Primary Graft Dysfunction after Lung...

199

Table 1. Characteristics of Selected Studies.

Author	Date of study (Year)	Country	Study Design	No. of Subjects (M/F)	Mean age, %	Definition of PGD	Quality Assessment
King et al,[7] 2000	1990–1998	USA	Retrospective, single-center chart review	100(NA)	49	Patients with a chest x-ray film (CXR) score of ≥ 6 and a PaO2/FiO2 gradient of less than 200 mm Hg	Fair
Thabut et al,[8] 2002	1988–2000	France	Retrospective multicenter cohort study	257 (169/88)	48	The presence of reperfusion pulmonary edema with or without early hemodynamic failure.	Fair
Christie et al,[9] 2003	199–2000	USA	Retrospective single-center cohort study	252(123/129)	49	The presence of a diffuse alveolar infiltrate and a PaO2/FiO2 gradient of less than 200 mm Hg	Good
Whitson et al,[10] 2006	1992–2004	USA	Retrospective, single-center chart review	402 (185/217)	50	ISHLT PGD Grading System	Fair
Burton et al,[11] 2007	1999–2004	Denmark	Retrospective	180 (82/98)	56	The presence of a unilateral diffuse radiological infiltrate of the lung allograft.	Fair
Krenn et al,[12] 2007	2003–2006	Austria	Prospective single-center cohort study	150 (76/74)	38	ISHLT PGD Grading System	Good
Kuntz et al,[13] 2009	1994–2002	USA	Secondary analysis of multicenter registry (UNOS/ISHLT)	6984 (4315/2669)	—	A PaO2/FiO2 ratio less than 200, with evidence of radiographic infiltrates, and absence of secondary causes of allograft dysfunction.	Good
Felten et al,[14] 2011	2006–2008	France	Retrospective, multicenter cohort study	122 (63/59)	25	ISHLT PGD Grading System	Good
Fang et al,[15] 2011	2002–2007	USA	Prospective multicenter cohort study	126 (60/66)	56	ISHLT PGD Grading System	Good
Allen et al,[16] 2012	2002–2007	USA	Prospective, single-center cohort study	28 (12/16)	51	ISHLT PGD Grading System	Fair
Shah et al,[17] 2012	2006–2008	USA	Prospective multicenter cohort study	108(56/52)	37	ISHLT PGD Grading System	Good
Samano et al,[18] 2012	2003–2010	Brazil	Retrospective, single-center chart review	78 (46/32)	44	ISHLT PGD Grading System	Fair
Diamond et al,[19] 2013	2002–2010	USA	Prospective, multicenter cohort study (LTOG)	1255 (211/1044)	35	ISHLT PGD Grading System	Good

M, male; F, female; PGD, primary graft dysfunction; ISHLT, International Society for Heart and Lung Transplantation.

Table 2. The recipient-related risk factors examined in the original articles.

Author	Age	Gender	Race	Pulmonary Diagnosis	PAP	BLT vs SLT	BMI	CPB	Inhaled NO	Blood products transfusion	Mortality
King et al,[7]	√			√	√	√		√			√
Thabut et al,[8]	√	√		√		√		√			√
Christie et al,[9]	√	√	√	√	√	√			√		
Whitson et al,[10]		√		√		√		√			√
Burton et al,[11]	√	√		√			√	√			√
Krenn et al,[12]	√	√		√	√	√		√			√
Kuntz et al,[13]		√	√	√			√				
Felten et al,[14]	√	√					√		√	√	
Fang et al,[15]	√	√	√		√	√		√	√	√	
Allen et al,[16]	√	√		√	√	√		√	√		√
Shah et al,[17]	√	√	√	√		√	√	√			
Samano et al,[18]	√	√				√		√			√
Diamond et al,[19]	√	√	√	√	√	√		√		√	√

PAP, pulmonary artery pressure; BLT, bilateral lung transplant; SLT, single lung transplant; BMI, body mass index; CPB, cardiopulmonary bypass; NO, nitric oxide.

resolved by consensus or by a third party. For each study, the following data were extracted: first author's last name, publication year, study date, country, study design, sample size, patient characteristics (age and gender) and definition of PGD. Initially, we scrutinized in detail the literature about PGD after lung transplantation to identify all possible risk factors. The initial search yielded 18 possible risk factors. Following review by an expert panel (YL, LLS and SJJ), 10 factors that were considered to be easily measured in routine clinical practice and had been analyzed in at least 2 studies were selected for the full systematic review. These factors assessed including age, gender, race, pulmonary diagnosis, PAP, type of transplant (single lung transplant (SLT) vs bilateral lung transplant (BLT)), body mass index (BMI), cardiopulmonary bypass (CPB), intra-operative inhaled nitric oxide (NO), and blood products transfusion.

Study Quality Assessment

The Newcastle-Ottawa Scale was used to assess the quality of observational studies based on the following nine questions: (1) representativeness of the exposed cohort; (2) selection of the non-exposed cohort; (3) ascertainment of exposure; (4) demonstration that the outcome was not present at outset of study; (5) comparability; (6) assessment of outcome; (7) length of follow-up sufficient; (8) adequacy of participant follow-up; (9) total stars [26]. Maximum score on this scale is a total of 9. "Good" was defined as a total score of 7 to 9; "fair," a total score of 4–6; and "poor," defined as a total score of <4.

Statistical analyses

Our meta-analysis and statistical analyses were performed with Revman software (version 5.2; Cochrane Collaboration, Oxford, United Kingdom) and Stata software (version 11.0; Stata Corporation, College Station, TX, USA). The odds ratios (ORs)

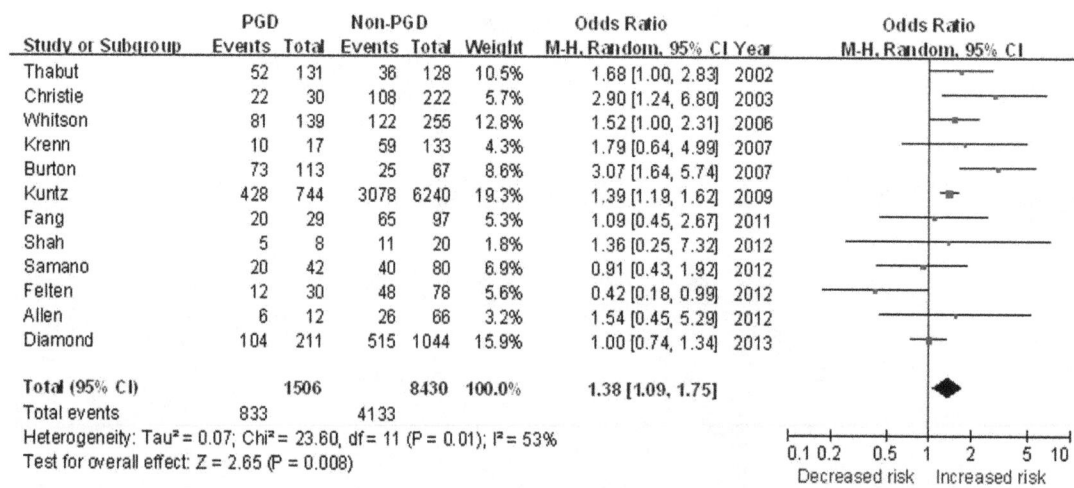

Study or Subgroup	PGD Events	PGD Total	Non-PGD Events	Non-PGD Total	Weight	Odds Ratio M-H, Random, 95% CI	Year
Thabut	52	131	38	128	10.5%	1.68 [1.00, 2.83]	2002
Christie	22	30	108	222	5.7%	2.90 [1.24, 6.80]	2003
Whitson	81	139	122	255	12.8%	1.52 [1.00, 2.31]	2006
Krenn	10	17	59	133	4.3%	1.79 [0.64, 4.99]	2007
Burton	73	113	25	67	8.6%	3.07 [1.64, 5.74]	2007
Kuntz	428	744	3078	6240	19.3%	1.39 [1.19, 1.62]	2009
Fang	20	29	65	97	5.3%	1.09 [0.45, 2.67]	2011
Shah	5	8	11	20	1.8%	1.36 [0.25, 7.32]	2012
Samano	20	42	40	80	6.9%	0.91 [0.43, 1.92]	2012
Felten	12	30	48	78	5.6%	0.42 [0.18, 0.99]	2012
Allen	6	12	26	66	3.2%	1.54 [0.45, 5.29]	2012
Diamond	104	211	515	1044	15.9%	1.00 [0.74, 1.34]	2013
Total (95% CI)		1506		8430	100.0%	1.38 [1.09, 1.75]	
Total events	833		4133				

Heterogeneity: Tau² = 0.07; Chi² = 23.60, df = 11 (P = 0.01); I² = 53%
Test for overall effect: Z = 2.65 (P = 0.008)

0.1 0.2   0.5   1   2   5   10
Decreased risk   Increased risk

Figure 2. The influence of recipient gender on PGD.

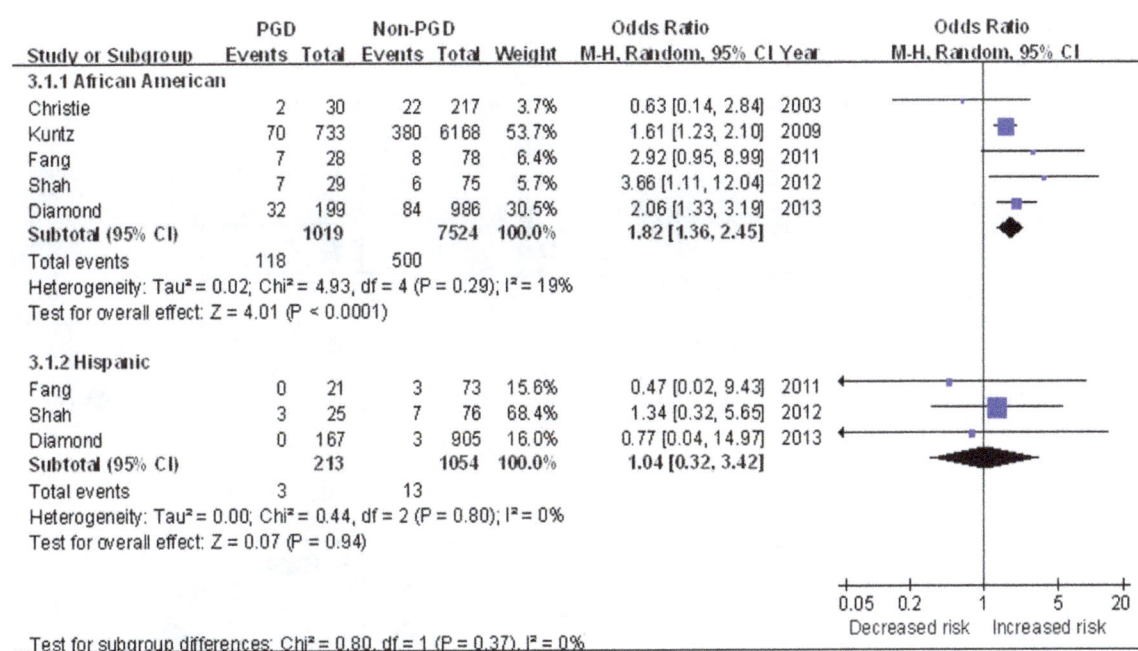

Study or Subgroup	PGD Events	Total	Non-PGD Events	Total	Weight	Odds Ratio M-H, Random, 95% CI	Year	Odds Ratio M-H, Random, 95% CI
3.1.1 African American								
Christie	2	30	22	217	3.7%	0.63 [0.14, 2.84]	2003	
Kuntz	70	733	380	6168	53.7%	1.61 [1.23, 2.10]	2009	
Fang	7	28	8	78	6.4%	2.92 [0.95, 8.99]	2011	
Shah	7	29	6	75	5.7%	3.66 [1.11, 12.04]	2012	
Diamond	32	199	84	986	30.5%	2.06 [1.33, 3.19]	2013	
Subtotal (95% CI)		1019		7524	100.0%	1.82 [1.36, 2.45]		
Total events	118		500					

Heterogeneity: Tau² = 0.02; Chi² = 4.93, df = 4 (P = 0.29); I² = 19%
Test for overall effect: Z = 4.01 (P < 0.0001)

3.1.2 Hispanic								
Fang	0	21	3	73	15.6%	0.47 [0.02, 9.43]	2011	
Shah	3	25	7	76	68.4%	1.34 [0.32, 5.65]	2012	
Diamond	0	167	3	905	16.0%	0.77 [0.04, 14.97]	2013	
Subtotal (95% CI)		213		1054	100.0%	1.04 [0.32, 3.42]		
Total events	3		13					

Heterogeneity: Tau² = 0.00; Chi² = 0.44, df = 2 (P = 0.80); I² = 0%
Test for overall effect: Z = 0.07 (P = 0.94)

Test for subgroup differences: Chi² = 0.80, df = 1 (P = 0.37), I² = 0%

Figure 3. The influence of African American and Hispanic race on PGD compared with white race.

and 95% confidence intervals (CIs) were calculated to estimate the association between binary factors and development of PGD. When mean values and SDs for a certain risk factor were provided, we calculated the mean differences (MDs) between patients with and without PGD. The statistical estimates of effect were derived using a random-effects (DerSimonian and Laird) model, which assumes that the true underlying effect varies among included studies, because of the different characteristics of study population, transplantation procedure, and the PGD definitions that were involved in the original trials.

The definitions of PGD may be a potential source of heterogeneity. In order to analyze the heterogeneity associated with different definitions, we performed subgroup analyses by comparing summary results obtained from subsets of studies grouped by "the International Society for Heart and Lung Transplantation (ISHLT) PGD Grading System [28]" or other definitions. Statistical heterogeneity of treatment effects between studies was formally tested with Cochran's $\chi 2$ statistics and with significance set at $P<0.10$. The I^2 statistic was used to quantify heterogeneity. Using accepted guidelines [27], an I^2 of 0% to 40% was considered to exclude heterogeneity, an I^2 of 30% to 60% to represent moderate heterogeneity, an I^2 of 50% to 90% to represent substantial heterogeneity, and an I^2 of 75% to 100% to represent considerable heterogeneity. Publication bias was assessed with funnel plots and the Begg's test.

Results

Literature search and study characteristics

The method used to select studies is shown in Figure 1. A total of 331 potentially eligible articles were initially identified, and 289 articles were excluded as they were not relevant to the purpose of the current meta-analysis. Therefore, 42 potentially relevant articles were selected for detailed evaluation. From the overall pool of full-text articles, 29 articles were excluded because they did not provide PGD data according to the risk factors we evaluated (n = 16), reported the risk factors in an unusable format (n = 3), did

not make any objective diagnosis of PGD (n = 4), or were duplicate studies (same cohort of patients with different endpoints measured) (n = 6). Thus, 13 studies were included in the meta-analysis with a total of 10042 patients [7–19]. Additional data were requested from the authors of three studies but didn't receive any reply.

Baseline characteristics of the studies included are shown in Table 1. The 13 included studies consisted of 5 prospective cohort studies [12,15–17,19], 7 retrospective analyses of cohort data or chart review [7–11,14,18], and 1 secondary analysis of multicenter registry [13]. Eight of the 13 studies involved American subjects [7,9,10,13,15–17,19], and the populations of the remaining five studies came from France [8,14], Denmark [11], Austria [12], and Brazil [18]. The studies varied in size from 28 to 6984 subjects, and the average age of the patients ranged from 25 to 56 years.

There were some variations in the definition of PGD. The ISHLT PGD grading schema was used in the majority of the studies. The other 5 studies also defined PGD based on the presence of infiltrates in the lung allograft on chest radiograph and/or the PaO2/FiO2 ratio [7–9,11,13]. PGD, as defined in the original articles, was present in 16.4% of the lung transplant patients. All studies were of high methodological quality (good or fair) as assessed by the Newcastle-Ottawa Scale [26] (Table 1). The risk factors examined in the 13 included studies are summarized in Table 2.

Outcomes and synthesis of results

Age. Ten studies investigated the influence of recipient age on the occurrence of PGD [7–9,11,12,14–18], including 434 patients with PGD and 969 controls. Findings from this analysis suggested no significant difference in mean age between patients with or without PGD (MD -0.75 y, 95% CI -2.12 to 0.63 y, $P=0.29$). Statistical heterogeneity among the studies was significant ($I^2 = 61\%$, $P=0.006$).

Gender. Twelve studies investigated the influence of recipient gender on the occurrence of PGD [8–19]. These studies included 1506 patients with PGD and 8430 controls. The proportion of

Study or Subgroup	PGD Events	Total	Non-PGD Events	Total	Weight	Odds Ratio M-H, Random, 95% CI	Year	Odds Ratio M-H, Random, 95% CI
4.1.1 Idiopathic pulmonary fibrosis								
King	5	12	8	43	1.7%	3.13 [0.79, 12.43]	2000	
Thabut	26	72	26	84	7.3%	1.26 [0.65, 2.46]	2002	
Christie	4	18	38	174	2.4%	1.02 [0.32, 3.29]	2003	
Whitson	19	94	27	195	7.8%	1.58 [0.83, 3.01]	2006	
Burton	9	94	3	42	1.8%	1.38 [0.35, 5.37]	2007	
Krenn	4	5	20	85	0.6%	13.00 [1.37, 123.08]	2007	
Kuntz	154	441	967	4328	74.9%	1.87 [1.51, 2.30]	2009	
Allen	4	5	7	14	0.6%	4.00 [0.35, 45.38]	2012	
Shah	11	19	30	58	3.0%	1.28 [0.45, 3.65]	2012	
Diamond	91	145	364	782	0.0%	1.94 [1.34, 2.79]	2013	
Subtotal (95% CI)		760		5023	100.0%	1.78 [1.49, 2.13]		
Total events	236		1126					
Heterogeneity: Tau² = 0.00; Chi² = 6.80, df = 8 (P = 0.56); I² = 0%								
Test for overall effect: Z = 6.26 (P < 0.00001)								
4.1.2 Sarcoidosis								
King	2	9	4	39	52.1%	2.50 [0.38, 16.41]	2000	
Allen	0	1	1	8	13.9%	1.67 [0.04, 64.08]	2012	
Shah	4	12	1	29	34.0%	14.00 [1.36, 143.59]	2012	
Subtotal (95% CI)		22		76	100.0%	4.25 [1.09, 16.52]		
Total events	6		6					
Heterogeneity: Tau² = 0.00; Chi² = 1.58, df = 2 (P = 0.45); I² = 0%								
Test for overall effect: Z = 2.09 (P = 0.04)								
4.1.3 Cystic fibrosis								
Thabut	19	65	20	78	14.7%	1.20 [0.57, 2.50]	2002	
Christie	5	19	18	154	8.1%	2.70 [0.87, 8.38]	2003	
Whitson	19	94	25	193	16.8%	1.70 [0.88, 3.28]	2006	
Krenn	5	6	21	86	2.5%	15.48 [1.71, 140.05]	2007	
Kuntz	109	396	1114	4475	32.3%	1.15 [0.91, 1.44]	2009	
Allen	1	2	2	9	1.3%	3.50 [0.14, 84.69]	2012	
Shah	3	11	17	45	5.3%	0.62 [0.14, 2.65]	2012	
Diamond	16	70	163	580	18.9%	0.76 [0.42, 1.36]	2013	
Subtotal (95% CI)		663		5620	100.0%	1.28 [0.89, 1.84]		
Total events	177		1380					
Heterogeneity: Tau² = 0.09; Chi² = 11.95, df = 7 (P = 0.10); I² = 41%								
Test for overall effect: Z = 1.33 (P = 0.18)								

0.05   0.2   1   5   20
Decreased risk   Increased risk

Test for subgroup differences: Chi² = 4.31, df = 2 (P = 0.12), I² = 53.6%

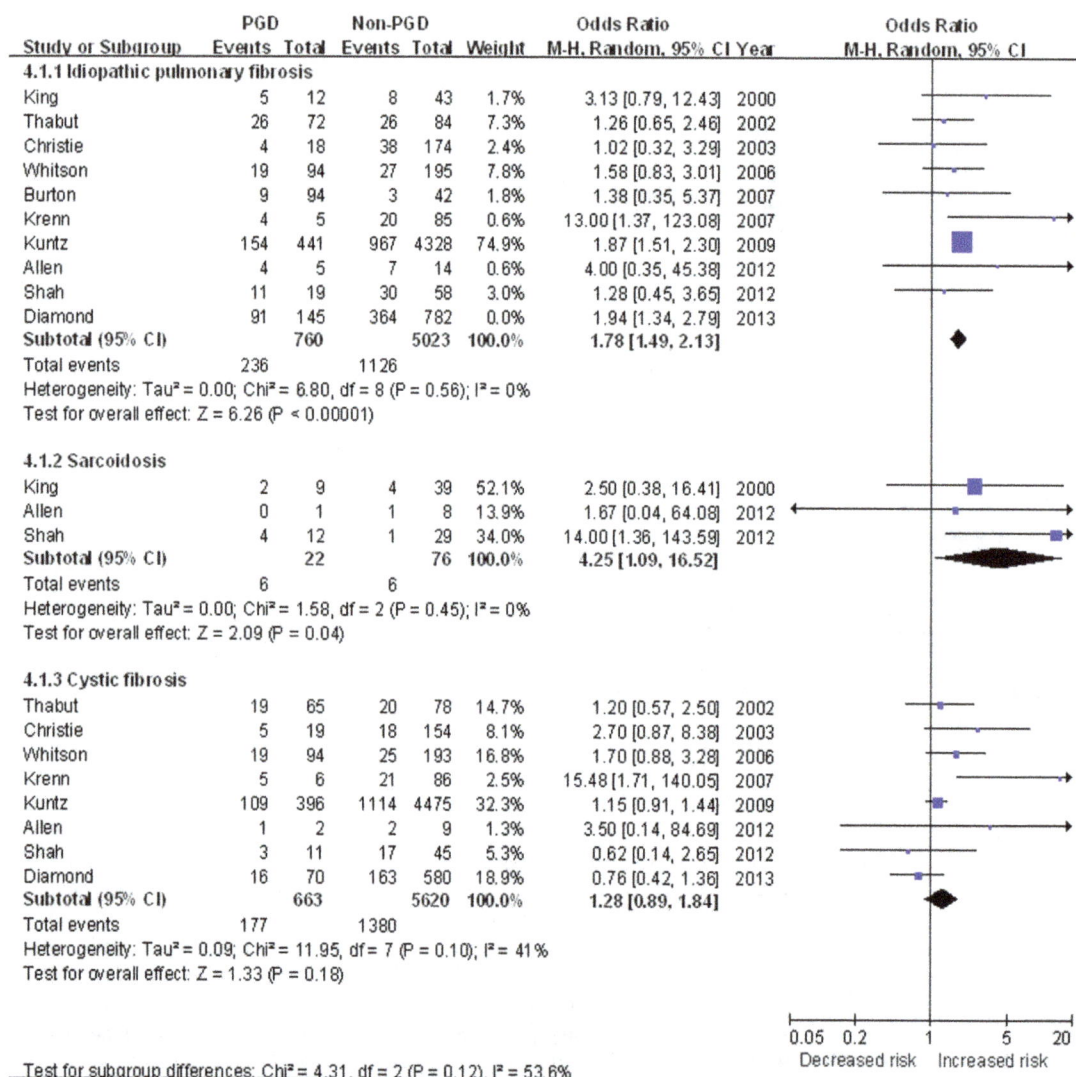

Figure 4. The influence of recipient pulmonary diagnosis on PGD. COPD was used as the reference group.

female recipients was 55.3% in patients with PGD compared with 49.0% in patients without. Analysis suggested female recipients had an increased risk of PGD (OR 1.38, 95% CI 1.09 to 1.75, P=0.008) (Figure 2).

Race. Five studies reported the influence of recipient race [9,13,15,17,19]. PGD was found in 11.4% of patients with white race, 19.1% of African American patients, and 18.7% of Hispanic patients. White race was used as the reference group given the lowest incidence of PGD. Analysis of these studies showed compared with white race, African American was associated with a significantly increased risk of PGD (OR 1.82, 95%CI 1.36 to 2.45, P<0.0001), while Hispanic race did not appear to affect the risk of PGD (OR 1.04, 95%CI 0.32 to 3.42, P=0.94) (Figure 3).

Pulmonary Diagnosis. The effect of recipient pulmonary diagnosis on PGD development was evaluated in 10 studies [7–13,16,17,19]. The incidence of PGD was 11.8% in patients with chronic obstructive pulmonary disease (COPD), 18.0% in patients with idiopathic pulmonary fibrosis (IPF), 50% in sarcoidosis and 12.4% in cystic fibrosis. For patients with pulmonary hypertension, PGD was observed in 30.3% of patients with PPH and 29.3% of secondary pulmonary hypertension (SPH).

Using COPD as the reference group (with the lowest incidence of PGD), IPF (OR 1.78, 95% CI 1.49 to 2.13, P<0.0001) [7–13,16,17,19] and sarcoidosis (OR 4.25, 95% CI 1.09 to 16.52, P=0.04) [7,16–17] were both associated with increased risk of PGD; while cystic fibrosis was non-significantly associated with PGD development (OR 1.28, 95% CI 0.89 to 1.84, P=0.18) [8–10,12,13,16,17,19] (Figure 4). PPH was also significantly associated with PGD, with a 3.73-fold increased risk of PGD was observed (OR 3.73, 95%CI 2.16 to 6.46, P<0.001) [7–10,12,13,16–17]; while unlike PPH, SPH did not confer an significantly increased risk of PGD (OR 2.23, 95%CI 0.65 to 7.69, P=0.20) [10,13] (Figure 5).

PAP. There were 7 studies compared the mean PAP between patients with and without PGD (325 PGD patients and 1093 controls) [7,9,12,15–17,19]. Findings from the meta-analysis showed a significant higher PAP was observed in the PGD patients as compared with the controls (MD 6.00 mmHg, 95% CI 3.91 to 8.09 mmHg, P<0.0001). Statistical heterogeneity was observed among the studies (I² = 77%, P=0.0003) (Figure 6).

BLT vs. SLT. Eleven studies evaluated the impact of BLT vs. SLT on PGD development, including 4554 patients undergoing

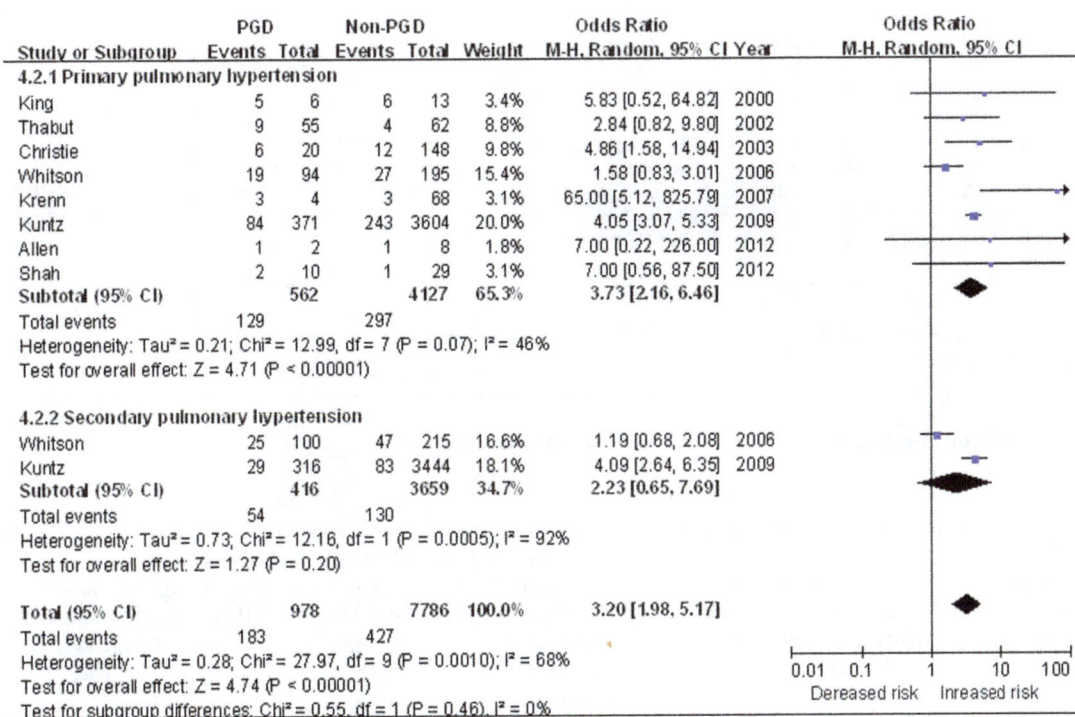

Study or Subgroup	PGD Events	Total	Non-PGD Events	Total	Weight	Odds Ratio M-H, Random, 95% CI	Year	Odds Ratio M-H, Random, 95% CI
4.2.1 Primary pulmonary hypertension								
King	5	6	6	13	3.4%	5.83 [0.52, 64.82]	2000	
Thabut	9	55	4	62	8.8%	2.84 [0.82, 9.80]	2002	
Christie	6	20	12	148	9.8%	4.86 [1.58, 14.94]	2003	
Whitson	19	94	27	195	15.4%	1.58 [0.83, 3.01]	2006	
Krenn	3	4	3	68	3.1%	65.00 [5.12, 825.79]	2007	
Kuntz	84	371	243	3604	20.0%	4.05 [3.07, 5.33]	2009	
Allen	1	2	1	8	1.8%	7.00 [0.22, 226.00]	2012	
Shah	2	10	1	29	3.1%	7.00 [0.56, 87.50]	2012	
Subtotal (95% CI)		562		4127	65.3%	3.73 [2.16, 6.46]		
Total events	129		297					

Heterogeneity: Tau² = 0.21; Chi² = 12.99, df = 7 (P = 0.07); I² = 46%
Test for overall effect: Z = 4.71 (P < 0.00001)

Study or Subgroup	PGD Events	Total	Non-PGD Events	Total	Weight	Odds Ratio M-H, Random, 95% CI	Year	
4.2.2 Secondary pulmonary hypertension								
Whitson	25	100	47	215	16.6%	1.19 [0.68, 2.08]	2006	
Kuntz	29	316	83	3444	18.1%	4.09 [2.64, 6.35]	2009	
Subtotal (95% CI)		416		3659	34.7%	2.23 [0.65, 7.69]		
Total events	54		130					

Heterogeneity: Tau² = 0.73; Chi² = 12.16, df = 1 (P = 0.0005); I² = 92%
Test for overall effect: Z = 1.27 (P = 0.20)

Total (95% CI)		978		7786	100.0%	3.20 [1.98, 5.17]		
Total events	183		427					

Heterogeneity: Tau² = 0.28; Chi² = 27.97, df = 9 (P = 0.0010); I² = 68%
Test for overall effect: Z = 4.74 (P < 0.00001)
Test for subgroup differences: Chi² = 0.55, df = 1 (P = 0.46), I² = 0%

Figure 5. The influence of recipient pulmonary hypertension on PGD. COPD was used as the reference group.

BLT and 5190 patients undergoing SLT [7–10,12,13,15–19]. The pooled analysis showed the incidence of PGD was 14.5% in BLT recipients, compared to 13.8% in SLT recipients. Findings from the meta-analysis showed an insignificant association between the transplant type (SLT or BLT) and PGD (OR 1.10, 95% CI 0.97 to 1.24, P = 0.14). No statistically significant heterogeneity was observed between studies (I² = 0%, P = 0.65).

BMI. Two studies evaluated the effect of BMI (as a continuous variable) on PGD [11,14], including 155 patients with PGD and 147 controls. The pooled analysis of the 2 studies showed patients with PGD had a higher mean BMI level than controls (MD 1.20 kg/m², 95% CI 0.13 to 2.27 kg/m², P = 0.03). Other 2 studies investigated the impact of elevated BMI (BMI ≥ 25 kg/m²) on PGD development [13,19]. The incidence of PGD was 15.2% in the 3105 patients with elevated BMI, compared to 9.4% in the 5091 patients with normal BMI. Analysis

of these studies showed a significant association between elevated BMI level and PGD (OR 1.83, 95% CI 1.26 to 2.64, P = 0.001).

CPB. Eleven studies evaluated the effect of CPB for PGD [7,8,10–12,14–19]. PGD was found in 263 of 813 patients (32.3%) use of CPB compared to 490 of 1984 patients (24.7%) without CPB. The pooled analysis of these studies showed a 2.29-fold increased risk of PGD was present for patients requiring CPB (OR 2.29, 95% CI 1.43 to 3.65, P = 0.0005), with statistical heterogeneity among the studies (I² = 69%, P = 0.0004).

Inhaled NO. Four studies investigated the influence of intra-operative use of inhaled NO on the occurrence of PGD [9,14–16]. The incidence of PGD was 23.4% (50 of 214 patients) and 18.8% (59 of 314 patients) in patients with and without use of inhaled NO, respectively. Findings from this analysis suggested there was no significant association between intra-operative inhaled NO use and development of PGD (OR 1.09, 95% CI 0.68 to 1.74,

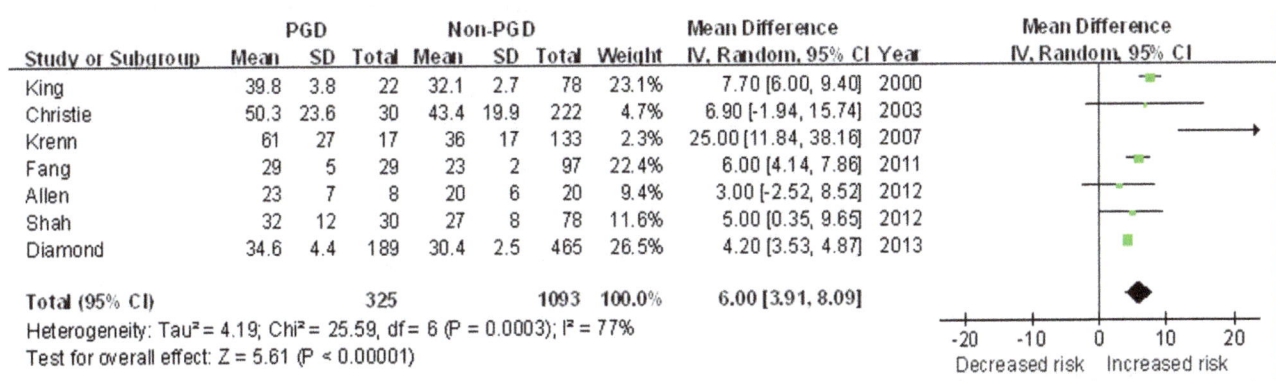

Study or Subgroup	PGD Mean	SD	Total	Non-PGD Mean	SD	Total	Weight	Mean Difference IV, Random, 95% CI	Year	Mean Difference IV, Random, 95% CI
King	39.8	3.8	22	32.1	2.7	78	23.1%	7.70 [6.00, 9.40]	2000	
Christie	50.3	23.6	30	43.4	19.9	222	4.7%	6.90 [-1.94, 15.74]	2003	
Krenn	61	27	17	36	17	133	2.3%	25.00 [11.84, 38.16]	2007	
Fang	29	5	29	23	2	97	22.4%	6.00 [4.14, 7.86]	2011	
Allen	23	7	8	20	6	20	9.4%	3.00 [-2.52, 8.52]	2012	
Shah	32	12	30	27	8	78	11.6%	5.00 [0.35, 9.65]	2012	
Diamond	34.6	4.4	189	30.4	2.5	465	26.5%	4.20 [3.53, 4.87]	2013	
Total (95% CI)			325			1093	100.0%	6.00 [3.91, 8.09]		

Heterogeneity: Tau² = 4.19; Chi² = 25.59, df = 6 (P = 0.0003); I² = 77%
Test for overall effect: Z = 5.61 (P < 0.00001)

Figure 6. The influence of mean pulmonary artery pressures (PAP) on PGD.

Study or Subgroup	PGD Events	PGD Total	Non-PGD Events	Non-PGD Total	Weight	Odds Ratio M-H, Random, 95% CI	Year	Odds Ratio M-H, Random, 95% CI
King	9	22	9	78	8.6%	5.31 [1.77, 15.91]	2000	
Thabut	38	131	14	128	18.9%	3.33 [1.70, 6.51]	2002	
Whitson	24	139	23	255	21.4%	2.11 [1.14, 3.89]	2006	
Krenn	2	17	8	133	4.1%	2.08 [0.40, 10.73]	2007	
Burton	16	113	2	67	4.9%	5.36 [1.19, 24.10]	2007	
Allen	3	8	2	20	2.7%	5.40 [0.70, 41.75]	2012	
Samano	8	12	18	66	6.2%	5.33 [1.43, 19.90]	2012	
Diamond	49	211	52	1044	33.3%	5.77 [3.78, 8.82]	2013	
Total (95% CI)		653		1791	100.0%	3.95 [2.80, 5.57]		
Total events	149		128					

Heterogeneity: Tau² = 0.05; Chi² = 8.66, df = 7 (P = 0.28); I² = 19%
Test for overall effect: Z = 7.83 (P < 0.00001)

0.05   0.2   1   5   20
Decreased risk   Increased risk

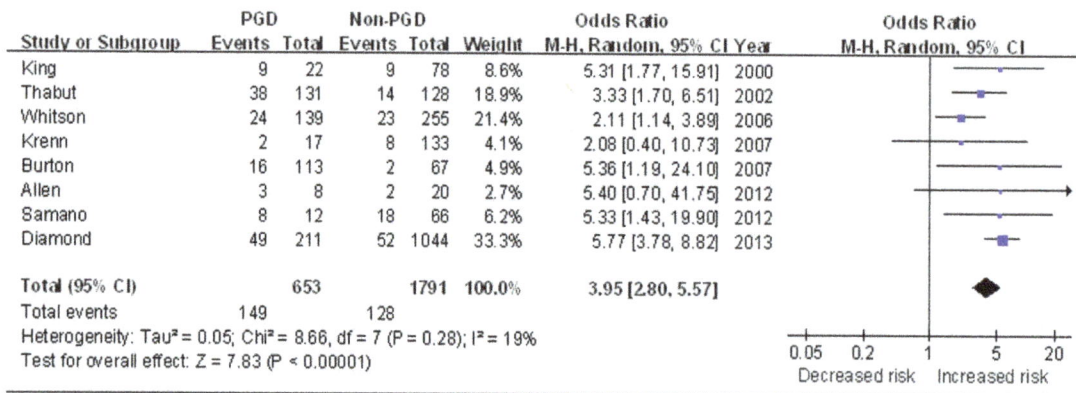

Figure 7. The influence of PGD on short-term mortality (mortality within 90 days).

$P = 0.72$). No statistical heterogeneity was observed between studies ($I^2 = 0\%$, $P = 0.95$).

Blood products transfusion. Three studies reported the amount of packed red blood cells (RBCs) and plasma used during the lung transplant procedure to evaluate the effect of intra-operative transfusion on PGD [14,15,19]. Findings from the meta-analysis showed a greater amount of packed RBCs and plasma transfused in patients with PGD compared with those without (RBCs: MD 341 ml, 95% CI 254 to 427 ml, $P < 0.001$; plasma: MD 131 ml, 95% CI 71 to 191 ml, $P < 0.001$). The χ^2 test for heterogeneities were also non-significant ($I^2 = 0\%$, $P = 0.84$ and $I^2 = 44\%$, $P = 0.17$).

Mortality risk for PGD. The impact of PGD on mortality (within 90 days) was reported in 8 studies [7,8,10–12,16,18,19]. All-cause mortality within 90 days was 22.8% for patients with PGD versus 7.1% for patients without. The pooled analysis suggested patients with PGD was associated with a nearly 4 fold increased risk of short-term mortality (OR 3.95, 95% CI 2.80 to 5.57, $P < 0.001$) compared with those without PGD. There was no statistical heterogeneity among the studies ($I^2 = 19\%$, $P = 0.28$) (Figure 7).

Subgroup analysis according to the definitions for PGD. In the subgroup meta-analysis, we compared the associations between above risk factors and PGD in subsets of studies grouped by ISHLT PGD grade or other definitions (Table 3). The results showed no matter which definition was used in the original studies, no significant difference was observed in the effects of age, gender, race, pulmonary diagnosis, mPAP, BLT vs SLT, use of CPB, or inhaled NO in PGD development (P for subgroup difference > 0.05).

Publication Bias

We performed funnel plot analysis and Begg's test to assess publication bias. Funnel plot analysis was performed using the recipient gender as an index, the funnel plot of the 12 studies appeared to be symmetrical (Figure 8), and the Begg's test of funnel plot suggested no publication bias ($P = 0.87$). Also no publication bias was detected by Begg's test for other outcomes analysis (all $P > 0.05$).

Discussion

Despite the significant morbidity and mortality in patients with PGD after lung transplantation, the recipient related risk factors contributing to this devastating syndrome remain controversial. Our meta-analysis comprehensively reviewed 13 studies involving

10042 lung transplantation recipients which addressed the clinical risk factors for PGD. The results showed recipient female gender, African American race, preoperative diagnosis of IPF, sarcoidosis, or PPH, elevated mean PAP and BMI, use of CPB and blood products transfusion were significantly and consistently associated with development of PGD. All of these factors are likely to be measured and monitored in the primary care setting. To the best of our knowledge, this is the first systematic review on this topic.

Among baseline variables, we have demonstrated that female gender and African-American race had increased risk of PGD, which have not been validated in previous studies. Female gender has been associated with a higher risk of development of acute respiratory distress syndrome (ARDS) in the Ibuprofen in Sepsis Study Group [29], as well as in a cohort study of trauma patients [30]. Similarly, donor female gender was also shown to have an independent impact on PGD [9]. Possible mechanisms for these findings are unclear. Some theories for the differential outcome based on gender differences have been advocated, including immunity and tolerance theories [31] and the influence of gender hormones [32]. However, as of now few data have been published that evaluate the effect of gender on graft function and survival. Similarly, mechanisms for the observed worse outcome of African-American race remain speculative, but may reflect differences in vascular endothelium (such as expression of angiotensin-converting enzyme) [33,34], which could potentially predispose African Americans to more severe ischemia reperfusion injury.

Elevated BMI was another risk factor for PGD in our meta-analysis. Prior studies have identified obesity as a risk factor for early mortality and increased intensive care unit stay after lung transplant [35,36]. Technical difficulties of performing a lung transplant operation in obese recipients may increase risk of PGD. Other possible explanations may be obesity affects the milieu of cytokines produced by adipose tissue during ischemia-reperfusion, such as leptin [37], which has been shown to be increased in patients with acute lung injury and play a role in the development of acute lung injury in animal model [38]. In the study by Lederer et al, higher plasma leptin levels were associated with PGD after lung transplantation [39]. In addition, modulation of lung inflammation by other adipokines, such as resistin, adiponectin, which produced by macrophages recruited to hypertrophic and hypoxic adipose tissue, could also be responsible [39–41]. Future studies of adipokines in lung tissue or bronchoalveolar lavage fluid and examination of their roles in the development of PGD should be pursued.

Table 3. Subgroup analysis according to the definitions for PGD.

	No.of studies	Test for association		Test for subgroup difference	
		OR (95% CI)	P	I²	P
Age				0%	0.72
ISHLT	5	−1.33 (−5.09 to 2.43)	0.49		
Othe definitions	5	−0.58 (−2.17 to 1.10)	0.48		
Female				0%	0.33
ISHLT	8	1.21 (0.82 to 1.77)	0.33		
Othe definitions	4	1.50 (1.23 to 1.83)	<0.001		
Race					
African-American				36%	0.21
ISPGS	3	2.28 (1.55 to 3.36)	<0.001		
Othe definitions	3	1.37 (0.68 to 2.74)	0.38		
Diagnosis					
IPF				0%	0.58
ISHLT	5	1.88 (1.40 to 2.54)	<0.001		
Othe definitions	5	1.65 (1.14 to 2.38)	0.0009		
Cystic fibrosis				0%	0.71
ISHLT	5	1.41 (0.63 to 3.18)	0.41		
Othe definitions	3	1.20 (0.93 to 1.55)	0.16		
PPH				0%	0.61
ISHLT	5	6.58 (1.04 to 41.59)	<0.001		
Othe definitions	3	4.04 (3.12 to 5.24)	0.05		
Mean PAP				0%	0.61
ISHLT	4	5.80 (1.65 to 9.94)	0.006		
Othe definitions	3	6.93 (5.69 to 8.17)	<0.001		
BLT vs SLT				0%	0.73
ISHLT	6	1.06 (0.84 to 1.33)	0.63		
Othe definitions	5	1.11 (0.96 to 1.28)	0.15		
CPB				0%	0.77
ISHLT	7	2.31 (1.23 to 4.33)	0.009		
Othe definitions	4	2.62 (1.47 to 4.66)	0.001		
Use of inhaled NO				0%	0.69
ISHLT	2	1.22 (0.59 to 2.51)	0.60		
Othe definitions	2	1.00 (0.54 to 1.85)	0.99		

PGD, primary graft dysfunction; ISHLT, International Society for Heart and Lung Transplantation; IPF, idiopathic pulmonary fibrosis; PPH, primary pulmonary hypertension; PAP, pulmonary artery pressure; BLT, bilateral lung transplant; SLT, single lung transplant; CPB, cardiopulmonary bypass; NO, nitric oxide.

In nearly all previous studies, diagnosis of PPH was the most significant risk factor for PGD [6,10,13,19], and our findings further support this, showing both PPH and elevated mPAP were strongly associated with PGD after lung transplant. Possible explanations are not fully understood. In PPH, right ventricular dysfunction is universally present, and the hypertrophied, failing right ventricle is acutely afterload reduced at transplantation, resulting in increased shear stress on the formerly hypoxic pulmonary vascular endothelium. Shear stress leads to capillary leak and worse graft function [42,43]. Christie et al showed diagnosis of PPH was even more strongly associated with an increased risk of PGD after adjustment for recipient PAP (adjusted RR = 9.24, P = 0.009) [9]. This implies it is the disease state of PPH that increases the risk, rather than just the presence or severity of pulmonary hypertension. Unlike PPH, our study suggested SPH did not confer an increased risk of PGD. In prior

studies, the association between SPH and PGD was controversial and the conclusions were inconsistent [10,13,15,18]. Fang et al demonstrated SPH in patients with IPF was independently associated with the development of PGD [15]. While for patients with CF, based on data from the ISHLT registry, no significant difference was observed in PGD incidence for patients with and without pulmonary hypertension [6]. These findings suggested that the association between pulmonary hypertension and PGD might depend on the underlying diagnoses to some extent. For studies included in this meta-analysis, SPH has been all-inclusive, regardless of cause [10,13,18]. Therefore, for further discussion, it is better to focus on the primary disease of SPH.

IPF was also identified as a risk factor with intermediate risk of PGD in our analysis. Previous observational studies reported patients undergoing transplantation for IPF had somewhat worse survival than for other indications, when matched on multiple

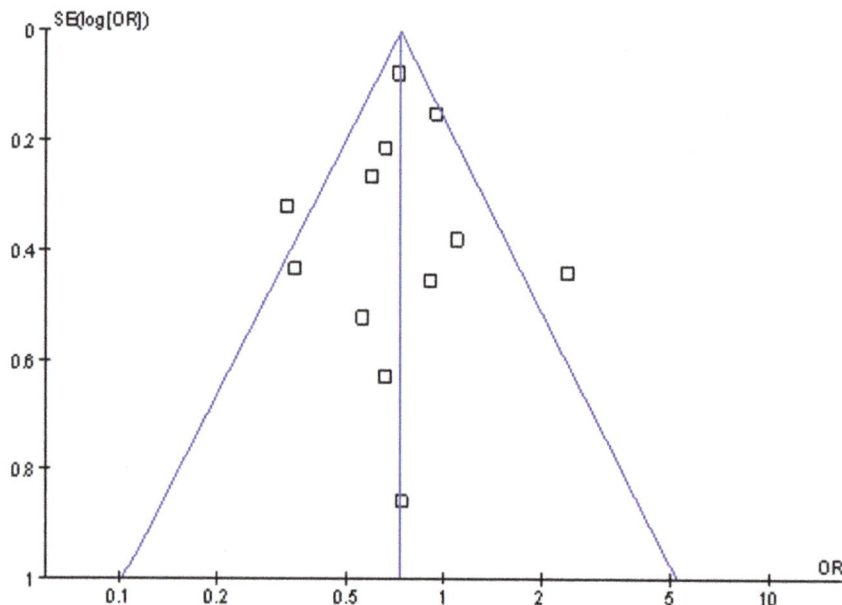

Figure 8. Funnel plot of the 12 studies evaluated the effect of the recipient gender on PGD.

variables [44,45]. Possible explanations may be related to the pathogenesis of IPF. IPF carries a progressive course of pulmonary dysfunction that is inhibited, but not eliminated, by transplantation. Vasoactive mediators such as endothelin-1, platelet-derived growth factor, transforming growth factor-β, and fibroblast growth factor have all been implicated in the pathogenesis of IPF, and also contribute to the development of lung injury [46]. Moreover, IPF patients have a restrictive pattern of pulmonary disease with smaller-than-predicted total lung capacity. Shrinking lung volume may have caused irreversible damage to pulmonary mechanics by contracting the chest wall (remodeling). This relative "oversize" donor lung within smaller chest may lead to worse graft function [45,47]. Nevertheless, at this point, reasons for the poor outcomes of IPF after transplantation remain elusive and warrant focused investigation.

The intra-operative use of CPB was another potential contributor to PGD in our meta-analysis. CPB causes a systemic, pro-inflammatory response with activation of cytokines, leukocytes and the complement cascade [48,49]. Patients requiring CPB have been shown to have more radiographic infiltrates, worse immediate graft function, longer intubation, and ultimately, decreased survival [50,51]. However, a notable difficulty in interpreting the data is the overall severity of the patient's illness or operative difficulty requiring the use of CPB. It is not possible to accurately differentiate planned use of CPB from emergent initiation intra-operatively because of deterioration in patient hemodynamics or oxygenation. As a result, independent of indication for CPB use, the association between PGD and CPB is still debatable. The type of transplant procedure (bilateral vs. single) was not identified as a significant risk factor for PGD in our study. Although the reported incidence of PGD was somewhat higher in BLT recipients, higher pre-transplant PAP and CPB use in BLT recipients likely confounded these results [5,10].

The finding of blood products transfusion as a risk factor for PGD has been shown in recent multicenter studies and our meta-analysis confirmed this tendency [19,52], but the exact relationship between the two processes is not yet clear. Blood products transfusion in-and-of-itself is associated with transfusion-related

lung injury, which results in an ARDS-like picture similar to that seen with PGD [53]. The transfusion-related lung injury might accentuate any underlying mild ischemia/reperfusion injury, resulting in the onset of clinically significant PGD [53]. Nonetheless, the need for blood products administration has been shown to collinear with other PGD risk factors, including PPH and the use of CPB, and unmeasured operative characteristics may also lead to transfusion requirements [54]. Therefore dissecting the independence of the relationship between blood transfusion and PGD is difficult.

Inhaled NO has been investigated as a potential agent for the prevention of PGD, given its effects on pulmonary vasodilation and capillary integrity. Although our analysis did not support use of inhaled NO to be effective in PGD prevention, it may be beneficial in clinical settings of established PGD. Several reports and case series have shown improved outcomes with inhaled NO administration [55,56]. However, there have also been studies that do not show efficacy in the setting of PGD [57]. Lack of randomized clinical trials showing survival benefit precludes widespread recommendation of inhaled NO for the treatment of PGD. Again, extrapolating from inhaled NO use in studies with ARDS, the beneficial effects of inhaled NO may be real, but also appear to be transient [58].

Limitations of the review

Although we believe that the current meta-analysis provided useful information, some potential limitations should be addressed. Firstly, heterogeneity in our study is substantial and may be attributed to differences in type of patients, study era, operative practice, and definition of PGD. Definition of PGD is a major cause of heterogeneity, and with potential for misclassification bias. As the ISHLT PGD criteria were first published in 2005, studies performed before 2005 did not use standard defining criteria; even for the studies defined PGD based on the ISHLT guidelines, the PGD grades were retrospectively assigned to those patients enrolled before 2005. To clarify the heterogeneity, subgroup analyses were performed by dividing studies according to ISHLT or other definitions, and the results suggested our findings were not significantly affected by varying definitions. Secondly, our analysis was by necessity restricted to individual risk factors. Therefore, the distinct possibility exists that the strength of association may be weaker with a multi-factorial regression analysis; for instance, the individual effects of CPB, use of blood products, and elevated PAP cannot be delineated since they are often apparent in the same patients. In the present meta-analysis, it was not possible to adjust or stratify for potential confounders, which restricted us doing more detailed relevant analysis and obtaining more comprehensive results. Finally, given that a proportion of studies included are retrospective, a possibility of residual confounding variables by unmeasured factors cannot be eliminated. This provided associative, not causal, evidence and mandates caution when interpreting these results.

Conclusion

Our systematic review and meta-analysis have identified several recipient-related risk factors for development of PGD, all of which are readily available in clinical settings. The identification of

higher-risk recipients has great clinical relevance with respect to individual screening, risk factor modification, selective management aimed at prevention of PGD, and ultimately improves the outcomes of patients undergoing lung transplantation. Further research into the underlying mechanisms responsible for these associations should be advocated.

Supporting Information

Checklist S1 The PRISMA Checklist for this Systematic Reviews and Meta-Analyses.

Author Contributions

Conceived and designed the experiments: Yao Liu Yi Liu LS SJJ. Performed the experiments: Yao Liu Yi Liu SJJ. Analyzed the data: Yao Liu LS SJJ. Contributed reagents/materials/analysis tools: Yao Liu Yi Liu LS SJJ. Wrote the paper: Yao Liu SJJ.

References

1. Arcasoy SM, Kotloff RM (1999) Lung transplantation. N Engl J Med 340:1081–1091.
2. Christie JD, Van Raemdonck D, de Perrot M, Barr M, Keshavjee S, et al; ISHLT Working Group on Primary Lung Graft Dysfunction (2005) Report of the ISHLT Working Group on Primary Lung Graft Dysfunction part I: introduction and methods. J Heart Lung Transplant 24:1451–1453.
3. King RC, Binns OA, Rodriguez F, Kanithanon RC, Daniel TM, et al. (2000) Reperfusion injury significantly impacts clinical outcome after pulmonary transplantation. Ann Thorac Surg 69:1681–1685.
4. Christie JD, Kotloff RM, Ahya VN, Tino G, Pochettino A, et al. (2005) The effect of primary graft dysfunction on survival after lung transplantation. Am J Respir Crit Care Med 171:1312–131.
5. Lee JC, Christie JD, Keshavjee S (2010) Primary graft dysfunction: definition, risk factors, short- and long-term outcomes. Semin Resp Crit Care Med 31:161–71.
6. Barr ML, Kawut SM, Whelan TP, Girgis R, Bottcher H, et al. (2005) Report of the ISHLT Working Group on Primary Lung Graft Dysfunction part IV: recipient-related risk factors and markers. J Heart Lung Transplant 24:1468–1482.
7. King RC, Binns OA, Rodriguez F, Kanithanon RC, Daniel TM, et al. (2000) Reperfusion injury significantly impacts clinical outcome after pulmonary transplantation. Ann Thorac Surg 69:1681–5.
8. Thabut G, Vinatier I, Stern JB, Lesèche G, Loirat P, et al. (2002) Primary graft failure following lung transplantation: predictive factors of mortality. Chest 121:1876–82.
9. Christie JD, Kotloff RM, Pochettino A, Arcasoy SM, Rosengard BR, et al. (2003) Clinical risk factors for primary graft failure following lung transplantation. Chest 124:1232–1241.
10. Whitson BA, Nath DS, Johnson AC, Walker AR, Prekker ME, et al. (2006) Risk factors for primary graft dysfunction after lung transplantation. J Thorac Cardiovasc Surg 131:73–80.
11. Burton CM, Iversen M, Milman N, Zemtsovski M, Carlsen J, et al. (2007) Outcome of lung transplanted patients with primary graft dysfunction. Eur J Cardiothorac Surg 31:75–82.
12. Krenn K, Klepetko W, Taghavi S, Lang G, Schneider B, et al. (2007) Recipient vascular endothelial growth factor serum levels predict primary lung graft dysfunction. Am J Transplant 7:700–6.
13. Kuntz CL, Hadjiliadis D, Ahya VN, Kotloff RM, Pochettino A, et al. (2009) Risk factors for early primary graft dysfunction after lung transplantation: a registry study. Clin Transplant 23:819–30.
14. Felten ML, Sinaceur M, Treilhaud M, Roze H, Mornex JF, et al. (2012) Factors associated with early graft dysfunction in cystic fibrosis patients receiving primary bilateral lung transplantation. Eur J Cardiothorac Surg 41:686–90.
15. Fang A, Studer S, Kawut SM, Ahya VN, Lee J, et al; Lung Transplant Outcomes Group (2011) Elevated pulmonary artery pressure is a risk factor for primary graft dysfunction following lung transplantation for idiopathic pulmonary fibrosis. Chest 139:782–7.
16. Allen JG, Lee MT, Weiss ES, Arnaoutakis GJ, Shah AS, et al (2012) Preoperative recipient cytokine levels are associated with early lung allograft dysfunction. Ann Thorac Surg 93:1843–9.
17. Shah RJ, Diamond JM, Lederer DJ, Arcasoy SM, Cantu EM, et al. (2012) Plasma monocyte chemotactic protein-1 levels at 24 hours are a biomarker of primary graft dysfunction after lung transplantation. Transl Res 160:435–42.
18. Samano MN, Fernandes LM, Baranauskas JC, Correia AT, Afonso JE Jr, et al. (2012) Risk factors and survival impact of primary graft dysfunction after lung transplantation in a single institution. Transplant Proc 44:2462–8.
19. Diamond JM, Lee JC, Kawut SM, Shah RJ, Localio AR, et al. (2013) Clinical risk factors for primary graft dysfunction after lung transplantation. Am J Respir Crit Care Med 187:527–34.
20. de Perrot M, Bonser RS, Dark J, Kelly RF, McGiffin D, et al. (2005) Report of the ISHLT Working Group on Primary Lung Graft Dysfunction part III: donor-related risk factors and markers. J Heart Lung Transplant 24:1460–1467.
21. Aeba R, Griffith BP, Kormos RL, Armitage JM, Gasior TA, et al. (1994) Effect of cardiopulmonary bypass on early graft dysfunction in clinical lung transplantation. Ann Thorac Surg 57: 715–22.
22. Shigemura N, Toyoda Y, Bhama JK, Gries CJ, Crespo M, et al. (2013) Donor smoking history and age in lung transplantation: a revisit. Transplantation 95:513–8.
23. Alvarez A, Moreno P, Illana J, Espinosa D, Baamonde C, et al. (2013) Influence of donor-recipient gender mismatch on graft function and survival following lung transplantation. Interact Cardiovasc Thorac Surg 16:426–35.
24. Stroup DF, Berlin JA, Morton SC, Olkin I, Williamson GD, et al. (2000) Meta-analysis of observational studies in epidemiology: a proposal for reporting. Meta-analysis Of Observational Studies In Epidemiology (MOOSE) group. JAMA 283: 2008–2012.
25. Moher D, Cook DJ, Eastwood S (1999) Improving the quality of reports of meta-analyses of randomized controlled trials: the QUOROM statement. Quality of reporting of meta-analyses. Lancet 354: 1896.
26. Wells G, Shea B, O'Connell D, Guyatt G, Peterson J, et al. (2006) The Newcastle-Ottawa Scale (NOS) for assessing the quality of nonrandomized studies in meta-analysis. Ottawa Health Research Institute (OHRI).
27. Higgins JPT, Green S, eds (2009) Cochrane handbook for systematic reviews of interventions. Version 5.0.2. New York, NY: Wiley. The Cochrane Collaboration. Available: www.cochrane-handbook.org. Accessed: 2008 June.
28. Christie JD, Carby M, Bag R, Corris P, Hertz M, et al. (2005) Report of the ISHLT working group on primary lung graft dysfunction, part II: definition. A consensus statement of the International Society for Heart and Lung Transplantation. J Heart Lung Transplant 24: 1454–9.
29. Mangialardi RJ, Martin GS, Bernard GR, Wheeler AP, Christman BW, et al. (2000) Hypoproteinemia predicts acute respiratory distress syndrome development, weight gain, and death in patients with sepsis: Ibuprofen in Sepsis Study Group. Crit Care Med 28:3137–3145.
30. Hudson LD, Milberg JA, Anardi D, Maunder RJ (1995) Clinical risks for development of the acute respiratory distress syndrome. Am J Respir Crit Care Med 151:293–301.
31. Simpson E, Scott D, Chandler P (1997) The male-specific histocompatibility antigen. Ann Rev Immunol 15:39–61.
32. Sweezey N, Tchepichev S, Cagnon S, Fertuck K, O'Brodovich H (1998) Female gender hormones regulate mRNA levels and function of the rat lung epithelial Na channel. Am J Physiol 274:379–86.
33. Hooper WC, Lally C, Austin H, Benson J, Dilley A, et al. (1999) The relationship between polymorphisms in the endothelial cell nitric oxide synthase gene and the platelet GPIIIa gene with myocardial infarction and venous thromboembolism in African Americans. Chest 116:880–886.
34. Jones DS, Andrawis NS, Abernethy DR (1999) Impaired endothelial dependent forearm vascular relaxation in black Americans. Clin Pharmacol Ther 65:408–412.

35. Kanasky WF Jr, Anton SD, Rodrigue JR, Perri MG, Szwed T, et al. (2002) Impact of body weight on long-term survival after lung transplantation. Chest 121:401–6.

36. Madill J, Gutierrez C, Grossman J, Allard J, Chan C, et al. (2001) Nutritional assessment of the lung transplant patient: body mass index as a predictor of 90-day mortality following transplantation. J Heart Lung Transplant 20:288–96.

37. Jain M, Budinger GS, Lo A, Urich D, Rivera SE, et al. (2011) Leptin promotes fibroproliferative ARDS by inhibiting peroxisome proliferator-activated receptor-γ. Am J Respir Crit Care Med 183:1490–1498.

38. Bellmeyer A, Martino JM, Chandel NS, Scott Budinger GR, Dean DA, et al. (2007) Leptin resistance protects mice from hyperoxia-induced acute lung injury. Am J Respir Crit Care Med 175:587–594.

39. Lederer DJ, Kawut SM, Wickersham N, Winterbottom C, Bhorade S, et al. (2011) Obesity and primary graft dysfunction after lung transplantation: the Lung Transplant Outcomes Group Obesity Study. Am J Respir Crit Care Med 184:1055–1061.

40. Medoff BD, Okamoto Y, Leyton P, Weng M, Sandall BP, et al. (2009) Adiponectin deficiency increases allergic airway inflammation and pulmonary vascular remodeling. Am J Respir Cell Mol Biol 41:397–406.

41. Summer R, Little FF, Ouchi N, Takemura Y, Aprahamian T, et al. (2008) Alveolar macrophage activation and an emphysema-like phenotype in adiponectin-deficient mice. Am J Physiol Lung Cell Mol Physiol 294:L1035–L1042.

42. Pierre AF, DeCampos KN, Liu M, Edwards V, Cutz E, et al. (1998) Rapid reperfusion causes stress failure in ischemic rat lungs. J Thorac Cardiovasc Surg 116:932–42.

43. Halldorsson AO, Kronon MT, Allen BS, Rahman S, Wang T (2000) Lowering reperfusion pressure reduces the injury after pulmonary ischemia. Ann Thorac Surg 69: 198–203.

44. Thabut G, Mal H, Castier Y, Groussard O, Brugière O, et al. (2003) Survival benefit of lung transplantation for patients with idiopathic pulmonary fibrosis. J Thorac Cardiovasc Surg 126:469–75.

45. Mason DP, Brizzio ME, Alster JM, McNeill AM, Murthy SC, et al. (2007) Lung transplantation for idiopathic pulmonary fibrosis. Ann Thorac Surg 84:1121–8.

46. Wahidi MM, Ravenel J, Palmer SM, McAdams HP (2002) Progression of idiopathic pulmonary fibrosis in native lungs after single lung transplantation. Chest 121:2072–6.

47. Khalil N, O'Connor R (2004) Idiopathic pulmonary fibrosis: current understanding of the pathogenesis and the status of treatment. CMAJ 171:153–60.

48. Wan S, LeClerc JL, Vincent JL (1997) Inflammatory response to cardiopulmonary bypass: mechanisms involved and possible therapeutic strategies. Chest 112:676–92.

49. Butler J, Rocker GM, Westaby S (1993) Inflammatory response to cardiopulmonary bypass. Ann Thorac Surg 55: 552–9.

50. Aeba R, Griffith BP, Kormos RL, Armitage JM, Gasior TA, et al. (1994) Effect of cardiopulmonary bypass on early graft dysfunction in clinical lung transplantation. Ann Thorac Surg 57:715–22.

51. Gammie JS, Cheul Lee J, Pham SM, Keenan RJ, Weyant RJ, et al. (1998) Cardiopulmonary bypass is associated with early allograft dysfunction but not death after double-lung transplantation. J Thorac Cardiovasc Surg 115:990–7.

52. Christie JD, Shah CV, Kawut SM, Mangalmurti N, Lederer DJ, et al.(2009) Plasma levels of receptor for advanced glycation end products, blood transfusion, and risk of primary graft dysfunction. Am J Respir Crit Care Med 180: 1010–1015.

53. Webert KE, Blajchman MA (2003) Transfusion-related acute lung injury. Transfus Med Rev 17:252–262.

54. Wang Y, Kurichi JE, Blumenthal NP, Ahya VN, Christie JD, et al. (2006) Multiple variables affecting blood usage in lung transplantation. J Heart Lung Transplant 25:533–538.

55. Adatia I, Lillehei C, Arnold JH, Thompson JE, Palazzo R, et al. (1994) Inhaled nitric oxide in the treatment of postoperative graft dysfunction after lung transplantation. Ann Thorac Surg 57:1311–1318.

56. Macdonald P, Mundy J, Rogers P, Harrison G, Branch J, et al. (1995) Successful treatment of life-threatening acute reperfusion injury after lung transplantation with inhaled nitric oxide. J Thorac Cardiovasc Surg 110:861–863.

57. Garat C, Jayr C, Eddahibi S, Laffon M, Meignan M, et al. (1997) Effects of inhaled nitric oxide or inhibition of endogenous nitric oxide formation on hyperoxic lung injury. Am J Respir Crit Care Med 155: 1957–1964.

58. Shargall Y, Guenther G, Ahya VN, Ardehali A, Singhal A, et al. (2005) Report of the ISHLT working group on primary lung graft dysfunction: Part VI. Treatment. J Heart Lung Transplant 24:1489–1500.

21

Sodium-Coupled Neutral Amino Acid Transporter 1 (SNAT1) Modulates L-Citrulline Transport and Nitric Oxide (NO) Signaling in Piglet Pulmonary Arterial Endothelial Cells

Anna Dikalova[1,2], Angela Fagiana[1,2], Judy L. Aschner[5], Michael Aschner[1,2,3], Marshall Summar[4], Candice D. Fike[1,2]*

1 Dept. of Pediatrics, Vanderbilt University Medical Center, Nashville, Tennessee, United States of America, 2 Monroe Carell Jr. Children's Hospital at Vanderbilt, Nashville, Tennessee, United States of America, 3 Vanderbilt Center for Molecular Toxicology, Nashville, Tennessee, United States of America, 4 Division of Genetics and Metabolism, Children's National Medical Center, Washington, District of Columbia, United States of America, 5 Dept of Pediatrics, Albert Einstein College of Medicine and the Children's Hospital at Montefiore, New York, New York, United States of America

Abstract

Rationale: There is evidence that impairments in nitric oxide (NO) signaling contribute to chronic hypoxia-induced pulmonary hypertension. The L-arginine-NO precursor, L-citrulline, has been shown to ameliorate pulmonary hypertension. Sodium-coupled neutral amino acid transporters (SNATs) are involved in the transport of L-citrulline into pulmonary arterial endothelial cells (PAECs). The functional link between the SNATs, L-citrulline, and NO signaling has not yet been explored.

Objective: We tested the hypothesis that changes in SNAT1 expression and transport function regulate NO production by modulating eNOS coupling in newborn piglet PAECs.

Methods and Results: A silencing RNA (siRNA) technique was used to assess the contribution of SNAT1 to NO production and eNOS coupling (eNOS dimer-to-monomer ratios) in PAECs from newborn piglets cultured under normoxic and hypoxic conditions in the presence and absence of L-citrulline. SNAT1 siRNA reduced basal NO production in normoxic PAECs and prevented L-citrulline-induced elevations in NO production in both normoxic and hypoxic PAECs. SNAT1 siRNA reduced basal eNOS dimer-to-monomer ratios in normoxic PAECs and prevented L-citrulline-induced increases in eNOS dimer-to-monomer ratios in hypoxic PAECs.

Conclusions: SNAT1 mediated L-citrulline transport modulates eNOS coupling and thus regulates NO production in hypoxic PAECs from newborn piglets. Strategies that increase SNAT1-mediated transport and supply of L-citrulline may serve as novel therapeutic approaches to enhance NO production in patients with pulmonary vascular disease.

Editor: Tim Lahm, Indiana University, United States of America

Funding: This work was supported by HL97566 to CDF from NIH (www.NIH.gov). The funders had no role in study design, data collection and analysis, decision to publish, or preparation of the manuscript.

Competing Interests: The authors have read the journal's policy and have the following conflicts: CF, JA, and MS are listed as inventors on a patent application to treat lung diseases with intravenous citrulline.

* E-mail: Candice.fike@vanderbilt.edu

Introduction

Infants with chronic cardiopulmonary disorders associated with persistent or episodic hypoxia develop pulmonary hypertension. Impairments in nitric oxide (NO) signaling may contribute to the development of chronic hypoxia-induced pulmonary hypertension [1,2]. NO production from endothelial nitric oxide synthase (eNOS) is regulated in part by the availability of the substrate, arginine, and the cofactor, tetrahydrobiopterin (BH_4) [3,4,5]. In the absence of sufficient arginine or BH_4, eNOS activation generates superoxide ($O_2^{\bullet-}$) instead of NO, a process known as NOS uncoupling [3,4,5]. Mechanisms that drive NOS re-coupling are poorly defined but provide potentially powerful therapeutic targets. Since L-arginine promotes eNOS coupling, strategies that

effectively increase intracellular L-arginine availability to eNOS could prove beneficial. While there is evidence that direct L-arginine supplementation may be effective treatment in some experimental models of pulmonary hypertension [5,6,7] detrimental effects of L-arginine supplementation have also been reported and results from L-arginine treatment have been variable [8,9,10,11]. Thus, alternate means for driving NOS re-coupling and increasing NO production merit further exploration.

The L-arginine-NO precursor, L-citrulline, provides an alternate approach to deliver bioavailable L-arginine for NO production. There is evidence that in endothelial cells, L-citrulline is converted by a two-step enzymatic process to L-arginine which is directly channeled to eNOS for efficient NO production [9,12].

Surprisingly, little is known about the transport of L-citrulline into pulmonary arterial endothelial cells (PAECs). This knowledge could provide another means to manipulate NO production.

We recently showed that sodium-coupled neutral amino acid transporters (SNATs) are involved in transporting L-citrulline into PAECs under both normoxic and hypoxic conditions [13]. Expression of SNAT1 is increased in PAECs cultured under hypoxic conditions [13]. However, the link between SNAT1 expression, L-citrulline uptake, and NO signaling has not been explored. The major purpose of this study was to test the hypothesis that changes in SNAT1 expression and transport function regulate NO production by modulating eNOS coupling in newborn piglet PAECs.

Methods

Ethics statement

Use of animals conformed to the Guide for the Care and Use of Laboratory Animals published by the US National Institutes of Health (NIH Publication No. 85-23) and was approved by the Institutional Animal Care and Use Committee of Vanderbilt University Medical Center, which is fully accredited by the Association for Assessment and Accreditation of Laboratory Animal Use.

PAEC isolation

Using previously published methods [13], the main pulmonary artery was isolated from the lungs of 5-day-old York-Landrace mixed breed piglets, flushed with PBS, then filled with 0.25% trypsin-EDTA and incubated for 5 min. To remove the endothelial cells, the pulmonary artery was gently flushed with endothelial growth medium (EGM-2, Lonza). Harvested endothelial cells were cultured in EGM-2 in 100 mm plates in a humidified, normoxic incubator (21% O_2, 5% CO_2) at 37°C. PAECs were identified by their cobblestone morphology and eNOS-positive staining. Cells were subcultured at near confluence and used at passages 4–10.

Modulation of SNAT1 expression

Using a modification of methods previously described [14], PAECs were transfected with non-targeting (control) oligonucleotides (siGENOME Non-targeting siRNA #5) or SNAT1 targeting oligonucleotides (sense, 5′-ACGAACAGCCAUUUG-GAAAUU-3′; anti-sense, 5′-UUUCCAAAUGGCUGUUC-GUUU-3′; sense, 5′-CCGGAAGAUGAUAACAUUAUU-3′ anti-sense, 5′-UAAUGUUAUCAUCUUCCGGUU-3′; anti-sense, 5′-UAAUGUUAUCAUCUUCCGGUU-3′; sense, 5′-CA-GUAACACUUCUGUCUAUUU-3′ anti-sense, 5′-AUAGACA-GAAGUGUUACUGUU-3′) purchased from Thermo Scientific. For transfection, EGM-2 was replaced with OPTI-MEM (Gibco). PAECs were transfected with a 300–600 pmol suspension of either non-targeting or SNAT1 oligonucleotides (100–200 pmol for each of the 3 different SNAT1 targeting oligonucleotides) using lipofectamine (Invitrogen) in OPTI-MEM. After 4 hours, the medium was replaced with EGM-2 and 10% FBS.

L-Citrulline uptake

After 48 hours in normoxic (21% O_2, 5% CO_2) or hypoxic (4% O_2, 5% CO_2) conditions, PAECs were prepared for measuring L-citrulline uptake using methods previously described [13]. PAEC were washed with 2 mL fresh sodium-HEPES buffer composed of the following: 2 mol/L NaCl, 2 mol/L KCl, 0.3 mol/L $MgSO_4$, 0.325 mol/L $CaCl_2$, 0.3 mol/L KH_2PO_4 and 1 mol/L HEPES adjusted to pH of 7.4 with 1 mol/L NaOH. Cells were incubated under normoxic conditions (21% O_2, 5% CO_2, 37°C) with

0.25 µCi/mL ^{14}C-L-citrulline (specific activity: 56.3 mCi/mmol; Perkin Elmer, Norwalk, CT, USA) in the presence of a saturating concentration (200 µmol/L) of unlabeled L-citrulline. Incubations were stopped after 5–10 min by washing three times with 2 mL ice-cold sodium-HEPES buffer. All cells were lysed with 450 µL 1 mol/L NaOH for 30 min at 37°C. A 400 µL aliquot of each lysate was transferred to a scintillation vial, LSC cocktail (Fisher Scientific, Pittsburgh, PA, USA) was added and radioactivity was measured in a scintillation counter (Beckman LS 6500; Brea, CA, USA). The remainder of the lysate was used for protein determination by bicinchoninic acid protein assay (Pierce, Rockford, IL, USA). Uptake of L-citrulline was expressed as radioactive counts per minute (CPM) per mg of protein.

NO measurement by ESR

PAECs were incubated under normoxic (21% O_2, 5% CO_2) or hypoxic (4% O_2, 5% CO_2) conditions for 48 hours in basal media (EGM-2), which contains 4 µmol/L L-citrulline. During the final hour of the 48-hour incubation period, L-citrulline was added to the medium of some cells to achieve a final conc. of 1 mmol/L. Cells were washed with chilled Krebs-HEPES buffer and incubated with calcium ionophore, A-23187 (10 µmol/L) and 200 µmol/L Fe(DETC)$_2$ at 37°C for 1 hour. The cells were then scraped in 0.5 ml of Krebs-HEPES buffer and snap-frozen in liquid nitrogen and stored at −80°C until assessed for NO production by electron spin resonance (ESR) as previously described [14]. The amount of detected NO was determined from the calibration curve for integral intensity of the ESR signal of NO-Fe^{2+}(MGD)$_2$ prepared at various concentrations of the NO-donor MAHMA-NONOate (ENZO Life Sciences Inc. NY, USA).

Superoxide measurement using dihydroethidium and an HPLC-based assay

Superoxide was measured using dihdroethidium (DHE) and an HPLC-based assay as previously described [14]. PAECs were cultured under normoxic or hypoxic conditions for 48 hours in basal media (EGM-2), which contains 4 µmol/L L-citrulline. During the final hour of the 48-hour incubation period, L-citrulline was added to the medium of some cells to achieve a final conc. of 1 mmol/L. PAECs were washed three times with chilled Krebs-HEPES buffer and then incubated with 25 µmol/L dihydroethidium for 20 min at 37°C in Krebs-HEPES buffer. The cells were harvested in 0.3 ml of methanol, homogenized and filtered through 0.22 µm filters and stored at −80°C until analyzed by HPLC. Protein measurements by Bradford assay were done in aliquots of homogenates collected prior to filtration. Separation of ethidium, 2-hydroxyethidium, and dihydroethidium was performed using a Beckman HPLC System Gold model with a C-18 reverse phase column (Nucleosil 250, 4.5 mm; Sigma-Aldrich, St. Louis, MO) equipped with both UV and fluorescence detectors. Fluorescence detection at 580 nm (emission) and 480 nm (excitation) was used to monitor 2-hydroxyethidium production. UV absorption at 355 nm was used for the detection of dihydroethidium. The mobile phase was composed of a gradient containing 60% acetonitrile and 0.1% trifluoroacetic acid. Dihydroethidium, ethidium and 2-hydroxyethidium were separated by a linear increase in acetonitrile concentration from 37 to 47% over 23 min at a flow rate of 0.5 mL/min. Hydroxyethidium was expressed per milligram protein.

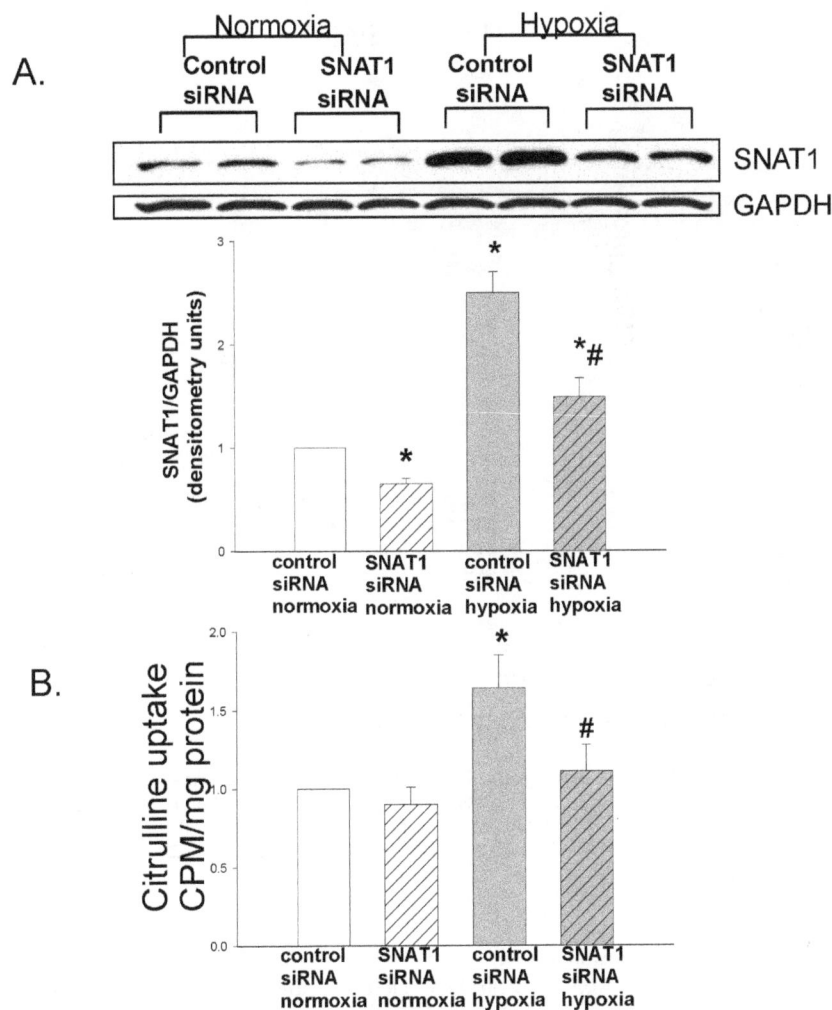

Figure 1. SNAT1 expression and L-citrulline uptake in PAECs cultured under normoxic or hypoxic conditions. Hypoxia increased both the expression of the amino acid transporter, SNAT1 (A), and the uptake of ^{14}C-L-citrulline (B) in PAECs (n = 11) from newborn piglets. In normoxic PAECs (n = 11), SNAT1 siRNA reduced SNAT1 expression (A) without having a detectable impact on ^{14}C-L-citrulline uptake (B: L-citrulline uptake in normoxic PAECs treated with SNAT1 siRNA was 0.9±0.11; p = 0.4). *different from normoxia control siRNA, #different from hypoxia control siRNA; P<0.05.

Immunoblot analysis of SNAT1, eNOS, and eNOS dimers and monomers

PAECs were washed with PBS, then collected and stored at −80°C. Frozen PAECs were crushed under liquid N_2 into a fine powder, transferred to a tube containing homogenization buffer with protease inhibitors, and then sonicated. Protein concentrations for all homogenates were determined by the protein assay (Bradford). For SNAT1 and eNOS analysis, using previously described methods [13], supernatants were applied to tris-glycine pre-cast 4–20% polyacrylamide gels (Invitrogen, Carlsbad, CA, USA) so that equal amounts of protein were loaded. Electrophoresis was carried out and the proteins were transferred from the gel to a nitrocellulose membrane. The membrane was incubated at room temperature in PBS containing 7.5% non-fat dried milk and 0.1% Tween-20 to block non-specific protein binding. To detect SNAT1 or eNOS, the nitrocellulose membrane was incubated overnight with the primary antibody (SNAT1 1:800, ABCAM; eNOS 1:2000, eNOS antibody from BD-Transduction Laboratory, San Diego, CA) diluted in PBS containing 0.1% Tween-20 and 1% non-fat dried milk (carrier buffer); followed by incubation with a horseradish peroxidase-conjugated secondary antibody (Zymed) diluted in the carrier buffer (1:5000). Using non-sonicated and nonboiled lysates and low-temperature SDS-PAGE, eNOS dimers/monomers were immunoblotted (1:2000, eNOS antibody, BD-Transduction Laboratory, San Diego, CA) as described elsewhere [15]. The membranes were developed using enhanced chemiluminescence reagents (ECL, Amersham) and the chemiluminescent signal was captured on X-ray film (ECL Hyperfilm, Kodak). Similar procedures were followed to reprobe the membranes for β-actin (Sigma-Aldrich, St. Louis, MO) or GAPDH (ABCAM, 1:1000). The bands for each protein were quantified using densitometry.

Statistical Analysis

Data are presented as mean ± SEM. Data were compared by unpaired t-test or one-way ANOVA with Fisher's protected least significant difference (PLSD) post hoc comparison test as appropriate. P-values <0.05 were considered significant.

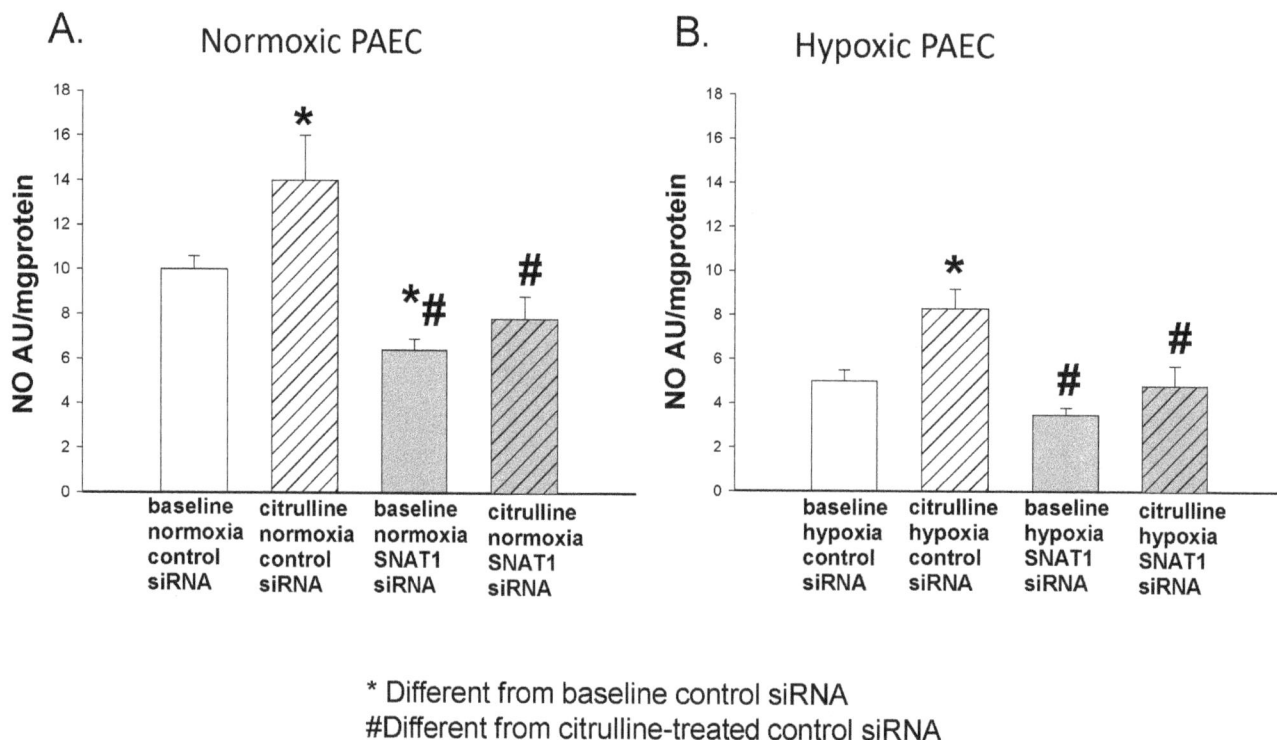

A. Normoxic PAEC

B. Hypoxic PAEC

* Different from baseline control siRNA
#Different from citrulline-treated control siRNA

Figure 2. NO production in PAECs cultured under normoxic or hypoxic conditions. SNAT1 siRNA prevented L-citrulline-induced increases in NO production in both normoxic (A, n = 5) and hypoxic (B, n = 5) PAECs from newborn piglets. A: for SNAT1 siRNA treated normoxic PAECs in the absence *vs* presence of L-citrulline NO production was respectively, 6.4±0.5 and 7.8±1.0 AU/mg protein, p = 0.4. B: for SNAT1 siRNA treated hypoxic PAECs in the absence *vs* presence of L-citrulline, NO production was respectively, 3.5±0.3 and 4.8±0.9 AU/mg protein, p = 0.21. *different from baseline control siRNA, #different from citrulline-treated control siRNA, P<0.05.

Results

Hypoxia increased SNAT1 expression (p<0.001; Fig. 1A) and L-citrulline uptake (p = .003; Fig. 1B) in PAECs. In normoxic PAECs, SNAT1 siRNA reduced SNAT1 expression (p = 0.04; Fig. 1A) without having a detectable impact on L-citrulline uptake (p = 0.4; Fig. 1 B). More importantly, SNAT1 siRNA inhibited the hypoxia-induced elevation in SNAT1 expression (p<0.001; Fig. 1A) and concomitantly prevented the hypoxia-induced increase in L-citrulline uptake (p = 0.01; Fig. 1B). These findings indicate that hypoxia increases L-citrulline uptake in PAECs via SNAT1 and demonstrate an association between SNAT1 and the transport of the L-arginine-NO substrate, L-citrulline, in PAECs of newborn piglets.

To explore the role of L-citrulline and SNAT1 in modulating NO signaling in PAECs, we determined the effects of L-citrulline treatment and SNAT1 depletion by siRNA on NO production in normoxic and hypoxic PAECs. L-citrulline significantly increased NO production in both normoxic (p = 0.03; Fig. 2A) and hypoxic (p = 0.005; Fig. 2B) PAECs. SNAT1 siRNA prevented the L-citrulline-induced increase in NO production in both normoxic (Fig. 2A; p = 0.4) and hypoxic PAECs (Fig. 2B, p = 0.21). These findings show that L-citrulline-induced NO production is modulated by SNAT1.

NO production is influenced by the state of eNOS coupling. Uncoupled eNOS can be demonstrated as a loss of eNOS dimer formation and an increase of eNOS monomers. We determined the effects of L-citrulline treatment and SNAT1 siRNA on eNOS dimer-to-monomer ratios in normoxic and hypoxic PAECs. L-citrulline had no effect on the eNOS dimer-to-monomer ratio in normoxic PAECs transfected with control siRNA (Fig. 3A and 3B; p = 0.97). L-citrulline increased the eNOS dimer-to-monomer ratio in normoxic PAECs transfected with SNAT1 siRNA (Fig. 3A and 3B; p = 0.001). SNAT1 siRNA decreased both baseline eNOS dimer-to-monomer ratios (Fig. 3A and 3B; p<0.001) and baseline NO production (Fig. 2A; p = 0.03) in normoxic PAECs. Neither L-citrulline nor SNAT1 siRNA altered total eNOS expression in normoxic PAECs (Figure 4; p = 0.7). These data suggest that SNAT1 knockdown reduced baseline NO production in normoxic PAECs, at least in part, by uncoupling eNOS.

In hypoxic PAECs, L-citrulline increased eNOS dimer-to-monomer ratios (Fig. 3A and 3C; p = 0.002), an effect that was abolished by SNAT1 siRNA (Fig. 3A and 3C; p = 0.3). Total eNOS expression was unchanged by L-citrulline and SNAT1 siRNA (Figure 4; p = 0.7). In conjunction with the NO data in Figure 2 B, these findings suggest that L-citrulline and SNAT1 modulate NO production in hypoxic PAECs by influencing the state of eNOS coupling.

We also determined the effects of L-citrulline treatment and SNAT1 siRNA on $O_2^{\cdot-}$ production in normoxic and hypoxic PAECs in the absence and presence of the NOS inhibitor, L-NAME. L-citrulline had no effect on $O_2^{\cdot-}$ production in normoxic PAECs transfected with control siRNA in either the presence or absence of L-NAME, (Fig. 5A, p = 0.5 and 5C, p = 0.08). In contrast, L-citrulline reduced $O_2^{\cdot-}$ production in normoxic PAECs transfected with SNAT1 siRNA in the absence of L-NAME (Fig. 5A, p = 0.036) but not the presence of L-NAME (Fig. 5C, p = 0.9). Moreover, SNAT1 siRNA increased baseline $O_2^{\cdot-}$ production in normoxic PAEC in the absence of L-NAME (Fig. 5A; p = 0.008) but not the presence of L-NAME (Fig. 5C,

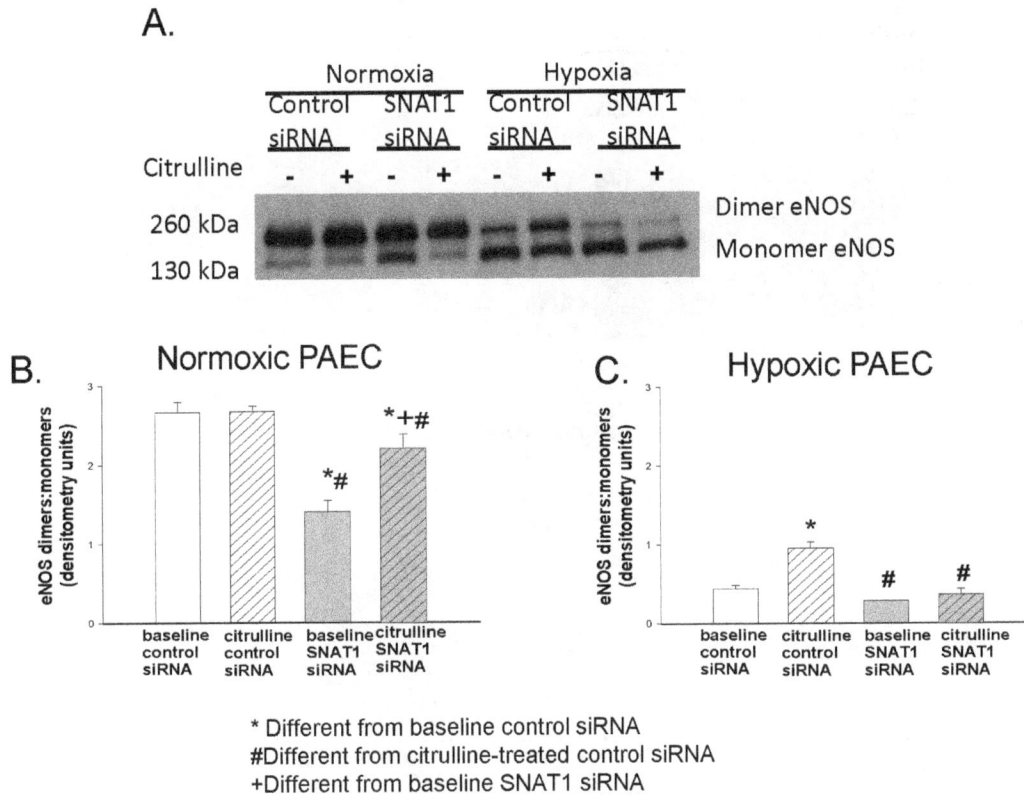

Figure 3. eNOS dimers/monomers in PAECs cultured under normoxic or hypoxic conditions. Representative western blot (A); densitometry for normoxic (B, n = 5) and hypoxic (C, n = 5) PAECs. In normoxic PAECs, L-citrulline had no effect on the eNOS dimer-to-monomer ratio when transfected with control siRNA (A and B: in the absence vs presence of L-citrulline eNOS dimer-to-monomer ratio was respectively: 2.7 ± 0.13 and 2.7 ± 0.07, p = 0.97) but increased the eNOS dimer-to-monomer ratio when transfected with SNAT1 siRNA. In hypoxic PAECs, L-citrulline increased eNOS dimer-to-monomer ratios when transfected with control siRNA but did not increase the eNOS dimer-to-monomer ratio when transfected with SNAT1 siRNA (A and C: in the absence vs presence of L-citrulline, eNOS dimer-to-monomer ratio was respectively: 0.28 ± 0.003 vs 0.37 ± 0.07, p = 0.3). *different from baseline control siRNA, #different from L-citrulline-treated control siRNA, +different from baseline SNAT1 siRNA; P<0.05.

p = 0.08). That is, in the presence of L-NAME (Fig. 5C), neither L-citrulline nor SNAT1 siRNA caused changes in $O_2^{\bullet-}$ production in normoxic PAECs. In addition, changes in $O_2^{\bullet-}$ production in normoxic PAEC in the absence of L-NAME (Fig. 5A) were concordant with changes in eNOS dimer-to-monomer ratios (Fig. 3A and 3B). Taken together, these findings show that both L-citrulline and SNAT1 modulate $O_2^{\bullet-}$ production in normoxic PAECs in a NOS-dependent fashion that reflects the state of eNOS coupling.

In the absence of L-NAME (Fig. 5 B), L-citrulline reduced $O_2^{\bullet-}$ production in hypoxic PAECs transfected with either control siRNA (p = 0.01) or SNAT1 siRNA (p = 0.001). In the presence of L-NAME, L-citrulline had no effect on $O_2^{\bullet-}$ production in hypoxic PAECs transfected with control siRNA (Fig. 5D, p = 0.8). However, in the presence of L-NAME, reductions in $O_2^{\bullet-}$ production with L-citrulline persisted in hypoxic PAECs transfected with SNAT1 siRNA (p = 0.001; Fig. 5D). An increase in baseline $O_2^{\bullet-}$ production occurred with SNAT1 siRNA in hypoxic PAECs both in the absence (p = <0.001; Fig. 5B) and presence (p = <0.001; Fig. 5D) of L-NAME. In the latter case, the magnitude of increase in $O_2^{\bullet-}$ production was reduced by the presence of L-NAME (increase in $O_2^{\bullet-}$ production was $44 \pm 4\%$ vs $25 \pm 5\%$ respectively in the absence vs the presence of L-NAME, p<0.05). These findings show that both L-citrulline and SNAT1 modulate $O_2^{\bullet-}$ production in hypoxic PAECs in a NOS-dependent fashion.

Discussion

Our studies reveal a number of novel findings regarding L-citrulline and NO signaling in PAECs. We show for the first time that the neutral amino acid transporter, SNAT1, modulates L-citrulline-induced increases in NO production. Moreover, we provide important new evidence that L-citrulline supplementation increases NO production by re-coupling eNOS in a SNAT1-dependent manner in hypoxic PAECs.

There are limited data on the transport of the amino acid, L-citrulline, by neutral amino acid transporters in vascular cells [16]. Information about the impact of hypoxia on neutral amino acid transporters, including SNAT1, in cells from vascular beds is also scarce [17]. L-citrulline uptake was reported to remain unchanged in PAECs from adult pigs cultured for up to 24 hours in hypoxia [18]. However, we previously found that L-citrulline uptake was increased in PAECs from newborn piglets cultured under hypoxic conditions for 24, 48, or 72 hours [13]. Moreover, we provided evidence that the hypoxia-induced increase in L-citrulline transport involved the System A family of sodium-coupled neutral amino acid transporters [13]. We confirm our previous findings and extend them by identifying SNAT1 as the System A transporter that is responsible for the enhanced ability to transport L-citrulline in hypoxic PAECs.

To our knowledge, we are the first to provide evidence of an important functional link between SNAT1, L-citrulline, and NO

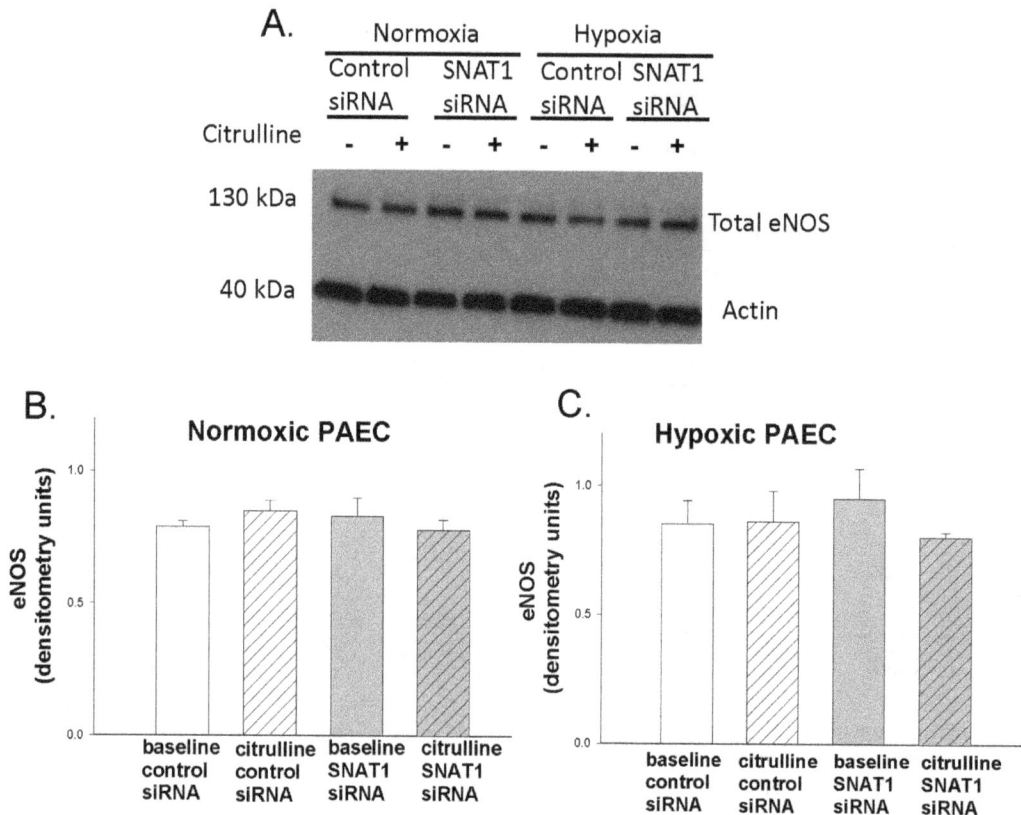

Figure 4. Total eNOS measured under baseline conditions and with L-citrulline treatment in PAECs cultured under normoxic or hypoxic conditions. A: representative western blot: B: densitometry for normoxic PAECs, n = 5; C: densitometry for hypoxic PAECs, n = 5. Neither L-citrulline nor SNAT1 siRNA altered total eNOS expression in either normoxic or hypoxic PAECs.

signaling in PAECs. Others have shown that L-citrulline can increase NO production in endothelial cells [19]. However, our findings provide the first mechanistic evidence that SNAT1 is integral to the effect of L-citrulline on NO production in both normoxic and hypoxic PAECs. Furthermore, we are the first to show that SNAT1 is involved in modulating eNOS uncoupling and $O_2^{\bullet-}$ production in PAECs.

The role of SNAT1 in modulating eNOS re-coupling and $O_2^{\bullet-}$ production. differs between normoxic and hypoxic PAECs. SNAT1 siRNA reduced baseline eNOS dimer formation and also increased $O_2^{\bullet-}$ production in normoxic PAECs indicating that SNAT1 is essential for either maintaining or promoting eNOS dimerization under basal conditions, thereby impacting basal $O_2^{\bullet-}$ and NO production. However, despite transfection with SNAT1 siRNA, L-citrulline increased eNOS dimer-to-monomer ratios in normoxic PAECs, suggesting that other transporters are involved in the mechanism by which L-citrulline re-couples eNOS in normoxic PAECs. In contrast, SNAT1 is integral to the ability of L-citrulline to re-couple eNOS in hypoxic PAECs.

Findings in this study reveal additional novel information on the mechanisms underlying L-citrulline-induced increases in NO production. We have shown previously in an *in vivo* model that L-citrulline supplementation increases pulmonary vascular NO production and attenuates chronic hypoxia-induced pulmonary hypertension in newborn piglets [20]. Findings herein provide additional insight into the mechanisms by which L-citrulline might alleviate pulmonary hypertension. We show that when hypoxic

PAECs are treated with L-citrulline there is a significant increase in the eNOS dimer:monomer ratio, indicating that L-citrulline reduces eNOS uncoupling. Consistent with eNOS re-coupling, $O_2^{\bullet-}$ generation is reduced and NO production is increased in hypoxic PAECs treated with L-citrulline. In addition, we demonstrate that the decrease in $O_2^{\bullet-}$ seen with L-citrulline supplementation is abolished by treatment with L-NAME, further supporting that L-citrulline works in a NOS-dependent fashion.

Augmentation of NO production in normoxic PAECs occurs without a change in the state of eNOS coupling. Under normoxic conditions, eNOS dimers predominate making it biologically unlikely and technically difficult to demonstrate that greater eNOS coupling is driving enhanced NO production. The likely explanation for the increase in NO production with L-citrulline in normoxic PAECs is that, once transported into PAECs by SNAT1, L-citrulline is enzymatically converted to L-arginine by argininosuccinate synthetase (ASS) and argininosuccinate lyase (ASL), increasing the intracellular pool of L-arginine that is available to eNOS [9]. There is evidence that ASS-ASL-eNOS are co-localized in plasmalemmal caveolae of endothelial cells [19]. Hence, instead of equilibrating with bulk intracellular levels, L-citrulline induced increases in L-arginine could be directly channeled to eNOS thereby driving NO production [12].

Our study has some limitations that merit discussion. All studies were performed with PAECs isolated from the main pulmonary artery of newborn piglets. Whether our findings reflect endothelial cells from other species, other postnatal ages, all segments of the

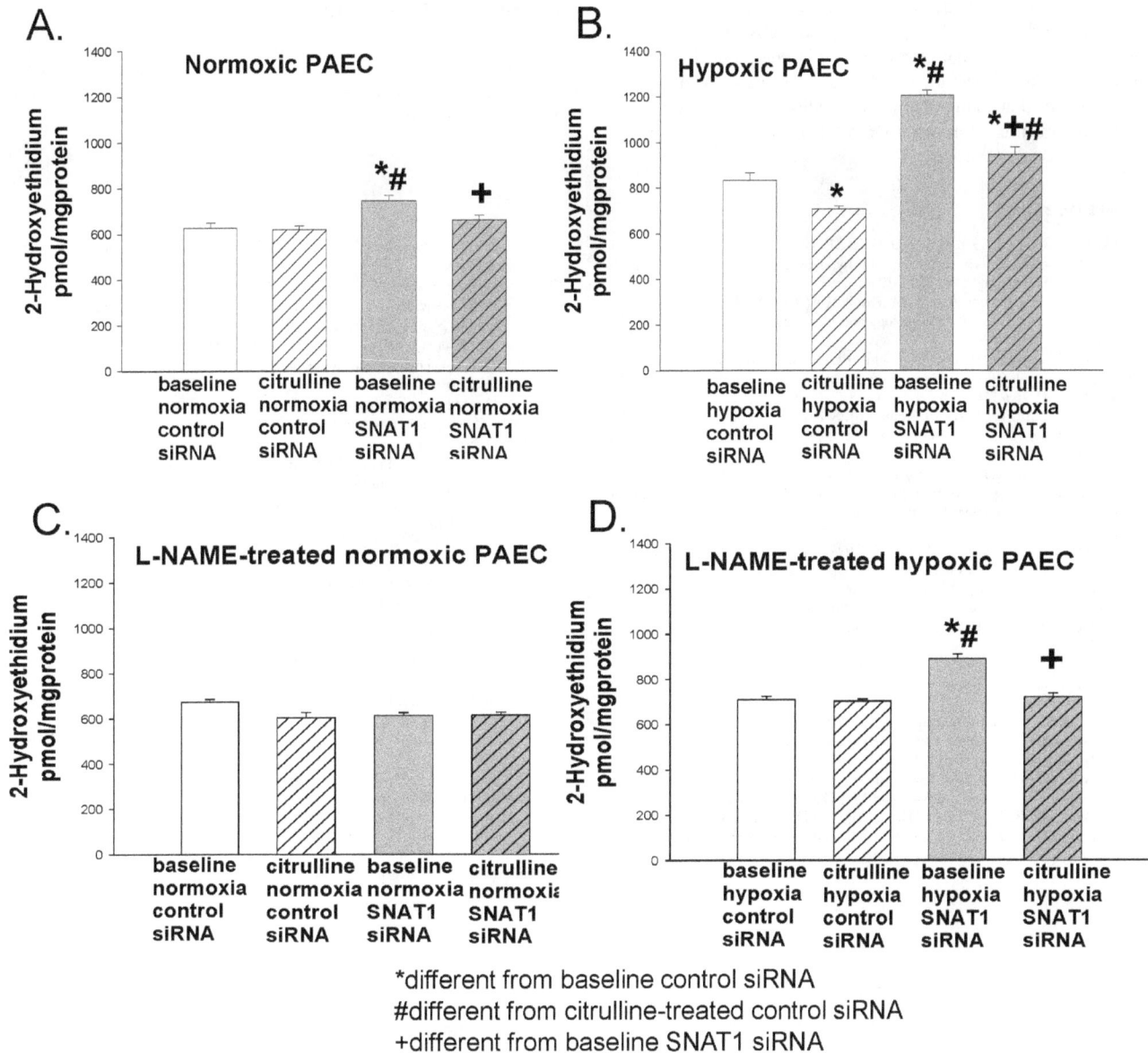

*different from baseline control siRNA
#different from citrulline-treated control siRNA
+different from baseline SNAT1 siRNA

Figure 5. Superoxide production, as assessed by the formation of 2-hydroxyethidium, in PAECs cultured under normoxic or hypoxic conditions. Normoxic PAECs (n = 5) in the absence (A) or presence (C) of L-NAME; Hypoxic PAECs (n = 5) in the absence (B) or presence (D) of L-NAME. In normoxic conditions, L-citrulline had no effect on superoxide production in PAECs transfected with control siRNA in either the presence (C) or absence (A) of L-NAME (A: $O_2^{\bullet-}$ production in the absence vs presence of L-citrulline was respectively, 625 ± 23 and 603 ± 28 pmol/mg protein, p = 0.5 and C: $O_2^{\bullet-}$ production in the absence vs presence of L-citrulline was respectively, 670 ± 12 and 610 ± 28 pmol/mg protein, p = 0.08). L-citrulline reduced superoxide production in PAECs transfected with SNAT1 siRNA in the absence (A) but not the presence (C) of L-NAME (C: $O_2^{\bullet-}$ production in the absence vs presence of L-citrulline was respectively, 613 ± 12 and 614 ± 13 pmol/mg protein, p = 0.9). Moreover, SNAT1 siRNA increased baseline $O_2^{\bullet-}$ production in normoxic PAEC in the absence (A) but not the presence (C) of L-NAME (C: $O_2^{\bullet-}$ production for control siRNA vs SNAT1 siRNA was respectively, 670 ± 12 and 613 ± 12 pmol/mg protein, p = 0.08). In hypoxic conditions, L-citrulline reduced superoxide production in PAECs transfected with control siRNA in the absence (B) but not the presence of L-NAME (D: $O_2^{\bullet-}$ production in the absence vs presence of L-citrulline was respectively, 711 ± 14 and 703 ± 9 pmol/mg protein, p = 0.8). L-citrulline reduced superoxide production in PAECs transfected with SNAT1 siRNA in both the presence (D) and the absence (B) of L-NAME. *different from baseline control siRNA; #different from L-citrulline-treated control siRNA; +different from baseline SNAT1 siRNA; P<0.05.

pulmonary circulation, or other vascular beds will require future exploration. We were unable to detect a significant reduction in L-citrulline uptake in normoxic PAECs treated with SNAT1 siRNA. Given the overlap of substrate specificity of amino acid transporters, SNAT1 would not be expected to be the only L-citrulline transporter. The presence of other transporters, which could compensate for SNAT1 knockdown, likely led to an undetectable net change in L-citrulline uptake in normoxic PAECs.

In summary, we provide novel, mechanistic data supporting an integral role for SNAT1 in modulating L-citrulline-induced changes in NO signaling in PAECs of newborn piglets. Our findings have potential therapeutic significance and support a role for L-citrulline supplementation as a means to reduce $O_2^{\bullet-}$ generation and increase NO production thereby ameliorating the development of pulmonary hypertension in newborns. In addition, our findings provide the impetus for future research to investigate the possibility that manipulating L-citrulline transport could be a viable therapeutic approach to modulate NO production in a variety of vascular diseases.

References

1. Fike CD, Aschner JL, Zhang Y, Kaplowitz MR (2004) Impaired NO signaling in small pulmonary arteries of chronically hypoxic newborn pigs. Am J Physiol Lung Cell Mol Physiol 286: 1244–1254.
2. Tonelli AR, Haserodt S, Aytekin M, Dweik RA (2013) Nitric oxide deficiency in pulmonary hypertension: Pathobiology and implications for therapy. Pulm Circ 3: 20–30.
3. Gielis JF, Lin JY, Wingler K, Schil PEYV, Schmidt HH, et al. (2011) Pathogenetic role of eNOS uncoupling in cardiopulmonary disorders. Free Rad Biol Med 50: 765–776.
4. Martasek P, Miller RT, Liu Q, Roman LJ, Salerno JC, et al. (1998) The C331A mutant of neuronal nitric-oxide synthase is defective in arginine binding. J Biol Chemistry 273: 34799–34805.
5. Ou Z-J, Wei W, Huang D, Luo D, Wang Z, et al. (2010) L-arginine restores endothelial nitric oxide coupled activity and attenuates monocrotaline-induced pulmonary artery hypertension in rats. Am J Physiol Endocrinol Metab 298: E1131–E1139.
6. Mitani Y, Maruyama K, Minoru S (1997) Prolonged administration of L-arginine ameliorates chronic pulmonary hypertension and pulmonary vascular remodeling in rats. Circulation 96: 689–697.
7. Sasaki S, Asano M, Ukai T, Nomura N, Maruyama K, et al. (2004) Nitric oxide formation and plasma L-arginine levels in pulmonary hypertensive rats. Respir Med 98: 205–212.
8. Hoet PH, Nemery B (2000) Polyamines in the lung: polyamine uptake and polyamine-linked pathological or toxicological conditions. Am J Physiol Lung Cell Mol Physiol 278: L417–L433.
9. Solomonson LP, Flam BR, Pendleton LC, Goodwin BL, Eichler DC (2003) The caveolar nitric oxide synthase/arginine regneration system for NO production in endothelial cells. J Exp Biol 206: 2083–2087.
10. Boger RH (2008) L-arginine therapy in cardiovascular pathologies: beneficial or dangerous? Curr Opin Clin Nutr and Met Care 11: 55–61.
11. Schulman SP, Becker LC, Kass DA, Champion HC, Terrin ML, et al. (2006) L-arginine therapy in acute myocardial infarction: the vascular interaction with age in myocardial infarction (VINTAGE MI) randomized clinical trial. JAMA 295: 58–64.
12. Erez A, Nagamani SC, Shchelochkov OA, Premkumar MH, Campeau PM, et al. (2011) Requirement of argininosuccinate lyase for systemic nitric oxide production. Nature Medicine 17: 1619–1626.
13. Fike CD, Sidoryk-Wegrzynowicz M, Aschner M, Summar M, Prince LS, et al. (2012) Prolonged hypoxia augments L-citrulline transport by System A in the newborn piglet pulmonary circulation. Cardiovasc Res 95: 375–384.
14. Dikalova AE, Bikineyeva AT, Budzyn K, Nazarewicz RR, McCann L, et al. (2010) Therapeutic targeting of mitochondrial superoxide in hypertension. Circ Res 107: 106–116.
15. Klatt P, Schmidt K, Lehner D, Glatter O, Bachinger HP, et al. (1995) Structural analysis of porcine brain nitric oxide synthase reveals a role for tetrahydrobiopterin and L-arginine in the formation of an SDS-resistant dimer. EMBO J 14: 3687–3695.
16. Bahri S, Zerrouk N, Aussel C, Moinard C, Crenn P, et al. (2013) Citrulline: From metabolism to therapeutic use. Nutrition 29: 479–484.
17. Mann GE, Yudilevich DL, Sobrevia L (2003) Regulation of amino acid and glucose transporters in endothelial and smooth muscle cells. Physiol Rev 83: 183–252.
18. Su Y, Block ER (1995) Hypoxia inhibits L-arginine synthesis from L-citrulline in porcine pulmonary artery endothelial cells. Am J Physiol Lung Cell Mol Physiol 269: 581–587.
19. Flam BR, Hartmann PJ, Harrell-Booth M, Solomonson LP, Eichler DC (2001) Caveolar localization of arginine regeneration enzymes, argininosuccante synthase, and lyase, with endothelial nitric oxide synthase. Nitric Oxide 5: 187–197.
20. Ananthakrishnan M, Barr FE, Summar ML, Smith HA, Kaplowitz M, et al. (2009) L-Citrulline ameliorates chronic hypoxia-induced pulmonary hypertension in newborn piglets. Am J Physiol Lung Cell Mol Physiol 297: 506–511.

Author Contributions

Conceived and designed the experiments: AD AF JLA MA MS CDF. Performed the experiments: AD AF. Analyzed the data: AD AF CDF. Contributed reagents/materials/analysis tools: AD AF JLA MA CDF. Wrote the paper: AD AF JLA MA CDF.

22

Analysis of Volatile Compounds in Exhaled Breath Condensate in Patients with Severe Pulmonary Arterial Hypertension

J. K. Mansoor[1], Edward S. Schelegle[2]*, Cristina E. Davis[3], William F. Walby[2], Weixiang Zhao[3], Alexander A. Aksenov[3], Alberto Pasamontes[3], Jennifer Figueroa[2], Roblee Allen[4]

1 Department of Physical Therapy, University of the Pacific, Stockton, California, United States of America, **2** Department of Anatomy, Physiology and Cell Biology, University of California Davis, Davis, California, United States of America, **3** Department of Mechanical and Aerospace Engineering, University of California Davis, Davis, California, United States of America, **4** Department of Medicine, University of California Davis Medical Center, Sacramento, California, United States of America

Abstract

Background: An important challenge to pulmonary arterial hypertension (PAH) diagnosis and treatment is early detection of occult pulmonary vascular pathology. Symptoms are frequently confused with other disease entities that lead to inappropriate interventions and allow for progression to advanced states of disease. There is a significant need to develop new markers for early disease detection and management of PAH.

Methodolgy and Findings: Exhaled breath condensate (EBC) samples were compared from 30 age-matched normal healthy individuals and 27 New York Heart Association functional class III and IV idiopathic pulmonary arterial hypertenion (IPAH) patients, a subgroup of PAH. Volatile organic compounds (VOC) in EBC samples were analyzed using gas chromatography/mass spectrometry (GC/MS). Individual peaks in GC profiles were identified in both groups and correlated with pulmonary hemodynamic and clinical endpoints in the IPAH group. Additionally, GC/MS data were analyzed using autoregression followed by partial least squares regression (AR/PLSR) analysis to discriminate between the IPAH and control groups. After correcting for medicaitons, there were 62 unique compounds in the control group, 32 unique compounds in the IPAH group, and 14 in-common compounds between groups. Peak-by-peak analysis of GC profiles of IPAH group EBC samples identified 6 compounds significantly correlated with pulmonary hemodynamic variables important in IPAH diagnosis. AR/PLSR analysis of GC/MS data resulted in a distinct and identifiable metabolic signature for IPAH patients.

Conclusions: These findings indicate the utility of EBC VOC analysis to discriminate between severe IPAH and a healthy population; additionally, we identified potential novel biomarkers that correlated with IPAH pulmonary hemodynamic variables that may be important in screening for less severe forms IPAH.

Editor: Masataka Kuwana, Keio University School of Medicine, Japan

Funding: Research supported by contracts from Gilead Sciences, Inc. The funders had no role in study design, data collection and analysis, decision to publish, or preparation of the manuscript.

Competing Interests: Dr. Roblee Allen is a member of the advisory board, speaker's bureau and has contracts for pharmaceutical development from Gilead Sciences, Inc., Bayer AG, and United Therapeutics Corporation. He also has contracts for pharmaceutical development with Actelion Pharmaceuticals, Inc., Aires Pharmaceuticals, Inc. and GeNO, LLC. None of the other authors have any financial or other conflicts of interest to disclose regarding this publication.

* E-mail: esschelegle@ucdavis.edu

Introduction

An important challenge to pulmonary arterial hypertension (PAH) diagnosis and treatment is the early detection of occult pulmonary vascular pathology. Despite recognized risk factors for the disease, patients often present clinically only after a prolonged interval of symptoms. These symptoms are frequently confused with other disease entities, sometimes leading to inappropriate interventions and further progression to advanced states of disease. Even with proper diagnosis and therapy, the ability to judge the effectiveness of intervention is limited by the lack of assessment tools and biological markers.

Assessment tests such as the New York Heart Association (NYHA) Functional Classification and the 6 minute walk distance (6MWD) and biomarkers such as brain natriuretic peptide (BNP), though helpful, are limited in their ability to show PAH disease progression or quiescence. There is an unmet need to develop new markers for PAH disease detection and management that are valid, reliable and simple to obtain. Analysis of exhaled breath has been used to detect and monitor diverse pulmonary and systemic diseases such as oxidant-induced airway injury [1], aspirin-induced asthma [2], lung cancer [3,4] COPD [5], tuberculosis [6], lung transplant rejection [7], breast cancer [8], heart transplant rejection [9], diabetes mellitus [10], and unstable angina [11].

Investigation in our laboratory using non-invasive exhaled breath condensate (EBC) analysis has shown that vascular endothelial growth factor, leukotriene B$_4$, prostaglandin E$_2$, isoprostane, nitrates and nitrites can be isolated from EBC in humans exposed to altitude [12] and ozone [1]. The purpose of this study was to analyze the metabolic signature of volatile organic compounds (VOC) in EBC in patients with class 3 and 4 idiopathic PAH (IPAH) using gas chromatography/mass spectrometry (GC/MS). We compared this metabolic signature against age-matched healthy controls. It is hoped that this analysis is a first step in identifying new markers that can potentially be used to screen for less severe IPAH (classes I and II).

Methods And Materials

Ethics Statement

This study was approved by the University of California, Davis, Office of Human Research Protection Institutional Review Board (protocol #200917227-1). Written informed consent was obtained from participants and the study was conducted according to principles expressed in the Declaration of Helsinki.

Subjects

A total of 60 subjects ages 32–78 were recruited, with 30 healthy control subjects (8 males, 22 femlaes) and initially 30 functional class 3/4 IPAH who had undergone diagnostic right heart catheterization. The data from 3 IPAH subjects were insufficient for analysis reducing the final the IPAH group to 8 males and 19 females. Potential IPAH subjects were excluded if they were classified as functional class I/II IPAH or had anorexic drug-induced PAH, were HIV positive, were pregnant, had congenital heart disease, were currently smoking or had collagen-vascular disease. Control subjects were all non-smokers and pregnant women were excluded. An attempt was made to match age and body mass index (BMI).

Research Design and Data Collection

Subjects had their exhaled nitric oxide (ExNO) measured followed by collection of EBC. ExNO was measured with a chemiluminescence nitric oxide analyzer (Sievers, Boulder, CO) using the restricted breath technique at flow rate of 50 ml/s [13]. Historical 6MWD, New York functional class, BNP, hemodynamic measures and pulmonary function data was extracted from IPAH patients' medical records for correlation analysis.

EBC samples were collected as subjects sat quietly with a nose clip on breathing into the Jaeger EcoScreen (Viasys Healthcare, Conshohocken, PA) apparatus [12]. 0.5 mL EBC samples were stored at $-80°C$ in borosilicate vials and analyzed for VOC in a single batch using solid-phase microextraction (SPME). For SPME, EBC samples were thawed, 0.5 mL saturated NaCl solution added and sample vials placed on a chilled tray of a autosampler in randomized fashion. VOCs were sampled from the headspace using carboxen/polydimethylsiloxane df 75 μm (partially crosslinked [black hub]) SPME fibers (Supelco, St. Louis, MO) [14]. For analysis, EBC samples were transferred into a heater and agitated at 90°C with SPME tip exposed to the headspace. After sampling, the SPME was inserted into the heated inlet of a Varian 3800 GC with a 4000 Ion Trap MS (scanned mass-to-charge ratio (m/z) range 35–600 Th) equipped with an electron ionization source and a VF-5 ms 5% phenol/95% PDMS GC column (Varian, Walnut Creek, CA). The GC oven cycle was optimized for separation of benchmark human EBC samples.

Data Analysis

Exhaled Breath Condensate Gas Chromatograms/Mass Spectra Analysis. In order to compare EBC GC/MS profiles of control and IPAH subjects, whole chromatogram analysis and specific peak comparisons were used to test for statistically significant differences ($p<0.05$) between groups. Baseline correction was applied to remove the shifted regions of all chromatograms. A peak was defined as a minimum height of 500 ion counts. GC column bleed peaks (siloxanes) or extraneous contaminats (e.g. phtalates) were excluded. The height values of all peaks in the chromatogram were summed for each individual chromatogram (Σh_i) and the average was calculated (h). A correction coefficient r was then calculated as $r_i = \Sigma h_i / h$. Each chromatogram was corrected by dividing the peak height value by r_i in order to detect possible outliers and/or minimize the error in the sampling step. Then, peaks were normalized based on the height of the same peak of each sample to make the comparison on the same scale. Peaks with unacceptably low signal-to-noise ratios were not used. Across all of the chromatograms, 2668 peaks were identified using this approach.

To be considered unique, chromatograms of 70% of the subjects in a given group had to contain a given peak, while chromatograms of subjects in the other group did not contain the same peak. Peaks were considered in-common if chromatograms of subjects in both groups contained a given peak. We identified 62 unique peaks from the control group, 48 unique peaks from the IPAH group and 19 in-common peaks. In order to control for peaks that may have been affected by medications and/or dietary supplements being taken by the IPAH subjects, medications/dietary supplements were tabulated (see Table S1); 112 unique medications/dietary supplements were identified. A MANOVA was run using each medication/dietary supplement that was taken by 4 or more IPAH subjects as a grouping factor; if there was a statistically significant drug effect for a given peak, peak height data for the subjects taking that drug were removed from the database. After this, 5 peaks no longer met our criteria for an in-common peak and were removed from the original 19 in-common peaks for a total of 14 in-common peaks, and 16 peaks no longer met our criteria for a unique IPAH peaks and were removed from the original 48 unique IPAH peaks for a total of 32 unique IPAH peaks. MANOVA was used to determine if any of the 14 remaining in-common peaks were significantly different between groups.

GC/MS Autoregression/Partial Least Squares Regression Analysis. GC/MS data were converted into total ion count versus time. Each GC profile was composed of approximately 15,000 time points which covered 255 minutes. Baseline correction was applied to remove humps/plateaus in some of the chromatograms [15]. Auto-regression (AR) analysis was then used to reduce the number of variables needed to describe chromatograms from the original time scan number to one hundred AR coefficients [16,17]. Auto-regression analysis has the advantage of reducing the dimensionality of chromatography data while reducing the effects of possible signal misalignment within different profiles [16,17]. To visually and quantitatively compare the chromatography data of control and IPAH subjects, partial least square regression (PLSR) using AR coefficients was employed. PLSR further reduced the dimensionality from one hundred AR coefficients to two latent variables (PLSR components). The two PLSR components were then plotted against each other to examine separation within the data. This analysis was performed using Matlab software (MathWorks, Inc.; Natick, MA). This model was validated using the leave-one-out validation process. The results of this validation was used to calculate the sensitivity, specificity and positive and negative likelihood ratios.

Chemical Identification. Chemical identities of the 15 peaks unique to the control group with the highest ion counts and all of the unique IPAH and in-common peaks were explored. Where necessary, the Automated Mass Spectral Deconvolution and Identification System GC/MS analysis software (National Institute of Standards and Technology {NIST} v.2.64) was used to remove background noise and deconvolve peaks for co-eluting compounds. The MS spectra were compared against the NIST 2005 and Wiley 2009 MS libraries of deconvolve peaks for co-eluting compounds using NIST Mass Spectral Search Software v.2.0. The highest probability matches were considered and putative chemical identity was determined empirically by examining representative MS data and m/z in the data set. If the search produced a match with a probability greater than 80%, that match was considered to be the unknown compound (high confidence match). In some cases, no match was found or multiple chemical matches with very similar mass spectral fragmentation patterns and close match probability values (e.g., for isomers) were found. These were considered to be low confidence matches.

Correlation Analysis. The IPAH criteria endpoints of mean pulmonary arterial pressure (mPAP), pulmonary arterial wedge pressure (PAWP) and pulmonary vascular resistance (PVR) were correlated with all in-common or unique normalized peak heights of the IPAH group using Pearson-product moment correlation in order to identify peaks for inclusion in stepwise linear regression. mPAP, PAWP and PVR were also correlated with BNP and ExNO. All statistical analysis was performed using SPSS software version 21 (IBM Corp, Armonk, NY).

Results

Subject Characteristics

Table 1 shows the characteristics of the control and IPAH groups. The IPAH group mean values for PVR, PAWP, D_{LCO}, CI and 6MWD (Table 2) met or exceeded the minimal criteria for IPAH [18]. The groups were similar in the distribution of males and females. There was no difference in age and height between the two groups, however, the IPAH group was significantly heavier and had greater BMIs than the control group. Additionally, the IPAH group had significantly lower exhaled nitric oxide values.

EBC GC/MS Analysis

Figure 1A shows a representative gas chromatogram for a control and an IPAH subject superimposed on one-another. Unique peaks found in the IPAH subject but not in the control subject and a peak found in the control subject but not in the IPAH subject are shown in figures 1B and 1C, respectively.

Table 1. Subject characteristics.

	Control (n = 30)	PAH (n = 27)
Gender (n): Male	8	8
Female	22	19
Age (yrs)	52.5±6.8	51.6±11.0
Height (m)	1.68±0.08	1.67.3±0.08
Weight (kg)	80.0±20.7	96.2±29.4*
BMI (kg/m²)	28.4±6.7	34.3±9.8*
Exhaled Nitric Oxide	32.4±26.7	16.3±11.8*

Values are means ± standard deviation;
* significantly different from control $p \leq 0.05$; BMI = body mass index.

Table 2. Hemodynamic and clinical endpoints for IPAH subjects.

Endpoints	Values	n
MAP (mm Hg)	91.7±10.9	27
SBP (mm Hg)	123.0±14.9	27
DBP (mm Hg)	76.3±11.0	27
mPAP (mm Hg)	49.4±11.0	26
PAP$_{SYS}$ (mm Hg)	74.1±15.2	26
PAP$_{DIA}$ (mm Hg)	35.2±10.3	26
PAWP (mmHg)	10.6±4.2	26
PVR (mmHg/L/min)	705.2±295.6	26
P$_{RA}$ (mm Hg)	10.2±5.1	25
Cardiac Index (L/min/m²)	2.32±0.53	26
Brain Naturetic Peptide (pg/mL)	207.1±245.9	24
6 Minute Walk Distance (m)	342.6±112.3	23
D$_{LCO}$ (ml/min/mmHg)	20.4±7.7	21

Values are means ± standard deviation; MAP = mean arterial pressure; SBP = systolic blood pressure; DBP = diastolic blood pressure; mPAP = mean pulmonary artery pressure; PAP$_{SYS}$ = systolic pulmonary artery pressure; PAP$_{DIA}$ = diastolic pulmonary artery pressure; PAWP = pulmonary arterial wedge pressure; PVR = pulmonary vascular resistance; D$_{LCO}$ = lung cabon monoxide diffusing capacity. Note the high pulmonary arterial pressure and pulmonary vascular resistance characteristic of pulmonary arterial hypertension.

GC/MS Autoregression/Partial Least Squares Regression Analysis

The results of the GC/MS AR/PLSR analysis is shown in Figure 2. This analysis of the EBC metabolic signature shows that based on cross validation, the separation acurracy obtained by applying PLSR to AR coefficients is 75%. Using the pertinent information extracted from the whole spectra, the classification results suggest a good and robust seperability. Additionally, 22 out of 27 disease (positive) samples were confirmed as positive (sensitivity = 81.5%) and 21 out of 30 control (negative) samples were confirmed as negative (specificity = 70.0%). The positive likelihood ratio was 2.76 while the negative likelihood ratio was 0.368.

Chemical Identification

Two peaks unique to the control group, 10 peaks unique to the IPAH group and 4 peaks common to both groups were identified chemically with high confidence (Table 3). An in-common peak at retention time of 75.479 min. had significantly greater ion counts (p = 0.011) in the control group compared to the IPAH group. This peak was identified as benzene, 1-methyl-4-(1-methylethyl)-, a volatile organic compound produced by gut microbiota [19].

Correlation and Regression Analysis

Six of the 32 IPAH unique peaks were correlated with mPAP, PVR or PAWP (Table 4). There were no significant correlations between BNP or ExNO and mPAP, PVR and PAWP (Table 4). mPAP, PVR, and PAWP were used in the step-wise linear regression analysis and are shown in Figure 3.

Discussion

Currently, pulmonary hemodynamics along with 6MWD are common clinical measures used for the evaluation and diagnosis of

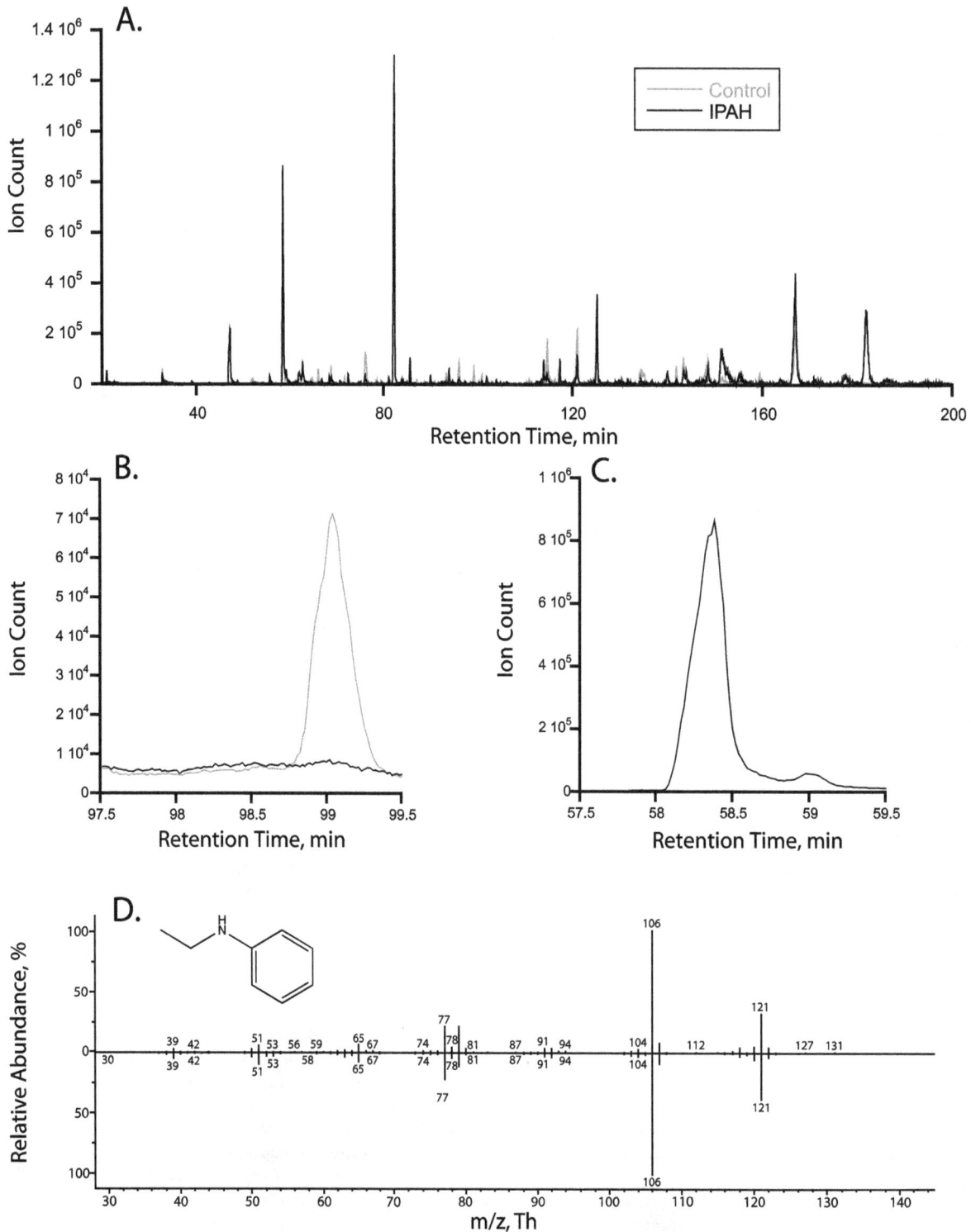

Figure 1. Representative gas chromatograms from a control subject (black line) and IPAH subject (grey line) (A) showing significantly different (p≤0.05) unique peaks for the control subject (B) and IPAH subject (C). An example of a head-to-tail comparison of an experimental mass spectrum (D) of one of the identified significantly different peaks unique for the IPAH group at a retention time of 81.436 min. (top) with a NIST/Wiley 2009 database search hit (bottom) identifying N-ethyl-Benzeneamine as giving the best match for the experimental spectrum.

IPAH [18]. In the current study the EBC metabolic signature was discriminatory in delineating severe IPAH subjects from age-matched controls. This in large part was due to the 48 peaks only present in IPAH subjects' gas chromatograms, and 62 peaks only present in control subjects' gas chromatograms. In addition, AR/PLSR analysis conserves these distinguishing features while greatly reducing the dimensionality of the data. This metabolomic approach provides a means to compare the complex information

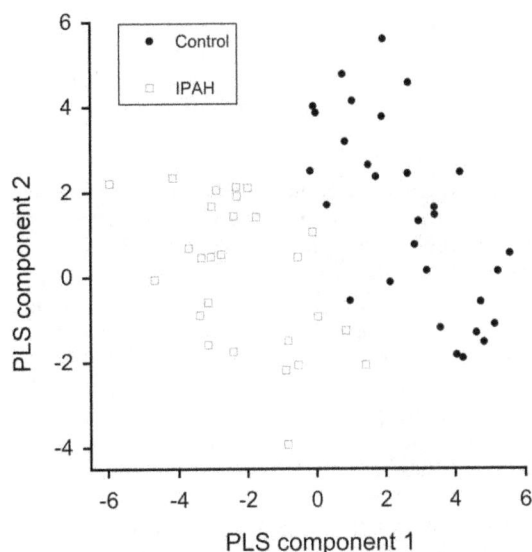

Figure 2. Plot of the results of autoregression and partial least squares analysis-weighted components of control subjects (dark circles) and IPAH subjects (open squares). 22 out of 27 disease (positive) samples were confirmed as positive (sensitivity =81.5%) and 21 out of 30 control (negative) samples were confirmed as negative (specificity =70.0%). The positive likelihood ratio was 2.76 while the negative likelihood ratio was 0.368.

presence or absence of a number of these compounds. However, the development and testing of such an index and the metabolomics approach based on AR/PLRS analysis requires further screening of a larger population of controls and individuals with diverse forms of pulmonary hypertension, as well as, individuals with other forms of lung disease to insure that the markers and chromatogram features identified are specific to IPAH.

The gas chromatograms obtained from IPAH samples would be expected to be affected by not only the underlying disease process but also the numerous medications the IPAH subjects were taking during the study. Of the 112 medications taken, 16 were taken by 4 or more of the IPAH subjects, indicating that most of the medications would not be expected to affect a large enough number of the 27 chromatograms studied to influence the group metabolic signature. The overall pattern is consistent with a metabolic signature that is unique to IPAH and is modified depending on the medications being taken. If any of the 48 IPAH unique peaks were a direct or indirect result of a medication or its metabolites, one would expect the height of those peaks to be different in subjects taking the medications compared with subjects not taking the medications. The data show that 30 of 48 IPAH unique peaks and 9 of 19 in-common peaks were affected by medication use; after eliminating peaks for individuals on given medications, 32 IPAH unique peaks and 14 in-common peaks contained a sufficient number of data points for subsequent correlation and regression analysis. Correlation and multiple linear regression analysis showed significant relationships between pulmonary hemodynamic PAH criteria and specific peaks from our GC/MS analysis (Table 4 and Figure 3). Although unknown at this point, it is possible that some medications affected peak heights in IPAH subjects and may have affected metabolic pathways important in the underlying mechanisms of IPAH.

Another factor that may have influenced our results is the significantly greater BMI in the IPAH group. This difference in BMI can be attributed to 4 subjects that had a mean BMI of 54.1. Removing these 4 subjects data from the dataset did not alter the

contained in the gas chromatograms and discriminate divergent groups, such as control and IPAH subjects in the current study. In total, these findings highlight the potential predictive value of VOCs in EBC for the evaluation and diagnosis of IPAH. This is supported by a positive likelihood ratio of 2.76 and a negative likelihood ratio of 0.37. Alternatively, the large number of unique compounds in both the control and IPAH groups suggests that an index for the screening of IPAH might be generated based on the

Table 3. Chemicals identified with "high confidence" for peaks found in all groups.

Peak Retention Time (min)	Present In	Proposed Chemical
18.843	IPAH	methyl isobutyl ketone
29.003	IPAH	furan, tetrahydro-2, 2, 4, 4-tetramethyl
52.031	Control	oxime-, methoxy-phenyl
55.271	In-common	benzaldehyde
58.237	IPAH	aniline
58.730	Contol	p-menth- 3 - ene
60.262	IPAH	2-menthene or other menthene isomers
65.244	IPAH	m-cymene or o-cymene
71.801	In-common	ethanone, 2,2-dihydroxy-1-phenyl-
75.479	In-common	benzene, 1-methyl-4-(1-methylethenyl)-
81.436	IPAH	benzenamine, N-ethyl-
83.224	IPAH	p-menthone
96.547	IPAH	benzothiazole
124.314	In-common	propanoic acid, 2-methyl-, 3-hydroxy-2, 4, 4-trimethylpentyl ester
127.194	IPAH	propanoic acid, 2-methyl-, 3-hydroxyhexyl ester
157.789	IPAH	1, 6-dioxacyclododecane-7, 12-dione

All peaks were identified with "high confidence", i.e., these structures were more likely to be the correct match than other potential candidate compounds.

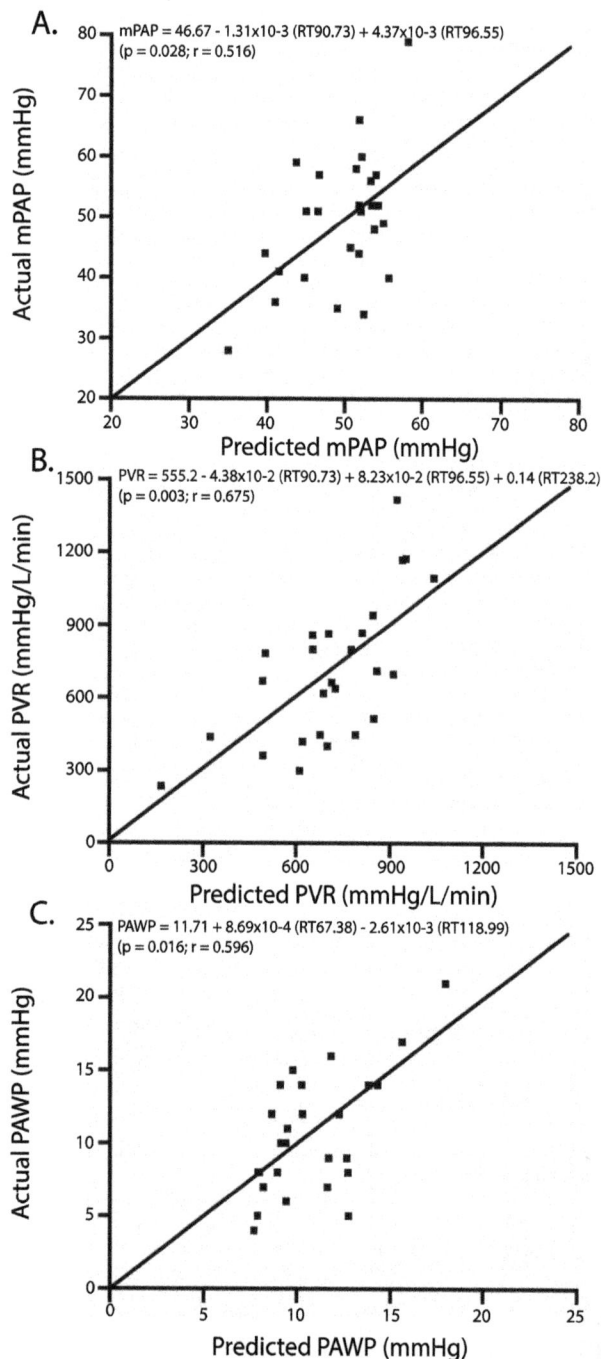

A. mPAP = 46.67 - 1.31x10-3 (RT90.73) + 4.37x10-3 (RT96.55)
(p = 0.028; r = 0.516)

B. PVR = 555.2 - 4.38x10-2 (RT90.73) + 8.23x10-2 (RT96.55) + 0.14 (RT238.2)
(p = 0.003; r = 0.675)

C. PAWP = 11.71 + 8.69x10-4 (RT67.38) - 2.61x10-3 (RT118.99)
(p = 0.016; r = 0.596)

Figure 3. Plots of step-wise linear regression analysis of actual vs. predicted values for mPAP, PVR, and PAWP. There were significant associations between mPAP and peak heights at retention times of 90.733 and 96.547 minutes (A); PVR and peak heights at retention times of 90.733, 96.547 and 238.247 minutes (B); PAWP and peak heights at retention times of 67.380 and 118.995 minutes (C).

outcomes of the AR/PLSR, correlation and regression analyses. This finding indicates that differences in BMI do not affect the unique characteristics of the chromatograms and individual peaks identified in our study groups using GC/MS.

The peak-by-peak analysis of GC/MS chromatograms provided insights into potential new biomarkers of disease severity and progression. Six peaks that were unique to the IPAH group

significantly correlated with pulmonary hemodynamics (Table 4). Interestingly, many identified biomarker compounds exhibited definite structural similarities: a number of compounds differed by only one functional group or could be formed from one another by common cellular chemical reactions. Overall, the identified IPAH group specific compounds appear to be more oxidized than specific compounds identified in the control group. For example, several substituted arenes presented in Table 3 (benzenamine; N-ethyl-, aniline, oxime-; methoxy-phenyl, benzaldehyde; ethanone, 2,2-dihydroxy-1-phenyl-; benzene, 1-methyl-4-(1-methylethenyl)-) could easily be converted to each other or result from common precursors such as phenylalanine, tryptophan or tyrosine due to bacterial degradation. Of note, benzene, 1-methyl-4-(1-methy-lethenyl)- is found in both the control and IPAH groups and is significantly lower in the IPAH group. Also of particular interest is benzothiazole (RT = 96.547 min), that is unique to the IPAH group and is significantly correlated with mPAP and PVR (Table 4).

Recently, Cikach et al. [20] analyzed expired breath in patients with NYHA class I-IV PAH using selected ion flow tube-mass spectrometry. They identified low molecular mass compounds (ammonia, propanol and alkenes) that discriminated between their control and PAH groups and that correlated with clinical markers of disease. These authors carried out a quantitative assessment of 21 pre-specified VOCs that were selected based on being previously described in association to or in the context of PAH disease. These chemical species also needed to be suitable for analysis using SIFT MS. The common restrictions of the SIFT MS method are an upper limit of mass of usually 240 Th and the need for multiple reactive ions for tentative compound identification [21]. More importantly, the SIFT MS method does not allow for unambiguous identification of unknown species, especially those of higher molecular mass that can have greater number of isomers. In Cikach et al. [20], mass scanning of ion products for H3O+, O2+, and NO+ from 14 to 200 atomic mass units was performed. Thus, to accommodate molecular ions such as NO+M, the parent's mass could not be higher than approximately 170 Th. In the present study, the SPME sorbent (carboxen/polydimethylsi-loxane) used for pre-concentration was optimized for molecular weight compounds of 30–225 Da. However, many compounds outside of this range can also be trapped. Additionally, the m/z range of the ion trap in the current study was set at 35–1000 Th ensuring inclusion of higher molecular weight biomarkers. By using this untargeted approach, the current study was able to identify several compounds not previously described and merit further investigation (Table 3). These structurally more complex molecules may convey more information regarding their source of origin and are less likely to result from background contamination [22]. Our subjects were NYHA class III and IV indicating that the metabolic profile of expired breath is altered in advanced IPAH. Additional studies that include NYHA functional class I and II patients would address whether the metabolites detected in the current study could be used in early detection of PAH.

The use of ExNO as a biomarker of IPAH has not always been successful partially due to variability seen in ExNO. ExNO has been reported to be decreased [23–25], normal [26], or increased [27] in PAH patients. In the current study, ExNO was significantly lower in IPAH patients compared to control subjects. ExNO was not correlated with any pulmonary hemodynamic endpoints in the current study. The present study included data on two previously described biomarkers of IPAH severity, plasma BNP and ExNO. Elevated plasma BNP or n-terminal proBNP has been shown to be correlated with the severity of right ventricular dysfunction in pulmonary hypertension [28–30]. In addition, BNP has been

Table 4. Correlations with pulmonary hemodynamic variables.

RT (min) or Biomarker	mPAP	PVR	PAWP
67.380			0.429 (26; 0.029)
81.436^	0.554 (14; 0.040)		
90.733	−0.423 (26; 0.031)	−0.476 (26; 0.014)	
96.547^	0.475 (26; 0.014)	0.427 (26; 0.029)	
118.995			−0.497 (26; 0.019)
238.247		0.483 (26; 0.012)	
ExNO	−0.132 (25; 0.530)	−0.242 (25; 0.243)	−0.181 (25; 0.386)
BNP	−0.204 (23; 0.351)	−0.159 (23; 0.468)	0.273 (23; 0.208)

Pearson correlation coefficients r (number of subjects; p value); ^ identified chemically with high confidence; RT = retention time; mPAP = mean pulmonary arterial pressure; PVR = pulmonary vascular resistance; PAWP = pulmonary arterial wedge pressure; ExNO = exhaled nitric oxide; BNP = brain naturetic peptide.

shown to be valuable as a prognostic indicator of IPAH [31] and is responsive to endothelin receptor antagonist treatment [32]. In contrast, our results show that BNP was not significantly correlated with any hemodynamic endpoints, including right atrial pressure. Given our restricted sampling of severe IPAH the lack of significant correlation with mPAP or any other hemodynamic measure should not be interpreted to mean that there is no relationship to BNP and the IPAH disease process. If a boarder range of diseases was present in our group or if BNP and hemodynamic values were available in our controls, then BNP may well have correlated with hemodynamic measures.

Our findings indicate the utility of EBC VOC analysis to discriminate between individuals with severe IPAH and age-matched healthy individuals and provides a means for identifying novel biomarkers significantly correlated with IPAH pulmonary hemodynamics. This novel metabolomics approach of analyzing VOCs in EBC in patients with IPAH using GC/MS provides a potential diagnostic tool for classification of disease severity and progression and will need to be confirmed in other subgroups of PAH that differ in severity and etiology to clarify its utility in disease management and detection.

Supporting Information

Table S1 Concomitant medication/supplements list for IPAH subjects. Number of subjects taking each medication in parentheses.

Acknowledgments

The authors would like to thank Ms. Macey Kelly for her assistance in recruiting subjects into the trial and the colation of the concomitant medication data.

Author Contributions

Conceived and designed the experiments: JKM ESS CED WFW RA. Performed the experiments: JKM ESS CED WFW WZ AAA AP JF RA. Analyzed the data: JKM ESS CED WFW WZ AAA AP JF RA. Contributed reagents/materials/analysis tools: ESS CED. Wrote the paper: JKM ESS CED WFW WZ AAA AP JF RA.

References

1. Alfaro MF, Walby WF, Adams WC, Schelegle ES (2007) Breath condensate levels of 8-isoprostane and leukotriene B4 after ozone inhalation are greater in sensitive versus nonsensitive subjects. Exp Lung Res 33:115–133.

2. Carpagnano GE, Resta O, Gelardi M, Spanevello A, Di Gioia G, et al. (2007) Exhaled inflammatory markers in aspirin-induced asthma syndrome. Am J Rhinology 21(5): 542–547.

3. Conrad DH, Goyette J, Thomas PS (2008) Proteomics as a method for early detection of cancer: a review of proteomics, exhaled breath condensate, and lung cancer screening. J Gen Int Med (suppl 1): 78–84.

4. Phillips M, Altorki N, Austin J, Cameron RB, Cataneo RN, et al. (2007) Prediction of lung cancer using volatile biomarkers in breath. Cancer Biomarkers 3(2): 95–109.

5. O'Reilly P, Bailey W (2007) Clinical use of exhaled biomarkers in COPD. Int J Chron Obstr Pulm Dis 2: 403–408.

6. Phillips M, Cataneo RN, Condos R, Ring Erickson GA, Greenberg J, et al. (2007) Volatile biomarkers of pulmonary tuberculosis in the breath. Tuberculosis 87(1): 44–52.

7. Van Muylem A, Knoop C, Estenne M (2007) Early detection of chronic pulmonary allograft dysfunction by exhaled biomarkers. Am J Respir Crit Care Med 175(7): 731–736.

8. Phillips M, Cataneo RN, Ditkoff BA, Fisher P, Greenberg J, et al. (2006) Prediction of breast cancer using volatile biomarkers in the breath. Breast Cancer Res and Treat 99(1): 19–21.

9. Phillips M, Boehmer JP, Cataneo RN, Cheema T, Eisen HJ, et al. (2004) Prediction of heart transplant rejection with a breath test for markers of oxidative stress. Am J Cardio 94(12): 1593–1594.

10. Phillips M, Cataneo RN, Cheema T, Greenberg J (2004) Increased breath biomarkers of oxidative stress in diabetes mellitus. Clinica Chimica Acta 344(1–2): 189–194.

11. Phillips M, Cataneo RN, Greenberg J, Grodman R, Salazar M (2003) Breath markers of oxidative stress in patients with unstable angina. Heart Disease 5(2): 95–99.

12. Mansoor JK, Morrissey BM, Walby WF, Yoneda KY, Juarez M, et al. (2005) L-arginine supplementation enhances exhaled NO, breath condensate VEGF, and headache at 4,342 m. High Alt Med Biol 6(4): 289–300.

13. American Thoracic Society (1999) Recommendations for standardized procedures for the online and offline measurement of exhaled lower respiratory nitric oxide and nasal nitric oxide in adults and children. Am. J. Respir Crit Care Med 160:2104–2117.

14. Molina M, Zhao W, Sankaran S, Schivo M, Kenyon NJ, et al. (2008) Design-of-experiment optimization of exhaled breath condensate analysis using a miniature differential mobility spectrometer (DMS). Analytica Chimica Acta 628:155–161.

15. Andrade L, Manolakos ES (2003) Signal backgound estimatin and baseline correction algorithms for accurate DNA sequencing. J VLSI Signal Process 35:229–243.

16. Zhao WX, Davis CE (2009) Autoregressive model based feature extraction method for time shifted chromatography data. Chemom Intell Lab Syst 96:252–257.

17. Zhao W, Morgan JT, Davis CE (2008) Gas chromatography data classification based on complex coefficients of an autoregressive model. J Sensors [serial online]. Available at: http://www.hindawi.com/journals/js/2008/262501/ via the Internet. Accessed 11 Feb 2011.

18. Hoeper MM, Bogaard HJ, Condliffe R, Frantz R, Khanna D, et al. (2013) Definitions and diagnosis of pulmonary hypertension. JACC 62:SupplD 42–50.

19. Windey K, De Preter V, Louat T, Schuit F, Herman J, et al. (2012) Modulation of protein fermentation does not affect fecal water toxicity: a randomized cross-over study in healthy subjects. PLoS One [serial online]. Dec. 20.

20. Cikach F, Tonelli A, Barnes J, Paschke K, Newman J, et al. (2013) Breath analysis in pulmonary arterial hypertension. Chest [Epub ahead of print]. Available: http://journal.publications.chestnet.org/article.aspx?articleid = 1745983 via the internet. Accessed 22 Nov 2013.

21. Smith D, Spaněl P (2011) Ambient analysis of trace compounds in gaseous media by SIFT-MS. Analyst 36:2009–2032.

22. Kwak J, Petri G (2011) Volatile disease biomarkers in breath: a critique. Curr Pharm Biotechnol 12:1067–1074.

23. Girgis RE, Champion HC, Diette GB, Johns RA, Permutt S, et al. (2005) Decreased exhaled nitric oxide in pulmonary arterial hypertension. Am J Respir Crit Care Med 172:352–357.

24. Cremona G, Higenbottam T, Borland C, Mist B (1994) Mixed expired nitric oxide in primary pulmonary hypertension in relation to lung diffusion capacity. QJM 87:547–551.

25. Kaneko FT, Arroliga AC, Dweik RA, Comhair SA, Laskowski D, et al. (1998) Biochemical reaction products of nitric oxide as quantitative markers of primary pulmonary hypertension. Am J Respir Crit Care Med 158:917–923.

26. Riley MS, Pórszász J, Miranda J, Engelen MP, Brundage B, et al. (1997) Exhaled nitric oxide during exercise in primary pulmonary hypertension and pulmonary fibrosis. Chest 111:44–50.

27. Archer SL, Djaballah K, Humbert M, Weir KE, Fartoukh M, et al. (1998) Nitric oxide deficiency in fenfluramine- and dexfenfluramine-induced pulmonary hypertension. Am J Respir Crit Care Med 158:1061–1067.

28. Nagaya N, Nishikimi T, Okano Y, Uematsu M, Satoh T, et al. (1998) Plasma brain natriuretic peptide levels increase in proportion to the extent of right ventricular dysfunction in pulmonary hypertension. J Am Coll Cardiol 31:202–208.

29. Leuchte HH, Holzapfel M, Baumgartner RA, Ding I, Neurohr C, et al. (2004) Clinical significance of brain natriuretic peptide in primary pulmonary hypertension. J Am Coll Cardiol 43:764–770.

30. Fijalkowsha A, Kurzyna M, Torbicki A, Szewczyk G, Florczyk M, et al. (2006) Serum n-terminal brain natriuretic peptide as a prognostic parameter in patients with pulmonary hypertension. Chest 129:1313–1321.

31. Nagaya N, Nishikimi T, Uematsu M, Satoh T, Kyotani S, et al. (2001) Plasma brain natriuretic peptide as a prognostic indicator in patients with primary pulmonary hypertension. Circulation 102:865–870.

32. Droste AS, Rohde D, Voelkers M, Filush A, Bruckner T, et al. (2009) Endothelin receptor antagonist and airway dysfunction in pulmonary arterial hypertension. Respir Res 10:129–136.

23

Identification of a New Intronic BMPR2-Mutation and Early Diagnosis of Heritable Pulmonary Arterial Hypertension in a Large Family with Mean Clinical Follow-Up of 12 Years

Katrin Hinderhofer[1,9], Christine Fischer[1,9], Nicole Pfarr[1,2]*, Justyna Szamalek-Hoegel[1], Mona Lichtblau[2], Christian Nagel[2], Benjamin Egenlauf[2], Nicola Ehlken[2], Ekkehard Grünig[2]*

1 Institute of Human Genetics, University of Heidelberg, Heidelberg, Germany, 2 Centre for pulmonary hypertension of the Thoraxclinic, University Hospital of Heidelberg, Heidelberg, Germany

Abstract

Background: Mutations in the bone morphogenetic protein receptor 2 (*BMPR2*) gene can lead to hereditary pulmonary arterial hypertension (HPAH) and are detected in more than 80% of cases with familial aggregation of the disease. Factors determining disease penetrance are largely unknown.

Methods: A mean clinical follow-up of 12 years was accomplished in 46 family members including echocardiography, stress-Dopplerechocardiography and genetic analysis of TGF-β pathway genes. Right heart catheterization and RNA-analysis was performed in members with pathological findings.

Results: Manifest HPAH was diagnosed in 8 members, 4 were already deceased, two died during the follow-up, two are still alive. Normal pulmonary artery systolic pressure at rest but hypertensive response to exercise has been identified in 19 family members. Analysis of *BMPR2* transcripts revealed aberrant splicing due to an insertion of an intronic Alu element adjacent to exon 6. All HPAH patients and 12 further asymptomatic family members carried this insertion. During follow-up two family members carrying hypertensive response and the Alu insertion developed manifest HPAH.

Conclusion: This is the first report of an intronic BMPR2 mutation due to an Alu element insertion causing HPAH in a large family which has been confirmed on RNA-level. Only those members that carried both hypertensive response and the mutation developed manifest HPAH during follow-up. Our findings highlight the importance of including further methods such as RNA analysis into the molecular genetic diagnostic of PAH patients. They suggest that at least in some families hypertensive response may be an additional risk factor for disease manifestation and penetrance.

Editor: James West, Vanderbilt University Medical Center, United States of America

Funding: The authors have no support or funding to report.

Competing Interests: CN receives lecture and/or consultancy fees from Actelion, GlaxoSmithKline, Pfizer, BayerHealthCare, Takeda/Nycomed, BerlinChemie, and Boehringer Ingelheim. BE receives lecture fees from Actelion. NE receives lecture fees from BayerHealthCare, Pfizer. EG receives lecture and/or consultancy fees from Actelion, Bayer, Gilead, GlaxoSmithKline, Lilly, Miltenyi, Novartis, Pfizer, RotexMedica, Alexion and received honoraria for clinical studies from Actelion, Bayer, GSK, Encysive, Lilly, United Therapeutics and Pfizer. He is member of the expert committees of BayerHealthCare, GlaxoSmithKline, Actelion, and Pfizer. There are no patents, products in development, or marketed products to declare.

* E-mail: ekkehard.gruenig@thoraxklinik-heidelberg.de

9 These authors contributed equally to this work.

Introduction

Pulmonary arterial hypertension (PAH) can be idiopathic (IPAH), heritable (HPAH) or associated with other conditions (APAH) [1] and is usually not detected before patients are severely affected with symptoms according to WHO-functional class III–IV and reduced prognosis [2]. Therefore, it might be of great value to identify the disease at an early stage.

Since 2000 in HPAH-patients and families several mutations of genes of the transforming growth factor beta (TGF-β) superfamily of receptors have been found as in the bone morphogenetic

protein receptor 2 (*BMPR2*) gene [3–5], *Activin A receptor type II-like 1* (*ACVRL1*, also called *ALK1*) [6], *Endoglin* [7], and *SMAD9* [8] (also called SMAD8).

However, the major genetic determinant underlying HPAH are germline heterozygous mutations of the *BMPR2* gene on chromosome 2q33 that account for approximately 80% of patients with a known family history of PAH and 20% of apparently sporadic cases [9,10]. More than 300 independent *BMPR2* mutations have been detected so far which are widely distributed across the 13 exons of the gene [5]. Today, standard genetic screening methods focus on the sequencing of the exonic coding regions of the *BMPR2*, *Alk1*, *Endoglin*, and *SMAD9* genes [11]. Intronic regions have not been studied systematically so far, though they might harbour disease causing mutations.

Although HPAH is a monogenetic disease with autosomal dominant inheritance [12] only ~20% of BMPR2-mutation carriers will develop the disease due to an incomplete age and gender related penetrance [12,13]. The underlying factors of the incomplete penetrance are yet unknown. Thus, in HPAH-families there are asymptomatic gene carriers with an approximately 20%-risk to develop manifest HPAH during their life span who might potentially be detected at an early stage of disease. Regular echocardiography and genetic counseling have been recommended in several PH-guidelines [1,14,15]. However, reports on follow-up assessments in these families analyzing the natural course of the disease and clinical signs of an early manifestation are lacking. So far there are no systematic prospective long-term follow-up studies which evaluated the usefulness of screening-assessments in these families. In one case, onset of HPAH was detected by follow-up cardiopulmonary exercise testing in an initially healthy relative with BMPR-2 mutation [16].

We previously described a large German family (S965) with 7 affected members in 3 generations [17]. This family had no identifiable mutations in *BMPR2* gene by exonic sequencing or multiple ligation-dependent probe amplification, although linkage to chromosome 2q32-33 has been detected [18]. At baseline, several members of this family with no signs of manifest PAH at rest showed hypertensive pulmonary artery systolic pressure (PASP) response to exercise (HR), measured by stress-Dopplerechocardiography [17,18]. In a large multicenter study similar findings have been obtained in other PAH-families. In this study HR during exercise and hypoxia was identified more frequently in relatives of PAH patients than in healthy controls and was associated with a significantly higher proportion of BMPR2-mutations [19]. It was hypothesized, that this phenotype might constitute a risk factor for the development of manifest PAH in some asymptomatic relatives.

The aim of this study was to extend the molecular genetic analyses in this family to the candidate genes *ALK1*, *ENG*, or *SMAD9* and to RNA analysis of the *BMPR2* gene and to explore if manifest PAH can be clinically detected at an early stage in further family members by regular non-invasive follow-up assessments. Furthermore, the natural clinical course of asymptomatic mutation carriers and HR-members should be analysed.

Materials and Methods

Study population and design

The study group consisted of a large German family (S965). A four generation pedigree has been drawn including 83 family members, 59 related to the founder couple (Figure 1).

All 48 living genetically related members were invited to participate in a clinical and genetic evaluation. After informed consent was obtained, 46 members underwent clinical assessment and genetic counseling. EDTA-blood and anticoagulated whole blood were taken for genetic analysis. All relatives were native-born residents of a low altitude area and were assessed in Heidelberg, Germany, at an altitude of ~100 meters. The study was approved by the Ethics Committee of the Medical Faculty of the University of Heidelberg. All patients gave written informed consent to the study. Informed consent was additionally obtained from the caretaker in case of enrolment of children.

Clinical procedures

Assessments consisted of recording the family and medical history, physical examination, laboratory parameters including N-type pro brain natriuretic peptide (NT-proBNP), 12-lead ECG, lung function test, arterial blood gases, echocardiography, stress-Dopplerechocardiography (SDE) and cardiopulmonary exercise testing. Manifest HPAH was diagnosed according to the current guidelines [1]. Left heart catheterization and/or CT-scan of the lungs were performed in all patients with suspected left heart or respiratory diseases and when clinically indicated. Right heart catheterization was performed in the living HPAH patients, in the first degree family members and in all family members with suspicion of PH during follow-up.

Echocardiography

Two-dimensional and Dopplerechocardiographic recordings were obtained using 2.5 MHz Duplex transducers and conventional equipment (Aloka Vario View 2200, Tokyo, Japan) as described previously [19]. Echocardiographic studies were performed by experienced cardiac sonographers (EG, CN), who had no knowledge of the molecular genetic data.

Stress-Dopplerechocardiography (SDE)

The participants were examined on a supine bicycle ergometer (model 8420; KHL Corp., Kirkland, Washington) as described previously [19]. Systolic pulmonary arterial pressure was estimated from peak tricuspid regurgitation jet velocities according to the equation: $PASP = 4 (V)^2 + 5$ mmHg, where V is the peak velocity (in m/s) of tricuspid valve regurgitant jet, and 5 mmHg is the estimated right atrial pressure. Maximal tricuspid velocity was measured at the highest coherent boundary on the spectral wave form. Signals were considered technically adequate if they had complete envelopes with well-defined borders. In subjects with inadequate Doppler-signals, SDE was repeated within 6–18 months. PASP<25 mmHg at rest and ≤40 mmHg during exercise were classified as normal.[19] Hypertensive PASP response was declared when maximal systolic pulmonary arterial pressure >40 mmHg was reached during low-dose exercise (up to 125 Watt) in at least one measurement under exclusion of causal hypertensive systemic blood pressure. In patients with hypertensive systemic blood pressure and diastolic dysfunction, treatment for arterial hypertension was initiated.

Measurements during Hypoxia

Measurements were performed in family members with no known manifest HPAH at baseline = initial visit and in some family members at the next control visit (n = 23). Measurements were performed in a hypoxia-room with a gas mixture of 12% oxygen and 88% nitrogen corresponding to an altitude of 4.500 m. The subjects were examined in supine position and oxygen saturation and heart rate were recorded continuously using a fingertip pulse oxymeter (Ohmeda Biox 3700, Louisville, Colorado, USA). Two-dimensional and Doppler-echocardiographic recordings were performed during baseline in normoxia and at 45, 90, and 120 minutes of hypoxia ($F_iO_2 = 12\%$). PASP was estimated as described. For all calculations the mean value of at least 3 TRV measurements was used. Right atrial pressure has been estimated from characteristics of the inferior vena cava [20].

Right heart catheterization

Right heart catheterization was carried out simultaneously with SDE in all living PAH patients and in 12 first degree family members, using a Swan-Ganz balloon tipped catheter (Baxter,

Family S965

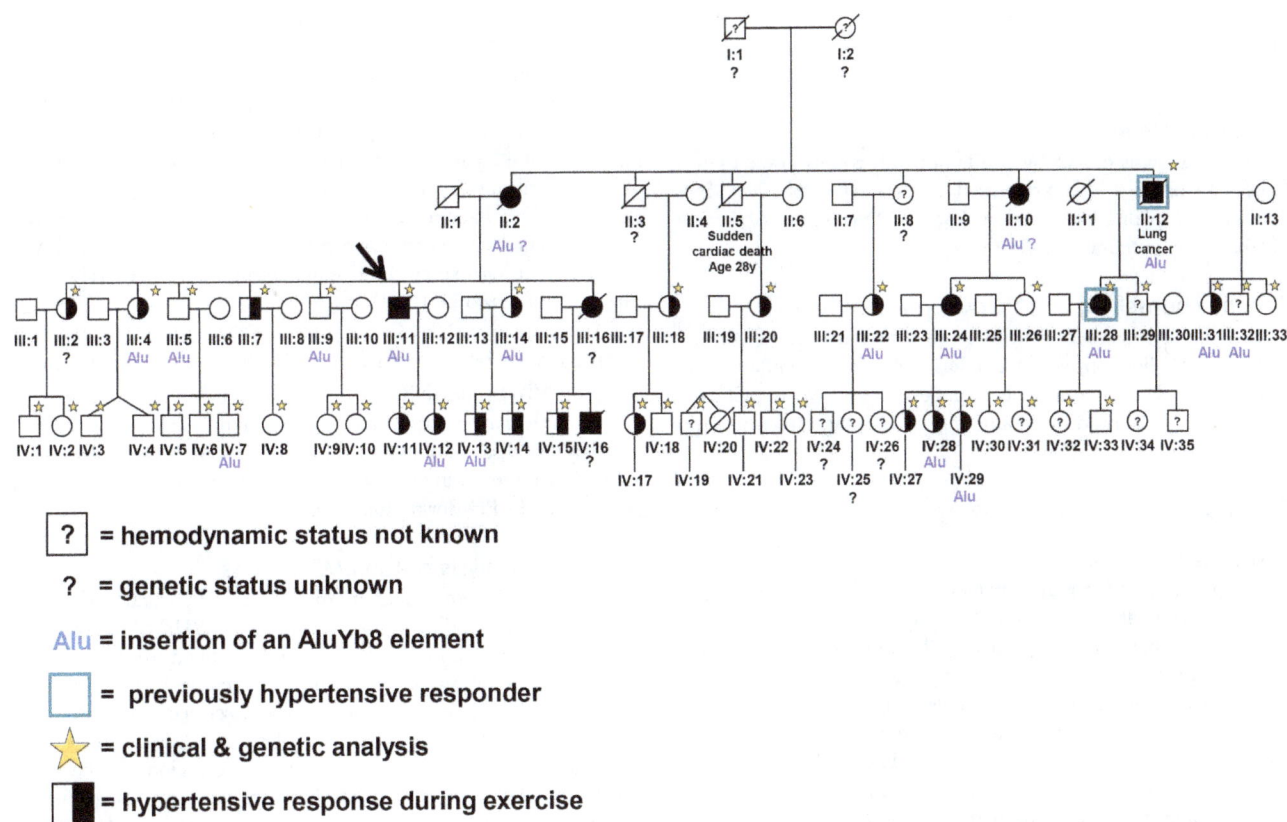

? = hemodynamic status not known

? = genetic status unknown

Alu = insertion of an AluYb8 element

☐ = previously hypertensive responder

★ = clinical & genetic analysis

◧ = hypertensive response during exercise

Figure 1. Pedigree of the large German family. This figure represents the pedigree tree of the German family analysed in this study. The index patient of the family is marked by an arrow. All family members with manifest PAH are shown in black. Healthy family members have open symbols and those who were heterozygous for the identified mutation are marked with "Alu". Those family members with hypertensive response due to exercise have half-filled symbols. Family members with unknown hemodynamic status have open symbols with a question mark inside. A question mark below the pedigree ID indicates that the genetic status in this family member is unknown. An open blue square marks the family members which presented at the beginning of the follow-up with hypertensive response due to exercise and changed their status to manifest PAH (II:12 and III:28). All family members who participated in the clinical and/or genetic analysis are marked by a star. The numbering of the individuals in the pedigree corresponds to the IDs of the family members in table 1.

Santa Ana, USA) placed in the pulmonary artery. Pressures at rest and during supine bicycle exercise were recorded using a polygraph (Hellige, Freiburg, Germany). Cardiac output and mixed venous oxygen saturation were obtained at rest and during exercise as described before [19].

Mutation analysis

Human genomic DNA was prepared from peripheral blood lymphocytes. The complete coding sequence and exon/intron boundaries of the *BMPR2* gene were amplified and analysed by direct sequencing according to Sanger. The complete 5′ untranslated region of the *BMPR2* gene (up to position c.-1270) and the complete intron 5 were also investigated. Primer sequences and PCR conditions are available upon request. Standard DNA sequencing reactions were performed using version 1.1 of Big Dye terminator cycle sequencing kit (Applied Biosystems Inc., Darmstadt) and were analysed on a 3100 Genetic Analyzer (Applied Biosystems Inc., Darmstadt). Screening for larger *BMPR2* rearrangements was performed with the SALSA Multiplex Ligation-dependent Probe Amplification (MLPA) P093-B1 HHT/PPH1 probe mix kit (MRC-Holland BV, Amsterdam, The Netherlands). Mutation nomenclature refers to the NCBI

human *BMPR2* nucleotide sequence (Accession number: NM_001204) with A of the ATG start codon denoted as +1 and initiator methionine as codon 1.

Furthermore, we analyzed the complete coding sequences of 5 other genes participating in the signalling pathway (*ALK1*, *ENG*, *SMAD1*, *SMAD5*, and *SMAD9*).

RNA analysis

Lymphocytes from the index patient (III:11) his healthy sister (III:14) were isolated from anticoagulated whole blood and exposed to Epstein - Barr virus (EBV) to induce cell immortalization as previously described [21,22]. Total RNA was isolated from peripheral blood lymphocytes from all family members and from the cultivated lymphocytes, respectively, by use of a phenol–chloroform method according to Chomczynski and Sacchi [23]. Synthesis of cDNA was performed using Superscript II reverse transcriptase (Life Technologies, Darmstadt) according to manufacturers' recommendation.

Reverse transcription was performed by use of the Transcriptor Reverse Trancriptase Kit according to the manufacturer's recommendations. The following PCR was performed by use of a forward primer located in the untranslated region of exon 1 and a set of reverse primers located in exons 2 to 7 (Roche Diagnostics GmbH, Mannheim; primer sequences and PCR conditions are available upon request). If necessary, RT-PCR products were subcloned by use of the TOPO-TA cloning kit (Life Technologies, Darmstadt). Positive clones were sequenced in both directions.

Statistical methods

For the analysis of two by two tables with counts lower than 5 Fishers Exact Test was performed using IBM SPSS 20 (SPSS Statistics V20, IBM Corporation, Somers, New York). A p-value <0.05 was counted as significant.

Genetic counselling and follow-up assessments

In all family members genetic counselling has been performed and clinical follow-up assessment has been recommended in all genetically related family members every 2–6 years. Clinical assessments comprised the same procedures at screening and during follow-up.

Results

Clinical assessment

The pedigree of the family includes 83 relatives (Figure 1, 2) of which 59 are related to the founder couple (I:1 and I:2). In 1996 when the initial screening started, 11 relatives were already deceased. In total 46 family members participated in the study (21 males, mean age 25.4±13.6 y). Follow-up examinations were performed every 2–6 years with a maximum of 17 years and a mean follow-up time of 12±6.6 years (Figure 2). In 5 family members, PASP during exercise was not measurable. Two patients were not able to perform the cardiopulmonary exercise testing, e.g. family member IV:19, born in the sixth month of pregnancy, presented with spastic tetraplegia and member III:32 could not perform stress echocardiography due to neurological defects. Three family members (III:29, IV:31, IV:32) had poor Doppler-echocardiographic signals. In two family members, elevated PASP response during at least one measurement occurred due to arterial hypertension (III:5, III:9). These patients were classified as normal, as PASP also showed normal increase during hypoxia (III:5, III:9).

Family members with manifest HPAH

Pulmonary arterial hypertension was already diagnosed in the index patient (III:11) and his female cousin (III:24). Four other family members, who also suffered from HPAH, were already deceased due to right heart failure (II:2, II:10, III:16, IV:16). The index patient died at the age of 57 due to right heart failure, 38 years after diagnosis. His female cousin (III:24) is still alive after initial diagnosis in 1989 (24 years of disease duration until today). Another member (III:28) is still alive after 8 years of PAH. Family members II:2, II:12, II:10, III:16 and IV:16 died within 1 to 5 years (mean: 2.2±1.6 years) after diagnosis, after a short period of disease duration. Family member II:12 died at the age of 69 after the development of lung cancer.

Family members with normal PASP at rest- hypertensive PASP-response to exercise and/or hypoxia (HR)

In 19 relatives with normal PASP at rest elevated PASP-response to exercise and/or hypoxia was observed (Table 1). Two of the 19 family members developed manifest HPAH during follow-up, four (II:12) and seven (III:28) years after the first screening (Figure 1, 2). Two further family members with HR (III:18 and III:20) developed secondary pulmonary hypertension

due to diastolic dysfunction of the left ventricle one year after primary assessments.

One family member (III:4) with HR status recently presented with diastolic dysfunction of the left ventricle. In her last follow-up examination in 2013, she presented with a maximal mean pulmonary arterial pressure of 42 mmHg at 125 Watts and an elevated systemic diastolic pressure of 100 mmHg.

In 11 of 12 patients with hypertensive response (92%), PASP response during hypoxia was equal to PASP response during exercise. One patient who showed normal values during hypoxia was classified as hypertensive responder due to elevated PASP increase during exercise and equal results during exercise right heart catheterization (III:4).

Family members with normal PASP at rest and during exercise/hypoxia (NR)

Twenty relatives presented with normal PASP response (NR) during exercise. Results of echocardiography were in-line with PASP-increase during hypoxia. No NR-members developed PAH or secondary PH during follow-up.

Genomic analysis of the BMPR2 gene

After direct sequencing in the index patient no pathogenic mutation in the coding regions for the genes BMPR2, ALK1, ENG, SMAD1, SMAD5, and SMAD9 could be identified. In exon 5 of the BMPR2 gene we found one known polymorphism c.600A>C (p.L200L). This sequence variant was described previously with the frequency of 2.4%.[5] MLPA analysis did also not reveal any large deletion or duplication in the coding regions of the genes BMPR2, ALK1 and ENG. Therefore, we performed screening of the 5′ untranslated region of BMPR2 exon 1 including the putative promoter region (up to position c.−1270). By this we found only one heterozygous single nucleotide insertion of a cytosine between the nucleotides at position −212 and −211 (c.-212_-211insC). This insertion occurred within a short C-mononucleotide tract consisting of 7 cytosines (Figure 3A). Although we could not confirm the presence of this variant in a cohort of unrelated German controls (n = 86) its polymorphic nature cannot be excluded. PCR experiments performed in relatives of the index patient indicated that both derived sequence variants, the C insertion in 5′ UTR and the A>C polymorphism in exon 5, are located on the same allele. We identified these two variants also in further unrelated patients with I/HPAH (n = 15).

Analysis of the BMPR2 transcript

For the investigation of the BMPR2 transcript in the index patient we used these two heterozygous sequence variants: c.600A>C and c.-212_-211insC as markers. The analyses were performed with the forward primer (Figure 3A, F2) located in the upstream 5′-untranslated region of exon 1 in combination with reverse primers located in exons 2 to 5. This resulted in PCR products containing a C insertion in heterozygous state. In the case of the primer from the distal part of exon 5 the A>C polymorphism was also detected heterozygous (data not shown). This observation indicates transcription of both BMPR2 alleles. By using a reverse primer located at the beginning of exon 6 (BMPR2-X6-1-RT-R) we could amplify only the wild type allele with respect to both polymorphic variants (Figure 3B, marked as R1 in figure 3b). Further analysis performed with primers located in exons 4 - 7 and 5 - 7, respectively, resulted in amplification of at least five PCR products of different size (Figure 3B). Cloning of the different PCR products and sequencing analysis revealed the presence of the wild type transcript with the entire exon 6, and of

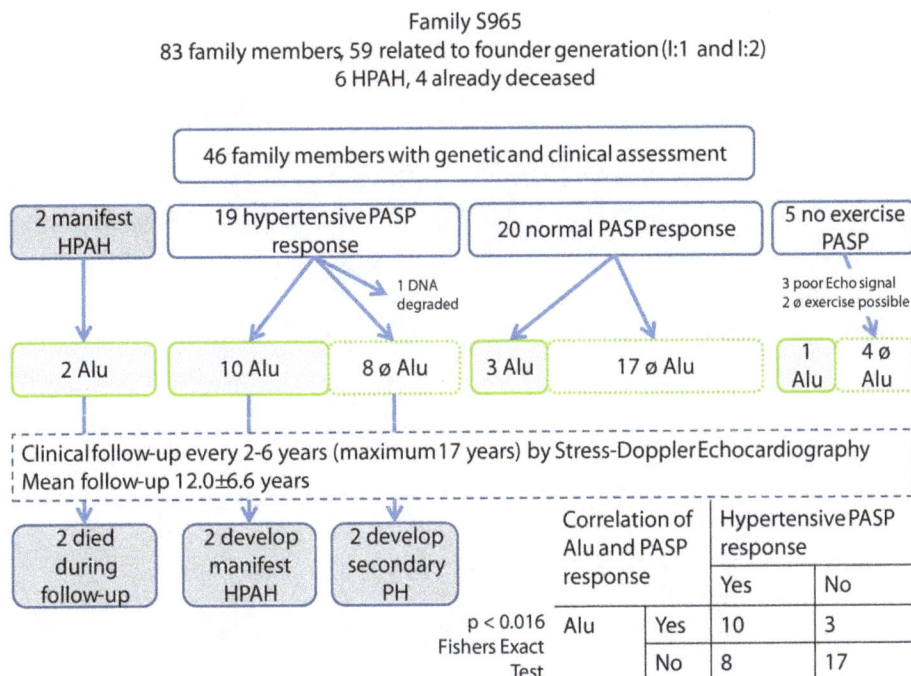

Figure 2. Genotype-phenotype correlations of Alu carriers and PASP during exercise. This figure shows the genotype-phenotype correlation between Alu insertion and PASP during exercise, classified as HR and NR. Only patients who carried both HR and Alu insertion developed manifest PAH during follow-up. Patients with the Alu insertion in the *BMPR2* gene show significantly more frequent Hypertensive response to exercise (10/13 vs. 8/25; Fishers exact test p = 0.016).

four aberrant transcripts. In one, the entire exon 6 was missing (231 bp, position c.622 to c.852, transcript 5) whereas in the second aberrant transcript only the distal fragment of exon 6 (position c.715 to c.852, transcript 4) could be detected. As inferred from the *BMPR2* structure, if translated, the loss of exon 6 does not lead to the change in frame but to the loss of 77 amino acids (amino acids p.208 to p.284). The loss of the first 93 bp of exon 6 in the second abnormal transcript results in deletion of amino acids p.209 to p.238 encompassing the complete ATP binding site of the serine/threonine kinase domain. The two larger products contained both the complete exon 6, 13 bases of the flanking sequence of intron 5 (splice acceptor site), and in addition parts of an Alu element of different length (Figure 3B, transcripts 1 and 2). All aberrant splice products contained the polymorphic c.600C variant whereas in the wild type product the c.600A variant was present indicating that the insertion lies on the same allele as the two polymorphic variants (c.600A>C and c.-212_-211insC). Transcripts 1 and 2 could not been amplified with primer set F1 and R1 presumably due to the AT rich regions close to the primer binding site of R1.

Screening of the intronic *BMPR2* regions

In order to search for the mutation which caused the aberrant splicing of exon 6, we sequenced the adjacent flanking intronic regions. In intron 6 we did not find any mutation. In contrast, with a forward primer located in intron 5 and the reverse primer situated in exon 6 we obtained two PCR products of different length. Sequencing of the longer, gel-extracted PCR product revealed an insertion of an Alu element (AluYb8) in antisense orientation to *BMPR2* 26 bp upstream of exon 6 (c.622-26_-27insAluYb8), which is flanked by a direct duplication of a CCTTGCTTTCTTT sequence (c.622-13_-26; Figure 4). The aberrant *BMPR2* allele is at least 329 bp longer than the normal

one. Because of polymerase slippage events during amplification of a long poly-T tract, which is present at the end of this insert, the exact length of the insert could not be estimated.

The Alu insertion was not found in 116 analysed control persons nor reported in the 1000 Genomes Project. Additionally, we did not find the insertion (data not shown).

Genotype-phenotype correlation

Clinical and molecular genetic information of the family are summarized in Figure 2. In 46 family members clinical assessment and genetic analysis was performed. We found the AluYb8 insertion in 16 family members, four of them with HPAH. According to the inheritance pattern, at least two further deceased family members with manifest PAH were carriers of this insertion (II:2 and II:10, see Figure 1). Additionally, person II:8 carried the insertion but her phenotype could not be determined. For two deceased patients with HPAH neither genetic analysis could be performed nor can the inheritance pattern be used to infer the genetic status. In total 6 of the 15 (13+2 deceased) AluYb8 carriers developed a manifest HPAH resulting in a penetrance of 0.40 (95% CI 0.163–0.677) for this family. If we use the pedigree information and hypothesize that the remaining two HPAH patients (II:2 and II:10) had the AluYb8 insertion as well, the penetrance is 0.47 (8/17, 95% CI 0.230–0.722).

Follow-up data from the echocardiographic measurement of the PASP during exercise was compared between family members carrying the AluYb8 insertion with those family members without the insertion. Ten carriers of the Alu insertion showed a hypertensive PASP response (HR; >40 mmHg) during exercise. A significantly smaller number presented with HR among Alu negative family members (8/25, p<0.016, Fishers exact test, Figure 2). BMPR2 genotype and the PASP status HR/NR were

Table 1. Clinical and genetic assessment in family members.

Pedigree ID	Age at first screening (years)	male/female	BMPR2 (AluYb8 insertion)	Classification due to PASP response during exercise	Echocardiography	Hypoxia	RHC
III:28	35	f	y/PAH	HR ⇨ PAH (age 44 y)	✓		✓
II:12	64	m	y/PAH	HR ⇨ PAH (age 69 y)	✓		✓
III:2	54	f	n.m.	HR	✓	✓	✓
III:4	48	f	y	HR	✓	✓	✓
III:7	44	m	n	HR	✓	✓	✓
III:14	40	f	y	HR	✓		✓
III:22	45	f	y	HR	✓		
III:31	18	f	y	HR	✓		
IV:15	26	m	n	NR	✓	✓	
IV:11	10	f	n	HR	✓	✓	
IV:12	15	f	y	HR	✓		✓
IV:13	13	m	y	HR	✓	✓	
IV:14	10	m	n	HR	✓		
IV:17	17	f	n	HR	✓		
IV:27	16	f	n	HR	✓	✓	
IV:28	13	f	y	HR	✓		
IV:29	10	f	y	HR	✓		
III:18	43	f	n	HR ⇨ sec. PH	✓		✓
III:20	58	f	n	HR ⇨ sec. PH	✓		✓
III:5	47	m	y	NR	✓	✓	✓
III:9	43	m	y	NR	✓	✓	
III:26	38	f	n	NR	✓		
III:33	16	f	n	NR	✓		
IV:1	20	m	n	NR	✓	✓	
IV:2	15	f	n	NR	✓		✓
IV:3	12	m	n	NR	✓		
IV:4	12	m	n	NR	✓	✓	
IV:5	17	m	n	NR	✓		
IV:6	14	m	n	NR	✓	✓	✓
IV:7	11	m	y	NR	✓	✓	
IV:9	15	f	n	NR	✓		
IV:10	19	f	n	NR	✓	✓	
IV:8	10	f	n	HR	✓	✓	
IV:18	15	m	n	NR			
IV:21	35	m	n	NR	✓		

Table 1. Cont.

Pedigree ID	Age at first screening (years)	male/female	BMPR2 (AluYb8 insertion)	Classification due to PASP response during exercise	Echocardiography	Hypoxia	RHC
IV-22	29	m	n	NR	✓		
IV-23	26	f	n	NR	✓		
IV-30	11	f	n	NR	✓		
IV-33	5	m	n	NR	✓		
III-29	30	m	n	n.m.	✓		
III-32	17	m	y	n. m. (seizures)	✓		
IV-19	36	m	n	n. m. (spastic tetraplegia)	✓		
IV-31	9	f	n	n.m.	✓		
IV-32	8	f	n	n.m.	✓		

f = female, m = male, n = no, y = yes, n.m. = not measurable, HR = hypertensive response, NR = normal response, PAH = pulmonary arterial hypertension, sec. PH = secondary pulmonary hypertension, RHC = right heart catheterization.

significantly associated. The BMPR2 gene causes PAH and seems also to be associated to hypertensive PASP response.

Both family members that developed manifest HPAH during follow up carried the Alu- insertion and had HR. In contrast, none of the relatives showing normal PASP values during exercise or without carrying the AluYb8 insertion developed manifest PAH during follow-up. Two Alu negative family members developed PH during follow-up due to diastolic dysfunction of the left ventricle which is associated with their left heart disease and systemic arterial hypertension.

Discussion

This study is the first description of an intronic Alu element insertion resulting in aberrant splicing of the *BMPR2* transcript as the underlying cause for the development of HPAH in a large family, which has been validated by RNA-analysis and was initially overseen by the standard DNA exon sequencing. This result indicates that the proportion of mutations in apparently negative families might be underestimated due to the fact that standard mutation screenings only analyse the exonic regions and short flanking intronic region on DNA level. It highlights the importance of including further methods such as RNA analysis into the molecular genetic work-up of PAH patients. Furthermore, this is the first report an a long-standing follow-up screening of relatives which revealed in this family that it is possible to detect manifest HPAH at an early stage in previously asymptomatic gene carriers. One of the family members who was diagnosed at an early stage responded excellent to PAH-targeted therapy and reminded stable over many years until today. In this family, only mutation-carriers with hypertensive PASP-response to exercise developed a manifest HPAH after several years. Thus, HR is possibly an additional risk factor at least if further underlying causes as high systemic blood pressure and left ventricular diastolic dysfunction have been ruled out.

Influence of an AluYb8 insertion on the splicing of *BMPR2* transcript

After initial screening of the *BMPR2* coding region [18,24] by standard screening methods (sequencing and MLPA technique) the family was initially assessed as *BMPR2* mutation negative. However, including the analysis on RNA level by RT-PCR experiments an aberrant splicing of exon 6 was observed which resulted from the insertion of an Alu element from the Y8b subfamily in Intron 5. The AluYb8 insertion in the *BMPR2* gene occurred close to the acceptor splice site, which had markedly increased the distance between this splice site and the branch point in intron 5. In transcript 4 and 5 exon 6 was missing which contains parts of the functionally important serine/threonine kinase domain. We assume, all aberrant splicing products caused either a dysfunctional BMPR2 protein or its complete loss leading to the development of HPAH in this family.

This is supported by reports of intronic Alu insertions causing aberrant splicing previously been published for other diseases [25–28]. Furthermore, the inserted Alu element lies in antisense orientation to the *BMPR2* gene. Antisense Alu elements are more likely to cause disease [29]. Lev-Maor et al. [30] previously described in their study a process termed Alu exonization, where retention of antisense Alu elements within the mature mRNA resulted from the introduction of new splice sites from the Alu sequences.

Alu repeats belong to the largest family of mobile elements, the so called short interspersed elements (SINEs), in the human genome. The human-specific subfamilies AluYa, Yb, and Yc

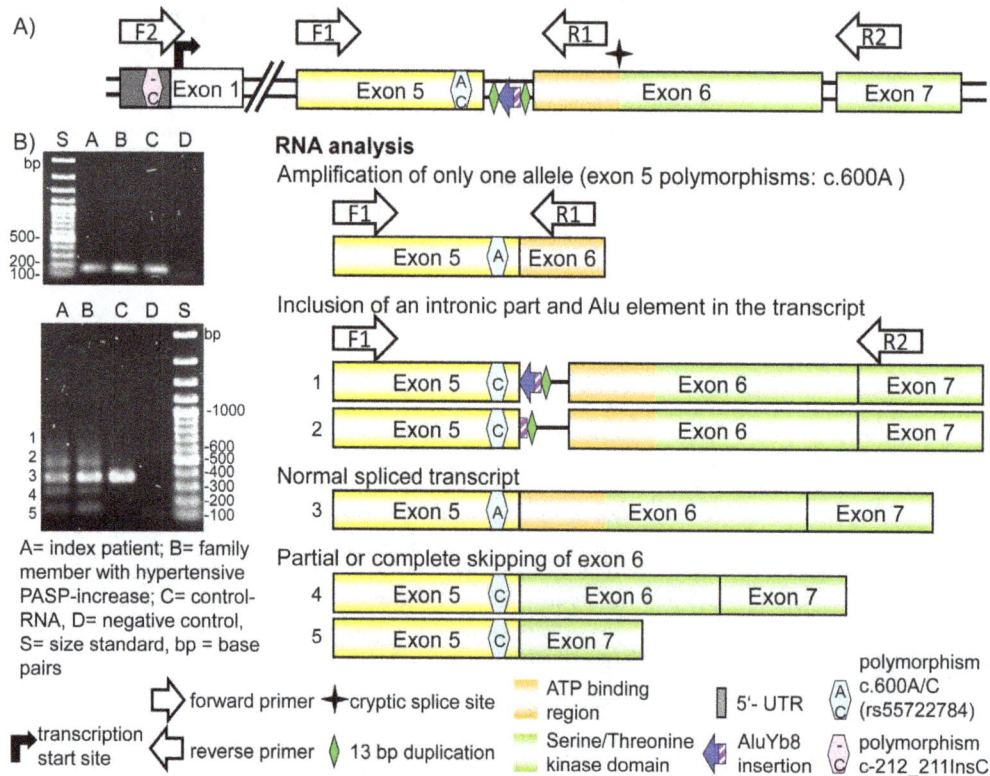

Figure 3. Results of the analysis on RNA level. A) Schematic representation of the genomic region from 5'-untranslated Region (5'-UTR) to exon 7 of *BMPR2*. Indicated are the identified polymorphisms (c.-212_-211insC and c.600A>C) used as markers for the analysis of the *BMPR2* transcript in the index patient, the primer used for the amplification, the location of the inserted Alu element, the duplicated 13 bp region and a potential cryptic splice site (marked by a star with four spikes). B) The upper part of this figure shows the amplified product using the forward primer located in exon 5 with the reverse primer located at the beginning of exon 6. The PCR with primers F1 and R1 resulted in amplification of a single transcript with the polymorphism in exon 5 in apparently homozygous state (c.600A). The other PCR with the same forward primer in exon 5 as above but with another reverse primer located in exon 7 (R2) resulted in amplification of at least five products of different length. Product #3 corresponds to the normally spliced wild type sequence with an apparently homozygous c.600A polymorphism in exon 5; the two larger products (#1 and #2) contained a complete and partial (only left arm) incorporated AluYb8 element, respectively. Furthermore, two smaller products were identified in which the 5' part of exon 6 (product #4) and the complete exon 6 (product #5) are missing. All aberrant spliced products (#1, 2, 4, and 5) contained apparently homozygous the C-allele of the polymorphism located in exon 5 (c.600C).

belong to the evolutionary youngest SINE elements and are supposed to be still active in terms of *de novo* retrotransposition in modern humans. The current Alu amplification rate is estimated to be in the range of one new insertion per 20–200 human births [31–33]. Commonly, the insertion of a new Alu element influences the splicing by changing the open reading frame of the gene. As a consequence, Alu insertions contribute to about 0.1% of human genetic disorders [29,31,34]. Alu elements create an approximately 300 bp insertion at any genomic insertion site as seen in our case flanked by a direct duplication of a short genomic region [34]. When an insertion occurs in the middle of an intron or between genes only a minimal effect on genes is observed. In contrast, if an insertion occurs in a coding exon, or near a splice site junction, they are likely to disrupt the proper expression or influence the splicing of a gene [31].

Genotype-phenotype correlation

The functional analysis of the AluYb8 insertion in the intronic region of the *BMPR2* gene and the clinical follow up show that the AluYb8 insertion is the major cause of HPAH in this family with a penetrance of at least 40–47%. Additionally, the significant association between the presence of the Alu insertion and the PASP status (HR/NR) indicates that the aberrant splicing of the

BMPR2 gene could also be a risk factor for hypertensive PASP response during exercise.

Early HPAH-diagnosis by regular clinical follow-up assessment

Familial PAH is associated with a worse prognosis. It occurs at an earlier age and progresses more rapidly than non-heritable PAH [35,36]. Often, healthy family members are interested whether they also have a higher risk to develop HPAH. If a causal mutation is detected in the family, healthy family members can be tested for the familial mutation. They can also be offered intensified medical care that allows early diagnosis and treatment as shown in our family.

Our study shows that HR status is associated to the Alu insertion. We suppose that HPAH and HR may share genetic risk factors.

However, HR should be interpreted with caution as it can also be caused by other diseases e.g. diastolic left ventricular dysfunction in patients with high systemic blood pressure as seen in this family. Thus, for interpretation of an HR, a causal systemic arterial hypertension has to be ruled out.

We observed that both family members that developed manifest HPAH during follow up carried the Alu- insertion and had HR.

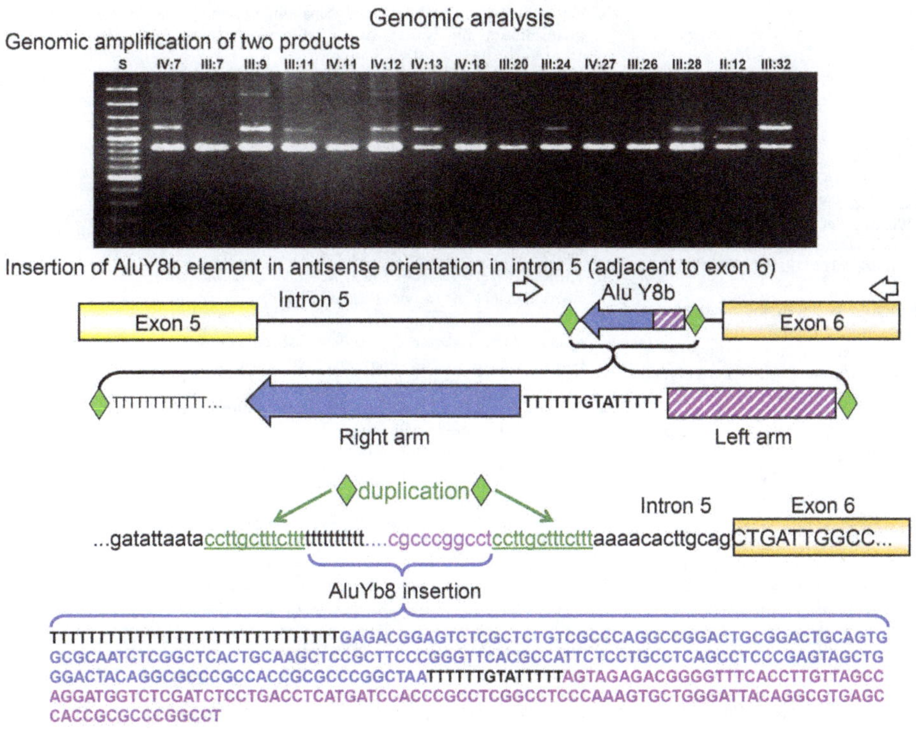

Figure 4. Genomic analysis of the intronic region. The genomic amplification with forward primer located in intron 5 and a reverse primer located in intron 6 resulted in two products of different length identified in several family members (shown is the result of 15 family members). Sequencing analysis of the larger products revealed the insertion of an AluYb8 element with an adjacent duplicated sequence motive in antisense orientation to *BMPR2* in intron 5 (adjacent to exon 6). A schematic representation of the region and the insertion of the Alu element on one allele and the complete sequence of the Alu element, the duplicated sequence and the beginning of exon 6 are shown.

This is in line with the hypothesis that HR might promote PAH development in mutation carriers, however more evidence from larger samples is needed. These results are also supported by the frequency of HR status in other European PAH-families, showing a significantly higher proportion of HR of 30% compared to 10% in the normal population [19].

However, the clinical course of the family members is still evolving and further cases of PAH and secondary PH may occur in the future. Therefore, further studies and on-going follow-up assessments of PAH families are needed to confirm these results.

Conclusions

This is the first report of an Alu insertion in an intronic sequence of the *BMPR2* gene leading to aberrant RNA splicing as cause for the development of HPAH in a large German family. Our findings show that analyses on the RNA level increase the rate of *BMPR2* mutation detection, highlight the involvement of aberrant pre-mRNA splicing in the pathogenesis of pulmonary arterial hypertension and extend the mutational spectrum of the *BMPR2* gene. The results support the hypothesis that HR and HPAH share genetic risk factors and additionally that HR promotes PAH development in mutation carriers.

Author Contributions

Conceived and designed the experiments: KH NP JSH EG. Performed the experiments: KH NP JSH ML CN BE NE EG. Analyzed the data: CF NE. Contributed reagents/materials/analysis tools: KH NP JSH EG. Wrote the paper: KH CF NP JSH ML CN BE NE EG.

References

1. Galiè N, Hoeper MM, Humbert M, Torbicki A, Vachiery JL, et al. (2009) ESC Committee for Practice Guidelines (CPG). Guidelines for the diagnosis and treatment of pulmonary hypertension: the Task Force for the Diagnosis and Treatment of Pulmonary Hypertension of the European Society of Cardiology (ESC) and the European Respiratory Society (ERS), endorsed by the International Society of Heart and Lung Transplantation (ISHLT). Eur Heart J 30:2493–537.

2. Hoeper MM, Huscher D, Ghofrani HA, Delcroix M, Distler O, et al. (2013) Elderly patients diagnosed with idiopathic pulmonary arterial hypertension: Results from the COMPERA registry. Int J Cardiol 168:871–80.

3. Lane KB, Machado RD, Pauciulo MW, Thomson JR, Phillips JA 3rd, et al. (2000) Heterozygous germline mutations in BMPR2, encoding a TGF-beta receptor, cause familial primary pulmonary hypertension. Nat Genet 26:81–4.

4. Deng Z, Morse JH, Slager SL, Cuervo N, Moore KJ, et al. (2000) Familial primary pulmonary hypertension (gene PPH1) is caused by mutations in the bone morphogenetic protein receptor-II gene. Am J Hum Genet 67:737–44.

5. Machado RD, Aldred MA, James V, Harrison RE, Patel B, et al. (2006) Mutations of the TGF-beta type II receptor BMPR2 in pulmonary arterial hypertension. Hum Mutat 27:121–32.

6. Trembath RC (2001) Mutations in the TGF-beta type 1 receptor, ALK1, in combined primary pulmonary hypertension and hereditary haemorrhagic telangiectasia, implies pathway specificity. J Heart Lung Transplant 20:175.

7. Chaouat A, Coulet F, Favre C, Simonneau G, Weitzenblum E, et al. (2004) Endoglin germline mutation in a patient with hereditary haemorrhagic telangiectasia and dexfenfluramine associated pulmonary arterial hypertension. Thorax 59:446–8.

8. Shintani M, Yagi H, Nakayama T, Saji T, Matsuoka R (2009) A new nonsense mutation of SMAD8 associated with pulmonary arterial hypertension. J Med Genet 46:331–7.

9. Machado RD, Eickelberg O, Elliott CG, Geraci MW, Hanaoka M, et al. (2009) Genetics and genomics of pulmonary arterial hypertension. J Am Coll Cardiol 30:S32–42.

10. Pfarr N, Szamalek-Hoegel J, Fischer C, Hinderhofer K, Nagel C, et al. (2011) Hemodynamic and clinical onset in patients with hereditary pulmonary arterial hypertension and BMPR2 mutations. Respir Res 12:99.

11. Austin ED, Loyd JE (2013) Heritable forms of pulmonary arterial hypertension. Semin Respir Crit Care Med 34:568–80.

12. Loyd JE, Primm RK, Newman JH (1984) Familial primary pulmonary hypertension: clinical patterns. Am Rev Respir Dis 129:194–7.

13. Loyd JE, Butler MG, Foroud TM, Conneally PM, Phillips JA 3rd, et al. (1995) Genetic anticipation and abnormal gender ratio at birth in familial primary pulmonary hypertension. Am J Respir Crit Care Med 152:93–7.

14. Grünig E, Barner A, Bell M, Claussen M, Dandel M, et al. (2011) Non-invasive diagnosis of pulmonary hypertension: ESC/ERS Guidelines with Updated Commentary of the Cologne Consensus Conference 2011. Int J Cardiol 154 Suppl 1:S3–12.

15. Olschewski H (2006) Current recommendations for the diagnosis and treatment of pulmonary hypertension. Dtsch Med Wochenschr. 131:S334–7.

16. Trip P, Vonk-Noordegraaf A, Bogaard HJ (2012) Cardiopulmonary exercise testing reveals onset of disease and response to treatment in a case of heritable pulmonary arterial hypertension. Pulm Circ 387–389.

17. Grunig E, Janssen B, Mereles D, Barth U, Borst MM, et al. (2000) Abnormal pulmonary artery pressure response in asymptomatic carriers of primary pulmonary hypertension. Circulation 102:1145–50.

18. Janssen B, Rindermann M, Barth U, Miltenberger-Miltenyi G, Mereles D, et al. (2002) Linkage analysis in a large family with primary pulmonary hypertension: genetic heterogeneity and a second primary pulmonary hypertension locus on 2q31–32. Chest 121:54S–56S.

19. Grunig E, Weissmann S, Ehlken N, Fijalkowska A, Fischer C, et al. (2009) Stress Doppler echocardiography in relatives of patients with idiopathic and familial pulmonary arterial hypertension: results of a multicenter European analysis of pulmonary artery pressure response to exercise and hypoxia. Circulation 119:1747–57.

20. Ommen SR, Nishimura RA, Hurrell DG, Klarich KW (2000) Assessment of right atrial pressure with 2-dimensional and Doppler echocardiography: a simultaneous catheterization and echocardiographic study. Mayo Clin Proc. 75:24–9.

21. Bird AG, McLachlan SM, Britton S (1981) Cyclosporin A promotes spontaneous outgrowth in vitro of Epstein-Barr virus-induced B-cell lines. Nature 289:300–1.

22. Oh HM, Oh JM, Choi SC, Kim SW, Han WC, et al. (2003) An efficient method for the rapid establishment of Epstein-Barr virus immortalization of human B lymphocytes. Cell Prolif 36:191–7.

23. Chomczynski P, Sacchi N (1987) Single-step method of RNA isolation by acid guanidinium thiocyanate-phenol-chloroform extraction. Anal Biochem 162:156–9.

24. Rindermann M, Grunig E, von Hippel A, Koehler R, Miltenberger-Miltenyi G, et al. (2003) Primary pulmonary hypertension may be a heterogeneous disease with a second locus on chromosome 2q31. J Am Coll Cardiol 41:2237–44.

25. Ferlini A, Muntoni F (1998) The 5′ region of intron 11 of the dystrophin gene contains target sequences for mobile elements and three overlapping ORFs. Biochem Biophys Res Commun 242:401–6.

26. Ganguly A, Dunbar T, Chen P, Godmilow L, Ganguly T (2003) Exon skipping caused by an intronic insertion of a young Alu Yb9 element leads to severe hemophilia A. Hum Genet 113:348–52.

27. Ricci V, Regis S, Di Duca M, Filocamo M (2003) An Alu-mediated rearrangement as cause of exon skipping in Hunter disease. Hum Genet 112:419–25.

28. Wallace MR, Andersen LB, Saulino AM, Gregory PE, Glover TW, Collins FS (1991) A de novo Alu insertion results in neurofibromatosis type 1. Nature 353:864–6.

29. Kaer K, Speek M (2013) Retroelements in human disease. Gene 518:231–41.

30. Lev-Maor G, Sorek R, Shomron N, Ast G (2003) The birth of an alternatively spliced exon: 3′ splice-site selection in Alu exons. Science 300:1288–91.

31. Deininger PL, Batzer MA (1999) Alu repeats and human disease. Mol Genet Metab 67:183–93.

32. Li X, Scaringe WA, Hill KA, Roberts S, Mengos A, et al. (2001) Frequency of recent retrotransposition events in the human factor IX gene. Hum Mutat 17:511–9.

33. Xing J, Zhang Y, Han K, Salem AH, Sen SK, et al. (2009) Mobile elements create structural variation: analysis of a complete human genome. Genome Res 19:1516–26.

34. Batzer MA, Deininger PL (2002) Alu repeats and human genomic diversity. Nat Rev Genet 3:370–9.

35. Chida A, Shintani M, Yagi H, Fujiwara M, Kojima Y, et al. (2013) Outcomes of childhood pulmonary arterial hypertension in BMPR2 and ALK1 mutation carriers. Am J Cardiol 110:586–93.

36. Benza RL, Miller DP, Gomberg-Maitland M, Frantz RP, Foreman AJ, et al. (2010) Predicting Survival in Pulmonary Arterial Hypertension - Insights From the Registry to Evaluate Early and Long-Term Pulmonary Arterial Hypertension Disease Management (REVEAL). Circulation 122:164–172.

Permissions

All chapters in this book were first published in PLOS ONE, by The Public Library of Science; hereby published with permission under the Creative Commons Attribution License or equivalent. Every chapter published in this book has been scrutinized by our experts. Their significance has been extensively debated. The topics covered herein carry significant findings which will fuel the growth of the discipline. They may even be implemented as practical applications or may be referred to as a beginning point for another development.

The contributors of this book come from diverse backgrounds, making this book a truly international effort. This book will bring forth new frontiers with its revolutionizing research information and detailed analysis of the nascent developments around the world.

We would like to thank all the contributing authors for lending their expertise to make the book truly unique. They have played a crucial role in the development of this book. Without their invaluable contributions this book wouldn't have been possible. They have made vital efforts to compile up to date information on the varied aspects of this subject to make this book a valuable addition to the collection of many professionals and students.

This book was conceptualized with the vision of imparting up-to-date information and advanced data in this field. To ensure the same, a matchless editorial board was set up. Every individual on the board went through rigorous rounds of assessment to prove their worth. After which they invested a large part of their time researching and compiling the most relevant data for our readers.

The editorial board has been involved in producing this book since its inception. They have spent rigorous hours researching and exploring the diverse topics which have resulted in the successful publishing of this book. They have passed on their knowledge of decades through this book. To expedite this challenging task, the publisher supported the team at every step. A small team of assistant editors was also appointed to further simplify the editing procedure and attain best results for the readers.

Apart from the editorial board, the designing team has also invested a significant amount of their time in understanding the subject and creating the most relevant covers. They scrutinized every image to scout for the most suitable representation of the subject and create an appropriate cover for the book.

The publishing team has been an ardent support to the editorial, designing and production team. Their endless efforts to recruit the best for this project, has resulted in the accomplishment of this book. They are a veteran in the field of academics and their pool of knowledge is as vast as their experience in printing. Their expertise and guidance has proved useful at every step. Their uncompromising quality standards have made this book an exceptional effort. Their encouragement from time to time has been an inspiration for everyone.

The publisher and the editorial board hope that this book will prove to be a valuable piece of knowledge for researchers, students, practitioners and scholars across the globe.

List of Contributors

Christine Wandall-Frostholm, Lykke Moran Skaarup, Elise Røge Hedegaard, Susie Mogensen and Ulf Simonsen
Department of Biomedicine, Aarhus University, Aarhus, Denmark

Veeranjaneyulu Sadda
Department of Biomedicine, Aarhus University, Aarhus, Denmark
Institute for Molecular Medicine, Cardiovascular and Renal Research, University of Southern Denmark, Odense, Denmark

Gorm Nielsen
Institute for Molecular Medicine, Cardiovascular and Renal Research, University of Southern Denmark, Odense, Denmark

Ralf Köhler
Institute for Molecular Medicine, Cardiovascular and Renal Research, University of Southern Denmark, Odense, Denmark
Aragon Institute of Health Sciences I+CS and ARAID, Zaragoza, Spain

Michael L. Paffett, Selita Lucas and Matthew J. Campen
Department of Pharmaceutical Sciences, University of New Mexico Health Sciences Center, Albuquerque, New Mexico, United States of America

Jacob Hesterman and Jack Hoppin
inviCRO, Boston, Massachusetts, United States of America

Gabriel Candelaria, Daniel Irwin, Jeffrey Norenberg and Tamara Anderson
Radiopharmaceutical Sciences Program, College of Pharmacy and Keck-UNM Small-Animal Imaging Resource, University of New Mexico Health Sciences Center, Albuquerque, New Mexico, United States of America

Xia Tian, Christina Vroom, Hossein Ardeschir Ghofrani, Norbert Weissmann, Ewa Bieniek, Friedrich and Grimminger
Medical Clinic II/V, University Hospital, Giessen, Germany

Werner Seeger, Ralph Theo Schermuly and Soni Savai Pullamsetti
Medical Clinic II/V, University Hospital, Giessen, Germany

Max-Planck-Institute for Heart and Lung Research, Bad Nauheim, Germany

Chris Cheadle, Alan E. Berger, Tonya N. Watkins, Yumiko Sugawara, Sangjucta Barkataki, Jinshui Fan, Meher Boorgula, Michael A and Kathleen C. Barnes
Division of Allergy and Clinical Immunology, Johns Hopkins University School of Medicine, Baltimore, Maryland, United States of America

Stephen C. Mathai, Ari L. Zaiman, Reda Girgis and Paul M. Hassoun
Division of Pulmonary/Critical Care Medicine, Johns Hopkins University School of Medicine, Baltimore, Maryland, United States of America

Dmitry N. Grigoryev
Medical Genetic Core, Children's Mercy Hospitals and Clinics, Kansas City, Missouri, United States of America

Frederick Wigley and Laura Hummers
Division of Rheumatology, Johns Hopkins University School of Medicine, Baltimore, Maryland, United States of America

McDevitt
Division of Hematology, Johns Hopkins University School of Medicine, Baltimore, Maryland, United States of America

Roger A. Johns
Department of Anesthesiology and Critical Care Medicine, Johns Hopkins University School of Medicine, Baltimore, Maryland, United States of America

Guillermo Pousada and Diana Valverde
Department of Biochemistry, Genetics and Immunology, Faculty of Biology, University of Vigo, Instituto de Investigación Biomédica de Vigo (IBIV), Vigo, Spain

Adolfo Baloira
Respiratory Division, Complejo Hospitalario Universitario de Pontevedra, Pontevedra, Spain

Carlos Vilariño
Respiratory Division, Complejo Hospitalario Universitario de Vigo, Vigo, Spain

Jose Manuel Cifrian
Respiratory Division, Hospital Universitario Marqués de Valdecilla, Santander, Spain

Christian Nagel, Felix Prange, Jochen Herb, Nicola Ehlken and Ekkehard Grünig
Centre for Pulmonary Hypertension, Thoraxclinic at University Hospital Heidelberg, Heidelberg, Germany

Stefan Guth and Eckhard Mayer
Department of Thoracic Surgery, Kerckhoff-Klinik Bad Nauheim, Bad Nauheim, Germany

Christine Fischer
Department of Human Genetics, University of Heidelberg, Heidelberg, Germany

Frank Reichenberger
Department of Pneumology, University Gießen-Marburg, Gießen, Germany

Stephan Rosenkranz
Department of Cardiology, University of Cologne, Cologne, Germany

Hans-Juergen Seyfarth
Department of Pneumology, University of Leipzig, Leipzig, Germany

Michael Halank
Department of Pneumology, University of Dresden, Dresden, Germany

Stefan Pabst, Christoph Hammerstingl, Georg Nickenig and Dirk Skowasch
The Department of Internal Medicine II – Cardiology/Pneumology, University of Bonn, Bonn, Germany

Rainer Woitas and Felix Hundt
The Department of Internal Medicine I - Nephrology, University of Bonn, Bonn, Germany

Thomas Gerhardt
Praxis für Nieren- und Hochdruckkrankheiten Bonn, Bonn, Germany

Christian Grohé
The Lungenklinik Berlin-Buch, Berlin, Germany

Min Yu, Dapeng Gong and Anna Arutyunyan
Section of Molecular Carcinogenesis, Division of Hematology/Oncology, and The Saban Research Institute of Children's Hospital, Los Angeles, California, United States of America

John Groffen and Nora Heisterkamp
Section of Molecular Carcinogenesis, Division of Hematology/Oncology, and The Saban Research Institute of Children's Hospital, Los Angeles, California, United States of America
Departments of Pediatrics and Pathology, Keck School of Medicine, University of Southern California, Los Angeles, California, United States of America

Min Lim
Departments of Pediatrics and Pathology, Keck School of Medicine, University of Southern California, Los Angeles, California, United States of America

Tanya Hartney, Rahul Birari, Sujatha Venkataraman and Maylyn Martinez
Department of Pediatrics, University of Colorado Denver, Aurora, Colorado, United States of America

Leah Villegas, Kurt R. Stenmark and Eva Nozik-Grayck
Department of Pediatrics, University of Colorado Denver, Aurora, Colorado, United States of America
Cardiovascular Pulmonary Research Laboratory, University of Colorado Denver, Aurora, Colorado, United States of America

Stephen M. Black
Georgia Health Sciences University, Augusta, Georgia, United States of America

Enrico Novelli
Vascular Medicine Institute, University of Pittsburgh, Pittsburgh, Pennsylvania, United States of America

Mark T. Gladwin and Mariana Hildesheim
Vascular Medicine Institute, University of Pittsburgh, Pittsburgh, Pennsylvania, United States of America
Division of Pulmonary Allergy and Critical Care Medicine, University of Pittsburgh Medical Center, Pittsburgh, Pennsylvania, United States of America

Lakshmanan Krishnamurti
Vascular Medicine Institute, University of Pittsburgh, Pittsburgh, Pennsylvania, United States of America
Children's Hospital of Pittsburgh, Pittsburgh, Pennsylvania, United States of America

Robyn J. Barst and Erika Berman Rosenzweig
Columbia University, New York, New York, United States of America

J. Simon R. Gibbs
National Heart and Lung Institute, Imperial College London, London, United Kingdom

Vandana Sachdev, Gregory J. Kato and James G. Taylor VI
Cardiovascular Branch, NHLBI, Bethesda, Maryland, United States of America

Mehdi Nouraie and Oswaldo L. Castro
Howard University, Washington, DC, United States of America

Kathryn L. Hassell and David B. Badesch
University of Colorado HSC, Denver, Colorado, United States of America

Jane A. Little
Case Western Reserve University, Cleveland, Ohio, United States of America

Dean E. Schraufnagel, Victor R. Gordeuk and Roberto F. Machado
University of Illinois, Chicago, Illinois, United States of America

Reda E. Girgis
Johns Hopkins University, Baltimore, Maryland, United States of America

Claudia R. Morris
Emory University School of Medicine, Atlanta, Georgia, United States of America

Jonathan C. Goldsmith
National Heart Lung and Blood Institute/NIH, Bethesda, Maryland, United States of America

Zhibin Yuan, Jian Chen, Dewei Chen, Gang Xu and Yuqi Gao
Department of Pathophysiology and High Altitude Physiology, College of High Altitude Military Medicine, Third Military Medical University, Chongqing, China
Key Laboratory of High Altitude Medicine, Ministry of Education, Third Military Medical University, Chongqing, China
Key Laboratory of High Altitude Medicine, PLA, Third Military Medical University, Chongqing, China

Minjie Xia and Yong Xu
Key Lboratory of Cardiovascular Disease, Department of Pathophysiology, Nanjing Medical University, Nanjing, Jiangsu
China

Dennis Rottlaender, Lukas J. Motloch, Sara Reda and Robert Larbig
Department of Internal Medicine II, Paracelsus Medical University, Salzburg, Austria

Uta C. Hoppe
Department of Internal Medicine II, Paracelsus Medical University, Salzburg, Austria
Department of Internal Medicine III, University of Cologne, Cologne, Germany
Center of Molecular Medicine Cologne, University of Cologne, Cologne, Germany

Daniel Dumitrescu, Erland Erdmann and Daniela Schmidt
Department of Internal Medicine III, University of Cologne, Cologne, Germany

Stephan Rosenkranz
Department of Internal Medicine III, University of Cologne, Cologne, Germany
Center of Molecular Medicine Cologne, University of Cologne, Cologne, Germany

Martin Wolny
Center of Molecular Medicine Cologne, University of Cologne, Cologne, Germany

Pi-Ou Tseng, Jean Hertzberg and Wei Tan
Department of Mechanical Engineering, University of Colorado at Boulder, Boulder, Colorado, United States of America

Yan Tan
Department of Mechanical Engineering, University of Colorado at Boulder, Boulder, Colorado, United States of America
Department of Pediatrics, University of Colorado at Denver, Aurora, Colorado, United States of America

Daren Wang, Hui Zhang, Kendall Hunter and Kurt R. Stenmark
Department of Pediatrics, University of Colorado at Denver, Aurora, Colorado, United States of America

Scott H. Visovatti, Diane Bouis, Vallerie V. McLaughlin and David J. Pinsky
Division of Cardiology, Department of Medicine, University of Michigan, Ann Arbor, Michigan, United States of America

Matthew C. Hyman
Department of Medicine, University of Pennsylvania, Philadelphia, Pennsylvania, United States of America

Richard Neubig
Department of Pharmacology, University of Michigan, Ann Arbor, Michigan, United States of America

Jonas D. Baandrup, Lars H. Markvardsen, Nils E., Magnusson and Ulf Simonsen
Department of Pharmacology, Aarhus University, Aarhus, Denmark

Christian D. Peters and Uffe K. Schou
The Water and Salt Research Center, Department of Anatomy, Aarhus University, Aarhus, Denmark

Jens L. Jensen
Department of Theoretical Statistics, Institute of Mathematics, Aarhus University, Aarhus, Denmark

Torben F. Ørntoft and Mogens Kruhøffer
Molecular Diagnostic Laboratory, Department of Clinical Biochemistry, Aarhus University Hospital, Aarhus, Denmark

Hui-Li Gan, Jian-Qun Zhang, Qi-Wen Zhou, Lei Feng, Fei Chen and Yi Yang
Department of Cardiac Surgery, Beijing Anzhen Hospital, Capital Medical University, Beijing Institute of Heart, Lung and Blood Vessel Diseases, Beijing, China

Ella M. Poels, Nicole Bitsch, Leon J. de Windt and Paula A. da Costa Martins
Department of Cardiology, CARIM School for Cardiovascular Diseases, Faculty of Health, Medicine and Life Sciences, Maastricht University, Maastricht, The Netherlands

Jos M. Slenter and M. Eline Kooi
Department of Radiology, CARIM School for Cardiovascular Diseases, Maastricht University Medical Centre, Maastricht, The Netherlands

Chiel C. de Theije
Department of Respiratory Medicine, NUTRIM School Nutrition, Toxicology and Metabolism, Maastricht University Medical Centre, Maastricht, The Netherlands

Vanessa P. M. van Empel
Department of Cardiology, Heart Vessel Center, Maastricht University Medical Centre, M aastricht, The Netherlands

Michael Pienn and Zoltán Bálint
Ludwig Boltzmann Institute for Lung Vascular Research, Graz, Austria

Michael Helmberger
Ludwig Boltzmann Institute for Lung Vascular Research, Graz, Austria
Institute for Computer Graphics and Vision, Graz University of Technology, Graz, Austria

Horst Olschewski and Gabor Kovacs
Ludwig Boltzmann Institute for Lung Vascular Research, Graz, Austria
Division of Pulmonology, Department of Internal Medicine, Medical University of Graz, Graz, Austria

Andrea Olschewski
Ludwig Boltzmann Institute for Lung Vascular Research, Graz, Austria
Experimental Anesthesiology, Department of Anesthesia and Intensive Care Medicine, Medical University of Graz, Graz, Austria

Martin Urschler
Institute for Computer Graphics and Vision, Graz University of Technology, Graz, Austria
Ludwig Boltzmann Institute for Clinical Forensic Imaging, Graz, Austria

Peter Kullnig
DiagnostikZentrum Graz, Graz, Austria

Rudolf Stollberger
Institute for Medical Engineering, Graz University of Technology, Graz, Austria

Daniela Farkas, Donatas Kraskauskas, Jennifer I. Drake, Aysar A. Alhussaini, Vita Kraskauskiene, Norbert F. Voelkel and Laszlo Farkas
Victoria Johnson Center for Obstructive Lung Research, Department of Internal Medicine, Division of Respiratory Disease and Critical Care Medicine, Virginia
Commonwealth University, Richmond, Virginia, United States of America

Harm J. Bogaard
Department of Pulmonary Medicine, VU University Medical Center, Amsterdam, The Netherlands

Carlyne D. Cool
Department of Pathology, University of Colorado at Denver and Health Sciences Center, Denver, Colorado, United States of America

Yao Liu, Yi Liu, Lili Su and Shu-juan Jiang
Department of Respiratory Medicine, Provincial Hospital Affiliated to Shandong University, Jinan, Shandong, China

Anna Dikalova, Angela Fagiana and Candice D. Fike
Dept. of Pediatrics, Vanderbilt University Medical Center, Nashville, Tennessee, United States of America
Monroe Carell Jr. Children's Hospital at Vanderbilt, Nashville, Tennessee, United States of America

Michael Aschner
Dept. of Pediatrics, Vanderbilt University Medical Center, Nashville, Tennessee, United States of America
Monroe Carell Jr. Children's Hospital at Vanderbilt, Nashville, Tennessee, United States of America
Vanderbilt Center for Molecular Toxicology, Nashville, Tennessee, United States of America

Marshall Summar
Division of Genetics and Metabolism, Children's National Medical Center, Washington, District of Columbia, United States of America

Judy L. Aschner
Dept of Pediatrics, Albert Einstein College of Medicine and the Children's Hospital at Montefiore, New York, New York, United States of America

J. K. Mansoor
Department of Physical Therapy, University of the Pacific, Stockton, California, United States of America

Edward S. Schelegle, William F. Walby and Jennifer Figueroa
Department of Anatomy, Physiology and Cell Biology, University of California Davis, Davis, California, United States of America

Cristina E. Davis, Weixiang Zhao Alexander A. Aksenov and Alberto Pasamontes
Department of Mechanical and Aerospace Engineering, University of California Davis, Davis, California, United States of America

Roblee Allen
Department of Medicine, University of California Davis Medical Center, Sacramento, California, United States of America

Katrin Hinderhofe, Christine Fischer and Justyna Szamalek-Hoegel
Institute of Human Genetics, University of Heidelberg, Heidelberg, Germany

Nicole Pfarr
Institute of Human Genetics, University of Heidelberg, Heidelberg, Germany
Centre for pulmonary hypertension of the Thoraxclinic, University Hospital of Heidelberg, Heidelberg, Germany

Mona Lichtblau, Christian Nagel, Benjamin Egenlauf, Nicola Ehlken and Ekkehard Grünig
Centre for pulmonary hypertension of the Thoraxclinic, University Hospital of Heidelberg, Heidelberg, Germany

Index

www.ingramcontent.com/pod-product-compliance
Lightning Source LLC
Chambersburg PA
CBHW080511200326
41458CB00012B/4163